Pathologic Myopia

Richard F. Spaide · Kyoko Ohno-Matsui
Lawrence A. Yannuzzi

Editors

Pathologic Myopia

Second Edition

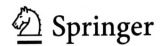 Springer

Editors
Richard F. Spaide
Vitreous, Retina, Macula Consultant
New York, NY
USA

Lawrence A. Yannuzzi
LuEsther T. Mertz Retinal Research
Columbia University School of Medicine
New York, NY
USA

Kyoko Ohno-Matsui
Department of Ophthalmology and Visual Science
Tokyo Medical and Dental University
Bunkyo-Ku, Tokyo
Japan

ISBN 978-3-030-74336-9   ISBN 978-3-030-74334-5   (eBook)
https://doi.org/10.1007/978-3-030-74334-5

This Springer imprint is published by the registered company Springer Nature Switzerland AG
The registered company address is: Gewerbestrasse 11, 6330 Cham, Switzerland

To my family Chang, Ted, Chris, and Emily and also to all of the teachers I have had over the years.

Richard F. Spaide

I would like to thank my mentor Emeritus Professor Takashi Tokoro, and my family, Seiji and Kyoka.

Kyoko Ohno-Matsui

I would like to thank my wife, children, and grandchildren.

Lawrence A. Yannuzzi

Foreword I

A quarter of a century ago, I dedicated a significant amount of my professional career to the study of pathologic myopia. At that time, I realized the importance of this ocular disease worldwide, specifically, in terms of its prevalence and severe impact on visual disabilities. In an attempt to meet the need of the eye care community with a comprehensive clinical and scientific study of the disorder, I wrote a comprehensive text in 1985. This was based on the accumulated knowledge of the subject at the time. It included the history and significance of myopia on the refractive state of the eye, the prevalence of the disorder, the related pathophysical and clinical factors that affected the visual prognosis, the hereditary and environmental causes, and the optical considerations. Back then, there was very little available to clinicians to help them provide meaningful management and visual rehabilitation. The same was true for the evaluation of these eyes. All that existed was ophthalmoscopy and limited imaging with fundus photography, ultrasonography, and fluorescein angiography.

Today multimodal imaging, including high-speed fundus autofluorescence, angiographic studies of the two ocular circulations, optical coherence tomography, and 3-dimensional MRI imaging, has assisted in incorporating basic science knowledge of the disease in the clinical setting. At this time of my life, it is such a great pleasure to witness these developments, which now provide great promise towards unraveling many of the diagnostic and therapeutic mysteries of the disease. Yet today, pathologic myopia is still clearly the critical aspect of the near-sighted eye. It has intensified in its clinical importance and impact in the eye care community, especially with an increase in its prevalence and the expected longevity of the population.

It should be mentioned that pathologic myopia can occur in all stages of life, from the newborn to the elderly. Congenital developmental abnormalities such as coloboma, retinopathy of prematurity, anisometropia, and amblyopia rival the adult nemesis, the posterior staphyloma and its clinical implications and consequences. It is my hope that this new text will lead to a better appreciation of the great importance of the posterior staphyloma in pathologic myopia and the need for physicians to monitor closely all of the clinical features of the disease that are major factors in its visual prognosis.

Several years ago, I invited one of my inquisitive, industrious, and, I might add, intellectually gifted students to revise my text. He promised to do so, since he was also a dear friend and I was, as he put it, one of his principal mentors. I am pleased that he (LAY) keeps his promises and, in this case, collaborated with two additional editors (distinguished colleagues and friends) whom he has stated, "know more about pathologic myopia than I." These three editors have managed to recruit contributing authors and to assimilate their combined knowledge and experience in pathologic myopia into a comprehensive and current text and atlas. The contributing authors represent an elite corps of clinical scientists who are leaders in the field. Each has devoted a large part of his or her career to the study of certain aspects of this disease. Their combined effort represents a labor of love by the editors and the authors, all of whom are true experts with encyclopedic knowledge of the disease and an accurate vision of the future research needed to provide the necessary advances in its management. I am sure that their combined efforts will be rewarded by the gratitude of clinicians, scientists, ophthalmologists, retinal specialists, ophthalmologists, students, and patients by the incalculable pleasure that will result on the part of the casual as well as the discerning reader of this, in my opinion, masterpiece in pathologic myopia.

New York, NY, USA   Brian J. Curtin

Foreword II

A book dedicated to myopia has long been expected. In 1985, Dr. Curtin published his book *The Myopias* in response to such expectations. In the original version of *The Myopias*, Dr. Curtin described the details about myopia from basic knowledge to clinical management with a huge number of cited literatures on myopia. For a long period of time, *The Myopias* has been the only book dedicated to myopia and has been a kind of bible for many researchers. However, recent advances in myopia research have been outstanding, and this great book is now in need of a revision, 30 years after its original publication.

Myopia is generally divided into simple myopia and pathologic myopia. Simple myopia is within a normal variation of refractive error and the patients obtain a good vision by appropriate optical correction. In contrast, the patients with pathologic myopia could show a decrease of corrected visual acuity. Recently, the rate of myopia has been increasing worldwide, and pathologic myopia is currently a major cause of blindness in various countries. In general, progression of pathologic myopia is slow; however, patients sometimes develop acute visual loss. It is required to treat complications due to pathologic myopia; however, prediction of the natural course and preventive management are also necessary. Thanks to the recent advances in clinical examinations as well as in experimental procedures, some of the underlying features of pathologic myopia have been clarified and new insights have been obtained for prevention and treatment against pathologic myopia.

The recent examinations include optical measurements of axial length, indocyanine green angiography, optical coherence tomography (OCT) of the anterior and posterior segment of the eye, fundus imaging using adaptive optics, and the analysis of eye shape using three dimensional magnetic resonance imaging (3D MRI). Using these new modalities, novel insights on the eye shape characteristic to pathologic myopia and new findings of the myopic fundus lesions have been clarified.

Both genetic and environmental factors are causes of developing myopia; however, the genetic influence is considered more important for pathologic myopia. Thus, gene analysis for pathologic myopia has been actively performed. Also, animal models of experimental myopia induced by form deprivation or induced by optical lens have contributed to the research investigating the pathogenesis of myopia development.

The interventions to prevent myopia progression include progressive multifocal glasses, the glass lens or contact lens which is designed specifically to decrease peripheral defocus, and orthokeratology. Long-term data are necessary to confirm whether these treatments are effective in preventing the progression to pathologic myopia.

Myopic choroidal neovascularization, which is a major cause of visual decrease in the patients with pathologic myopia, can now be treated by anti-VEGF agents to at least some extent. Glaucoma or myopic optic neuropathy, both of which are common problems in eyes with pathologic myopia, are still being treated by decreasing the intraocular pressure by eye drops, which are not fundamental treatments. Thus, the modalities to treat the features of pathologic myopia, an increase of axial length and staphyloma formation, have been expected.

Due to many new findings in myopia research, prevention and treatments for myopia have been obtaining a lot more attention in the world.

In such circumstances, the publishing of the revised version of *The Myopias* edited by Dr. Spaide, Dr. Ohno-Matsui, and Dr. Yannuzzi is very timely. In this book, the first set of chapters are assigned for the basic aspects of myopia including the definition, epidemiology, genetics, and animal models. The second set of chapters are for the analysis of human eye shape, and the third set of chapters cover the pathologies and possible therapies for pathologic myopia. The final set of chapters mention the treatment strategies to prevent myopia progression. Along with the three editors, world leaders in each field have contributed to the chapters as well. I believe that this book will be an essential book for many researchers and clinicians who would like to study myopia.

Finally, I would like to greatly expect that this book will be the fundamental step for future research of pathologic myopia.

Tokyo, Japan   Takashi Tokoro

Preface

Poorly understood, highly prevalent, and vastly under researched, myopia is a leading worldwide cause of severe vision loss, transcending gender, age, and racial boundaries. Furthermore, the incidence of myopia is increasing worldwide, especially in East Asian countries. There is estimated to be 400,000,000 myopes in China alone. The portion of the population that is highly myopic is also increasing in these same countries. The prevalence of high myopia in the United States is said to be approximately 1–2%, lower in that range for African-Americans and higher for Caucasians. High myopia in Japan affects 5–6% of the population; in Singapore 15% of military recruits are highly myopic. An astounding 38% of university students in Taiwan have high myopia. The magnitude of change in myopia in East Asian countries followed their transitions from agrarian to modern highly technical societies and suggests that, in addition to environmental factors, genetic and epigenetic factors may play a role in susceptibility. There does not seem to be anywhere in the world where the desire for socioeconomic progress will abate, so the environmental factors contributing to the development of myopia are not likely to change. That is, unless we come to understand, and control, the precise mechanisms by which myopia develops.

Myopia is the second largest cause of blindness in the world, following cataracts. With increasing progress and delivery of modern medical care around the world, cataracts seem to be a surmountable problem. Myopia presents numerous challenges because it affects every important structure related to eye function. We have little information about the frequency or severity of any of these component changes and even less about their pathophysiology. The interconnectedness of all of constituent transformations occurring in the development of myopia makes these same changes difficult to research. The goal in science is often reductionist; we try to isolate clean-cut questions and hypotheses to evaluate through experiment. In myopia, any one change is associated with numerous confounding alterations. As one example, the expansion of the eye wall in myopia is associated with choroidal thinning and eventual atrophy, stretching of the retina, distortion of normal vitreoretinal interface interactions, alteration in the regional shape of the eye, and induction of various potential stresses on the optic nerve, so determining why visual function in any one given patient is affected can be challenging. Determining these factors and their interactions in populations of patients with high myopia is multiplicatively harder. There isn't a simple way to isolate any one problem to study it, and there is a lack of suitable animal models for many of the problems seen in human myopia.

Progress in the understanding of myopia, its pathologic consequences, and the development of effective treatment has been the result of hard work by ophthalmologists and scientists around the world. The number of publications related in some way to high myopia, ranging from basic science investigations such as scleral morphogenesis or the biomechanics of the optic nerve to clinical application of new imaging modalities or the development of biologic agents directed against growth factors promoting new vessel growth, has grown exponentially. The range, sophistication, and expertise evident in these publications are amazing, but with each passing year, the scope and complexity of the information becomes increasingly difficult to take in. Because of the complexity and interconnectedness of the problems induced by myopia, the solutions are likely to require interconnected networks of knowledgeable researchers. It is a purpose of this text on pathologic myopia to report on the current status of our understanding of these eyes with regard to converging lines of experimental and clinical advances in virtually every aspect of the disease: its epidemiology, genetics, molecular biological basis, clinical manifestations, and potential therapeutic approaches to management. Obviously no single investigator has the ability to excel in all of these clinical scientific areas. Accordingly, we have assembled an elite corps of contributors, indisputable experts in their specialized study of pathologic myopia. Each has also surveyed the ophthalmic literature to assimilate the contributions of others in conjunction with his or her investigations, knowledge, experience, and perspectives.

Myopia is rapidly increasing worldwide, establishing it as one of the most prevalent abnormalities found in humans and a major cause of severe vision loss worldwide. Converging lines of clinical and scientific research are currently under investigation by clinicians and researchers alike, across a broad spectrum of disciplines. Meaningful therapeutic concepts are now being tested in a broad range of areas to advance our management of the disease. Hopefully our text and illustrations will serve in the delineation of the natural course of the disease, identification of potential risk factors, codify our understanding of the pathophysiology of disease, and highlight the management of currently treatable manifestations. We realize that most of the road lies ahead of us and that we have made insufficient progress so far. In that, we hope that the text will also inspire the eye care field, from the casual observer to the discerning investigator, to devote time and talent to the understanding of its pathogenesis and to the development of new methods of prevention and treatment in the future.

New York, NY, USA   Richard F. Spaide
Bunkyo-Ku, Tokyo, Japan   Kyoko Ohno-Matsui
New York, NY, USA   Lawrence A. Yannuzzi

Contents

Part III   Sequella of Pathologic Myopia and Their Potential Treatments

Part IV   Treatment of Pathologic Myopia

Contributors

Regan S. Ashby, PhD Centre for Research into Therapeutic Solutions, Faculty of Science and Technology, University of Canberra, Bruce, ACT, Australia

Chiu Ming Gemmy Cheung, MBBS Singapore Eye Research Institute, Singapore National Eye Centre, Singapore, Singapore

DUKE-NUS Medical School, Singapore, Singapore

Sung Chul (Sean) Park, MD Department of Ophthalmology, Manhattan Eye, Ear and Throat Hospital and Lenox Hill Hospital, New York, NY, USA

Department of Ophthalmology, Donald and Barbara Zucker School of Medicine at Hofstra/Northwell, Hempstead, NY, USA

Jeffrey Cooper, MS, OD SUNY-State College of Optometry, New York, NY, USA

Jack M. Dodick, MD Department of Ophthalmology, NYU Langone Health, New York, NY, USA

Michael Engelbert, MD, PhD Vitreous Retina Macula Consultants of New York, New York, NY, USA

Yuxin Fang, MD Department of Ophthalmology and Visual Science, Tokyo Medical and Dental University, Bunkyo-Ku, Tokyo, Japan

Eva Fenwick, MA, PhD Singapore Eye Research Institute, Singapore National Eye Centre, Singapore, Singapore

DUKE-NUS Medical School, Singapore, Singapore

Takashi Fujikado, MD, PhD Osaka University Graduate School of Frontier Bioscience, Osaka, Japan

Hans E. Grossniklaus, MD, MBA L.F Montogomery Laboratory, Department of Ophthalmology, Emory University School of Medicine, Atlanta, GA, USA

Quan V. Hoang, MD, PhD Singapore Eye Research Institute, Singapore, Singapore

Department of Ophthalmology, Duke-NUS, Singapore, Singapore

Singapore National Eye Centre, Singapore, Singapore

Department of Ophthalmology, Edward S. Harkness Eye Institute, Columbia University Medical Center, New York, NY, USA

Jost B. Jonas, MD Department of Ophthalmology, Medical Faculty Mannheim of the Ruprecht-Karls-University of Heidelberg, Mannheim, Germany

Jonathan B. Kahn, MD Department of Ophthalmology, NYU Langone Health, New York, NY, USA

Eugene Yu-Chuan Kang, MD Department of Ophthalmology, Chang Gung Memorial Hospital, Linkuo Medical Center, Kuei Shan, Taoyuan, Taiwan

Shoji Kishi, MD Department of Ophthalmology, Gunma University School of Medicine, Gunma University Hospital, Maebashi, Gunma, Japan

Ecosse L. Lamoureux, MSc, PhD Singapore Eye Research Institute, Singapore National Eye Centre, Singapore, Singapore

Essilor Centre for Innovation and Technologies AMERA, Singapore, Singapore

DUKE-NUS Medical School, Singapore, Singapore

National University of Singapore, Singapore, Singapore

Carla Lanca, PhD Singapore Eye Research Institute, Singapore, Singapore

Gerardo Ledesma-Gil, MD Vitreous Retina Macula Consultants of New York, New York, NY, USA

Jeffrey M. Liebmann, MD Bernard and Shirlee Brown Glaucoma Research Laboratory, Edward S. Harkness Eye Institute, Columbia University Irving Medical Center, New York, NY, USA

Ryan Eyn Kidd Man, BSc (Hons), PhD Singapore Eye Research Institute, Singapore National Eye Centre, Singapore, Singapore

DUKE-NUS Medical School, Singapore, Singapore

Seang Mei Saw, MPH, MBBS, PhD Singapore Eye Research Institute, Singapore National Eye Centre, Singapore, Singapore

National University of Singapore, Singapore, Singapore

Singapore Eye Research Institute, Singapore, Singapore

Saw Swee Hock School of Public Health, National University of Singapore, Singapore, Singapore

Duke-NUS Medical School, Singapore, Singapore

Ian G. Morgan, PhD Research School of Biology, Australian National University, Canberra, ACT, Australia

Muka Moriyama, MD, PhD Department of Ophthalmology and Visual Science, Tokyo Medical and Dental University, Tokyo, Japan

Sarah Mrejen, MD 15-20 Ophthalmologic National Hospital, Paris, France

Kyoko Ohno-Matsui, MD, PhD Department of Ophthalmology and Visual Science, Tokyo Medical and Dental University, Bunkyo-Ku, Tokyo, Japan

Department of Ophthalmology and Visual Science, Tokyo Medical and Dental University Graduate School of Medical and Dental Sciences, Bunkyo-Ku, Tokyo, Japan

Chen-Wei Pan, MD, PhD School of Public Health, Medical College of Soochow University, Suzhou, China

Songhomitra Panda-Jonas, MD Department of Ophthalmology, Medical Faculty Mannheim of the Ruprecht-Karls-University of Heidelberg, Mannheim, Germany

Institute of Clinical and Scientific Ophthalmology and Acupuncture Jonas & Panda, Heidelberg, Germany

Alia Rashid, MBChB L.F Montogomery Laboratory, Department of Ophthalmology, Emory University School of Medicine, Atlanta, GA, USA

Robert Ritch, MD Einhorn Clinical Research Center, New York Eye and Ear Infirmary of Mount Sinai, New York, NY, USA

Kathryn A. Rose, PhD School of Orthoptics, Graduate School of Health, University of Technology Sydney, Ultimo, NSW, Australia

Kosei Shinohara, MD, PhD Department of Ophthalmology and Visual Science, Tokyo Medical and Dental University, Tokyo, Japan

Richard F. Spaide, MD Vitreous, Retina, Macula Consultants of New York, New York, NY, USA

Jody A. Summers, PhD Department of Cell Biology, Oklahoma Center of Neuroscience, University of Oklahoma Health Science Center, Oklahoma City, OK, USA

Ramin Tadayoni, MD, PhD Department of Ophthalmology, Université de Paris, AP-HP, Hôpital Lariboisière, Hôpital Fondation Adolphe de Rothschild, Paris, France

Hiroyuki Takahashi, MD Department of Ophthalmology and Visual Science, Tokyo Medical and Dental University Graduate School of Medical and Dental Sciences, Bunkyo-Ku, Tokyo, Japan

Jun Takeuchi, MD, PhD Department of Ophthalmology, Nagoya University Hospital, Nagoya, Aichi, Japan

Hiroko Terasaki, MD, PhD Department of Ophthalmology, Nagoya University Hospital, Nagoya, Aichi, Japan

Nan-Kai Wang, MD, PhD Department of Ophthalmology, Chang Gung Memorial Hospital, Linkuo Medical Center, Kuei Shan, Taoyuan, Taiwan

Department of Ophthalmology, Edward S. Harkness Eye Institute, Columbia University, New York, NY, USA

C. P. Wilkinson, MD Department of Ophthalmology, Greater Baltimore Medical Center, Baltimore, MD, USA

Department of Ophthalmology, Johns Hopkins University, Baltimore, MD, USA

Tien-Yin Wong, MD, PhD Singapore Eye Research Institute, Singapore, Singapore

Duke-NUS Medical School, Singapore, Singapore

Yee Ling Wong, BSc (Hons), PhD Singapore Eye Research Institute, Singapore National Eye Centre, Singapore, Singapore

Essilor Centre for Innovation and Technologies AMERA, Singapore, Singapore

Chee Wai Wong, MBBS, PhD Singapore Eye Research Institute, Singapore National Eye Centre, Singapore, Singapore

Duke-NUS Medical School, Singapore, Singapore

Singapore National Eye Centre, Singapore, Singapore

Yong Loo Lin School of Medicine, National University of Singapore, Singapore, Singapore

Lawrence A. Yannuzzi LuEsther T. Mertz Retinal Research, Columbia University School of Medicine, New York, NY, USA

Tsuranu Yokoyama, MD, PhD Department of Pediatric Ophthamology, Osaka City General Hospital Children's Medical Center, Miyakojima-ku, Osaka, Japan

Daryle Jason G. Yu, MD Singapore Eye Research Institute, Singapore, Singapore

Qingjiong Zhang, MD, PhD State Key Laboratory of Ophthalmology, Zhongshan Ophthalmic Center, Sun Yat-sen University, Guangzhou, China

Part I

Basic Science of Pathologic Myopia

Myopia: A Historical Perspective

Eugene Yu-Chuan Kang and Nan-Kai Wang

The word "myopia" is thought to be derived from New Latin, original Greek word "mŭopia" (μυωπία, from myein "to shut" + ops [gen. opos] "eye"), which means contracting or closing the eye. This is a description of the typical facial expression of the uncorrected myopia when a patient attempts to obtain clear distance vision. Before the introduction of spectacles, squinting the eyelids resulting in a horizontal stenopeic slit was the only practical way to achieve clearer distance vision. In ancient times, the myope was reliant upon others with normal vision for the spoils of the hunt and protection in war. In prehistoric times, this dependency must have been even greater. With the advent of civilization, the emergence of agricultural handicrafts, and the written word, the nearsighted at least found a place of more worth in society. As knowledge and fine skills have become increasingly important in our advancing culture, this place of the myopia has been continually expanded.

For tracing the historical perspectives of pathologic myopia in the ophthalmic literature, the first to consider is the evolution of our knowledge of myopia, which has been marked by occasional giant strides based on numerous careful investigations. However, conflicting observations on this subject have been bewildering by their varied and complex protocols and their results and conclusions. A tendency toward advocacy rather than investigatory curiosity can be seen to influence the early literature. Yet, myopia remains one of the major causes of visual disability and blindness to this day. As a result, myopia continues to be one of the major perplexing problems worldwide. Table 1.1 lists some historical landmarks in myopia.

E. Y.-C. Kang
Department of Ophthalmology, Chang Gung Memorial Hospital,
Linkuo Medical Center, Kuei Shan, Taoyuan, Taiwan

N.-K. Wang (✉)
Department of Ophthalmology, Chang Gung Memorial Hospital,
Linkuo Medical Center, Kuei Shan, Taoyuan, Taiwan

Department of Ophthalmology, Edward S. Harkness Eye Institute,
Columbia University, New York, NY, USA

1.1 Pre-ophthalmoscopic Historical Landmarks in Myopia

Pre-ophthalmoscopic development in myopia started from light, optics, and anatomical studies. There are many reviews of the history of myopia [1–6]. Aristotle (384–321 BC) was generally thought to be the first to consider the problem seriously (Fig. 1.1). He described the difference between "long sight" and "short sight" and noted the tendency of the myopia to blink the lids and write in small script [7]. Galen's (138–201 AD, Fig. 1.2) concepts dominated the early years of medicine. Galen thought that ocular refraction was dependent upon both the composition and quantity of the eye fluids (animal spirit), and he was the first to use the term myopia [7]. From Aristotle's time, it was believed that the eye itself was a source of vision rays, an idea finally dismissed by Alhazin (AD 1100) [8]. Optical correction and myopia evolved very slowly. Although Nero is believed to have watched gladiator battles through a concave ruby, correcting spectacles did not make their appearance until near the end of the thirteenth century, and the myopia had to wait a few more centuries before the introduction of minus lenses.

The optics and image formation of refraction were poorly understood in those times. Porta (1558–1593) believed that the image fell on the anterior surface of the lens, whereas his contemporary, Maurolycus (1575), thought that the lens was involved in focusing the image and that it was more convex in myopia and flatter in hyperopia [9]. He did not mention the retina and believed the focal plane was on the optic nerve. Adding to the confusion was the problem of obtaining an upright image in the eye, an accomplishment that early workers considered indispensable for normal vision. A dramatic step forward was made by Kepler (Fig. 1.3), who seemed appropriate to address the subject because of his background in mathematics. In 1604, Kepler demonstrated the image formation of the eye and the role played by the cornea and lens. He placed the inverted image at the retina and defined the action of convex and concave lenses upon this system [10]. Later, Kepler noted that parallel rays of light fell in front of

Table 1.1 Historical landmarks in myopia

Year	Author	Description
384–321 BC	Aristotle	Difference between nearsighted and farsighted
138–201	Galen	First used the term "myopia" from the original Greek word: myein "to shut" + ops (gen. opos) "eye" Ocular refraction was dependent upon the composition and quantity of the eye fluids
1604	Johannes Kepler	Described the retina as the site of vision, not the lens Demonstrated concave lenses correct myopia and convex lenses correct hyperopia
1801	Antonio Scarpa	First anatomical description of posterior staphyloma, but did not make the link to myopia
1813	James Ware	Noted that people who were educated were often myopic
1854	Von Graefe	First postulated the association between myopia and axial length
1856	Carl Ferdinand Ritter von Arlt	First connected staphyloma and myopic refraction
1861	Eduard Jäger von Jaxtthal	First described and illustrated myopia "conus" and enlarged subarachnoid space around the nerve
1862	Carl Friedrich Richard Förster	First observed sub-retinal pigment epithelium choroidal neovascularization; "Forster spot"
1887	Adolf Eugen Fick	First used the term "contact lens" and designed glass contact lenses
1901	Ernst Fuchs	"Central black spot in myopia"; "Fuchs' spot"
1902	Maximilian Salzmann	First described defect in lamina vitrea (Bruch's membrane); was later coined as "lacquer crack"
1913	Adolf Steiger	Myopic refraction depends on corneal refraction and axial length
1938	Rushton, R.H.	Measured axial length by X-rays
1965	Gernet, H	Measured axial length by ultrasonography
1970	Brian J. Curtin and David B. Karlin	Discovered the relationship between axial length and chorioretinal atrophy First used "lacquer crack" in this article
1977	Brian J. Curtin	Classification scheme for staphyloma
1988	Takashi Tokoro	Classification of chorioretinal atrophy in the posterior pole in pathologic myopia Definition of pathologic myopia
1996	Brancato R. et al.	Indocyanine green angiography (ICGA) in pathologic myopia
1999	Morito Takano and Shoji Kishi	First illustrated foveal retinoschisis using optical coherence tomography (OCT) in eyes with posterior staphyloma

Table 1.1 (continued)

Year	Author	Description
2001	Verteporfin in Photodynamic Therapy Study Group	Treated myopic choroidal neovascularization with photodynamic therapy
2002	Baba T. et al.	First described different stages of myopic choroidal neovascularization using OCT
2005	Nguyen QD. et al.	Treated myopic choroidal neovascularization with bevacizumab
2008	Spaide RF. et al.	Enhanced depth imaging spectral domain OCT for choroidal imaging
2012	Ohno-Matsui K. et al.	Relationship between myopic retinochoroidal lesions with shape of sclera using 3D-magnetic resonance imaging (MRI) and intrachoroidal cavitation in pathologically myopic eyes using OCT
2013	Ohno-Matsui K.	Classification of posterior staphyloma based on MRI and wide-field fundus photos
2018	Panda-Jonas et al.	Hypothesis of myopization caused by production of Bruch's membrane

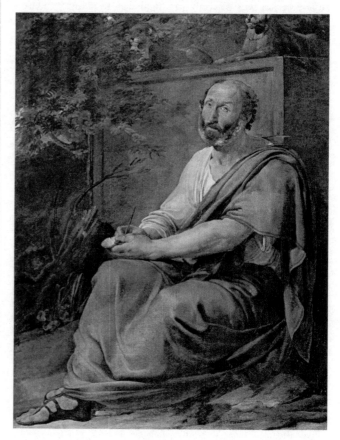

Fig. 1.1 Painting of Aristotle by Francesco Hayez (1791–1882)

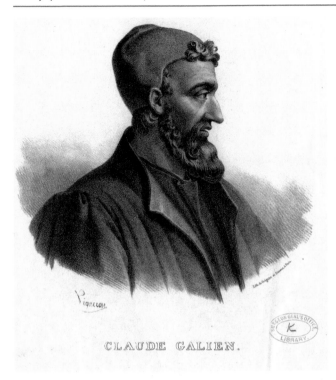

Fig. 1.2 A portrait of Galen by Pierre Roche Vigneron. (Paris: Lith de Gregoire et Deneux, ca. 1865). (Courtesy of the National Library of Medicine)

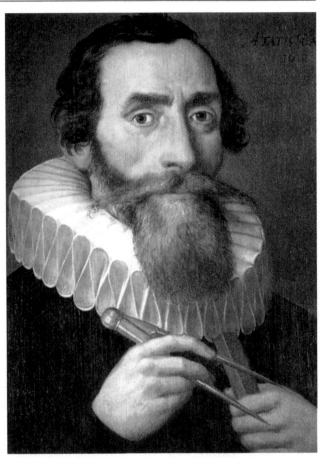

Fig. 1.3 A 1610 portrait of Johannes Kepler by an unknown artist

the retina in myopic eyes [11]. Kepler further attributed the ability to see clearly at both distance and near to alterations in the shape of the eye. He went on to propose the "near-work" hypothesis for myopia by stating that study and fine work in childhood rapidly accustoms the eye to near objects [11]. With aging, this adaptive mechanism produces a permanent, finite far point such that distant objects were seen poorly, a theory that is still accepted today [9].

Newton (1704) wrote about the concept of hyperopia as a condition due to parallel rays of light converging behind the retina and set the stage for the acceptance of axial length of the eye as the sole determinant of refraction. Plempius (1632) [9] provided anatomical proof of increased axial lengthening of the eye, and Boerhaave (1708) confirmed this lengthening and also reported the other cause of myopia: increased convexity of the refractive surfaces [12].

In the absence of the instruments necessary to measure corneal and lenticular variables, there were some studies confirming the variability of axial length. These included the studies of Morgagani (1761) [9], Guerin (1769) [9], Gendron (1770) [5], and Pichter (1790) [5]. Scarpa (Fig. 1.4 upper) is the first to describe anatomically posterior staphyloma (Fig. 1.4 lower) in two female eyes in 1801 [13]. He coined

the Greek word "*staphylos*" which literally means "a bunch of grapes." It is of note that Scarpa described staphyloma but did not link it to myopia. Von Ammon (1832) noted that posterior staphyloma was due to a distention of the posterior pole and was not a rare entity. However, he did not make a link either from posterior staphyloma to myopia [14].

1.2 Post-ophthalmoscopic Historical Landmarks in Myopia (1851)

Post-ophthalmoscopic development in myopia started from observations of the optic nerve, macula, and chorioretinal changes. Von Graefe (1854) first postulated the association between myopia and axial length in a combined ophthalmoscopic and anatomical study of two eyes measuring 29 mm and 30.5 mm in length [15]. However, it was Arlt's (1856) (Fig. 1.5) anatomical studies that convinced the scientific world of the intimate association of myopia with axial elon-

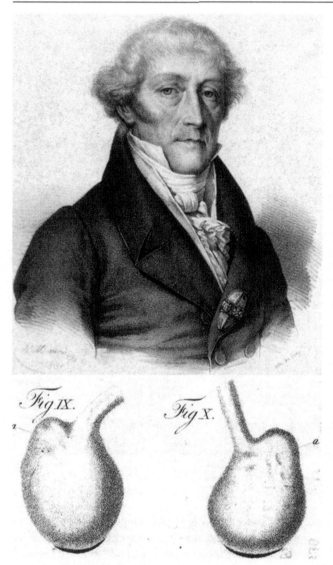

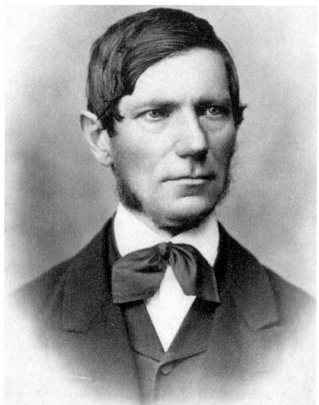

Fig. 1.5 A portrait of Carl Ferdinand Ritter von Arlt by Fritz Luckhardt. The anatomical studies of Carl Ferdinand Ritter von Arlt convinced the scientific world of the intimate association of myopia with axial elongation of the globe at the expense of the posterior pole

Fig. 1.4 Upper: Portrait of Antonio Scarpa; Lower: The earliest depiction of posterior staphyloma as contained in the text of Antonio Scarpa [13]

gation of the globe at the expense of the posterior pole [16]. After Arlt made the connection between staphyloma and myopic refraction [16], clinical findings in pathologic myopia were investigated.

Von Jaeger (Fig. 1.6) was the first to describe and illustrate myopic conus and enlarged subarachnoid space around the nerve in 1861 [17]. He found that the choriocapillaris was sometimes absent within the limits of the conus and that in extensive staphyloma the choroid over the conus presented the appearance of a glass-like membrane which was exceedingly fine and delicately striated and contained a few vessels [17]. In 1862, Carl Friedrich Richard Förster (Fig. 1.7, upper) first observed sub-RPE choroidal neovascularization (CNV) (Fig. 1.7, lower) [18], and this is what we called "Forster spots." In 1901, Ernst Fuchs (Fig. 1.8, left) later discovered

"central black spot in myopia" [19] (Fig. 1.8, right) [20], and this is what we called "Fuchs' spots." Fuchs concluded that the choroid is not destroyed, but is either converted into, or covered by, a callosity. It starts with sudden visual disturbances in the form of metamorphoses or positive scotomas, which in the course of years become more marked. Anatomically, there is an intense proliferation of the pigment epithelium covered by a gelatinous acellular exudation (coagulum of fibrin), adherent to the retina, but the etiology was obscure [12]. Henry Wilson described atrophy of choroidal epithelium in 1868 [21]. In 1902, Salzmann (Fig. 1.9, left) noted that cleft-shaped or branched defects were found in atrophic areas in the lamina vitrea that were concentric with the optic disc (Fig. 1.9, Right) [22, 23]. The lamina vitrea is also referred to as "Bruch's membrane." He felt that these defects seemed to be the result of purely mechanical stretching. Later, the term "lacquer cracks" was used by Curtin and Kerlin to describe this lesion, which typically occurs as yellowish to white lines in the posterior segment of highly myopic eyes, resulting from progressive eyeball elongation. Salzmann believed that atrophic changes noted in the myopic choroid followed inflammation and the primary process driving this was stretching of the choroidal stroma [24].

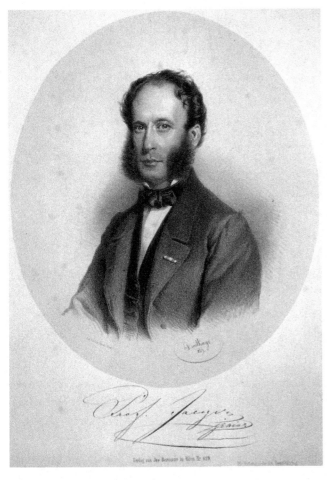

Fig. 1.6 A portrait of Eduard Jäger von Jaxtthal by Adolf Dauthage in 1859

1.3 Modern Historical Landmarks in Myopia

Modern historical landmarks include studies dedicated to exploring the individual optical elements of myopia, axial length measurement (X-ray and ultrasound), and the development of contact lenses.

The greatest efforts of the ophthalmologic community were concentrated on a search for the causes of increased axial length of the eye. Donders [1] appreciated that axial length was not the sole determinant of refraction. Schanbe and Harrneiser (1895) had found axial lengths varying from 22.25 to 26.24 mm in 35 emmetropic eyes and hypothesized that emmetropia could be determined by axial length and total refraction [25]. Ludwig Hein (1899) thought that myopia was due to elongation of the globe [8]. Steiger (1913), in a large statistical study of corneal power in children, deemphasized the importance of axial length as the only determinant of refraction. His biomathematical study was large (5000 children), but his experimental method was somewhat faulty in that he assumed lens power to be a constant and

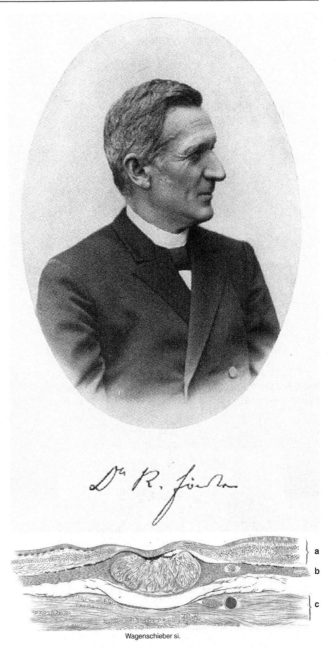

Wagenschieber si.

Fig. 1.7 Upper: A portrait of Carl Friedrich Richard Förster. (Reprinted with permission from The Royal Library, The National Library of Denmark and Copenhagen University Library); Lower: Cross-section of the retina, choroid, and sclera from a myopic eye shows a circumscript inclusion in the choroidal stroma which encroaches into the anterior layer of the choroid. (Förster [18])

therefore calculated the axial length of the eye from total refraction in this manner [9]. The variability of lens power had been alluded to as early as 1575 by Maurolycus [5], and variations in lens thickness, refractive index, and position had been considered as possible causes of myopia prior to Donder's time [1]. In addition, actual lens power measurements, albeit in small samples, had been demonstrated by von Reuss (1887–1890), Awerbach (1900), and Zeeman

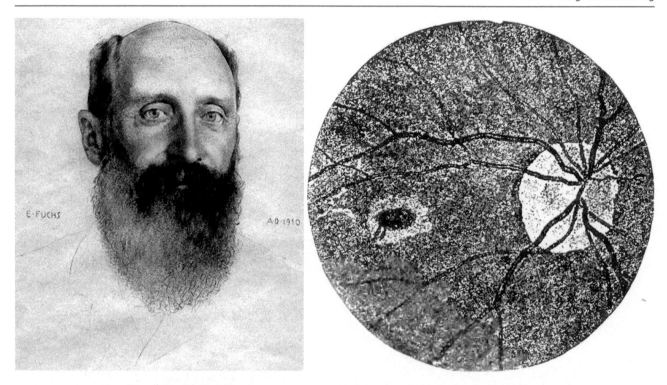

Fig. 1.8 Left: Portrait of Ernst Fuchs. Original etching by Emil Orlik, 1910. (Reprinted with permission from the Medical University of Vienna, Austria); Right: The earliest figure of "Fuchs' spot," which was described by Dr. Ernst Fuchs as "The central black spot in myopia." (Fuchs [20])

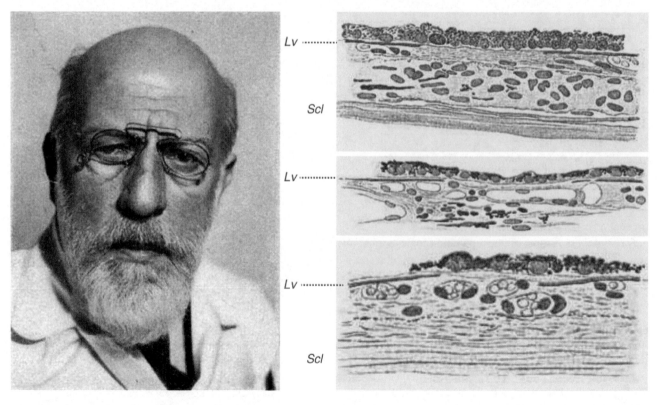

Fig. 1.9 Left: Photograph of Maximilian Salzmann, M.D. (Reprinted with permission from The Royal Library, The National Library of Denmark and Copenhagen University Library); Right: Top: Break in lamina of Bruch covered with the epithelium. Middle: Changes in the epithelium. Bottom: Break in lamina with epithelial covering and hyaline membrane. (Salzmann [23])

(1911) to show considerable variations [7]. Steiger's corneal measurements gave a Gaussian curve extending from 39 D to 48 D [26]. He did not note any set value of corneal power in emmetropia. He further made a distribution curve of +7 D to −7D using his corneal values and calculated axial lengths found in emmetropia (21.5–25.5 mm). Steiger viewed emmetropia and refractive errors as points on a normal distribution curve, with corneal power and axial lengths as free and independent variables [26]. Tscherning (1854–1939) was crucial in the understanding of optics in pathologic myopia [27], and he made many contributions in this area. In addition, he wrote a thesis about the frequency of myopia in Denmark [28]. Schnabel, Fuchs, Siegrest, and Elschnig were important to the studies of histopathology in myopic eyes, especially in relation to optic nerve changes in pathologic myopia [9]. These concepts brought an entirely new approach to the study of myopia.

Tron (1934–1935) followed with a study of 275 eyes and carefully avoided the pitfalls of Steiger's work [29, 30]. In his study, the only optical element not measured directly was axial length, which was calculated from the refraction, corneal power, lens power, and anterior chamber depth. Tron confirmed the wide range of axial lengths in emmetropia (22.4–27.3 mm) [29]. He also deduced that axial length was the determining factor for refraction only in the range beyond +4 D and −6 D [29]. He obtained essentially binomial curves for all the elements of refraction except for axial length. With the elimination of myopic eyes of more than 6 D, the curve for axial length also assumed a normal distribution [7]. Stenstrom (1946) [31] directly measured axial length by using X-rays contributed by the development of this technique by Rushton (1938) [32]. Stenstrom studied 1000 right eyes and confirmed the results Tron had obtained in his smaller series. Both biometric studies found essentially normal distribution curves for corneal power, anterior chamber depth, lens power, and total refraction. Both also showed a peaking (excess) for axial length above the binomial curve as well as an extension of the limb toward increased axial length (skewness) [29, 31]. Stenstrom noted that the distribution curve of refraction had basically the same disposition as that of axial length, featuring both a positive excess at emmetropia and a skewness toward myopia [5].

This deviation in the population refraction curve had been noted previously by Scheerer and Betsch (1928–1929) [7], who had attributed this to the incorporation of eyes with crescent formation at the optic nerve. When these eyes were deleted from the data, a symmetric curve was obtained for the distribution of refraction. In the analysis of these data, it was pointed out that a positive excess persisted in the "corrected" curve. Stenstrom's refractive curve [7] after the removal of eyes with crescent also demonstrated an excess.

This central peaking was attributed to two factors: the first was the effect of the component correlation in the emmetropic range as postulated by Wibaut (1928) [5] and Berg (1931) [5] and the second was the direct effect of axial length distribution upon the curve of refraction [7]. Sorsby (1957) [9] later confirmed again the results of both Tron and Stenstrom and further explored the variables in the correlations between the optical components in various refractions. This had been done to a limited extent by Berg [5]. Sorsby and co-workers demonstrated conclusively in their study of 341 eyes the "emmetropization" effect that was noted in distribution curves of refraction as a result of a correlation of corneal power and axial length. In ametropia +4 D and above, this correlation appeared to break down. Their study also indicated that neither the lens nor the chamber depth was an effective emmetropization factor [2]. Gernet (1965) proposed the use of ultrasound to measure the ocular axial length [33] after ultrasonography was pioneered in ophthalmology by Mundt and Hughes in 1956 [34].

In 1887, Adolf Eugen Fick submitted a very original paper entitled "Eine Contactbrille" (A contact spectacle) to the *Archiv für Augenheilkunde*. This was a report on his work, which led to the development of contact lenses. He published his paper in 1888 and coined the term "contact lens" [35]. Fick designed glass contact lenses to correct myopia and irregular astigmatism using lenses that were specially ground by Abbe, of Jena [36]. There were many early contact lens designs, but the first one to allow circulation of tear film was made by Tuohy in 1948; the lens was made by plastic.

1.4 Recent Historical Landmarks in Myopia

There are many recent contributors to pathologic myopia. No work has influenced and inspired the eye care field more than the published comprehensive textbook on myopia in 1985 by Brian J. Curtin, M.D. [7] (Fig. 1.10): *The Myopias: Basic Science and Clinical Management*. It increased the evidence that pathologic myopia represented an important cause for severe vision loss worldwide, particularly in selected racial populations. Curtin's textbook was an awakening on the importance of the disease and made clinical scientists to accelerate and intensify their research to expand our knowledge of the related embryological, epidemiological, molecular, biological, genetic, and clinical aspects of pathologic myopia. Curtin has many scientific contributions, and some of these will be briefly described here. Curtin and Karlin first used "lacquer cracks" and described the association between axial length and chorioretinal atrophy in 1970 [37]. In addi-

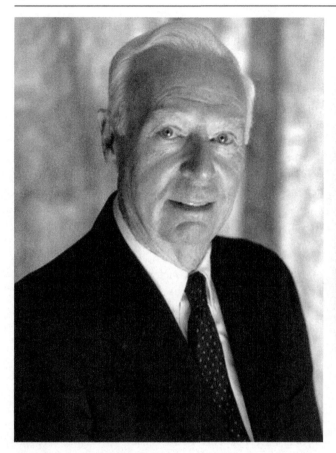

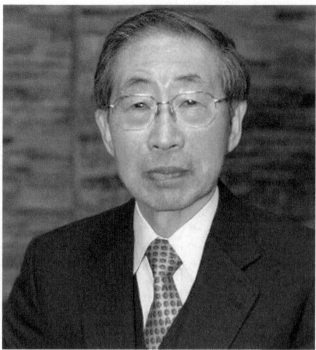

Fig. 1.11 Photograph of Takashi Tokoro, M.D.

Fig. 1.10 Photograph of Brian Curtin, M.D.

tion, Klein and Curtin discovered the formation of subretinal hemorrhage caused by lacquer cracks without choroidal neovascularization (CNV) in 1975 [38]. In 1977, Curtin created a classification scheme for staphyloma [39]. His textbook emphasized the importance of the posterior staphyloma which was incriminated in the clinical manifestations associated with severe visual decline. In addition, Curtin helped to identify the optic nerve as an important cause of visual changes in myopia and described the ocular changes putting myopic patients at risk for retinal detachment, early cataract formation, glaucoma, and a myriad of macular manifestations as its complications leading to severe vision loss [1].

The other important figure is Tokoro, (Fig. 1.11), and some of his accomplishments will be mentioned here. Tokoro described the mechanism of axial elongation and chorioretinal atrophy in high myopia [40]. In 1988, Tokoro defined pathologic myopia [41], which has been used for many myopic studies. Afterward, Tokoro classified chorioretinal atrophy in the posterior pole in pathologic myopia as tessellated fundus, diffuse chorioretinal atrophy, small patch atrophy, and small macular hemorrhage [42].

Some other recent landmarks in myopia were attributed to advanced technology and new treatments. Although fluorescein angiography (FA) is the main tool for diagnosing myo-

pic CNV, indocyanine green angiography (ICGA) may better identify the CNV when large hemorrhages are present. ICGA also allows a better definition of lacquer cracks than FA [43, 44]. Optical coherence tomography (OCT) is a powerful real-time imaging modality. Since its introduction, it has been utilized in understanding the ocular structure in many eye diseases. In 1999, Takano and Kishi reported foveal retinoschisis and retinal detachment in severely myopic eyes with posterior staphyloma [45]. Three years later, Baba et al. first used OCT to demonstrate characteristic features at each stage of myopic CNV [46]. As for other findings investigated using OCT, Spaide invented enhanced depth imaging spectral domain OCT to obtain images of choroid [47] and found thinner choroids in highly myopic eyes [48]. Excessive thinning of the choroid eventually leads to chorioretinal atrophy. Ohno-Matsui and Moriyama have furthered our understanding of the shape of pathologically myopic eyes and posterior staphyloma using high-resolution 3D magnetic resonance images and ultrawide-field fundus photos [49–51]. With the advent of swept-source OCT (SS-OCT), structural changes in myopic eyes could be studied more clearly. Ohno-Matsui et al. described intrachoroidal cavitation using SS-OCT [52]. Recently, Dr. Ohno-Matsui and her group used ultrawide-field SS-OCT and found that the sites of posterior staphyloma and myopic macular retinoschisis are spatially related to each other in high myopic eyes [53]. In 2017, Jonas et al. hypothesized that axial elongation is caused by production of Bruch's membrane in the retro-equatorial region, which plays an important role in myopization [54]. Because of potential of visual loss from myopic CNV, several treatments have been tried, for example, thermal laser photocoagulation [55] and photodynamic therapy (PDT) with Visudyne [56]. In 2005, Nguyen et al. reported the effectiveness of bevacizumab in treating CNV secondary to pathologic myopia. After that, ophthalmologists started to use anti-vascular endothelial growth factor to treat myopic CNV. Many details of diagnosis and treatment for myopic patients will be mentioned in later chapters.

Acknowledgment: Dr. Brian J Curtin The early documentation of the history of myopia was based on his work. The update was incorporated in this perspective with his full consent.

References

1. Donders FC. On the anomalies of accommodation and refraction of the eye. London: The New Sydenham Society; 1864.
2. Sorby A, Benjamin B, Davey J, Sheridan M, Tauner J. Emmetropia and its aberrations. MRC special report series no 293. London: HMSO; 1957.
3. Alphen GWHMV. On emmetropia and ametropia. Basel, New York: S. Karger; 1961.
4. Blach RK. The nature of degenerative myopia: a clinico-pathological study. Master thesis. University of Cambridge; 1964.
5. Duke-Elder S. In: Duke-Elder S, editor. System of ophthalmology, vol. 1–15. St. Louis: Mosby; 1970.
6. Roberts J, Slaby D. Refraction status of youths 12–17 years, United States. Vital Health Stat. 1974;11(148):1–55.
7. Curtin BJ. The myopias: basic science and clinical management. Philadelphia: Harper & Row; 1985.
8. Wood CA. The American encyclopedia and dictionary of ophthalmology, vol. 11. Chicago: Cleveland Press; 1917.
9. Albert DM, Edwards DD. The history of ophthalmology. Cambridge, MA: Blackwell Science; 1996.
10. Kepler J. Ad Vitellionem Paralipomena (A Sequel to Witelo). C. Marnius & Heirs of J. Aubrius: Frankfurt; 1604.
11. Kepler J. Dioptrice. Augsburg; 1611.
12. Wood CA. The American encyclopedia and dictionary of ophthalmology, vol. 10. Chicago: Cleveland Press; 1917.
13. Scarpa A. Saggio di osservazioni e d'esperienze sulle principali malattie degli occhi. Pavia: Presso Baldessare Comino; 1801.
14. Ammon FAV. Histologie des Hydrophthalmus und des Staphyloma scleroticae posticum et laterale. Zeitschrift für die Ophthalmologie. 1832;2:247–56.
15. Graefe AV. Zwei Sektionsbefunde bei Sclerotico-chorioiditis posterior und Bemerkungen uber diese Krankheit. Arch Ophthalmol. 1854;1(1):390.
16. Arlt FV. Die Krankheiten des Auges. Prag Credner & Kleinbub; 1856.
17. Jaeger E. Ueber die Einstellungen des dioptrischen Apparates Im Menschlichen Auge. Kais. Kön. Hof- und Staatsdruckerei; 1861.
18. Förster R. Ophthalmologische Beiträge. Berlin: Enslin; 1862.
19. Fuchs E. Der centrale schwarze Fleck bei Myopie. Zeitschrift für Augenheilkunde. 1901;5:171–8.
20. Fuchs E. Text-book of ophthalmology. 5th ed. Philadelphia & London: Lippincott; 1917.
21. Wilson H. Lectures on the theory and practice of the ophthalmoscope. Dublin: Fannin & Co.; 1868.
22. Salzmann M. The choroidal changes in high myopia. Arch Ophthalmol. 1902;31:41–2.
23. Salzmann M. Die Atrophie der Aderhaut im kurzsichtigen Auge. Albrecht von Graefes Archiv fur Ophthalmologie. 1902;54:384.
24. Sym WG. Ophthalmic review: a record of ophthalmic science, vol. 21. London: Sherratt and Hughes; 1902.
25. Schnabel I, Herrnheiser I. Ueber Staphyloma Posticum, Conus und Myopie. Fischer's Medicinische Buchhandlung; 1895.
26. Steiger A. Die Entstehung der sphärischen Refraktionen des menschlichen Auges. Berlin: Karger; 1913.
27. Tscherning MHE. Physiologic optics: dioptrics of the eye, functions of the retina, ocular movements and binocular vision. Philadelphia: The Keystone Publishing Co.; 1920.
28. Norn M, Jensen OA. Marius Tscherning (1854–1939): his life and work in optical physiology. Acta Ophthalmol Scand. 2004;82(5):501–8.
29. Tron E. Uber die optischen Grundlagen der Ametropie. Albrecht Von Graefes Arch Ophthalmol. 1934;132:182–223.
30. Tron E. Ein Beitrag zur Frage der optischen Grundlagen der Anisound Isometropie. Albrecht Von Graefes Arch Ophthalmol. 1935;133:211–30.
31. Stenstrom SLHV. Untersuchungen über die Variation und Kovariation der optischen Elemente des menschlichen Auges. Uppsala: Appelbergs Boktr; 1946.
32. Rushton RH. The clinical measurement of the axial length of the living eye. Trans Ophthalmol Soc UK. 1938;58:136–42.
33. Gernet H. Biometrie des Auges mit Ultraschall. Klin Monatsbl Augenheilkd. 1965;146:863–74.
34. Mundt GH, W. Ultrasonics in ocular diagnosis. Am J Ophthalmol. 1956;41:488–98.
35. The "Kontaktbrille" of Adolf Eugen Fick; 1887.
36. Dor H. On contact lenses. Ophthal Rev. 1893;12(135):21–3.
37. Curtin BJ, Karlin DB. Axial length measurements and fundus changes of the myopic eye. I. The posterior fundus. Trans Am Ophthalmol Soc. 1970;68:312–34.
38. Klein RM, Curtin BJ. Lacquer crack lesions in pathologic myopia. Am J Ophthalmol. 1975;79(3):386–92.
39. Curtin BJ. The posterior staphyloma of pathologic myopia. Trans Am Ophthalmol Soc. 1977;75:67–86.
40. Tokoro T. Mechanism of axial elongation and chorioretinal atrophy in high myopia. Nippon Ganka Gakkai Zasshi. 1994;98(12):1213–37.
41. Tokoro T. On the definition of pathologic myopia in group studies. Acta Ophthalmol Suppl. 1988;185:107–8.
42. Tokoro T. Atlas of posterior fundus changes in pathologic myopia. 1st ed. Tokyo: Springer-Verlag; 1998. p. 5–22.
43. Brancato R, Trabucchi G, Introini U, Avanza P, Pece A. Indocyanine green angiography (ICGA) in pathological myopia. Eur J Ophthalmol. 1996;6(1):39–43.
44. Ohno-Matsui K, Morishima N, Ito M, Tokoro T. Indocyanine green angiographic findings of lacquer cracks in pathologic myopia. Jpn J Ophthalmol. 1998;42(4):293–9.
45. Takano M, Kishi S. Foveal retinoschisis and retinal detachment in severely myopic eyes with posterior staphyloma. Am J Ophthalmol. 1999;128(4):472–6.
46. Baba T, Ohno-Matsui K, Yoshida T, Yasuzumi K, Futagami S, Tokoro T, Mochizuki M. Optical coherence tomography of choroidal neovascularization in high myopia. Acta Ophthalmol Scand. 2002;80(1):82–7.
47. Charbel Issa P, Finger RP, Holz FG, Scholl HP. Multimodal imaging including spectral domain OCT and confocal near infrared reflectance for characterization of outer retinal pathology in pseudoxanthoma elasticum. Invest Ophthalmol Vis Sci. 2009;50(12):5913–8.
48. Fujiwara T, Imamura Y, Margolis R, Slakter JS, Spaide RF. Enhanced depth imaging optical coherence tomography of the choroid in highly myopic eyes. Am J Ophthalmol. 2009;148(3):445–50.
49. Ohno-Matsui K, Akiba M, Modegi T, Tomita M, Ishibashi T, Tokoro T, Moriyama M. Association between shape of sclera and

myopic retinochoroidal lesions in patients with pathologic myopia. Invest Ophthalmol Vis Sci. 2012;53(10):6046–61.

50. Moriyama M, Ohno-Matsui K, Modegi T, Kondo J, Takahashi Y, Tomita M, Tokoro T, Morita I. Quantitative analyses of high-resolution 3D MR images of highly myopic eyes to determine their shapes. Invest Ophthalmol Vis Sci. 2012;53(8):4510–8.

51. Ohno-Matsui K. Proposed classification of posterior staphylomas based on analyses of eye shape by three-dimensional magnetic resonance imaging and wide-field fundus imaging. Ophthalmology. 2014;121(9):1798–809.

52. Ohno-Matsui K, Akiba M, Moriyama M, Ishibashi T, Hirakata A, Tokoro T. Intrachoroidal cavitation in macular area of eyes with pathologic myopia. Am J Ophthalmol. 2012;154(2):382–93.

53. Shinohara K, Tanaka N, Jonas JB, Shimada N, Moriyama M, Yoshida T, Ohno-Matsui K. Ultrawide-field OCT to investigate relationships between myopic macular retinoschisis and posterior staphyloma. Ophthalmology. 2018;125(10):1575–86.

54. Jonas JB, Ohno-Matsui K, Jiang WJ, Panda-Jonas S. Bruch membrane and the mechanism of myopization: a new theory. Retina (Philadelphia, PA). 2017;37(8):1428–40.

55. Secretan M, Kuhn D, Soubrane G, Coscas G. Long-term visual outcome of choroidal neovascularization in pathologic myopia: natural history and laser treatment. Eur J Ophthalmol. 1997;7(4):307–16.

56. Verteporfin in Photodynamic Therapy Study Group. Photodynamic therapy of subfoveal choroidal neovascularization in pathologic myopia with verteporfin. 1-year results of a randomized clinical trial--VIP report no. 1. Ophthalmology. 2001;108(5):841–52.

Definition of Pathologic Myopia (PM)

Kyoko Ohno-Matsui

Myopia is a significant public health concern worldwide [1–3]. It is estimated that by 2050, there will be 4.8 billion people with myopia which is approximately one-half (49.8%) of the world population. Of these, 938 million individuals will have high myopia which is 9.8% of the world population [4].

Although most myopic patients obtain good vision with optic correction of refractive error, the exception is pathologic myopia (PM). Eyes with PM develop different types of fundus lesions, called myopic maculopathy, which can lead to a significant reduction of central vision [5, 6]. In fact, myopic maculopathy in eyes with PM is a major cause of blindness worldwide, especially in East Asian countries [7–11].

The definitions of myopia and pathologic myopia have not been standardized, and the term "pathologic myopia" is often confused with "high myopia." However, these two are distinctly different. "High myopia" is defined as an eye with a high degree of myopic refractive error, and "pathologic myopia" is defined as myopic eyes with the presence of pathologic lesions in the posterior fundus. Duke-Elder defined "pathologic myopia," as "that type of myopia which is accompanied by degenerative changes occurring especially in the posterior pole of the globe" [12].

Myopia is defined as a refractive condition of the eye in which parallel rays of light entering the eye are brought to a focus in front of the retina when the ocular accommodation is relaxed [13]. This refractive status is dependent on the axial length, and a disproportionate increase of the axial length of the eye can lead to myopia, called axial myopia, or a disproportionate increase in the refractive power of the eye can also lead to myopia, called refractive myopia. The WHO Report defines myopia as "a condition in which the refractive error (spherical equivalent) is ≤ -0.50 diopter (D) in either eye" [3].

Myopia is classified into low myopia, moderate myopia, and high myopia. The cutoff values for the different degrees have not been consistent among studies. The WHO Report defined "high myopia" as "a condition in which the objective refractive error (spherical equivalent) is ≤ -5.00 D in either eye" [3]. Very recently, Flitcroft on behalf of the International Myopia Institute (IMI) proposed a set of standards to define and classify myopia [13]. Low myopia is defined as a refractive error of ≤ -0.50 and > -6.00, and high myopia is defined as refractive error of ≤ -6.00 D [13]. The Japan Myopia Society proposed a category of "moderate myopia" between "low myopia" and "high myopia" (http://www.myopiasociety.jp/member/guideline/index.html). According to this society, low myopia was defined as a refractive error of ≤ -0.50 and > -3.00 D, moderate myopia is ≤ -3.00 and > -6.00 D, and high myopia is ≤ -6.00 D. Table 2.1 shows a modified summary of the classification of different degrees of myopia and PM.

As mentioned above, PM is classified as being present when myopic eyes have characteristic lesions in the posterior fundus. The changes are the presence of myopic macu-

Table 2.1 Summary of definitions of various types of myopia

Term	Definition
Myopia	A condition in which the spherical equivalent refractive error of an eye is ≤ -0.50 D when ocular accommodation is relaxed
Low myopia	A condition in which the spherical equivalent refractive error of an eye is ≤ -0.50 D and > -3.00 D when ocular accommodation is relaxed
Moderate myopia	A condition in which the spherical equivalent refractive error of an eye is ≤ -3.000 D and > -6.00 D when ocular accommodation is relaxed
High myopia	A condition in which the spherical equivalent refractive error of an eye is ≤ -6.000 D when ocular accommodation is relaxed
Pathologic myopia	Myopia that accompanies characteristic myopic fundus changes (the presence of myopic maculopathy equal to or more serious than diffuse choroidal atrophy or the presence of posterior staphyloma)

Revised from Flicott et al. in IOVS 2019

K. Ohno-Matsui (✉)
Department of Ophthalmology and Visual Science, Tokyo Medical and Dental University, Bunkyo-Ku, Tokyo, Japan
e-mail: k.ohno.oph@tmd.ac.jp

© Springer Nature Switzerland AG 2021
R. F. Spaide et al. (eds.), *Pathologic Myopia*, https://doi.org/10.1007/978-3-030-74334-5_2

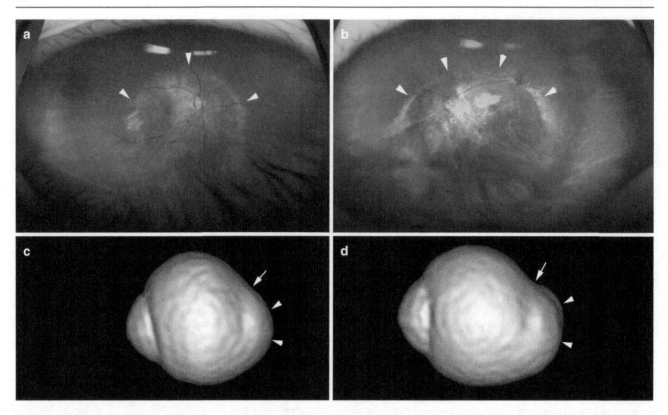

Fig. 2.1 Three-dimensional magnetic resonance images (3D MRI) of an eye with unilateral high myopia. (Modified and cited with permission from Ref. [15]). The axial length was 24 mm in the right eye and 28 mm in the left. Ultra-widefield fundus images show the upper edge of the staphylomas (**a** and **b** outlined by arrowheads). In 3D MRI images viewed nasally, a posterior protrusion (arrowheads) due to a staphyloma is seen in both eyes (**c** and **d**), although the degree is milder in the right eye (**c**). The upper edge is observed as a notch (**c** and **d** arrows)

lopathy equal to or more serious than diffuse choroidal atrophy (equal to Category 2 in the META-PM classification [5]) and/or the presence of a posterior staphyloma [14]. The cutoff values of the myopic refractive error and axial length should not be set for the definition of pathologic myopia because a posterior staphyloma has been reported to occur in eyes with normal axial length (Fig. 2.1) [15] and even in eyes with axial lengths <26.5 mm [16]. This suggested that PM occurs independently of the axial length of the eye.

References

1. Morgan IG, Ohno-Matsui K, Saw SM. Myopia. Lancet. 2012;379(9827):1739–48.
2. Resnikoff S, Jonas JB, Friedman D, et al. Myopia – a 21st century public health issue. Invest Ophthalmol Vis Sci. 2019;60(3):Mi–Mii.
3. Institute WHO-BHV. The impact of myopia. The impact of myopia and high myopia report of the joint World Health Organization – Brien Holden Vision Institute Globa Scientific Meeting on Myopia. Available at: https://www.visionuk.org.uk/download/WHO_Report_Myopia_2016.pdf.2016.
4. Holden BA, Fricke TR, Wilson DA, et al. Global prevalence of myopia and high myopia and temporal trends from 2000 through 2050. Ophthalmology. 2016;123(5):1036–42.
5. Ohno-Matsui K, Kawasaki R, Jonas JB, et al. International photographic classification and grading system for myopic maculopathy. Am J Ophthalmol. 2015;159(5):877–83.
6. Fang Y, Yokoi T, Nagaoka N, et al. Progression of myopic maculopathy during 18-year follow-up. Ophthalmology. 2018;125(6):863–77.
7. Iwase A, Araie M, Tomidokoro A, et al. Prevalence and causes of low vision and blindness in a Japanese adult population: the Tajimi Study. Ophthalmology. 2006;113(8):1354–62.
8. Xu L, Wang Y, Li Y, et al. Causes of blindness and visual impairment in urban and rural areas in Beijing: the Beijing Eye Study. Ophthalmology. 2006;113(7):1134 e1–11.
9. Buch H, Vinding T, La Cour M, et al. Prevalence and causes of visual impairment and blindness among 9980 Scandinavian adults: the Copenhagen City Eye Study. Ophthalmology. 2004;111(1):53–61.
10. Cotter SA, Varma R, Ying-Lai M, et al. Causes of low vision and blindness in adult Latinos: the Los Angeles Latino Eye Study. Ophthalmology. 2006;113(9):1574–82.
11. Varma R, Kim JS, Burkemper BS, et al. Prevalence and causes of visual impairment and blindness in Chinese American adults: the Chinese American Eye Study. JAMA Ophthalmol. 2016;134(7):785–93.
12. Duke-Elder S, editor. Pathological refractive errors. St. Louis: Mosby; 1970.

13. Flitcroft DI, He M, Jonas JB, et al. IMI – defining and classifying myopia: a proposed set of standards for clinical and epidemiologic studies. Invest Ophthalmol Vis Sci. 2019;60(3): M20–30.

14. Ohno-Matsui K, Lai TYY, Cheung CMG, Lai CC. Updates of pathologic myopia. Prog Retin Eye Res. 2016;52(5): 156–87.

15. Moriyama M, Ohno-Matsui K, Hayashi K, et al. Topographical analyses of shape of eyes with pathologic myopia by high-resolution three dimensional magnetic resonance imaging. Ophthalmology. 2011;118(8):1626–37.

16. Wang NK, Wu YM, Wang JP, et al. Clinical characteristics of posterior staphylomas in myopic eyes with axial length shorter than 26.5 mm. Am J Ophthalmol. 2016;162:180–90.

Epidemiology of Myopia, High Myopia, and Pathological Myopia

3

Carla Lanca, Chen-Wei Pan, Seang Mei Saw, and Tien-Yin Wong

3.1 Introduction

Myopia (spherical equivalent [SE] < −0.5 D) is a significant global public health concern with a rapid increase in prevalence in recent decades worldwide [1–4]. It is estimated that globally 153 million people over 5 years of age are visually impaired as a result of uncorrected myopia and other refractive errors, and of these 8 million are blind [5]. The economic costs of myopia to individuals and society have been estimated to be $250 million/year in the USA alone [6]. Nevertheless, myopia is often perceived to be an unimportant condition, because visual impairment (VI) resulting from myopia can often be "corrected" with simple optical aids, such as glasses and contact lenses, or refractive surgery [7]. However, uncorrected and under-correction of myopia and other refractive error is still the major cause of VI worldwide, accounting for at least 33% of cases [8]. As an eye condition, myopia is more common than major diseases such as glaucoma, cataract, or diabetic retinopathy (DR) in East Asian populations. Early myopia onset is especially concerning as myopia progress fast for younger children and with longer duration, increasing the risk of having high myopia [9, 10].

High myopia (SE ≤ −5 or −6 D) poses an even more significant impact because of the higher risks of macular and retinal complications [11–14]. When high myopia is associated with significant retinal or optic nerve changes, the condition is known as pathological myopia or myopic macular degeneration (MMD), a common cause of irreversible VI and blindness in Asian populations [15, 16]. A systematic review comprising 137,514 participants estimated that 10.0 million people had VI from MMD in 2015 with 3.3 million of whom were blind [17]. By 2050, VI from MMD is expected to grow to 55.7 million people with 18.5 million of whom will be blind.

The cause of myopia is unknown, but myopia is a complex multifactorial trait driven by both genetic and environmental factors [2, 18–20]. Environmental exposures play a major role [1, 2]. This is supported by animal experiments which showed that manipulation of the environment can be achieved by making animals wear negative lenses, which would place the images of distant objects behind photoreceptors (hyperopic defocus), or form-deprivation myopia [21]. Macaque monkeys with surgically fused eyelids, i.e., form deprivation, experienced excessive axial length (AL) elongation and eventually develop myopia [22]. In addition, the environmental impact on myopia is also supported by the rapid increases in the prevalence of myopia over the past few decades that cannot be attributed to changing gene pools [1].

3.2 East–West Patterns in the Prevalence of Myopia

In 2000, 1406 million people from the world population were estimated to have myopia (22.9%; 95% confidence interval [CI], 15.2–31.5%) and 163 million people to have high myopia (2.7%; 95% CI, 1.4–6.3%) [23]. The prediction for 2050 is that there will be an increase to 4758 million people with

C. Lanca
Singapore Eye Research Institute, Singapore, Singapore
e-mail: carla.lanca@seri.com.sg

C.-W. Pan
School of Public Health, Medical College of Soochow University, Suzhou, China

S. M. Saw (✉)
Singapore Eye Research Institute, Singapore, Singapore

Saw Swee Hock School of Public Health, National University of Singapore, Singapore, Singapore

Duke-NUS Medical School, Singapore, Singapore
e-mail: ephssm@nus.edu.sg

T.-Y. Wong
Singapore Eye Research Institute, Singapore, Singapore

Duke-NUS Medical School, Singapore, Singapore

Singapore National Eye Centre, Singapore, Singapore

Yong Loo Lin School of Medicine, National University of Singapore, Singapore, Singapore
e-mail: ophwty@nus.edu.sg

© Springer Nature Switzerland AG 2021
R. F. Spaide et al. (eds.), *Pathologic Myopia*, https://doi.org/10.1007/978-3-030-74334-5_3

myopia (49.8%; 95% CI, 43.4–55.7%) and 938 million people with high myopia (9.8%; 95% CI, 5.7–19.4%).

Myopia prevalence has been reported to be high in middle-aged to elderly Chinese adults in urban Asian cities. The prevalence of myopia was reported to be 35.7% (n = 8716) in Singaporeans [24] and 38.7% in Singapore Chinese aged over 40 years (n = 1232) [25], similar to a Hong Kong study in Chinese over 40 years (40%, n = 355) [26]. However, prevalence of myopia was reported to be significantly lower in the rural area of China in the Handan Eye Study [27] (26.7%, n = 7557, aged over 30 years), urban city in the Beijing Eye Study [28] (22.9%, n = 4319, aged over 30 years), Yunnan province in Southwest China (26.35%, n = 1626, aged 40–80 years) [29], and Weitang town in East China (21.1%, n = 5613, aged over 60) [30].

Comparing Chinese with other East Asians such as Japanese and Koreans of similar age, the prevalence of myopia was higher. For example, myopia prevalence of urban Japanese adults aged 40–49 years was 70% in men and 68% in women in Tajimi City [31], whereas it was 45.2% in men and 51.7% in women in Singapore Chinese, although there may be secular trends as the Japanese studies were conducted more recently [25]. In Kumejima island, rural Japan, the prevalence was reported to be lower (29.5%, n = 2383 aged over 40) [32].

Although differences in sampling strategies, possible confounding factors such as preferred immigration to large cities (myopes are more likely to move to big cities due to higher educational levels), and study participant characteristics may partially contribute to the observed difference in myopia rates between Chinese living in and outside the mainland of China, the difference may still reflect country-specific environmental impact on the risk of myopia. However, compared to the current prevalence rates in younger birth cohorts in these areas, none of these rates are particularly high.

Myopia prevalence in childhood is higher in East Asian countries and can reach 69% at 15 years of age with 86% among Singaporean-Chinese [33]. Among Chinese children in the urban region of China such as Guangzhou, the prevalence of myopia was 30.1–78.4% in 10–15-year-olds [34]. Among children of similar age in Singapore, the prevalence of myopia was 29.0%, 34.7%, and 53.1% in 7-, 8-, and 9-year-olds [35]. In older children, there is an increase in the prevalence figures. Children from grade 12 in Fenghua, Eastern China, have a very high myopia prevalence (79.5%, n = 43,858) [36]. Similar results were reported in Beijing, China (70.9%, n = 35,745, 6–18 years), [37] and Korea (64.6%, n = 3862, aged 5–18 years) [38]. In younger cohorts, the prevalence remains lower. In a population-based study with Singaporean preschool children, the prevalence of myopia was reported to be 6.4% in children aged 5–6 years [39]. Reports from China and other Asian countries have not always revealed a high prevalence of myopia (0.8–13.7% in children aged 5–15 years) [40–46]. These low figures contrast with the higher prevalence of myopia in children with similar age observed in Southeast Asian countries with higher socioeconomic levels such as

Singapore. The trends show that myopia prevalence in children is increasing even in Europe. The proportion of myopes in the UK has more than doubled over the last 50 years in children aged between 10 and 16 years, and children are becoming myopic at a younger age [47]. Nevertheless, the trend is not the same in every European country. Lower prevalence has been reported in the Netherlands [2.4–12% in children aged 6 (n = 5711) [48] and 9 (n = 4734)] [49].

A meta-analysis found that myopia is most prevalent in Koreans aged 19 years (96.5%; 95% CI, 96.3–96.8) [50]. A report on Korean male conscripts (n = 23,616, age = 19 years) in Seoul reported extremely high myopia prevalence (96%) [51], while 82% of Singapore Chinese male conscripts (n = 15,095, ages = 17–19 years) were reported to have myopia [52]. Chinese were always considered the most myopic due to ethnic genetic differences. However, comparison among Chinese, Koreans, and Japanese indicates that this may not in fact be true. Recent reports on Korean prevalence still show considerable high prevalence of 51–53% in conscripts aged 18–35 years (n = 1,784,619) [53] and 70.6% in adults aged 19–49 years (n = 3398) [54].

In the Indian state of Andhra Pradesh, the prevalence of myopia in adults aged over 40 years was 34.6% (n = 3723) [55], while it was 31.0% in rural Chennai (n = 2508) [56]. Similar results were found in South India (35.6%, n = 4351 aged over 40) [57]. Although the overall prevalence of myopia was reported to be lower among Singapore Indians (28%; n = 2805) [58] than Indians of a similar age range residing in southern India, myopia was more prevalent in Singapore Indians than India Indians aged 40–49 years, reflecting a potentially "myopigenic" environment in Singapore. In adults aged more than 50 years, India Indians exceeded Singapore Indians in the prevalence of myopia due to earlier onset and more severity of nuclear cataract among India Indians. The Singapore Indian Eye Study also found a major difference in myopia rates between Indians born in and outside Singapore, which is a powerful evidence of impact of environmental factors [59]. However, myopia rates between Singapore Indians and Singapore Chinese did not show a significant difference in younger cohorts, albeit a bit higher in Chinese (82.2% vs. 68.7%) [52].

Myopia prevalence was reported to be significantly associated with ethnicity in several countries: non-White/European in Ireland (odds ratio [OR] = 3.7; 95% CI, 2.5, 5.3; p < 0.001), the Netherlands (OR = 2.95; 95% CI 2.30, 3.80; p < 0.001) [49, 60], and Asian/Pacific Islanders in the USA (OR = 1.64; CI, 1.58–1.70) [61]. However, the implication that the prevalence of myopia is always higher in East Asian than Western countries due to ethnic differences is debatable. There is a rapid increase in the prevalence of myopia of any amount in Whites in the USA. The 1999–2004 National Health and Nutrition Examination Survey (NHANES) reported that 33% of the Whites aged over 40 years in the USA have been affected by myopia using a more stringent criterion of −1 D [62, 63], which was not lower than the figures reported in most Asian studies. The difference in the prevalence of myopia in older cohorts between Singapore and the USA is not high. Younger cohorts also show an increase in prevalence with 41.9% of children aged 5–19 years old (n = 60,789) in southern California having myopia (SE $\leq$ −1 D) that might reflect the impact of new education practices [61].

Table 3.1 summarizes the evidence published on prevalence of myopia for the last 5 years. Comparability between studies is an important factor, especially the myopia definition. A British study analyzed population-based refraction data (n = 1985) from the 1958 British Birth Cohort Study and demonstrated that small variations (±0.25 D) in the threshold for defining myopia can significantly alter the conclusions drawn regarding associations with risk factors [64]. Also, not all the studies used cycloplegic refraction which can inflate myopia rates.

Data from Singapore, Hong Kong, China, and Southeast Asian countries indicated that Asia is not conceptually "myopigenic," and there are large variations in myopia rates in Asia associated with urbanization and environmental factors, such as education and time outdoors. Furthermore, myopia rates in the USA are not much lower than in Singapore but significantly higher than in Southeast Asian countries such as Laos and Cambodia, indicating that urbanization and education rather than geographic variation may play more important roles in myopia etiology. The role of education in myopia will be described in Sect. 3.5, "Environmental Risk Factors for Myopia."

3.3 Prevalence of High Myopia

It is important to document the variations in the prevalence of high myopia in addition to myopia as individuals with high myopia have an increased susceptibility to visual loss and blindness. Data from the Netherlands show that the cumulative risk of visual impairment was 5.7% (1.3) for participants aged 60 years and 39% (4.9) for those aged 75 years with SE of −6 D or less [73].

High myopia in young adults in East and Southeast Asia is reaching epidemic proportions, and environmental factors have major influence compared with the genetic background [74]. In Singapore, the prevalence of high myopia defined as SE at least −5 D in Indians (n = 2805) was 4.1% [58], which is significantly lower than that of Chinese in Singapore (9.1%) (n = 1113) [25] but slightly higher than Malays in Singapore (3.9%) (n = 2974) [75] of the same age range. A subsequent study reported a prevalence of 6% in Singaporeans aged over 40 [24]. However, non-cycloplegic refraction was used, which may imply that high myopia prevalence stabilized. In Korea, high myopia defined as SE of at least −6 D (n = 11,703) in participants aged 25–49 years was 7.0 ± 0.3% [76] and ranged from 11.3% to 12.9% (n = 1,784,619) in conscripts aged 18–35 years [53] (Table 3.1).

The prevalence rates of high myopia (SE < −6 D) were reported in Whites and Blacks aged over 40 years in the Baltimore Eye Study (1.4%, n = 5028) [77], Whites aged 49–97 years in the Blue Mountains Study (3.0%, n = 3654) [78], and Hispanics (2.4%, n = 5927) [79] aged over 40 years in the Los Angeles Latino Eye Study. The rates of high myopia are especially concerning in children. In Fenghua, Eastern China, the prevalence rate (SE < −6 D) was reported to range between 7.9% and 16.6% in children from grade 12 (n = 43,858) [36]. Similar results were found in Beijing, China (8.6%, n = 35,745 aged 6–18 years) [37].

Although the prevalence of high myopia has been documented in several population-based cohorts with higher values in Asia, the pattern is difficult to interpret. First, these studies were conducted in different years, and secular trends should not be neglected, considering the rapid increase in prevalence. Today's 85-year-olds were born in the 1930s, and 45-year-olds were born in the 1970s. Thus, the age range values are hard to interpret. In addition, most studies did not exclude the subjects with cataract, which is known to be highly correlated with myopia, especially high myopia [80, 81]. However, there is no doubt that the prevalence of high myopia is increasing as well as myopia, at least in East Asians. In the last report, about 12.9% of the Korean male conscripts have been reported to be affected by high myopia. This finding has an important implication, because the increase may represent an extension to extreme levels of acquired myopia, rather than the arguably more genetic high myopia of earlier generations.

3.4 Prevalence of Pathological Myopia

The most common complication of high myopia is pathological myopia (PM) or myopic macular degeneration (MMD). PM or MMD is a major cause of irreversible vision loss and blindness. MMD in older studies was sometimes called myopic retinopathy [82]. MMD is characterized by the presence of posterior staphyloma, lacquer cracks, Fuchs' spot, myopic choroidal thinning, and atrophy. The new classification for PM (META-PM classification) was developed in 2015. Myopic lesions were divided into five categories: no myopic retinal lesions (0), tessellated fundus only (1), diffuse chorioretinal atrophy (2), patchy chorioretinal atrophy (3), and macular atrophy (4), and plus lesions (lacquer cracks, myopic choroidal neovascularization, and Fuchs' spot) [83].

In Japan, MMD was reported to be the leading cause of blindness (22.4%) in the Tajimi Study [84]. In the Beijing Eye Study, MMD was also the second most common cause of low vision (32.7%) and blindness (7.7%) among adult Chinese aged 40 years and above [85]. In the Shihpai Eye Study among Taiwan elderly Chinese population 65 years of age or older, it was the second most frequent cause of visual impairment (12.5%) [86]. In Western countries, MMD was found to be the most frequent cause of visual impairment in subjects aged between 55 and 75 years in the Rotterdam Study [87].

In the Singapore Epidemiology of Eye Diseases (SEED) Study, the age-standardized prevalence of MMD using the

Table 3.1 Summary of evidence published on prevalence of myopia for the last 5 years

Study	Type	Country	Age (y)	Sample size	Myopia (SE in D)	Prevalence
Adults						
Wang et al., 2019 [29]	Cross-sectional	Yunnan Province, Southwest China	40–80	1626	M $\leq$ −0.50 HM $\leq$ −6.0	Age-adjusted[b] M: 26.35% (95% CI 24.01, 28.70%) HM: 2.64% (95% CI 1.75, 3.53%)
Han et al., 2019 [54]	Cross-sectional	Korea	19–49	3398	M $\leq$ −0.50 HM $\leq$ −6.0	M[b]: 70.6 ± 1.1% HM[b]: 8.0 ± 0.6%
Lee et al., 2018 [53]	Cohort (5-year)	Korea	18–35 (conscripts)	1,784,619	M $\leq$ −0.50 HM $\leq$ −6.0	M[b]: 50.6–53.0% HM[b]: 11.3–12.9%
Nakamura et al., 2018 [32]	Cross-sectional	Kumejima island, Japan	$\geq$40	2383	M $\leq$ −0.50 HM $\leq$ −5.0	M[b]: 29.5% HM[b]: 1.9%
Wong et al., 2018 [24]	Cohort	Singapore	$\geq$40	8716	M $\leq$ −0.50 HM $\leq$ −5.0	M[b]: 35.7% HM[b]: 6.0%
Joseph et al., 2018 [57]	Cross-sectional	South India	$\geq$40	4351	M $\leq$ −0.75	Age-standardized M[b]: 35.6% (95% CI 34.7, 36.6)
Xu et al., 2017 [30] Weitang Geriatric Diseases Study	Cross-sectional	Weitang town, East China	$\geq$60	5613	$M_1 \leq$ −0.50 $M_2 \leq$ −0.75 $M_3 \leq$ −1.0 $HM_1 \leq$ −5.0 $HM_2 \leq$ −6.0	Age-adjusted[b] M_1: 21.1% (95% CI 19.9, 22.2) M_2: 17.2% (95% CI 16.2, 18.3) M_3: 14.2% (95% CI 13.3, 15.2) HM_1: 2.5% (95% CI 2.1, 2.9) HM_2 2.0% (95% CI 1.6, 2.4)
Children						
Tideman et al., 2019 [49]	Cohort	Rotterdam, the Netherlands	9	4734	M $\leq$ −0.50	M[a]: 12.0%
Ma et al., 2018 [65]	Cohort (4-year)	Baoshan District, Shanghai	Grades 1–3	1385	M $\leq$ −0.50	2-years incidence M[a]: 36.2% 30.0% – grade 1 29.2% – grade 2 33.2% – grade 3
Zeng et al., 2018 [66]	Cross-sectional	Hubei province, China	Grade 1–3	18,532	M $\leq$ −0.50	M[a]: 24.15%; 12.67% – grade 1 24.91% – grade 2 34.95% – grade 3
Yang et al., 2018 [67]	Cross-sectional	Waterloo Region, Canada	6–8 11–13	166	M $\leq$ −0.50	M[a]: 17.5% (95% CI 11.7, 23.2%) 6.0% (95% CI 0.9, 11.1%) – 6-8 28.9% (95% CI 19.2, 38.7%) – 11-13
Lim et al., 2018 [38]	Cross-sectional	Korea	5–18	3862	M $\leq$ −0.50 HM $\leq$ −6.0	M[b]: 64.6% HM[b]: 5.4%
Theophanous et al., 2018 [61]	Cross-sectional	Southern California, USA	5–19	60,789	M $\leq$ -1.0	M[b]: 41.9%
Sun et al., 2018 [68]	Cross-sectional	Qingdao, China	10–15	3753	M $\leq$ −0.50	M[a]: 52.02% 22.61% – 10 years old 56.93% – 13 years old 69.34% – 15 years old
Hagen et al., 2018 [69]	Cross-sectional	Norway	16–19	393	M $\leq$ −0.50	M[a]: 13%

(continued)

Table 3.1 (continued)

Study	Type	Country	Age (y)	Sample size	Myopia (SE in D)	Prevalence
Li et al., 2018 [46]	Cohort (1-year follow-up)	Southwest China	Grades 1 and 7	2310 – grade 1 2191 – grade 7	M ≤ −0.50	Baseline M^a: 2.20% – grade 1 M^a: 29.45% – grade 7 1-year incidence 33.6% (95% CI 31.7, 35.5) – grade 1 54.0% (95% CI 51.5, 56.5) – grade 7
Wang et al., 2018 [70]	Cohort (6-year follow-up)	Guangzhou, China	Grades 1 and 7 at baseline	1969 – grade 1 2663 – grade 7	M ≤ −0.50 HM ≤ −6.0 D	Baseline M^b: 12.0% – grade 1 ($n = 237$) M^b: 67.4% – grade 7 ($n = 1795$) Incidence M^b 20–30% each year throughout both grades Incidence HM^b 0.1% (95% CI 0.0%, 0.3%) – grade 1 2.3% (95% CI 1.0%, 3.7%) – grade 9
Chen et al., 2018 [36]	Population-based, retrospective study (15-year)	Fenghua, Eastern China	Grade 12	43,858	M ≤ −0.50 HM ≤ −6.0	M^b: 79.5–87.7% HM^b: 7.9–16.6%
Pan et al., 2018 [71]	Cohort	Mojiang, Southwestern China	Grade 1 and 7	2432 – grade 1 2346 – grade 7	M ≤ −0.50 HM ≤ −5.0	M^a: 2.4% – grade 1 M^a: 29.4% – grade 7 HM^a: 0.1% – grade 1 HM^a: 0.4% – grade 7
Tideman et al., 2018 [48] Generation R	Cohort	The Netherlands	6	5711	M ≤ −0.50	M^a: 2.4%
Guo et al., 2017 [37] Greater Beijing School Children Myopia Study	Cross-sectional	Beijing, China	6–18	35,745	M_1 ≤ −0.50 M_2 ≤ −1.00 HM_1 ≤ −6.0 HM_2 ≤ −8.0 HM_3 ≤ −10.0	M_1^b: 70.9% (95% CI 70.5, 71.4) M_2^b: 60.9% (95% CI 60.4, 61.4) HM_1^b: 8.6% (95% CI 8.4, 8.9) HM_2^b: 2.2% (95% CI 2.0, 2.4) HM_3^b: 0.3% (95% CI 0.3, 0.4)
Li et al., 2017 [72]	Cohort (10-year)	Haidian District of Beijing, China	14–16	37,424	Non-M ≤ −0.5 Low M − 3.0 ≤ to < −0.5 Moderate M − 6.0 ≤ to < −3.0 HM < −6.0	M^a: 55.95% in 2006 65.48% in 2015 ($P < 0.001$) Low M: 32.27% in 2006 20.73% in 2015 Moderate M: 19.72% in 2006 38.06% in 2015 HM: 3.96% in 2006 6.69% in 2015
Guo et al., 2017 [45] Shenzhen Kindergarten Eye Study	Cross-sectional	Shenzhen, China	3–6	1127	M ≤ −0.50 D	M^a: 0% – 3 M^a: 3.7% (95% CI 1.0, 6.5) – 6

Legend: CI confidence interval, *D* diopter, *Y* years, *HM* high myopia, *M* myopia, *SE* spherical equivalent
[a]cycloplegic refraction
[b]noncycloplegic refraction

META-PM classification was 3.8% (95% CI, 3.4, 4.3%) with 7.7% among low to moderate myopes and 28.7% among high myopes [24]. It was also reported in later publications a significant proportion of high myopes affected by myopic retinopathy [88, 89]. Figure 3.1 shows the retinal fundus photographs of the right eye of a 44-year-old Malaysian woman with SE of −11 D. Temporal parapapillary atrophy (PPA) and disc tilt were demonstrated with type II staphyloma (macula involved).

Figure 3.2 shows the left eye of a 47-year-old male of Chinese ethnicity with SE of −11.00 D. Temporal PPA was demonstrated with type III staphyloma (peripapillary). The impact of MMD on visual impairment is important because it is often bilateral and irreversible and frequently affects individuals during their productive years [90]. It has been

estimated that patients with MMD are legally blind for an average of 17 years, a figure that nearly matches the mean duration of blindness from diabetes (5 years), age-related maculopathy (5 years), and glaucoma (10 years) combined [91]. The reasons for the development of MMD are not clear, but may be due to excessive axial elongation, thinning of the retina and choroid, and weakening of the sclera [1]. The development of a posterior staphyloma might further stretch and thin the retina and choroid, leading to characteristic lesions.

Table 3.2 summarizes the prevalence of MMD in population-based studies. In the Blue Mountains Eye Study, myopic retinopathy was defined as the presence of staphyloma, lacquer cracks, Fuchs' spot, and chorioretinal thinning or atrophy. The overall prevalence of myopic retinopathy was 1.2%. Staphyloma was present in 0.7% of the participants, lacquer cracks were seen in 0.2%, Fuchs' spot was present in 0.1%, and chorioretinal atrophy was present in 0.2%. In addition, the Blue Mountains Eye Study showed a marked and highly nonlinear relationship between refraction and the prevalence of myopic retinopathy. Myopes of less than −5 D had a myopic retinopathy prevalence of 0.42% as compared to 25.3% for myopes with greater than −5 D [92].

In the Beijing Eye Study using the same definition of myopic retinopathy as the Blue Mountains Eye Study, myopic retinopathy was present in 3.1% of the total 4319 participants aged over 50 years. Chorioretinal atrophy at the posterior pole was the most commonly encountered feature of myopic retinopathy, being present in all eyes with myopic retinopathy. The prevalence of staphyloma, lacquer cracks, Fuchs' spot, and chorioretinal atrophy at the posterior pole were 1.6%, 0.2%, 0.1%, and 3.1%, respectively. The prevalence of myopic retinopathy increased significantly with increasing myopic refractive error, from 3.8% in eyes with a myopic refractive error of <−4.0 D to 89.6% in eyes with a myopic refractive error of at least −10.0 D [93]. In another study of 6603 adults aged over 30 years in rural China, the prevalence of myopic retinopathy was only 0.9%. Staphyloma was the most frequent myopic retinopathy sign (86.9%), followed by chorioretinal atrophy (56.0%), lacquer cracks (36.9%), and Fuchs' spot (14.3%) [94].

In a Japanese cohort of 1892 adults aged over 40 years, myopic retinopathy was defined as the presence of at least one of the following lesions: diffuse chorioretinal atrophy at the posterior pole, patchy chorioretinal atrophy, lacquer cracks, or macular atrophy. The prevalence of myopic retinopathy was 1.7% with 2.2% in women and 1.2% in men [95]. In Taiwan, myopic retinopathy was defined as the presence of lacquer cracks, focal area of deep choroidal atrophy and macular choroidal neovascularization, or geographic atrophy in the presence of high myopia. Signs of myopic retinopathy were present in 32 (72.7%) of the 44 high myopic adults, representing a prevalence of 3.0% [96].

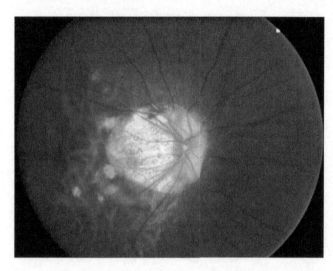

Fig. 3.1 Retinal fundus photograph of the right eye of a 44-year-old Malaysian female in the Singapore Epidemiology of Eye Diseases Study

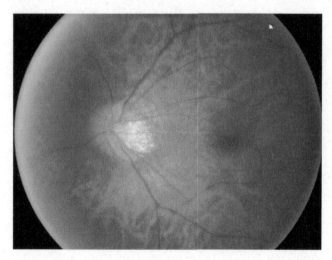

Fig. 3.2 Retinal fundus photograph of the left eye of a 47-year-old male of Chinese ethnicity in the Singapore Epidemiology of Eye Diseases Study

Table 3.2 Prevalence of myopic retinopathy and high myopia (SE < −5.0 D) in population-based studies

Study	n	Age	Definition of myopic retinopathy	Prevalence of myopic retinopathy (%)	Prevalence of high myopia (<−5 D) (%)
Blue Mountains Eye Study (Australia)	3653	≥49	Staphyloma Chorioretinal atrophy Fuchs' spot Lacquer cracks	1.2	2.2
Beijing Eye Study (China)	4139	≥40	Staphyloma Chorioretinal atrophy Fuchs' spot Lacquer cracks	3.7	3.3
Handan Eye Study (China)	6603	≥30	Staphyloma Chorioretinal atrophy Fuchs' spot Lacquer cracks	0.9	2.1
Shihpai Eye Study (Taiwan)	1058	≥65	Lacquer cracks, focal area of deep choroidal atrophy and macular choroidal neovascularization, or geographic atrophy in the presence of high myopia	3.0	2.3
Hisayama Study (Japan)	1892	≥40	Diffuse chorioretinal atrophy Patchy chorioretinal atrophy Lacquer cracks Macular atrophy	1.7	5.7

In Chinese American adults with myopia (SE < −0.5 D) aged 50 years and older, the prevalence of macular degeneration was 44.9% based on the presence of any degenerative lesion secondary to myopia. The prevalence was lower (32.2%) when MMD was defined by the modified version of the Meta-Analysis for Pathologic Myopia [97]. The prevalence of specific lesions was tessellation (31.7%), tilted disc (28.1%), peripapillary atrophy (7.0%), staphyloma (5.7%), diffuse atrophy (6.4%), lacquer cracks (2.6%), intrachoroidal cavitation (2.2%), patchy atrophy (0.9%), and end-stage MD (0.2%). The prevalence of MMD was also higher in older participants with more severe myopia and longer axial length ($p < 0.001$). In rural India, the Central India Eye and Medical Study (CIEMS) showed a much lower prevalence than other studies. High myopia defined as a refractive error ≤−8 D was present in 0.5% eyes, and myopic retinopathy was present in 0.24 ± 0.07% (95% CI, 0.01, 0.04) individuals with 30+ years old [98].

These studies cannot be directly compared primarily because the definitions of myopic retinopathy, myopic maculopathy, and MMD are different and there are variations in the characteristics of study participants (e.g., the age and proportion of either gender) and differences in the methodology or study design (e.g., the definition of myopic retinopathy) including sampling strategies and response rates. However, prevalence was similar between studies and varied between 0.9% and 3.7% using the myopic retinopathy definition and 3.8% using the META-PM adopted in 2015. Only one study reported a very high prevalence of 32.2% in Chinese Americans [97].

In the population-based studies reporting the prevalence of myopic retinopathy, the presence of high myopia was not a prerequisite for the definition of myopic retinopathy in most studies. Thus, in some studies, the prevalence of myopic retinopathy was even higher than high myopia as adults with low to moderate myopia may have pathologic changes in the retina. This may also lead to misclassification bias. For example, peripapillary atrophy was a criterion for myopic retinopathy in the Blue Mountains Eye Study, the Beijing Eye Study, and the Handan Eye Study, but peripapillary atrophy is also seen in glaucomatous and apparently otherwise normal retinas.

Visual prognosis for highly myopic patients with MMD is much poorer than for those without retinopathy. In a Japanese natural history study, 327 of the 806 highly myopic eyes (40.6%) showed progression of myopic retinopathy during the follow-up of 12.7 years. Only 13.4% of the eyes with a tessellated fundus showed a progression of myopic retinopathy during the follow-up period, whereas 69.3% of the eyes with lacquer cracks, 49.2% of the eyes with diffuse atrophy, 70.3% of the eyes with patchy atrophy, and 90.1% of the eyes with choroidal neovascularization showed progression of myopic retinopathy. The results indicated that the incidence and type of progression were different for the different types of fundus lesion [99].

In the Handan Eye Study (n = 5078), the 5-year incidence of myopic maculopathy was 0.05% (95% CI, 0.02–0.10%) in Chinese participants aged 30+ years. Progression occurred in 35.3% with new signs of patchy chorioretinal atrophy (21.6%), diffuse chorioretinal atrophy (13.7%), lacquer cracks (6.9%), macular atrophy (6.9%), and myopic choroidal neovascularization (3.9%) [100]. Myopic choroidal neovascularization is one of the most serious complications of PM that leads to progressive loss of central vision and visual impairment [16, 101].

3.5 Associations of Myopia with Other Age-Related Eye Diseases

3.5.1 Age-Related Macular Degeneration (AMD)

The association between refractive error and AMD was initially reported in several case–control studies [102–104] and then further assessed in population-based studies. For example, among White populations, the Rotterdam Study reported that increasing hyperopic refraction was associated with both prevalent and incident AMD [105]. The Blue Mountains Eye Study in Australia reported a weak association of hyperopic refraction with prevalent early AMD [106]. In Asians, both the Singapore Malay Eye Study and the Beijing Eye Study found a significant association between hyperopia and AMD in studies with cross-sectional designs [107, 108]. However, evidences from longitudinal population-based data have not supported this cross-sectional association. The US Beaver Dam Eye Study reported that baseline refraction was not associated with either incident early or late AMD [109, 110]. The Blue Mountains Eye Study also found no significant association between hyperopia and the 5-year incidence of early or late AMD [111]. It is possible, however, that longitudinal population-based studies which have assessed this association to date have lacked sufficient study power for incident AMD. Meanwhile, the impact of increasing age-related nuclear cataract with its secondary effect on refractive error (through induced index myopia) could also have confounded the ability to assess this longitudinal association using refractive measures rather than AL. Differences in study design and methods could possibly explain the inconsistent results observed among different ethnic groups as well. Examining the relationship between AL and AMD may provide further insights into possible mechanisms underlying the association of hyperopic refraction and AMD. However, only a few studies to date have evaluated the relationship between AMD and AL with inconsistent results. A Norwegian prevalence survey examined AL and AMD but found no relationship [112]. On the other hand, the Singapore Malay Eye Study found that each millimeter decrease in AL was associated with 29% increased odds of early AMD [107].

The idea that AMD may have a protective effect in myopic eyes in recent years has been attributed to the reduced ultraviolet exposure due to less time spent outdoors. However, recent evidence shows that older patients with high myopia have significant risk of dry and neovascular forms of AMD.

In Korean subjects over 55 years with high myopia (n = 442), the frequency of AMD was 11.9% (95% CI, 9.8–14.0%) [113]. Past studies have reported a lower prevalence in myopic patients. Nevertheless, the Korean study suggests that prevalence is similar with the data reported in the general population affected by AMD. Results must be analyzed carefully as the Korean study collected data from tertiary referral centers and prevalence may be overestimated. Another study using genome-wide data suggested that refractive error has very limited influence on the risk of AMD and that previously reported associations may be the result of confounding or selection bias [114].

3.5.2 Diabetic Retinopathy (DR)

The relationship between refractive errors and DR is not clear. In some clinic-based studies, myopic refraction was found to be associated with lower risk of DR [115–117]. However, clinic-based studies may be biased because myopic diabetics may undergo a routine eye examination. Only a few population-based studies assessed this association with inconsistent results. The Wisconsin Epidemiologic Study of Diabetic Retinopathy (WESDR) demonstrated that myopia was not associated with incident DR in univariate analyses, but showed a protective effect against progression to proliferative diabetic retinopathy in persons with younger-onset diabetes in multivariate models [118].

The Visual Impairment Project did not find any significant association between DR and myopia in a cross-sectional design [119]. In Malays living in Singapore, myopic refraction was associated with a lower risk of DR, particularly vision-threatening retinopathy, without any evidence of a threshold [120]. A cross-sectional, population-based study of the South Korean population (n = 13,424 participants who were 40 years and older) with mild myopia (−1.0 D to −2.99 D) and moderate to high myopia (≤−3.0 D) showed lower odds of diabetic retinopathy (OR, 0.42; 95% CI, 0.18–0.97 and OR, 0.14; 95% CI, 0.02–0.88, respectively) [121]. A systematic review was conducted using data from six population-based and three clinic-based studies. Myopic SE and each millimeter increase in AL were significantly associated with a decreased risk for DR (OR, 0.80 and 0.79, respectively; 95% CI, 0.67–0.95 and 0.73–0.86, respectively) [122]. Further longitudinal studies are required to examine the association between myopia and DR.

3.5.3 Age-Related Cataract

Cataract is the leading cause of blindness worldwide. In the USA, the Beaver Dam Eye Study of adults 43–84 years supported the cross-sectional association between myopia and nuclear cataract (OR, 1.67; 95% CI, 1.23, 2.27), but provide no evidence of a relationship between myopia and 5-year

Table 3.3 The association of myopia with age-related cataract in population-based studies

Author (year)	Study design	N	Age	Definition of myopia	OR (HR) of cataract for myopia (95% CI)		
					Nuclear	Cortical	PSC
Lim et al. (1999) [124]	Cross-sectional study	7308	49+	SE < −1.0 D	1.3 (1.0, 1.6)	1.2 (0.8, 1.6)	2.5 (1.6, 4.7)
McCarty (1999) [129]	Cross-sectional study	5147	40+	SE < −1.0 D	2.7 (1.9, 3.9)	1.8 (1.3, 2.4)	3.6 (2.5, 5.2)
Wong et al. (2001) [123]	Cohort study	4470	43–84	SE < −1.0 D	1.7 (1.3, 2.4)	0.9 (0.6, 1.2)	1.2 (0.8, 2.0)
Leske et al. (2002) [126].	Cohort study	2609	40–84	SE < −0.5 D	2.8 (2.0, 4.0)	–	–
Wong et al. (2003) [128]	Cross-sectional study	1029	40–79	−3 D < SE < −0.5 D	2.6 (1.5, 4.3)	1.1 (0.7, 1.8)	1.7 (0.9, 3.3)
Pan et al. (2012) [4]	Cross-sectional study	3400	40–84	SE < −0.5 D	1.6 (1.1, 2.2)	1.1 (0.8, 1.3)	1.7 (1.1, 2.7)

OR odds ratio, *HR* hazard ratio, *CI* confidence interval, *SE* spherical equivalent

incident cataract [123]. The Australian Blue Mountains Eye Study of adults aged over 49 years reported that posterior subcapsular cataract (PSC) was associated with low myopia (OR 2.1; 95% CI 1.4, 3.5), moderate myopia (OR 3.1; 95% CI 1.6, 5.7), and high myopia (OR 5.5; 95% CI 2.8, 10.9), while high myopia was associated with all three types of cataract [124]. Participants were re-examined after 5 and/or 10 years, and low (OR, 1.86; CI, 1.03–3.35) and high myopia (OR, 7.80; CI, 3.51–17.35) were significantly associated with higher incidence of posterior subcapsular cataract [125]. High myopia was also associated with increased incidence of nuclear cataract (OR, 3.01; 95% CI, 1.35–6.71).

The multivariate-adjusted OR of incident nuclear cataract in myopic adults (SE <−0.5 D) in the Barbados Eye Study of adults aged 40–84 years (*n* = 2609; follow-up = 4 years) was 2.8 (95% CI 2.0, 4.0) (PSC and cortical cataract results were not reported) [126]. In cross-sectional studies, refractive associations with PSC, cortical, and nuclear cataract were examined in the Visual Impairment Project in Australia (*n* = 5147) of adults 40 years and older. Only cortical cataract was found to be associated with myopia (SE < −1.0 D) [127]. A population-based study on Singapore Chinese supported the associations between nuclear cataract or PSC and myopia. This study also indicated that PSC is associated with deeper anterior chamber, thinner lens, and longer vitreous chamber, with vitreous chamber depth explaining most of the association between PSC and myopia [128] (Table 3.3).

3.5.4 Primary Open-Angle Glaucoma (POAG)

Glaucoma is a group of diseases, which have a final common pathway of progressive nerve fiber layer thinning and concomitant ganglion cell loss. Glaucomatous changes in a myopic eye are difficult to detect and can be confounded by myopia [130]. The association of glaucoma and myopia has been summarized in a systematic review and meta-analysis of 13 population-based studies [131]. We have summarized published studies in detail in Table 3.4. However, all these studies are case control or cross-sectional, which are limited to determine the casual relationship in nature.

3.6 Environmental Risk Factors for Myopia

3.6.1 Near Work and Education

Near work involving visual tasks at near distance including reading/writing and computer use has been found to be associated with myopia in several cross-sectional studies [145–147]. However, the association between near work and myopia might be stronger for intensity rather than the total duration or time spent on near work [145, 146]. For example, Australian children who read continuously for more than 30 min were 1.5-fold (OR 1.5; 95% CI 1.05, 2.1) more likely to develop myopia when compared to those who read less than 30 min continuously. Likewise, children who performed close reading distance of less than 30 cm were 2.5 times (OR 2.5; 95% CI 1.7, 4.0) more likely to have myopia than those who performed more than this distance [145]. However, this study concluded that near work per SE was not important. Similarly, a cross-sectional study among school children in Armenia (*n* = 1260) showed that myopia was significantly associated with continuous reading (OR 1.99, 95% CI 1.31–3.02), but not near work (OR 0.97, 95% CI 0.89–1.05). Continuous reading was defined by the average number of hours spent reading or on near work without a break [148]. Children from the second grade in Taipei with faster annual myopia progression were found to have a shorter eye–object distance when doing near work (OR, 1.45; 95% CI, 1.18–1.78) [149]. The Myopia Investigation Study in Taipei found that children from grade 2 (*n* = 6794) who spent ≥5 h every week on after-school tutoring programs (HR, 1.12; 95% CI, 1.02–1.22) had greater risk for incident myopia [150].

The Singapore Cohort Study of the Risk Factors for Myopia found that children who read more than two books per week were about three times more likely (OR, 3.05; 95% CI, 1.80–5.18) to have higher myopia (defined as SE at least −3.0 D) compared to those who read less than two books per week, after controlling for confounders [146]. However, the association is still inconsistent in cross-sectional studies.

Near work was not shown to be associated with myopia in several other studies. For example, Lu and coworkers [151] analyzed 998 Chinese school children aged 13–17 years

Table 3.4 The association of myopia with open-angle glaucoma

Author (year)	Study ethnicity	Study design	Study population (n)	Definition	Result (odds ratio/P-values)
Daubs and Crick (1981) [132]	White	Case–control study	General ophthalmology patients (n = 953)	OAG defined as eyes with open angles and characteristic VFD	OR of OAG 3.1 (95% CI 1.6–5.8) for high myopia compared with hyperopia, adjusted for age, IOP, sex, family history, season, blood pressure, astigmatism, urinalysis, and health
Ponte et al. (1994) [133]	White	Case–control study	40 years and older (n = 264)	Cases: IOP >24 mmHg or history of glaucoma or VF suggestive of glaucoma Controls: IOP <20 mmHg, CDR 0–0.2 and pink discs	OR of prevalent glaucoma for myopia (SE at least −1.5 D) was 5.56 (95% CI 1.85, 16.67), adjusted for diabetes, hypertension, steroid use, and iris texture
Mitchell et al. (1999) [134]	White	Cross-sectional study	49 years and older (n = 3654)	OAG defined as cup–disc ratio >0.7 or cup–disc asymmetry >0.3	OR of prevalent OAG was 3.3 (95% CI 1.7, 6.4) for moderate to high myopia (SE at least −3.0 D) and 2.3 (95% CI 1.3, 4.1) for patients with low myopia (SE < −3.0 D and >1.0 D), adjusted for sex, family history, diabetes, hypertension, migraine, steroid use, and pseudoexfoliation
Leske et al. (2001) [135]	African descent	Observational study of families of probands	230 probands and 1056 relatives (from 207 families)	OAG definition includes visual field criteria, optic disc criteria, and ophthalmologic criteria	OR of OAG for refractive error (<−0.5 D) is 2.82 (95% CI 1.5, 5.3)
Wong et al. (2003) [128]	White	Cross-sectional study	43–86 years (n = 4670)	POAG defined as VFD compatible with glaucoma, IOP >22 mmHg, CDR 0.8 or more, history of glaucoma treatment	The age- and gender-adjusted ORs of prevalent POAG for myopia (SE at least −1.0 D) were 1.6 (95% CI 1.1, 2.3)
Ramakrishnan et al. (2003) [136]	Indian	Cross-sectional study	40 years and older (n = 5150)	POAG was defined as angles open on gonioscopy and glaucomatous optic disc changes with matching visual field defects	OR of POAG for mild myopia was 2.9 (95% CI 1.3, 6.9), for moderate myopia was 2.1 (95% CI 1.0, 4.6), and for severe myopia was 3.9 (95% CI 1.6, 9.5)
Vijaya et al. (2005) [137]	Indian	Cross-sectional study	40 years and older (n = 3934)	Cases of glaucoma were defined according to the ISGEO classification	OR of POAG for myopia was 0.68 (95% CI 0.40, 1.17). There were no associations between POAG and myopia
Suzuki et al. (2006) [138]	Japanese	Cross-sectional study	119 POAG patients and 2755 controls	Diagnosis of glaucoma was made based on optic disc appearance, perimetric results, and other ocular findings	OR of POAG for low myopia (SE > −1.0 D and SE < −3.0 D) was 1.85 (95% CI 1.03–3.31) and for moderate to high myopia (SE > −3 D) was 2.60 [95% CI, 1.56–4.35]
Xu et al. (2007) [139]	Chinese	Cross-sectional study	40 years and older (n = 5324)	Optic disc glaucoma with structural optic disc abnormalities, perimetric glaucoma with optic disc abnormalities plus frequency doubling perimetry defects	In binary logistic regression analysis, presence of glaucoma was significantly associated with the myopic refractive error (P < 0.001)
Casson et al. (2007) [140]	Burmese	Cross-sectional study	40 years and older (n = 2076)	Primary open-angle glaucoma was diagnosed if the criteria for categories 1–3 were met and >90° of posterior TM was visible on static gonioscopy and no secondary cause for glaucoma was present	OR of POAG for myopia (SE < 0.5 D) was 2.82 (95% CI 1.28, 6.25) in univariate analysis and 2.74 (95% CI 1.0, 7.48) in multivariate analysis
Czudowska et al. (2010) [141]	White	Cohort study	55 years and older (n = 3939)	Glaucomatous visual field loss	RR of POAG for myopia (SE < 0.5 D) was 1.5 (95% CI 1.1, 2.0) in multivariate analysis
Perera et al. (2010) [142]	Malays	Cross-sectional study	40 years and older (n = 3109)	Optic disc abnormalities and glaucomatous visual field loss	OR of POAG for moderate myopia (SE < −4.0 D) was 2.8 (95% CI 1.1, 7.4) in multivariate analysis

(continued)

Table 3.4 (continued)

Author (year)	Study ethnicity	Study design	Study population (n)	Definition	Result (odds ratio/P-values)
Kuzin et al. (2010) [143]	Latinos	Cross-sectional study	40 years and older ($n = 5927$)	Optic disc abnormalities and glaucomatous visual field loss	OR of OAG for myopia (SE < −1.0 D) was 1.8 (95% CI 1.2, 2.8) in multivariate analysis
Tham et al. (2016) [144]	Malays, Indians, and Chinese	Cross-sectional study	40–80 years ($n = 9422$)	Cases of glaucoma were defined according to the ISGEO classification	OR of POAG for moderate to high myopia (<−3.0 D) was 4.27 (95% CI, 2.10–8.69) in multivariate analysis OR of POAG for AL of ≥25.5 mm was 16.22 (95% CI, 7.73 to 34.03) in multivariate analysis

AL axial length, *CDR* cup–disc ratio, *CI* confidence interval, *D* diopters, *IOP* intraocular pressure, *ISGEO* International Society of Geographical and Epidemiological Ophthalmology, *POAG* primary open-angle glaucoma, *OR* odds ratio, *SE* spherical equivalent, *VFD* visual field defect

from Xichang, China, and reported the multivariate-adjusted OR of myopia (SE at least −0.5 D) was 1.27 (95% CI, 0.75–2.14) for reading in hours per week. Similarly, Saw and coworkers recruited 128 children from one kindergarten in Singapore [152] and found that after adjusting for parental history of myopia and age, the OR of myopia was 1.0 (95% CI, 0.8–1.3) for near-work activity. Studies that have examined the risk factors for myopia in children below the age of 6 years old found no significant association between near work or outdoor time [153, 154]. In older children, similar results have been reported after adjustment of confounding variables [146, 155, 156]. However, contradictory findings have been reported. In Australian children who became myopic, it was found that the younger cohort (6 years old) performed significantly more near work than the older cohort (12 years old) [157].

In a recent prospective study, axial length-to-corneal radius ratio at baseline showed statistically significant interaction with number of books read per week ($P < 0.01$) and parental myopia ($P < 0.01$) [49]. In a cohort of urban students in Beijing ($n = 222$) after stratifying the near-work hours into quartile groups (3-year follow-up), students with a greater near-work load at baseline (trend $P = 0.03$) exhibited a greater myopic refractive change and had a higher risk to develop myopia (hazard ratio, 95% CI, 5.19, 1.49–18.13), after adjusting for confounders [158].

Longitudinal cohort studies establish the temporal sequence of prior exposure to environmental factors and subsequent increase in the risks of disease. However, evidence for the last years supporting near work as a risk factor for myopia in cohort studies was limited in both Asian [159] and non-Asian children [155]. Based on current evidence, it is still debatable to conclude that near work is an independent risk factor for myopia [160]. Table 3.5 provides a summary of evidence from studies on near work and myopia.

Korean children aged 5–18 years old with two myopic parents were more myopic than those with only one myopic parent [38]. Also, the risk of having myopia increased with the level of education of the mother in the presence of high myopia in one or both parents. Educational level and duration have been linked with higher prevalence of myopia and a more myopic SE in participants aged 20–85 years from the USA [161], 18–49 years from Korea [53, 54], and aged 35–79 from Gutenberg [162, 163].

A Singaporean ecological study of trends in myopia prevalence showed that the increased prevalence started in persons born after the 1970s which coincides with the changes in the education system in 1978 [164]. Another study concluded that the new high myopia cases are strongly associated with education and extrapolates that there might be two forms of high myopia that differ in age of onset and relationship with education [165]. Data from England, Scotland, and Wales in the UK Biobank cohort suggest that every additional year of education is associated with a more myopic refractive error of −0.18 D/y [166].

In a meta-analysis of population-based, cross-sectional studies from the European Eye Epidemiology (E(3)) Consortium, education was significantly associated with myopia [167]. The authors hypothesize that education may have an additive role, rather than explanatory.

Genetic factors may also play a role in mediating the relationship between education and myopia. One study showed that genetic predisposition of higher education was negatively associated with refractive error [168]. A study with Taiwanese children aged 7–12 years old showed that children attending cram schools (private classes outside the regular school system) ≥2 h/d (hazard ratio, 1.31; 95% confidence interval, 1.03–1.68) had a higher risk of incident myopia [169]. Although prevalence and severity of myopia are strongly associated with education, interethnic variation observed is not fully explained by differences in education level [52]. Ethnic differences in myopia and the effects of parental myopia seem more likely to be explained by environmental influences [170]. Higher myopia at baseline, higher myopic progression, and more time spent on reading and close work, as compared with time spent outdoors, were associated with high myopia in children between 8 and 13 years old from Finland [171].

Table 3.5 Summary of evidence from studies on near work and myopia

Study: authors, year	Study design	Participants: number, age Y, location	Study outcomes
Harrington et al., 2019 [60]	Cross-sectional	$n = 728$, 6–7 $n = 898$, 12–13	Myopia prevalence was significantly linked with frequent reading/writing (OR = 2.2, 95% CI 1.4–3.5, $p = 0.001$)
North India Myopia Study (NIM Study): Saxena et al., 2017 [175]	Prospective longitudinal (1 year)	$n = 9616$, 5–15, India, Delhi	Hours of reading/writing/week ($p < 0.001$) was a significant risk factor for progression of myopia ($n = 629$)
Handan Offspring Myopia Study (HOMS): Lin et al., 2017 [176]	Cross-sectional	$n = 572$, 6–18, China	Myopic children (5.0 ± 1.7 h) spent more time on near work as compared to non-myopic children (4.7 ± 1.6 h, $p = 0.049$). No association between near work and myopia was found after adjusting for age, gender, parental refractive error, parental educational level, and daily outdoor activity hours (OR = 95% CI, 1.10, 0.94–1.27)
Growing Up in Singapore Towards Healthy Outcomes (GUSTO): Chua et al., 2015 [153]	Cohort	$n = 572$, 3, Singapore	Children with two myopic parents were more likely to have a more myopic SE, longer AL, and myopia. Near work was not associated with SE, AL, and myopia
Anyang Childhood Eye Study (ACES): Li et al., 2015 [177]	Cross-sectional	$n = 1770$, grade 7, 10–15, China	Associations with > odds of myopia: continuous reading (>45 min, OR = 1.4; 95% CI, 1.1–1.8); head tilt when writing (OR = 1.3, 95% CI, 1.1–1.7). Reading more books for pleasure was significantly associated with greater myopia ($P = 0.03$) Close reading distance (≤20 cm) and close nib-to-fingertip distance (≤2 cm) were significantly associated with longer AL ($P < 0.01$) Reading distance and reading books for pleasure had significant interaction effects with parental myopia
Beijing Myopia Progression Study: Lin et al., 2014 [178]	Cross-sectional	$n = 317$, 6–17, Beijing, China	Children with more near work did not exhibit a significantly more myopic refraction after adjusting for gender, outdoor activity time, and average parental refractive error
Strabismus, Amblyopia and Refractive Error in Singaporean Children (STARS): Low et al., 2010 [154]	Cross-sectional	$n = 3009$, 6–72 months, Singapore	Children with two myopic parents were more likely to be myopic and to have a more myopic SE. Near work was not associated with preschool myopia
Lu et al., 2009 [151]	Cross-sectional	$n = 998$, 14.6, Xichang, China	Time and Dh spent on near activities did not differ between children with and without myopia. Time spent on near activities was unassociated with myopia, adjusting for age, sex, and parental education Girls spent significantly >time and Dh on homework and other reading ($P < 0.001$ for both) and were significantly more likely than boys to report any time spent during the last week doing homework or reading ($P < 0.001$)
Sydney Myopia Study: Ip et al., 2008 [145]	Cross-sectional	$n = 2339$, 12, Australia, Sydney	Time spent on reading (>30 m, OR = 1.5) and close reading distance (<30 cm, OR = 2.5) were associated with myopia after adjustment (P trend = 0.02) Time spent in near-work activities correlated poorly with SE (all $r ≤ 0.2$) and was not significant for myopia (SE ≤ −0.50 D). European Caucasian children reported spending less time in near work than East Asian children (26.0 h/wk vs. 32.5 h/wk, $P < 0.0001$)
Sydney Myopia Study: Rose et al., 2008 [156]	Cross-sectional	$n = 1735$, 6–12, Australia, Sydney	After adjusting, there was no overall association of near work and mean SER in the 6 years old ($p = 0.08$), although a significant association with mean SER was observed in children whose parents were not myopic ($p = 0.004$)
Orinda Longitudinal Study of Myopia: Jones et al., 2007 [155]	Cohort	$n = 514$, grade 1–8, USA, California	Three variables had predictive value: number of myopic parents, sports and outdoor activity h/w, and reading h/w. After adjustment, reading h/w was no longer a statistically significant factor
Singapore Cohort Study of the Risk Factors for Myopia (SCORM): Saw et al., 2002 [146]	Cross-sectional	$n = 1005$, 7–9, Singapore	OR for myopic children (at least −3.0 D) who read >2 books per week was 3.05 (95% CI, 1.80–5.18). OR for myopic children who read >2 h per day (1.50; 95% CI, 0.87–2.55) or >8 diopter hours[b] (1.04; 95% CI, 0.61–1.78,) was not significant, after adjustment
Orinda Longitudinal Study of myopia: Mutti et al. 2002 [147]	Cross-sectional	$n = 366$, grade 8, USA, California	Myopic children spent significantly > time studying and reading and scored higher on the Reading and Language subtests than emmetropic children ($p < 0.024$). OR (95% CI) for two compared with no parents with myopia was 6.40 (2.17–18.87) and 1.020 (1.008–1.032) for each diopter-h/w[a] of near work. Interactions between parental myopia and near work were not significant ($p = 0.67$)

Legend: AL axial length, *CI* confidence interval, *h/w* hours per week, *OR* odds ratio, *Y* years, *SE* spherical equivalent, *USA* United States of America

[a]Diopter-hours (Dh) variable was defined as Dh = 3 × (hours spent studying + hours spent reading for pleasure) + 2 × (hours spent playing video games or working on the computer at home) + 1 × (hours spent watching television)

[b]Weighted variable, diopter hours, was computed by adding three times reading, two times computer use, and two times video games use in hours per day for near-work activity outside school

Animal studies provided new insights into the role of near work. Smith et al. found that relatively long periods of form deprivation can be counterbalanced by quite short periods of unrestricted vision [172]. Norton et al. examine the ability of hyperopic defocus, minimal defocus, and myopic defocus to compete against a myopigenic −5 D lens in juvenile tree shrew eyes [173]. They found myopic defocus encoded by at tree shrew retinas as being different from hyperopic defocus, and myopic defocus can sometimes counteract the myopigenic effect of the −5 D lens (hyperopic defocus). Therefore, animal data indicated that whether the reading took place in many short periods or less frequent longer periods might have played an important role in myopia development.

Josh Wallman's work on chicks further indicated that the effects of episodes of defocus rise rapidly with episode duration to an asymptote and decline between episodes, with the time course depending strongly on the sign of defocus and the ocular component [174]. This finding has important implications on myopia prevention in children. The development of myopia in school-age children has been associated with the presumed hyperopic defocus that the eyes experience during reading. Given the distinctively different fall times of ocular compensation caused by positive and negative lens wear in chicks, it is likely that the total amount of near work does not capture all the temporal information used for integration of the defocus signals. It would not be possible to advise children in some Asian community such as Singapore and Hong Kong to spend less time in homework because of academic demands; it may be important to encourage children to take frequent breaks from reading and to view distant objects.

3.6.2 Screen Time

Screen time is emerging as a concerning environmental factor due to the increased time children spent using smartphones and mobile devices, either for pleasure or studying. Smartphones become popular 10 years ago, and research was not able to show the long-term effects of the increased use. A report from WHO provided guidelines to restrict sedentary screen time for children under 5 years old as some evidence suggest that screen time may increase sedentary behavior with negative impact for children's health [179]. Screen time has been less well documented compared with near work, and there is still no clear evidence of an association with myopia development [180]. Screen time is often classified as part of specific sedentary behaviors such as using the computer or playing video games, and correlations with total sedentary time have been found [181]. Screen time might be a behavioral risk factor that plays an important role in myopia development.

Few have examined the individual relationship between screen time as a risk factor for myopia (evidence is shown in Table 3.6) and frequently total near work (activities at short distance) which includes screen time such as computer use and playing games. Also, studies have limitations, some were conducted before screen time was common (e.g., 2002), or children's age was too young with insufficient screen time to cause myopia (e.g., 3 years old).

A study from Yunnan province, China, found that myopia in children aged 5–16 years old was associated with computer use (OR = 1.17) after adjustment, though the odds ratio was of modest effect size [182]. Similarly, in Singapore in school children (7–9 years old), the Singapore Cohort Study of the Risk Factors for Myopia found that computer use was statistically significantly different for higher myopes versus lower myopes and higher myopes versus non-myopes [146]. In contrast, other studies found that playing video games or working on a computer was not associated with myopia in American children from the first to eighth grade [147, 155]. At 3 years old, no association was found between computer use and myopia (≤−0.50 D) or SE in children from the GUSTO cohort [153]. Nonetheless, time using handheld devices was found to be associated with axial length [145, 153].

Screen time increased in the past few years due to an intensification in the use of computers and handheld devices (smartphones and tablets) by children. A study comparing screen time from GUSTO at 2 and 3 years old found an increase on average by 0.33 ± 2.42 h/day mainly due to an increase in handheld device viewing time [183]. In children with a mean age of 4.37 ± 0.01 years old from the Early Childhood Longitudinal Study–Birth Cohort in the USA, the average screen time was found to be similar (3.78 ± 0.06 h) [184]. Another study in 9–11-year-old children from 12 different countries found that 54.2% of the children were in contact with screens for 2 or more hours per day, failing the guidelines [181]. In Ireland, older ($p = 0.001$), urban ($p = 0.0005$), and myopic ($p = 0.04$) children spent significantly more time using digital screens compared to younger non-myopic children from a rural background [185].

LeBlanc et al. found that increased screen time is also associated with unhealthy behaviors, such as unhealthy eating pattern and reduced physical activity [181]. In the same study, children who spent more time outside were compensating with higher screen time when they were inside. Other authors found similar results with children who performed higher amounts of near work being protected from myopia if they also spent large amounts of time outdoors [145, 156, 186]. Outdoor time might be a confounding variable and needs to be adjusted when analyzing screen time and myopia. Screen time in children with myopia is

Table 3.6 Summary of evidence from studies on screen time and myopia

Study: authors, year	Study design	Participants: number, age (Y), location	Study outcomes
Harrington et al., 2019 [60]	Cross-sectional	$n = 728$, 6–7 $n = 898$, 12–13	Myopia prevalence was significantly linked with using screens >3 h per day (OR = 3.7, 95% CI 2.1–6.3, $p < 0.001$)
North India Myopia Study (NIM Study): Saxena et al., 2017 [175]	Prospective longitudinal (1 year)	$n = 9616$, 5–15, India, Delhi	Use of computers/video games ($P < 0.001$) was a significant risk factor for myopia progression ($n = 629$)
Qian et al., 2016 [182]	Cross-sectional	$n = 7681$, 5–16, Mangshi, rural China	Myopia prevalence = 39.1% (95% CI, 38.0, 40.2) and high myopia prevalence = 0.6% (95% CI, 0.4, 0.8) Myopia was associated with computer use (OR = 1.17; 95% CI, 1.03, 1.32) after adjusting for age, sex, and ethnicity
Growing Up in Singapore Towards Healthy Outcomes (GUSTO): Chua et al., 2015 [153]	Cohort	$n = 572$, 3, Singapore	Six percent had early-onset myopia. Children spent an average of 0.6 h/day (SD 0.8) using handheld devices and 0.1 h/day (SD 0.3) using a computer Computer (h/d) was not associated with SE ($p = 0.46$), AL ($p = 0.86$), or myopia ($p = 0.88$) Handheld devices (h/d) were associated with AL ($\beta = 0.07$; 95% CI, 0.01–0.23; $p = 0.03$), but not with SE ($p = 0.05$) and myopia ($p = 0.86$).
Sydney Myopia Study: Ip et al., 2008 [145]	Cross-sectional	$n = 2339$, 12, Australia, Sydney	Computer use ($p = 0.5$) and playing handheld console games ($p = 0.6$) were not associated with SE Time spent (h/w) playing handheld console games, although significant ($p = 0.01$), correlated poorly with AL (all $r = 0.05$) and was not significant for SE ($p = 0.5$)
Orinda Longitudinal Study of Myopia: Jones et al., 2007 [155]	Cohort	$n = 514$, grade 1–8, USA, California	Comparing non-myopes (78.4%) and myopes (21.6%) hours of computer/video games was not associated with myopia ($p > 0.05$)
Orinda Longitudinal Study of Myopia: Mutti et al. 2002 [147]	Cross-sectional	$n = 366$, grade 8, USA, California	Comparing myopes (18%), emmetropes (74%), and hyperopes (8%) playing video games/computer was not associated with myopia ($p > 0.05$)
Singapore Cohort Study of the Risk Factors for Myopia (SCORM): Saw et al., 2002 [146]	Cross-sectional	$n = 1005$, 7–9, Singapore	Myopia prevalence rates: 28% at age 7, 35% at age 8, and 43% at age 9 years Computer use (yes/no) was statistically significantly different for higher myopes versus lower myopes and higher myopes versus non-myopes in Chinese children ($p < 0.05$)

Legend: *AL* axial length, *CI* confidence interval, *h/d* hours per day, *h/w* hours per week, *OR* odds ratio, *Y* years, *SE* spherical equivalent, *USA* United States of America

poorly documented and its role is still unclear. Thus, there is the need to explore patterns of screen time in children and the association with myopia.

3.6.3 Time Outdoors

In cross-sectional studies, the association between time outdoors and myopia is well documented. In Singapore, the total time spent outdoors was associated with significantly less myopic refraction (regression coefficient, 0.17; 95% CI, 0.10–0.25; $P < 0.001$) and shorter axial length (regression coefficient, 20.06; 95% CI, 20.1–20.03; $P < 0.001$). Total sports was also significantly negatively associated with myopia ($P = 0.008$), but not indoor sports ($P = 0.16$) [187]. In the Sydney Myopia Study, a greater number of hours spent outdoors were associated with a more hyperopic refraction after multivariate adjustment. When hours spent on outdoor activities excluding sport were considered, the trends were highly

significant ($P = 0.0001$). In contrast, time spent on indoor sport had no significant effect on refractive error ($P = 0.9$) [156]. Using the same population-based study, a comparison of a younger cohort (6 years = 16.3 h/week) and an older cohort (12 years = 21 h/week) showed that more time outdoors is associated ($p = {<}0.001$) with a reduction in incident myopia [157]. In addition, the prevalence of myopia in children of Chinese ethnicity was significantly lower in Sydney (3.3%) than in Singapore (29.1%). The lower prevalence of myopia in Sydney was associated with increased hours of outdoor activities (13.75 vs. 3.05 h/week) [188]. Children of East Asian ancestry had higher incidence of myopia compared with European Caucasian ancestry and spent less time outdoors [157]. A study using wearable light sensors showed that Australian children (105 ± 42 min/d) are exposed to more daily outdoor light (>1000 lux) than Singaporean children (61 ± 40 min/d; $P = 0.005$), with longer duration on weekends [189]. In Beijing, less outdoor activity was also associated with longer ocular axial length in children from grades 1 to 4 [190]. However, in Canadian children aged 6–13 years old, outdoor time was the only statistically significant factor, with one additional hour of outdoor time per week lowering the odds of myopia by 14.3% (OR = 0.857; 95% CI, 0.766–0.959; p = 0.007) [67].

Sherwin et al. summarized the relationship between time spent outdoors and myopia in children and young adults by a systematic review and meta-analysis of observational studies [191]. They searched four databases (MEDLINE, Web of Science, Embase, and Cochrane) for studies that examined the association between time spent outdoors and the development or progression of myopia among children and adolescents aged 20 years or younger. The meta-analysis revealed that an additional hour spent outdoors per week was associated with a lower prevalence of myopia (pooled OR, 0.98; 95% CI, 0.97–0.99; P_{OR} < 0.001; I^2 = 44.3%; $P_{heterogeneity}$ = 0.09). In subgroup analysis, a stronger protective association was found between outdoor time and myopia risk in non-East Asian studies (OR, 0.97; 95% CI, 0.94–0.99; P_{OR} = 0.003) than in East Asian studies (OR, 0.99; 95% CI, 0.98–1.00; P_{OR} = 0.002). The limitations of the meta-analysis included the cross-sectional design of the included studies and the low number of studies included in the analysis. In another systematic review, time outdoors was found to have a protective effect on incident myopia (clinical trials: risk ratio (RR) = 0.536, 95% CI, 0.338–0.850; longitudinal cohort studies: RR = 0.574, 95% CI, 0.395–0.834) and prevalent myopia (cross-sectional studies: OR = 0.964, 95% CI, 0.945–0.982), but not for myopia progression [192]. Evidence suggests that time outdoors remains the most important factor in myopia, and there is no evidence that physical activity is an independent risk factor for myopia [193].

Longitudinal studies [155, 194] have provided evidence that time outdoors is associated with the onset of myopia. In a prospective cohort study of 1038 children with no myopia in the third grade of school (ages 8–9 years), Jones et al. followed the children for 5 years and found that the odds ratio of developing myopia for every 1 h of sport/outdoor activity per week was 0.91 (95% CI, 0.87–0.95). In the Collaborative Longitudinal Evaluation of Ethnicity and Refractive Error (CLEERE) Study, hours per week spent in outdoor/sports activities were significantly less for children who became myopic 3 years before onset through 4 years after onset by 1.1–1.8 h/week. A longitudinal study of 9109 children aged 7 years at baseline used survival analysis to investigate whether time spent outdoors or time spent in physical activity was predictive of myopia development, using a multidisciplinary data set from a birth cohort study. Children classified as spending a "low" amount of time outdoors at ages 8–9 years were about 40% more likely to have myopia between the ages of 11 and 15 years, compared to those classified as spending a "high" amount of time outdoors [195]. A

report from the CLEERE study examined 835 myopes to explore the relationship between time spent in various activities and the rate of myopia progression. This study showed that the performance of outdoor/sports activity was not associated with annual myopia progression following onset [196].

In the Avon Longitudinal Study of Parents and Children (ALSPAC), British children from age 2 to 15 years were included. Greater time outdoors was associated with a reduced risk of incident myopia (hazard ratio HR = 0.90 95% CI, 0.83–0.98; P = 0.012 at age 3 years; HR = 0.86 95% CI, 0.78–0.93, P = 0.001 at age 9 years), for each additional SD of time spent outdoors per day [197]. The Generation R birth cohort study from the Netherlands also found that myopic children aged 6 years old spent more time indoors than non-myopic children (p < 0.01) [48]. The Beijing Children Eye Study conducted a 4-year follow-up study in primary school children (n = 305) and found that greater axial elongation was associated with less time spent outdoors (P = 0.004; beta, −0.22), more time spent indoors studying (P = 0.02; beta, 0.18), and paternal myopia (P = 0.03; beta, 0.16) [198]. A prospective single-center study in Czech 12-year-old children (n = 398 eyes) showed that higher (p < 0.0001) axial length growth was observed during the winter period compared with spring [199]. The authors hypothesize that the eye grows more in the winter due to lack of daily light exposure that may predispose children to myopia.

In Taiwan, a longitudinal and interventional study was conducted to determine the effect of a class recess program of 80 min per day outdoors. The intervention had significant effect on myopia onset and myopia shift, especially in non-myopic children [200]. A similar study was conducted in northeast China adding two additional recess programs of 20 min. After the intervention, the authors concluded that increasing outdoor activities prevented myopia onset [201].

Randomized clinical trials (RCT) are important to test whether the association between time spent outdoors and myopia onset/progression is causal in nature. A few RCTs showed that increasing outdoor activities with interventions of 20–40 min during school time prevented myopia onset [201–203]. Findings from an RCT in Guangzhou, China, showed that a 40-min class of outdoor activities in school in children aged 6 years old (n = 952, intervention group) was able to reduce the myopia incidence rate (30.4% in the intervention group and 39.5% in the control group (difference of −9.1% [95% CI, −14.1% to −4.1%]; P < 0.001) [202]. In Taiwan, children were encouraged to go outdoors for up to 11 h weekly. The results showed a significant reduction in the myopic shift and axial elongation and progression [203].

In the 1-year Family Incentive Trial (FIT), 285 children were randomized to either the intervention (n = 147) or control (n = 138) arm. The intervention comprised of structured

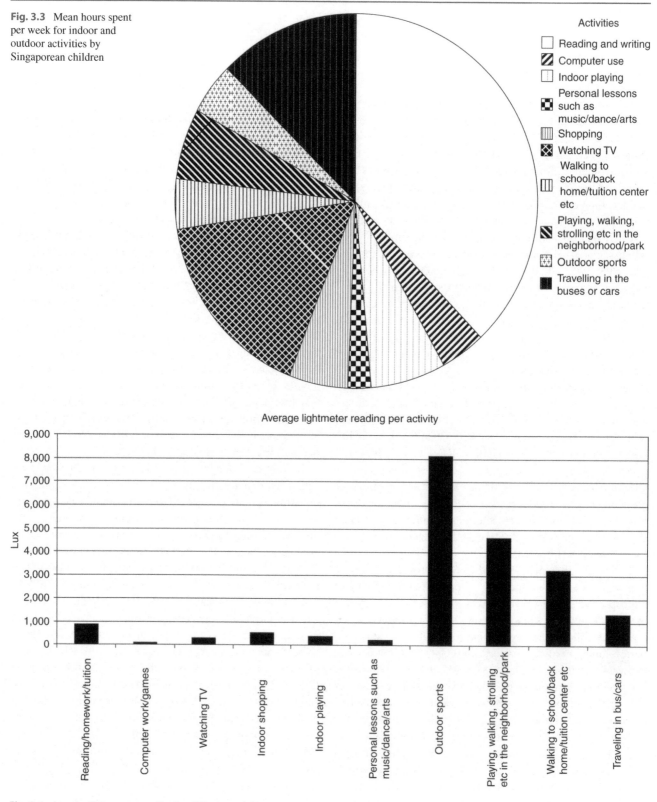

Fig. 3.3 Mean hours spent per week for indoor and outdoor activities by Singaporean children

Fig. 3.4 Average light meter reading by different activities

weekend outdoor activities in parks and incentives for children to increase their daily steps as measured via pedometers. Figure 3.3 demonstrates the mean hours children spent throughout the week in the control arm. In general, children in Singapore spent far more time doing indoor than outdoor activities. Figure 3.4 shows the average reading of light meter by different kinds of indoor and outdoor activities. The light meter readings varied significantly by outdoor activities. The mean light meter reading for outdoor activities including outdoor sports and walking in the park or on the way to school was much higher than indoor activities such as reading, watching TV, and indoor shopping or playing. In this study, the outdoor time increased by more 2.5 h/week for children in the intervention compared with the control arm, but the difference between the two groups decreased at the end of the trial (Saw et al. ARVO 2012 E-Abstract 2301). However, these preliminary results are difficult to justify, and further studies with larger sample size and longer follow-up periods may be warranted. In addition, more systematic monitoring of light exposures in epidemiological studies should be conducted by asking the participants to wear light meters and complete diaries of daily activities.

The role of outdoors in myopia progression is also not clear yet. The evidence suggests that greater time outdoors above 1000 lux is associated with slower axial elongation in non-myopic teenagers, but not in existing myopes [204]. Also, the best light cutoff was not settled yet. Participants exposed to 1000–3000 lux for 200 min show significantly less myopic shift [203]. However, in children who spent less time outdoors, levels of 10,000 lux might be needed to change the myopic shift. Also, there is a lack of knowledge of the light levels reaching the eye and exposure settings, including sun-protective measures. This is essential for producing recommendations for outdoor programs and myopia prevention. The FitSight tracker with its novel features may motivate children to increase time outdoors and play an important role in supplementing community outdoor programs to prevent myopia [205]. Objective measurements of light levels using wearable devices can give more accurate measurements of outdoor time in children (Figs. 3.5 and 3.6) and help further research to unveil the role of high lux intensities in myopia.

A public health approach is necessary to improve public knowledge about myopia and its relationship with vision impairment later in life. A study conducted in Ireland shows that compared to non-myopic parents, myopic parents viewed myopia as more of an optical inconvenience ($p < 0.001$), an expense ($p < 0.005$), and a cosmetic inconvenience ($p < 0.001$) [185]. In another study, Chinese parents' attitudes and behaviors towards children's visual care were also significantly associated with myopia risk in school-age children [206].

The role of UV exposure on myopia is also limited. A study on chicks was conducted to determine if emmetropization is possible in young chicks reared under higher luminance, UV lighting conditions. This study showed that the spatial resolving power of the UV cone photoreceptor network in the chick was sufficient to detect optical defocus and guided the emmetropization response, provided illumination was sufficiently high [207]. The effect of violet light (360–400 nm wave-

length) was also investigated in the chick myopia model showing suppression of axial length elongation and myopia progression [208]. A study showed that there was a protective association between the area of conjunctival ultraviolet autofluorescence and prevalent myopia. More direct measures of UV exposures may provide a surrogate measure of overall light exposures [209]. Chickens have four distinct spectral types of cones, one of which is sensitive to violet and ultraviolet light whereas humans have 3 spectral types opf cones and do not have ultraviolet sensitivity. In a multicountry European study, an SD increase in UVB exposure at age 14–19 years (OR, 0.81; 95% CI, 0.71–0.92) and 20–39 years (OR, 0.7; 95% CI, 0.62–0.93) was associated with a reduced adjusted OR of myopia [210]. The exact biological plausibility behind the observed association between time outdoors and myopia development has not been fully elucidated. The high ambient light level outdoors may be a potential mediator of the effects attributable to time outdoors. This has been supported by animal studies where ambient light levels have been found to influence the rate of visually induced form-deprivation myopia [211, 212], as well as the rate of compensation to monocularly imposed myopic and hyperopic defocus [212]. In animal models, chicks exposed to high illuminances (15,000 lx) for 5 h/day significantly slowed compensation for negative lenses compared with those under 500 lx. High illuminance also reduced deprivation myopia by about 60%, compared with that seen under 500 lx. This protective effect was abolished by the daily injection of spiperone, a dopamine receptor antagonist [211]. In addition, high-light-reared monkeys showed significantly lower average degrees of myopic anisometropia and average treated-eye refractive errors that were significantly more hyperopic than those observed in monocularly form-deprived monkeys reared under normal light levels [212]. Mehdizadeh and Nowroozzadeh have suggested an alternative possibility that the predominance of longer wavelength (red) light in the spectrum from incandescent lights, which would be in hyperopic defocus behind the retina, would promote greater axial elongation and more myopia [213].

However, this hypothesis was purely speculative and was not supported by a study on 3905 Polish students, where no differences in the use of light emitted by incandescent or fluorescent lamps on myopia were found ($P > 0.05$) [214]. In a review article, Flitcroft used computer-generated images to visualize the world in dioptric terms. The author found that the indoor world is essentially never optically flat, while the outdoor world dioptrically is much flatter than interior scenes. The three-dimensional structure of the environment may have impact in the patterns of defocus across the retina, thus resulting in a difference in the risk of myopia between indoor and outdoor [215]. However, this is an unproven hypothesis, and there is no evidence that a relatively more uniform dioptric environment would stabilize eye growth and prevent the development of myopia.

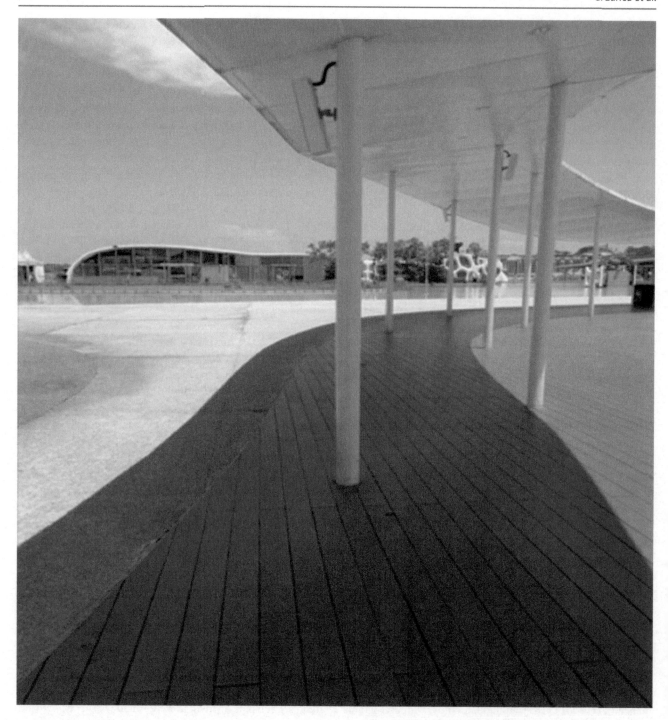

Fig. 3.5 Light intensity measured with the FitSight watch outside under a shelter in a sunny day at 1.30 pm (7573 lux)

In addition, vitamin D may be a link between time outdoors and myopia since time outdoors might create differences in vitamin D, while myopes appear to have lower average blood levels of vitamin D than non-myopes [216]. However, this theory is unlikely because of the lack of related evidence. Evidence supporting this idea comes from a case–control study, which showed that single-nucleotide polymorphisms within vitamin D receptor appear to be associated with low to moderate amounts of myopia. Data from the Korea National Health and Nutrition Examination Survey (KNHANES) V 2010–2012 ($n = 15,126$) showed that spherical equivalent from adults aged 20 years or older was significantly associated with serum 25(OH)D concentration after adjustment for confounding factors ($P = 0.002$) [217]. Low serum D levels and shorter daily sun exposure time may be independently associated with myopia. The same trend was

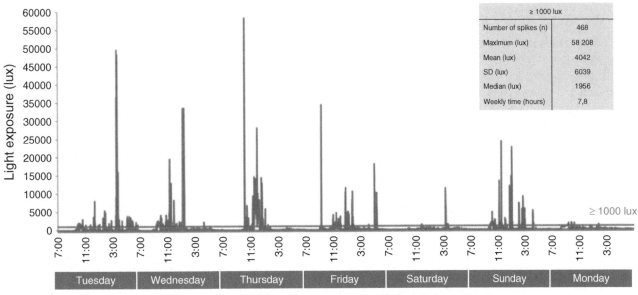

Fig. 3.6 Weekly daily light illuminance levels using the FitSight watch in one outdoor-centric child during school term

observed in Koreans ($n = 11,703$) that had sunlight exposure of ≥ 5 h/day (OR, 0.67) with higher serum 25-hydroxyvitamin D level (OR, 0.97 per 1 ng/mL) being protected against high myopia (SE ≤ -6 D) [76]. However, the evidence supporting that vitamin D plays a role in myopia development is still weak, and the mechanisms are unclear, mainly because vitamin D can be a biomarker for outdoor exposure and not an independent factor in myopia [218, 219]. Future studies, adjusting for confounders, should determine whether this finding can be replicated and should explore the biological significance of these variations with respect to myopia [220]. No independent associations between myopia and serum vitamin D3 concentrations nor variants in genes associated with vitamin D metabolism were found in a multicountry European study ($n = 3168$) [210]. Increasing evidence suggest that diurnal and circadian rhythms are related with eye growth and refractive error development [221]. However, more research needs to be further conducted.

concern with children exposure to UV light. More studies are needed on light exposure using UV protective measures and expand further on the impact of light on myopia.

There has long been a concern that increasing levels and severity of myopia will lead to a major increase in the number of people blind from myopia, but whether this will actually occur is still not known. The high myopia prevalence in young adults reported in Asia is of major concern as these adults will have more years of exposure to the disease and may become blind due to MMD. The number of people with visual impairment is expected to grow in 2050. Preventive strategies seem the best strategy to avoid blindness due to myopia.

The interactions of gene–environment mechanisms for etiology of myopia and axial length are still unknown. Further research on gene interactions with environment can elucidate on the last decades' changes in myopia prevalence with the newer generations having higher prevalence than older generations.

3.7 Answered and Unanswered Questions

Longitudinal studies are still necessary to unveil which optimal light exposure patterns are more protective from myopia. New questions need answers: (1) what is the amount of light exposure (threshold) necessary for avoiding myopia onset? (2) How intense and for how long needs to be the exposure to outdoor levels (e.g., 1000 lux, 5000 lux, or 10,000 lux)? (3) What wavelengths of light are optimal? (4) Which environmental factors can be changed to improve rates of myopia progression? While outdoor programs have been proved to be protective for myopia, there is an increased

3.8 Conclusions

New epidemiological data suggest the following. First, current studies do not support the concept that Asians are more susceptible to myopia. Second, there is a large variation in myopia rates in Asia associated with environmental factors (mainly education, near work, and time outdoors) of different countries. The prevalence of myopia is higher in new urbanized Asian societies such as Singapore and Hong Kong but lower in Cambodia, Nepal, and Laos. Third, pathological myopia, a major cause for low vision and blindness, affects about 1–4% of the general population. Since the visual prognosis for highly myopic patients with pathological myopia is poor, prevention of myopia, especially high myopia, is of utmost importance from a public health perspective. Fourth, outdoor time appears to be the most important modifiable factor related to myopia incidence. However, dose–response analysis did not find a relationship between time outdoors and myopic progression. Fifth, near-work activities including increasing screen time use in smartphones and devices may be a major factor for myopia. Therefore, combining health behavior programs aiming to increase outdoor time and decreasing screen time may prevent the onset of myopia, and interventions to slow the progression of low myopia to high myopia may prevent severe disease and associated pathological myopia complications. Considering the rapid increase in prevalence of myopia and high myopia in younger generations, there will be an epidemic of pathological myopia in the next few decades. This will be apparent when the young "myopic" generation in urban Asian cities age in the next few decades. However, it is possible that adults with acquired high myopia are less susceptible to myopic pathology than adults with a genetic predisposition to high myopia.

References

1. Morgan IG, Ohno-Matsui K, Saw S-M. Myopia. Lancet. 2012;379(9827):1739–48.
2. Morgan I, Rose K. How genetic is school myopia? Prog Retin Eye Res. 2005;24(1):1–38.
3. Saw S-M, Matsumura S, Hoang QV. Prevention and management of myopia and myopic pathology. Invest Ophthalmol Vis Sci. 2019;60(2):488.
4. Pan C-W, Ramamurthy D, Saw S-M. Worldwide prevalence and risk factors for myopia. Ophthalmic Physiol Opt. 2012;32(1):3–16.
5. Resnikoff S, Pascolini D, Mariotti SP, Pokharel GP. Global magnitude of visual impairment caused by uncorrected refractive errors in 2004. Bull World Health Organ. 2008;86(1):63–70.
6. Javitt JC, Chiang YP. The socioeconomic aspects of laser refractive surgery. Arch Ophthalmol. 1994;112(12):1526–30.
7. Chua J, Wong TY. Myopia-the silent epidemic that should not be ignored. JAMA Ophthalmol. 2016;134(12):1363–4.
8. McCarty CA. Uncorrected refractive error. Br J Ophthalmol. 2006;90(5):521–2.
9. Chua SYL, et al. Age of onset of myopia predicts risk of high myopia in later childhood in myopic Singapore children. Ophthalmic Physiol Opt. 2016;36(4):388–94.
10. Saw SM, Nieto FJ, Katz J, Schein OD, Levy B, Chew SJ. Factors related to the progression of myopia in Singaporean children. Optom Vis Sci. 2000;77(10):549–54.
11. Inhoffen W, Ziemssen F. Morphologische Charakteristika der myopen choroidalen Neovaskularisation. Der Ophthalmol. 2012;109(8):749–57.
12. Takeuchi K, Kachi S, Iwata E, Ishikawa K, Terasaki H. Visual function 5 years or more after macular translocation surgery for myopic choroidal neovascularisation and age-related macular degeneration. Eye. 2012;26(1):51–60.
13. Coco Martín MB, Arranz De La Fuente I, González García MJ, Cuadrado Asensio R, Coco Martín RM. Functional improvement after vision rehabilitation in low monocular vision after myopic macular degeneration and retinal detachment. Arch Soc Esp Oftalmol. 2002;77(2):95–8.
14. Rabb MF, Garoon I, LaFranco FP. Myopic macular degeneration. Int Ophthalmol Clin. 1981;21(3):51–69.
15. Wong TY, Ferreira A, Hughes R, Carter G, Mitchell P. Epidemiology and disease burden of pathologic myopia and myopic choroidal neovascularization: an evidence-based systematic review. Am J Ophthalmol. 2014;157(1):9–25, e12.
16. Neelam K, Cheung CMG, Ohno-Matsui K, Lai TYY, Wong TY. Choroidal neovascularization in pathological myopia. Prog Retin Eye Res. 2012;31(5):495–525.
17. Fricke TR, et al. Global prevalence of visual impairment associated with myopic macular degeneration and temporal trends from 2000 through 2050: systematic review, meta-analysis and modelling. Br J Ophthalmol. 2018;102(7):855–62.
18. Gilmartin B. Myopia: precedents for research in the twenty-first century. Clin Exp Ophthalmol. 2004;32(3):305–24.
19. Saw S-M. A synopsis of the prevalence rates and environmental risk factors for myopia. Clin Exp Optom. 2003;86(5):289–94.
20. Young TL. Complex trait genetics of refractive error. Arch Ophthalmol. 2007;125(1):38.
21. Wallman J, Winawer J. Homeostasis of eye growth and the question of myopia. Neuron. 2004;43(4):447–68.
22. Wiesel TN, Raviola E. Myopia and eye enlargement after neonatal lid fusion in monkeys. Nature. 1977;266(5597):66–8.
23. Holden BA, et al. Global prevalence of myopia and high myopia and temporal trends from 2000 through 2050. Ophthalmology. 2016;123(5):1036–42.
24. Wong Y-L, et al. Prevalence, risk factors, and impact of myopic macular degeneration on visual impairment and functioning among adults in Singapore. Invest Ophthalmol Vis Sci. 2018;59(11):4603.
25. Wong TY, et al. Prevalence and risk factors for refractive errors in adult Chinese in Singapore. Invest Ophthalmol Vis Sci. 2000;41(9):2486–94.
26. Van Newkirk MR. The Hong Kong vision study: a pilot assessment of visual impairment in adults. Trans Am Ophthalmol Soc. 1997;95:715–49.
27. Liang YB, et al. Refractive errors in a rural Chinese adult population the Handan Eye Study. Ophthalmology. 2009;116(11):2119–27.
28. Xu L, et al. Refractive error in urban and rural adult Chinese in Beijing. Ophthalmology. 2005;112(10):1676–83.
29. Wang M, et al. Prevalence and risk factors of refractive error: a cross-sectional Study in Han and Yi adults in Yunnan, China. BMC Ophthalmol. 2019;19(1):33.
30. Xu C, et al. Prevalence and risk factors for myopia in older adult east Chinese population. BMC Ophthalmol. 2017;17(1):191.
31. Sawada A, Tomidokoro A, Araie M, Iwase A, Yamamoto T. Refractive errors in an elderly japanese population. Ophthalmology. 2008;115(2):363–70, e3.
32. Nakamura Y, et al. Refractive errors in an elderly rural Japanese population: the Kumejima study. PLoS One. 2018;13(11):e0207180.
33. Rudnicka AR, et al. Global variations and time trends in the prevalence of childhood myopia, a systematic review and quantitative meta-analysis: implications for aetiology and early prevention. Br J Ophthalmol. 2016;100(7):882–90.
34. He M, Zeng J, Liu Y, Xu J, Pokharel GP, Ellwein LB. Refractive error and visual impairment in urban children in Southern China. Invest Ophthalmol Vis Sci. 2004;45(3):793.
35. Saw S-M, Carkeet A, Chia K-S, Stone RA, Tan DT. Component dependent risk factors for ocular parameters in Singapore Chinese children. Ophthalmology. 2002;109(11):2065–71.

36. Chen M, et al. The increasing prevalence of myopia and high myopia among high school students in Fenghua city, eastern China: a 15-year population-based survey. BMC Ophthalmol. 2018;18(1):159.

37. Guo Y, et al. High myopia in Greater Beijing School Children in 2016. PLoS One. 2017;12(11):e0187396.

38. Lim DH, Han J, Chung T-Y, Kang S, Yim HW. The high prevalence of myopia in Korean children with influence of parental refractive errors: The 2008–2012 Korean National Health and Nutrition Examination Survey. PLoS One. 2018;13(11):e0207690.

39. Dirani M, et al. Prevalence of refractive error in Singaporean Chinese children: the strabismus, amblyopia, and refractive error in young Singaporean Children (STARS) Study. Invest Ophthalmol Vis Sci. 2010;51(3):1348.

40. Gao Z, et al. Refractive error in school children in an urban and rural setting in Cambodia. Ophthalmic Epidemiol. 2012;19(1):16–22.

41. Casson RJ, Kahawita S, Kong A, Muecke J, Sisaleumsak S, Visonnavong V. Exceptionally low prevalence of refractive error and visual impairment in schoolchildren from Lao People's Democratic Republic. Ophthalmology. 2012;119(10):2021–7.

42. Pokharel GP, Negrel AD, Munoz SR, Ellwein LB. Refractive error study in children: results from Mechi Zone, Nepal. Am J Ophthalmol. 2000;129(4):436–44.

43. Zhao J, Pan X, Sui R, Munoz SR, Sperduto RD, Ellwein LB. Refractive error study in children: results from Shunyi District, China. Am J Ophthalmol. 2000;129(4):427–35.

44. Pi L-H, et al. Prevalence of eye diseases and causes of visual impairment in school-aged children in Western China. J Epidemiol. 2012;22(1):37–44.

45. Guo X, Fu M, Ding X, Morgan IG, Zeng Y, He M. Significant axial elongation with minimal change in refraction in 3- to 6-year-old Chinese preschoolers: the Shenzhen kindergarten eye study. Ophthalmology. 2017;124(12):1826–38.

46. Li L, Zhong H, Li J, Li C-R, Pan C-W. Incidence of myopia and biometric characteristics of premyopic eyes among Chinese children and adolescents. BMC Ophthalmol. 2018;18(1):178.

47. McCullough SJ, O'Donoghue L, Saunders KJ. Six year refractive change among white children and young adults: evidence for significant increase in myopia among white UK children. PLoS One. 2016;11(1):e0146332.

48. Tideman JWL, Polling JR, Hofman A, Jaddoe VW, Mackenbach JP, Klaver CC. Environmental factors explain socioeconomic prevalence differences in myopia in 6-year-old children. Br J Ophthalmol. 2018;102(2):243–7.

49. Tideman JWL, Polling JR, Jaddoe VWV, Vingerling JR, Klaver CCW. Environmental risk factors can reduce axial length elongation and myopia incidence in 6- to 9-year-old children. Ophthalmology. 2019;126(1):127–36.

50. Pan C-W, Dirani M, Cheng C-Y, Wong T-Y, Saw S-M. The age-specific prevalence of myopia in Asia: a meta-analysis. Optom Vis Sci. 2015;92(3):258–66.

51. Jung S-K, Lee JH, Kakizaki H, Jee D. Prevalence of myopia and its association with body stature and educational level in 19-year-old male conscripts in Seoul, South Korea. Invest Ophthalmol Vis Sci. 2012;53(9):5579.

52. Wu H-MM, et al. Does education explain ethnic differences in myopia prevalence? A population-based study of young adult males in Singapore. Optom Vis Sci. 2001;78(4):234–9.

53. Lee DC, Lee SY, Kim YC. An epidemiological study of the risk factors associated with myopia in young adult men in Korea. Sci Rep. 2018;8(1):511.

54. Han SB, Jang J, Yang HK, Hwang J-M, Park SK. Prevalence and risk factors of myopia in adult Korean population: Korea national health and nutrition examination survey 2013–2014 (KNHANES VI). PLoS One. 2019;14(1):e0211204.

55. Krishnaiah S, Srinivas M, Khanna RC, Rao GN. Prevalence and risk factors for refractive errors in the South Indian adult population: the Andhra Pradesh Eye disease study. Clin Ophthalmol. 2009;3:17–27.

56. Raju P, et al. Prevalence of refractive errors in a rural South Indian population. Invest Ophthalmol Vis Sci. 2004;45(12):4268–72.

57. Joseph S, et al. Prevalence and risk factors for myopia and other refractive errors in an adult population in southern India. Ophthalmic Physiol Opt. 2018;38(3):346–58.

58. Pan C-W, et al. Prevalence and risk factors for refractive errors in Indians: The Singapore Indian Eye Study (SINDI). Invest Ophthalmol Vis Sci. 2011;52(6):3166.

59. Pan C-W, et al. Variation in prevalence of myopia between generations of migrant Indians living in Singapore. Am J Ophthalmol. 2012;154(2):376–81, e1.

60. Harrington SC, Stack J, O'Dwyer V. Risk factors associated with myopia in schoolchildren in Ireland. Br J Ophthalmol. 2019;103(12):1803–9.

61. Theophanous C, Modjtahedi B, Batech M, Marlin D, Luong T, Fong D. Myopia prevalence and risk factors in children. Clin Ophthalmol. 2018;12:1581–7.

62. Vitale S, Ellwein L, Cotch MF, Ferris FL, Sperduto R. Prevalence of refractive error in the United States, 1999–2004. Arch Ophthalmol. 2008;126(8):1111–9.

63. Vitale S, Sperduto RD, Ferris FL. Increased prevalence of myopia in the United States between 1971–1972 and 1999–2004. Arch Ophthalmol. 2009;127(12):1632–9.

64. Cumberland PM, Bountziouka V, Rahi JS. Impact of varying the definition of myopia on estimates of prevalence and associations with risk factors: time for an approach that serves research, practice and policy. Br J Ophthalmol. 2018;102(10):1407–12.

65. Ma Y, et al. Cohort study with 4-year follow-up of myopia and refractive parameters in primary schoolchildren in Baoshan District, Shanghai. Clin Exp Ophthalmol. 2018;46(8):861–72.

66. Zeng CQ, et al. The epidemiology of myopia in primary school students of grade 1 to 3 in Hubei province. Zhonghua Yan Ke Za Zhi. 2018;54(10):756–61.

67. Yang M, et al. Myopia prevalence in Canadian school children: a pilot study. Eye (Lond). 2018;32(6):1042–7.

68. Sun JT, An M, Yan XB, Li GH, Wang DB. Prevalence and related factors for myopia in school-aged children in Qingdao. J Ophthalmol. 2018;2018:9781987.

69. Hagen LA, Gjelle JVB, Arnegard S, Pedersen HR, Gilson SJ, Baraas RC. Prevalence and possible factors of myopia in Norwegian adolescents. Sci Rep. 2018;8(1):13479.

70. Wang SK, et al. Incidence of and factors associated with myopia and high myopia in Chinese children, based on refraction without cycloplegia. JAMA Ophthalmol. 2018;136(9):1017.

71. Pan C-W, Wu R-K, Li J, Zhong H. Low prevalence of myopia among school children in rural China. BMC Ophthalmol. 2018;18(1):140.

72. Li Y, Liu J, Qi P. The increasing prevalence of myopia in junior high school students in the Haidian District of Beijing, China: a 10-year population-based survey. BMC Ophthalmol. 2017;17(1):88.

73. Tideman JWL, et al. Association of axial length with risk of uncorrectable visual impairment for europeans with myopia. JAMA Ophthalmol. 2016;134(12):1355.

74. Morgan IG, He M, Rose KA. epidemic of pathologic myopia: what can laboratory studies and epidemiology tell us? Retina. 2017;37(5):989–97.

75. Saw S-M, et al. Prevalence and risk factors for refractive errors in the Singapore Malay Eye Survey. Ophthalmology. 2008;115(10):1713–9.

76. Hwang HS, Chun MY, Kim JS, Oh B, Yoo SH, Cho B-J. Risk factors for high myopia in Koreans: the Korea National Health and Nutrition Examination Survey. Curr Eye Res. 2018;43(8):1052–60.

77. Katz J, Tielsch JM, Sommer A. Prevalence and risk factors for refractive errors in an adult inner city population. Invest Ophthalmol Vis Sci. 1997;38(2):334–40.

78. Attebo K, Ivers RQ, Mitchell P. Refractive errors in an older population: the Blue Mountains Eye Study. Ophthalmology. 1999;106(6):1066–72.

79. Tarczy-Hornoch K, Ying-Lai M, Varma R. Myopic Refractive Error in Adult Latinos: The Los Angeles Latino Eye Study. Invest Ophthalmol Vis Sci. 2006;47(5):1845.

80. Pan C-W, et al. Differential associations of myopia with major age-related eye diseases: the Singapore Indian Eye Study. Ophthalmology. 2013;120(2):284–91.

81. Saw S-M, Gazzard G, Shih-Yen EC, Chua W-H. Myopia and associated pathological complications. Ophthalmic Physiol Opt. 2005;25(5):381–91.

82. Ohno-Matsui K. Pathologic myopia. Asia-Pacific J Ophthalmol. 2016;5(6):415–23.

83. Ohno-Matsui K, et al. International photographic classification and grading system for myopic maculopathy. Am J Ophthalmol. 2015;159(5):877–83, e7.

84. Iwase A, Araie M, Tomidokoro A, Yamamoto T, Shimizu H, Kitazawa Y. Prevalence and causes of low vision and blindness in a Japanese adult population. Ophthalmology. 2006;113(8):1354–62, e1.

85. Xu L, et al. Causes of blindness and visual impairment in urban and rural areas in Beijing. Ophthalmology. 2006;113(7):1134. e1–1134.e11.

86. Hsu W-M, Cheng C-Y, Liu J-H, Tsai S-Y, Chou P. Prevalence and causes of visual impairment in an elderly Chinese population in Taiwan: the Shihpai Eye Study. Ophthalmology. 2004;111(1):62–9.

87. Klaver CC, Wolfs RC, Vingerling JR, Hofman A, de Jong PT. Age-specific prevalence and causes of blindness and visual impairment in an older population: the Rotterdam Study. Arch Ophthalmol. 1998;116(5):653–8.

88. Foong AWP, et al. Rationale and methodology for a population-based study of eye diseases in Malay people: the Singapore Malay Eye Study (SiMES). Ophthalmic Epidemiol. 2007;14(1):25–35.

89. Lavanya R, et al. Methodology of the Singapore Indian Chinese Cohort (SICC) Eye Study: quantifying ethnic variations in the epidemiology of eye diseases in Asians. Ophthalmic Epidemiol. 2009;16(6):325–36.

90. Steidl SM, Pruett RC. Macular complications associated with posterior staphyloma. Am J Ophthalmol. 1997;123(2):181–7.

91. Green JS, Bear JC, Johnson GJ. The burden of genetically determined eye disease. Br J Ophthalmol. 1986;70(9):696–9.

92. Vongphanit J, Mitchell P, Wang JJ. Prevalence and progression of myopic retinopathy in an older population. Ophthalmology. 2002;109(4):704–11.

93. Liu HH, Xu L, Wang YX, Wang S, You QS, Jonas JB. Prevalence and progression of myopic retinopathy in Chinese adults: the Beijing eye study. Ophthalmology. 2010;117(9):1763–8.

94. Gao LQ, et al. Prevalence and characteristics of myopic retinopathy in a rural Chinese adult population: the Handan Eye Study. Arch Ophthalmol. 2011;129(9):1199–204.

95. Asakuma T, et al. Prevalence and risk factors for myopic retinopathy in a Japanese population: the Hisayama Study. Ophthalmology. 2012;119(9):1760–5.

96. Chen S-J, et al. Prevalence and associated risk factors of myopic maculopathy in elderly Chinese: the Shihpai eye study. Invest Ophthalmol Vis Sci. 2012;53(8):4868–73.

97. Choudhury F, et al. Prevalence and characteristics of myopic degeneration in an adult Chinese American population: the Chinese American Eye Study. Am J Ophthalmol. 2018;187:34–42.

98. Jonas JB, Nangia V, Gupta R, Bhojwani K, Nangia P, Panda-Jonas S. Prevalence of myopic retinopathy in rural Central India. Acta Ophthalmol. 2017;95(5):e399–404.

99. Hayashi K, et al. Long-term pattern of progression of myopic maculopathy: a natural history study. Ophthalmology. 2010;117(8):1595–611, 1611.e1–4.

100. Lin C, et al. Five-year incidence and progression of myopic maculopathy in a rural Chinese adult population: the Handan Eye Study. Ophthalmic Physiol Opt. 2018;38(3):337–45.

101. Cheung CMG, et al. Myopic choroidal neovascularization: review, guidance, and consensus statement on management. Ophthalmology. 2017;124(11):1690–711.

102. The Eye Disease Case-Control Study Group. Risk factors for neovascular age-related macular degeneration. Arch Ophthalmol. 1992;110(12):1701–8.

103. Age-Related Eye Disease Study Research Group. Risk factors associated with age-related macular degeneration. A case-control study in the age-related eye disease study: age-related eye disease study report number 3. Ophthalmology. 2000;107(12):2224–32.

104. Chaine G, et al. Case-control study of the risk factors for age related macular degeneration. France-DMLA Study Group. Br J Ophthalmol. 1998;82(9):996–1002.

105. Ikram MK, van Leeuwen R, Vingerling JR, Hofman A, de Jong PTVM. Relationship between refraction and prevalent as well as incident age-related maculopathy: the Rotterdam Study. Invest Ophthalmol Vis Sci. 2003;44(9):3778–82.

106. Wang JJ, Mitchell P, Smith W. Refractive error and age-related maculopathy: the Blue Mountains Eye Study. Invest Ophthalmol Vis Sci. 1998;39(11):2167–71.

107. Lavanya R, et al. Hyperopic refractive error and shorter axial length are associated with age-related macular degeneration: the Singapore Malay Eye Study. Invest Ophthalmol Vis Sci. 2010;51(12):6247–52.

108. Xu L, Li Y, Zheng Y, Jonas JB. Associated factors for age related maculopathy in the adult population in China: the Beijing eye study. Br J Ophthalmol. 2006;90(9):1087–90.

109. Klein R, Klein BE, Jensen SC, Cruickshanks KJ. The relationship of ocular factors to the incidence and progression of age-related maculopathy. Arch Ophthalmol. 1998;116(4):506–13.

110. Wong TY, Klein R, Klein BEK, Tomany SC. Refractive errors and 10-year incidence of age-related maculopathy. Invest Ophthalmol Vis Sci. 2002;43(9):2869–73.

111. Wang JJ, Jakobsen KB, Smith W, Mitchell P. Refractive status and the 5-year incidence of age-related maculopathy: the Blue Mountains Eye Study. Clin Exp Ophthalmol. 2004;32(3):255–8.

112. Ulvik SO, Seland JH, Wentzel-Larsen T. Refraction, axial length and age-related maculopathy. Acta Ophthalmol Scand. 2005;83(4):419–23.

113. Corbelli E, et al. Prevalence and phenotypes of age-related macular degeneration in eyes with high myopia. Invest Ophthalmol Vis Sci. 2019;60(5):1394.

114. Wood A, Guggenheim JA. Refractive error has minimal influence on the risk of age-related macular degeneration: a Mendelian randomization study. Am J Ophthalmol. 2019;206:87–93.

115. Hövener G. The influence of refraction on diabetic retinopathy (author's transl). Klin Monatsbl Augenheilkd. 1975;167(5):733–6.

116. Grange JD, Leynaud JL. Diabetic retinopathy and severe myopia. Bull Soc Ophtalmol Fr. 1984;84(2):205–8.

117. Bazzazi N, Akbarzadeh S, Yavarikia M, Poorolajal J, Fouladi DF. High myopia and diabetic retinopathy: a contralateral eye study in diabetic patients with high myopic anisometropia. Retina. 2017;37(7):1270–6.

118. Moss SE, Klein R, Klein BE. Ocular factors in the incidence and progression of diabetic retinopathy. Ophthalmology. 1994;101(1):77–83.

119. McKay R, McCarty CA, Taylor HR. Diabetic retinopathy in Victoria, Australia: the visual impairment project. Br J Ophthalmol. 2000;84(8):865–70.

120. Lim LS, Lamoureux E, Saw SM, Tay WT, Mitchell P, Wong TY. Are myopic eyes less likely to have diabetic retinopathy? Ophthalmology. 2010;117(3):524–30.

121. Chao DL, Lin S-C, Chen R, Lin SC. Myopia is inversely associated with the prevalence of diabetic retinopathy in the South Korean population. Am J Ophthalmol. 2016;172:39–44.

122. Wang X, Tang L, Gao L, Yang Y, Cao D, Li Y. Myopia and diabetic retinopathy: a systematic review and meta-analysis. Diabetes Res Clin Pract. 2016;111:1–9.

123. Wong TY, Klein BE, Klein R, Tomany SC, Lee KE. Refractive errors and incident cataracts: the Beaver Dam Eye Study. Invest Ophthalmol Vis Sci. 2001;42(7):1449–54.

124. Lim R, Mitchell P, Cumming RG. Refractive associations with cataract: the Blue Mountains Eye Study. Invest Ophthalmol Vis Sci. 1999;40(12):3021–6.

125. Kanthan GL, Mitchell P, Rochtchina E, Cumming RG, Wang JJ. Myopia and the long-term incidence of cataract and cataract surgery: the Blue Mountains Eye Study. Clin Exp Ophthalmol. 2014;42(4):347–53.

126. Leske MC, Wu S-Y, Nemesure B, Hennis A, Barbados Eye Studies Group. Risk factors for incident nuclear opacities. Ophthalmology. 2002;109(7):1303–8.

127. Mukesh BN, Le A, Dimitrov PN, Ahmed S, Taylor HR, McCarty CA. Development of cataract and associated risk factors: the visual impairment project. Arch Ophthalmol. 2006;124(1):79–85.

128. Wong TY, Foster PJ, Johnson GJ, Seah SKL. Refractive errors, axial ocular dimensions, and age-related cataracts: the Tanjong Pagar survey. Invest Ophthalmol Vis Sci. 2003;44(4):1479–85.

129. McCarty CA, Mukesh BN, Fu CL, Taylor HR. The epidemiology of cataract in Australia. Am J Ophthalmol. 1999;128(4):446–65.

130. Tan NYQ, Sng CCA, Jonas JB, Wong TY, Jansonius NM, Ang M. Glaucoma in myopia: diagnostic dilemmas. Br J Ophthalmol. 2019;103(10):1347–55.

131. Marcus MW, de Vries MM, Junoy Montolio FG, Jansonius NM. Myopia as a risk factor for open-angle glaucoma: a systematic review and meta-analysis. Ophthalmology. 2011;118(10):1989–94, e2.

132. Daubs JG, Crick RP. Effect of refractive error on the risk of ocular hypertension and open angle glaucoma. Trans Ophthalmol Soc U K. 1981;101(1):121–6.

133. Ponte F, Giuffré G, Giammanco R, Dardanoni G. Risk factors of ocular hypertension and glaucoma. The Casteldaccia Eye Study. Doc Ophthalmol. 1994;85(3):203–10.

134. Mitchell P, Hourihan F, Sandbach J, Wang JJ. The relationship between glaucoma and myopia: the Blue Mountains Eye Study. Ophthalmology. 1999;106(10):2010–5.

135. Leske MC, Nemesure B, He Q, Wu SY, Fielding Hejtmancik J, Hennis A. Patterns of open-angle glaucoma in the Barbados Family Study. Ophthalmology. 2001;108(6):1015–22.

136. Ramakrishnan R, et al. Glaucoma in a rural population of southern India. Ophthalmology. 2003;110(8):1484–90.

137. Vijaya L, et al. Prevalence of open-angle glaucoma in a rural south Indian population. Invest Ophthalmol Vis Sci. 2005;46(12):4461.

138. Suzuki Y, et al. Risk factors for open-angle glaucoma in a Japanese population: the Tajimi Study. Ophthalmology. 2006;113(9):1613–7.

139. Xu L, Wang Y, Wang S, Wang Y, Jonas JB. High myopia and Glaucoma susceptibility. Ophthalmology. 2007;114(2):216–20.

140. Casson RJ, et al. Risk factors for primary open-angle glaucoma in a Burmese population: the Meiktila Eye Study. Clin Exp Ophthalmol. 2007;35(8):739–44.

141. Czudowska MA, et al. Incidence of glaucomatous visual field loss: a ten-year follow-up from the Rotterdam Study. Ophthalmology. 2010;117(9):1705–12.

142. Perera SA, Wong TY, Tay W-T, Foster PJ, Saw S-M, Aung T. Refractive error, axial dimensions, and primary open-angle glaucoma: the Singapore Malay Eye Study. Arch Ophthalmol. 2010;128(7):900–5.

143. Kuzin AA, Varma R, Reddy HS, Torres M, Azen SP. Ocular biometry and open-angle Glaucoma: the Los Angeles Latino Eye Study. Ophthalmology. 2010;117(9):1713–9.

144. Tham Y-C, et al. Joint effects of intraocular pressure and myopia on risk of primary open-angle Glaucoma: the Singapore Epidemiology of Eye Diseases Study. Sci Rep. 2016;6:19320.

145. Ip JM, et al. Role of near work in myopia: findings in a sample of Australian school children. Invest Ophthalmol Vis Sci. 2008;49(7):2903.

146. Saw S-M, et al. Nearwork in early-onset myopia. Invest Ophthalmol Vis Sci. 2002;43(2):332–9.

147. Mutti DO, Mitchell GL, Moeschberger ML, Jones LA, Zadnik K. Parental myopia, near work, school achievement, and children's refractive error. Invest Ophthalmol Vis Sci. 2002;43(12):3633–40.

148. Giloyan A, Harutyunyan T, Petrosyan V. Risk factors for developing myopia among schoolchildren in Yerevan and Gegharkunik Province, Armenia. Ophthalmic Epidemiol. 2017;24(2):97–103.

149. Hsu C-C, et al. Risk factors for myopia progression in second-grade primary school children in Taipei: a population-based cohort study. Br J Ophthalmol. 2017;101(12):1611–7.

150. Tsai D-C, et al. Myopia development among young schoolchildren: the myopia investigation study in Taipei. Invest Ophthalmol Vis Sci. 2016;57(15):6852–60.

151. Lu B, et al. Associations between near work, outdoor activity, and myopia among adolescent students in rural China: the Xichang pediatric refractive error study report no. 2. Arch Ophthalmol. 2009;127(6):769–75.

152. Saw SM, Chan B, Seenyen L, Yap M, Tan D, Chew SJ. Myopia in Singapore kindergarten children. Optometry. 2001;72(5):286–91.

153. Chua SYL, et al. Relative contribution of risk factors for early-onset myopia in young Asian children. Invest Ophthalmol Vis Sci. 2015;56(13):8101.

154. Low W, et al. Family history, near work, outdoor activity, and myopia in Singapore Chinese preschool children. Br J Ophthalmol. 2010;94(8):1012–6.

155. Jones LA, Sinnott LT, Mutti DO, Mitchell GL, Moeschberger ML, Zadnik K. Parental history of myopia, sports and outdoor activities, and future myopia. Invest Ophthalmol Vis Sci. 2007;48(8):3524.

156. Rose KA, et al. Outdoor activity reduces the prevalence of myopia in children. Ophthalmology. 2008;115(8):1279–85.

157. French AN, Morgan IG, Mitchell P, Rose KA. Risk factors for incident myopia in Australian schoolchildren. Ophthalmology. 2013;120(10):2100–8.

158. Lin Z, et al. The influence of near work on myopic refractive change in urban students in Beijing: a three-year follow-up report. Graefes Arch Clin Exp Ophthalmol. 2016;254(11):2247–55.

159. Saw S-M, et al. A cohort study of incident myopia in Singaporean children. Invest Ophthalmol Vis Sci. 2006;47(5):1839–44.

160. Mutti DO, Zadnik K. Has near work's star fallen? Optom Vis Sci. 2009;86(2):76–8.

161. Nickels S, Hopf S, Pfeiffer N, Schuster AK. Myopia is associated with education: results from NHANES 1999–2008. PLoS One. 2019;14(1):e0211196.

162. Mirshahi A, et al. Myopia and cognitive performance: results from the Gutenberg Health Study. Invest Ophthalmol Vis Sci. 2016;57(13):5230–6.

163. Mirshahi A, et al. Myopia and level of education: results from the Gutenberg Health Study. Ophthalmology. 2014;121(10):2047–52.

164. Sensaki S, et al. An ecologic study of trends in the prevalence of myopia in Chinese adults in Singapore born from the 1920s to 1980s. Ann Acad Med Singap. 2017;46(6):229–36.

165. Jonas JB, et al. Education-related parameters in high myopia: adults versus school children. PLoS One. 2016;11(5):e0154554.

166. Mountjoy E, et al. Education and myopia: assessing the direction of causality by Mendelian randomisation. BMJ. 2018;361:k2022.

167. Williams KM, et al. Increasing prevalence of myopia in Europe and the impact of education. Ophthalmology. 2015;122(7):1489–97.

168. Cuellar-Partida G, et al. Assessing the genetic predisposition of education on myopia: a Mendelian randomization study. Genet Epidemiol. 2016;40(1):66–72.

169. Ku P-W, et al. The associations between near visual activity and incident myopia in children. Ophthalmology. 2018;126(2):214–20.

170. Morgan IG, Rose KA. Myopia: is the nature-nurture debate finally over? Clin Exp Optom. 2019;102(1):3–17.

171. Pärssinen O, Kauppinen M. Risk factors for high myopia: a 22-year follow-up study from childhood to adulthood. Acta Ophthalmol. 2018;97(5):510–8.

172. Smith EL, Hung L-F, Kee C, Qiao Y. Effects of brief periods of unrestricted vision on the development of form-deprivation myopia in monkeys. Invest Ophthalmol Vis Sci. 2002;43(2):291–9.

173. Norton TT, Siegwart JT, Amedo AO. Effectiveness of hyperopic defocus, minimal defocus, or myopic defocus in competition with a myopiagenic stimulus in tree shrew eyes. Invest Ophthalmol Vis Sci. 2006;47(11):4687.

174. Zhu X, Wallman J. Temporal properties of compensation for positive and negative spectacle lenses in chicks. Invest Ophthalmol Vis Sci. 2009;50(1):37.

175. Saxena R, et al. Prevalence of myopia and its risk factors in urban school children in delhi: the North India Myopia Study (NIM Study). PLoS One. 2015;10(2):e0117349.

176. Lin Z, et al. Near work, outdoor activity, and myopia in children in rural China: the Handan offspring myopia study. BMC Ophthalmol. 2017;17(1):203.

177. Li S-M, et al. Near work related parameters and myopia in Chinese children: the Anyang childhood eye study. PLoS One. 2015;10(8):e0134514.

178. Lin Z, et al. Near work, outdoor activity, and their association with refractive error. Optom Vis Sci. 2014;91(4):376–82.

179. World Health Organization. WHO guidelines on physical activity, sedentary behaviour and sleep for children under 5 years of age. Geneva: World Health Organization; 2019.

180. Wu P-C, Huang H-M, Yu H-J, Fang P-C, Chen C-T. Epidemiology of myopia. Asia-Pacific J Ophthalmol. 2016;5(6):386–93.

181. LeBlanc AG, et al. Correlates of total sedentary time and screen time in 9–11 year-old children around the world: the international study of childhood obesity, lifestyle and the environment. PLoS One. 2015;10(6):e0129622.

182. Qian D-J, Zhong H, Li J, Niu Z, Yuan Y, Pan C-W. Myopia among school students in rural China (Yunnan). Ophthalmic Physiol Opt. 2016;36(4):381–7.

183. Bernard JY, et al. Predictors of screen viewing time in young Singaporean children: the GUSTO cohort. Int J Behav Nutr Phys Act. 2017;14(1):112.

184. Tandon PS, Zhou C, Christakis DA. Frequency of parent-supervised outdoor play of US preschool-aged children. Arch Pediatr Adolesc Med. 2012;166(8):707–12.

185. McCrann S, Flitcroft I, Lalor K, Butler J, Bush A, Loughman J. Parental attitudes: a key agent of change for myopia control? Ophthalmic Physiol Opt. 2018;38(3):298–308.

186. French AN, Ashby RS, Morgan IG, Rose KA. Time outdoors and the prevention of myopia. Exp Eye Res. 2013;114:58–68.

187. Dirani M, et al. Outdoor activity and myopia in Singapore teenage children. Br J Ophthalmol. 2009;93(8):997–1000.

188. Rose KA, Morgan IG, Smith W, Burlutsky G, Mitchell P, Saw S-M. Myopia, lifestyle, and schooling in students of Chinese ethnicity in Singapore and Sydney. Arch Ophthalmol. 2008;126(4):527–30.

189. Read SA, Vincent SJ, Tan C-S, Ngo C, Collins MJ, Saw S-M. Patterns of daily outdoor light exposure in Australian and Singaporean children. Transl Vis Sci Technol. 2018;7(3):8.

190. Guo Y, et al. Outdoor activity and myopia among primary students in rural and urban regions of Beijing. Ophthalmology. 2013;120(2):277–83.

191. Sherwin JC, Reacher MH, Keogh RH, Khawaja AP, Mackey DA, Foster PJ. The association between time spent outdoors and myopia in children and adolescents. Ophthalmology. 2012;119(10):2141–51.

192. Xiong S, et al. Time spent in outdoor activities in relation to myopia prevention and control: a meta-analysis and systematic review. Acta Ophthalmol. 2017;95(6):551–66.

193. Suhr Thykjaer A, Lundberg K, Grauslund J. Physical activity in relation to development and progression of myopia – a systematic review. Acta Ophthalmol. 2017;95(7):651–9.

194. Jones-Jordan LA, et al. Visual activity before and after the onset of juvenile myopia. Invest Ophthalmol Vis Sci. 2011;52(3):1841–50.

195. Guggenheim JA, et al. Time outdoors and physical activity as predictors of incident myopia in childhood: a prospective cohort study. Invest Ophthalmol Vis Sci. 2012;53(6):2856.

196. Jones-Jordan LA, et al. Time outdoors, visual activity, and myopia progression in juvenile-onset myopes. Invest Ophthalmol Vis Sci. 2012;53(11):7169.

197. Shah RL, Huang Y, Guggenheim JA, Williams C. time outdoors at specific ages during early childhood and the risk of incident myopia. Invest Ophthalmol Vis Sci. 2017;58(2):1158.

198. Guo Y, et al. Outdoor activity and myopia progression in 4-year follow-up of Chinese primary school children: the Beijing Children Eye Study. PLoS One. 2017;12(4):e0175921.

199. Rusnak S, Salcman V, Hecova L, Kasl Z. Myopia progression risk: seasonal and lifestyle variations in axial length growth in Czech Children. J Ophthalmol. 2018;2018:1–5.

200. Wu P-C, Tsai C-L, Wu H-L, Yang Y-H, Kuo H-K. Outdoor activity during class recess reduces myopia onset and progression in school children. Ophthalmology. 2013;120(5):1080–5.

201. Jin J-X, et al. Effect of outdoor activity on myopia onset and progression in school-aged children in northeast china: the Sujiatun eye care study. BMC Ophthalmol. 2015;15(1):73.

202. He M, et al. Effect of time spent outdoors at school on the development of myopia among children in China: a randomized clinical trial. JAMA. 2015;314(11):1142–8.

203. Wu P-CP-C, et al. Myopia prevention and outdoor light intensity in a school-based cluster randomized trial. Ophthalmology. 2018;125(8):1239–50.

204. Li S-YS-M, et al. Time outdoors and myopia progression over 2 years in Chinese children: the Anyang childhood eye study. Invest Ophthalmol Vis Sci. 2015;56(8):4734–40.

205. Verkicharla PK, et al. Development of the FitSight fitness tracker to increase time outdoors to prevent myopia. Transl Vis Sci Technol. 2017;6(3):20.

206. Zhou S, et al. Association between parents' attitudes and behaviors toward children's visual care and myopia risk in school-aged children. Medicine. 2017;96(52):e9270.

207. Hammond DS, Wildsoet CF. Compensation to positive as well as negative lenses can occur in chicks reared in bright UV lighting. Vis Res. 2012;67:44–50.

208. Torii H, et al. Violet light exposure can be a preventive strategy against myopia progression. EBioMedicine. 2017;15:210–9.

209. Sherwin JC, Hewitt AW, Coroneo MT, Kearns LS, Griffiths LR, Mackey DA. The association between time spent outdoors and myopia using a novel biomarker of outdoor light exposure. Invest Ophthalmol Vis Sci. 2012;53(8):4363–70.

210. Williams KM, et al. Association between myopia, ultraviolet B radiation exposure, serum vitamin D concentrations, and genetic polymorphisms in vitamin D metabolic pathways in a multicountry European study. JAMA Ophthalmol. 2017;135(1):47–53.

211. Ashby R, Ohlendorf A, Schaeffel F. The effect of ambient illuminance on the development of deprivation myopia in chicks. Invest Ophthalmol Vis Sci. 2009;50(11):5348–54.

212. Smith EL, Hung L-F, Huang J. Protective effects of high ambient lighting on the development of form-deprivation myopia in rhesus monkeys. Invest Ophthalmol Vis Sci. 2012;53(1):421–8.

213. Mehdizadeh M, Nowroozzadeh MH. Outdoor activity and myopia. Ophthalmology. 2009;116(6):1229–30; author reply 1230.

214. Czepita D, et al. Myopia and night lighting. Investigations on children with negative family history. Klin Ocz. 2012;114(1):22–5.

215. Flitcroft DI. The complex interactions of retinal, optical and environmental factors in myopia aetiology. Prog Retin Eye Res. 2012;31(6):622–60.

216. Mutti DO, Marks AR. Blood levels of vitamin D in teens and young adults with myopia. Optom Vis Sci. 2011;88(3):377–82.

217. Kwon J-W, Choi JA, La TY, Epidemiologic Survey Committee of the Korean Ophthalmological Society. Serum 25-hydroxyvitamin D level is associated with myopia in the Korea national health and nutrition examination survey. Medicine. 2016;95(46):e5012.

218. Pan C-W, Qian D-J, Saw S-M. Time outdoors, blood vitamin D status and myopia: a review. Photochem Photobiol Sci. 2017;16(3):426–32.

219. Guggenheim JA, et al. Does vitamin D mediate the protective effects of time outdoors on myopia? Findings from a prospective birth cohort. Invest Ophthalmol Vis Sci. 2014;55(12):8550–8.

220. Mutti DO, et al. Vitamin D receptor (VDR) and group-specific component (GC, vitamin D-binding protein) polymorphisms in myopia. Invest Ophthalmol Vis Sci. 2011;52(6):3818–24.

221. Chakraborty R, Ostrin LA, Nickla DL, Iuvone PM, Pardue MT, Stone RA. Circadian rhythms, refractive development, and myopia. Ophthalmic Physiol Opt. 2018;38(3):217–45.

Genetics of Pathologic Myopia

4

Qingjiong Zhang

4.1 Introduction

Pathologic myopia refers to a subgroup of high myopia with any myopic specific degenerative change in the retina, choroid, vitreous, sclera, and optic nerve [1, 2], in which high myopia is usually defined as refractive error of at least −6.00D or an axial length of 26 mm or more [3]. Pathologic myopia is also called as pathological myopia, degenerative myopia, malignant myopia, extreme myopia, severe myopia, or progressive myopia [4–9]. Pathologic myopia affects about 0.9–3.1% of the population [10]. It is ranked to be the first to third most common cause of legal blindness, accounting for 0.1–0.5% (European studies) or 0.2–1.4% (Asian studies) of the population [10].

Pathologic myopia is characterized by at least one of the three major signs: fundus degenerative changes, posterior staphyloma, and abnormal corrected visual acuity, which may not present concurrently at the early stage (Fig. 4.1). High myopia might be the first noticeable sign of pathologic myopia, and then the three major signs for pathologic myopia may present at the same time or developed/identified later. Myopic fundus degenerative changes usually include tessellated fundus appearance, tilted optic disc, circular or crescent peripapillary chorioretinal atrophy, vascular straightening, lacquer cracks, Fuchs spots, foveoschisis, spontaneous subretinal hemorrhages, macular or peripheral retinal holes, lattice degeneration in the peripheral retina, retinal white without pressure, snail track degeneration, vitreous opacities or liquefaction, posterior vitreous detachment, peripheral vitreous traction, etc. [1, 2, 11]. Progress of these changes may result in choroidal and retinal thinning or atrophy, photoreceptor loss, macular degeneration, macular choroidal neovascularization, retinal detachment, and finally blindness. Patients with pathologic myopia have high risk of developing glaucoma and cataracts. The myopic-specific fundus changes are considered to result from excessive elongation of the eyeball, which stretch the intraocular tissues, especially the retina, Bruch's membrane, and the choroid. Some of these changes may occur simultaneously.

Pathologic myopia generally appears in early childhood (preteen years) and is generally believed to be hereditary. Therefore, early-onset high myopia, presenting before school age and unrelated to excessive near work, is the most common form of pathologic myopia. A small portion of pathologic myopia may start from low or moderate myopia in preschool children and then quickly progresses to high myopia in a few years, which may or may not be accompanied with extensive near work. The most common form of high myopia, such as late-onset high myopia, is present in children who do not have myopia in preschool age but thereafter gradually become low, moderate to high myopia that is apparently associated with excessive near work. A few of late-onset high myopia, especially those with extreme high grade of myopia over −10.00D, may develop pathologic changes in the back of the eye.

Progress have been made in genetic study of myopia [12–16], including pathologic myopia. Genetic factors play a decisive role in those pathologic myopias that are derived from early-onset high myopia or early-onset myopia. Such type of pathologic myopia is mostly transmitted as Mendelian traits. Most of late-onset high myopia likely belong to the complex trait where both genetic and environmental factors are contributory. The Mendelian form of pathologic myopia may be independently inherited (nonsyndromic) or occurred as a significant sign of other hereditary ocular or systemic diseases (syndromic), such as Stickler syndrome (OMIM 108300), Marfan syndrome (OMIM 154700), familial exudative vitreoretinopathy (OMIM 133780), Ehlers-Danlos syndrome (OMIM 225400), ocular albinism (OMIM 300500), Knobloch syndrome (OMIM 267750), Wagner syndrome (OMIM 143200), and many others [12]. Mutations in a number of genes have been reported to be responsible for the

Q. Zhang (✉)
State Key Laboratory of Ophthalmology, Zhongshan Ophthalmic Center, Sun Yat-sen University, Guangzhou, China
e-mail: zhangqji@mail.sysu.edu.cn; zhangqingjiong@gzzoc.com

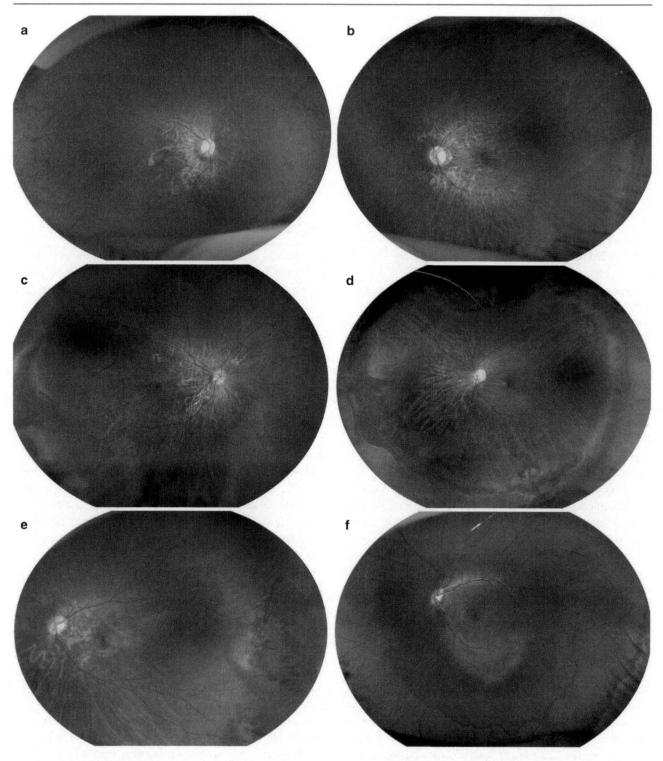

Fig. 4.1 Representative fundus photos of pathologic myopia taken by scanning laser ophthalmoscope. Clinical data from six unrelated patients with pathologic myopia demonstrated fundus degenerative changes, posterior staphyloma, and abnormal corrected visual acuity.

Fundus photos were from patients with *ARR3* mutation (**a**), *NYX* mutation (**b**), Stickler syndrome (**c** and **d**), or familial exudative vitreoretinopathy (**e** and **f**), respectively

Mendelian form of pathogenic myopia [12]. As for the complex form of pathogenic myopia, the exact molecular basis is largely unknown although a number of related genetic studies have been performed. In this chapter, the progress in genetics of pathologic myopia will be discussed.

4.2 Genetic Contribution in Pathologic Myopia

Evidence supporting genetic contribution to high myopia is also applied to pathologic myopia since it refers to a subgroup of high myopia with myopic-specific degenerative changes. Such evidence includes its onset in early childhood independent of extensive near work, family aggregation, families with Mendelian inheritance, as well as molecular genetic studies from genome-wide linkage scan, genome-wide association study, candidate gene sequencing, whole exome sequencing, and whole genome sequencing. If pathologic myopia a hereditary component, genetic factors should play a key role in its onset, progress, and prognosis. It is yet unclear that the proportion of pathologic high myopia belongs to Mendelian inheritance or complex inheritance. It is also unclear that the proportion of pathologic myopia with identifiable pathogenic mutations in genes is responsible for the Mendelian form of high myopia. However, Mendelian inheritance is more likely in early-onset high myopia than late-onset (or acquired) high myopia. Pathologic myopia is more frequently seen in early-onset high myopia than late-onset high myopia. Therefore, mutations in genes responsible for high myopia, especially early-onset high myopia, should be the important cause of pathologic myopia. So far, most early-onset high myopia with identified mutations could be considered as pathologic myopia due to the associated changes in the posterior portion of the eye. In some of these early-onset high myopia, pathologic myopia might be the first noticeable sign or the only temporal diagnosis at some time points although they may finally be recognized as an accompanying sign of other ocular or systemic diseases that might wholly develop later in life. However, in other children with early-onset high myopia, the myopic-specific degenerative changes in the posterior portion of the eye may not be prominent at early stage but may develop gradually with time. Therefore, pathologic myopia might be considered as a stage of simple high myopia or as a sign of other diseases, and it might be replaced by gene-based diagnosis in the era of genome medicine. Due to the close correlation of high myopia and pathologic myopia, genetic loci or genes responsible for high myopia are naturally considered in the analysis of pathologic myopia.

4.3 Genetic Loci and Genes Associated with Complex Pathologic Myopia

Genetic loci or genes for common myopia may be reasonable loci for high myopia as well as pathologic myopia. The exact genes for common myopia have not been identified so far. Some genetic loci for common myopia may not really contribute to pathologic myopia, while genetic loci for pathologic myopia may also not necessarily shared with common myopia. However, variable expression is a common phenomenon in hereditary diseases, so that mutations in genes responsible for pathologic myopia may also contribute to common myopia due to variable expression of the same mutation or due to different mutations with different functional consequences. In these sessions and other following sessions, only genetic loci or genes for high myopia are described as the genetic loci or genes for pathologic myopia.

A number of single nucleotide polymorphisms (SNPs) in the genome or close to specific candidate genes have been reported to be associated with refractive error or myopia based on genome-wide association study or candidate gene association study [12], in which SNPs at about 19 loci are also associated with complex high myopia (Table 4.1) [17–34]. However, the exact genetic defects in most of these loci or genes as well as the underlying molecular mechanism have not been identified. Since most results from association study are underpowered, only those loci or genes with p value less than 10^{-5} are listed in Table 4.1, and a full list of them is available in a previous review [12]. These loci or genes may also be considered as candidate loci or genes for pathologic myopia. However, SNPs or other variants inside or close to these loci or genes are not suitable to be used in clinical gene test at this stage.

4.4 Genetic Loci and Genes for Nonsyndromic Mendelian Pathologic Myopia

Mendelian high myopia is usually early-onset high myopia as compared with late-onset high myopia. So far, 28 loci or genes have been reported to be responsible for high myopia in human beings [30, 35–63], including 21 loci with assigned number and 7 genes without assigned number (Table 4.2). Pathologic myopia may be transmitted as autosomal dominant, autosomal recessive, X-linked recessive, and X-linked female-limited patterns of inheritance (Fig. 4.2). Of the 21 loci, causative genes were identified in 9 but were unknown in 12. In total, mutations in at least 16 genes have been reported to be responsible for high myopia (Table 4.2). Some of the 16 genes may need to be validated further as the reported evidence might be too weak or controversial. Variants in all these genes may only explain less than 10% of early-onset high myopia, even included those genes of uncertainty. The following genes are discussed further.

OPN1LW (OMIM 300822) and *OPN1MW* (OMIM 300821) genes encoding red and green visual pigments are the first genes identified to be responsible for the most common form of hereditary eye disorder, i.e., red-green color blindness, due to nonhomologous pairing and unequal crossing-over between *OPN1LW* and *OPN1MW* [64]. In 2013, rare exon 3 haplotype in *OPN1LW* has been identified to be responsible for most families with Bornholm eye dis-

Table 4.1 Loci or genes associated with complex high myopia

CHR	Location/loci	SNP or gene	Gene flanked	Method	Best p value	First author, year	PMID
1	1q41	rs4373767	LYPLAL1	Meta	4.38E-07	Fan Q, 2012	22685421
1	1q41	rs4373767	SLC30A10	Meta	4.38E-07	Fan Q, 2012	22685421
1	1q41	rs4373767	ZC3H11B	Meta	4.38E-07	Fan Q, 2012	22685421
1	1q24.3	rs235858	MYOC	A	4.00E-06	Tang WC, 2007	17438518
2	2q22.3	rs13382811	ZFHX1B	Meta	5.79E-10	Khor CC, 2013	23933737
4	4q25/MYP11	rs10034228	ESTs-BI480957	GWAS	7.70E-13	Li Z, 2011	21505071
5	5p15.2	rs6885224	CTNND2	A	5.29E-06	Lu B, 2011	21911587
5	5p15.2	rs12716080	CTNND2	GWAS	1.14E-05	Li Y, 2011	21095009
7	7q36.3	rs2730260	VIPR2	GWAS-Meta	8.95E-14	Shi Y, 2013	23406873
8	8p23/MYP10	rs55864141	MIR124-1/MSRA	GWAS	1.30E-07	Meng W, 2012	23049088
8	8p23/MYP10	rs17155227	MIR4660/PPP1R3B	GWAS	1.07E-10	Meng W, 2012	23049088
8	8q24.12	rs6469937	SNTB1	Meta	2.01E-09	Khor CC, 2013	23933737
8	8q24.12	rs4455882	SNTB1	GWAS-Meta	2.13E-11	Shi Y, 2013	23406873
10	10q21.1/MYP15	rs3107503	ZWINT/MIR3924	GWAS	1.54E-07	Meng W, 2012	23049088
11	11q24.1	rs577948	BLID/LOC399959	GWAS	2.22E-07	Nakanishi H, 2009	19779542
11	11q12.3	rs542269	CHRM1	A	2.38E-08	Lin H, 2009	19753311
11	11p13/MYP7	Haplotypes	PAX6	A	6.28E-23	Jiang B, 2011	21589860
12	12q23.2	Haplotypes	IGF1	A	3.70E-09	Mak JY, 2012	22332214
12	12q21–23	rs17306116	PPFIA2	A	2.65E-05	Hawthorne F, 2013	23422819
13	13q12.12/MYP20	rs9318086	MIPEP/C1QTNF9B	GWAS	1.91-E16	Shi Y, 2011	21640322
13	13q32.3	rs8000973	ZIC2	A	7.16E-07	Oishi M, 2013	24150758
15	15q14	rs634990	NA	A	p < 8.81E-7	Jiao X, 2012	23170057
15	15q14	rs524952	NA	A	8.78E-07	Hayashi H, 2011	21436269
15	15q25.1	rs4778879	RASGRF1	A	3.40E-07	Oishi M, 2013	24150758
22	22q12/MYP6	rs2009066	CRYBA4	A	1.54E-05	Ho DW, 2012	22792142

Some of these loci were originally identified to be associated with refractive error or common myopia and then were found to be responsible for high myopia, in which references for high myopia were listed in this table

CHR chromosome, *A* association study, *GWAS* genome-wide association study, *Meta* meta-analysis, *NA* not available

ease, a cone dysfunction syndrome with dichromacy and myopia [65]. Subsequently, the unique LVAVA haplotype in *OPN1LW* was found to be responsible for X-linked nonsyndromic high myopia mapped to MYP1 [35, 66]. These results have been further confirmed by additional studies [67–69]. The specific haplotypes of *OPN1LW*, LVAVA or LIAVA, would result in aberrant splicing or a reduced amount of transcript that may contribute to the development of myopia [69–71]. Unique exon 3 haplotype in *OPN1LW* may account for about 1% probands with early-onset high myopia.

Retinal arrestin 3 (*ARR3*, OMIM 301770) is a well-known gene with cone photoreceptor-specific expression. Heterozygous mutations in *ARR3* cause female-limited early-onset high myopia (MYP26, OMIM 301010) [53], a unique form of X-linked female-limited inheritance that is completely different from X-linked recessive or dominant trait. Almost all truncation mutations and part of missense mutations in *ARR3* are causative. Mutations in *ARR3* likely contribute to 2–3% of probands with early-onset myopia, the most common cause of Mendelian high myopia with identified pathogenic variants among the 16 genes.

Truncation mutations in *SCO2*, *SLC39A5*, and *BSG* are very rare in general population so that such mutations may

be a rare cause for autosomal dominant high myopia [39, 51, 56] although additional evidence are needed to confirm the correlation. The phenotype associated with truncation mutations in SLC39A5 may need to be further clarified except for high myopia. Mutations in these three genes may totally account for about 1% of probands with early-onset high myopia.

Biallelic truncation mutations in *LRPAP1* as well as *LOXL3* are responsible for autosomal recessive early-onset high myopia [50, 55, 72]. Mutations in the two genes may affect about 0.5% of probands with early-onset high myopia. Some patients with biallelic *LOXL3* mutations had phenotypes similar to Stickler syndrome.

Additional evidence is expected to confirm the pathogenicity of mutations in the genes described above as well as other genes listed in Table 4.2, especially what type of mutations are causative and what role of the variants may play (monogenic or association?). In addition, understanding the molecular mechanism of the high myopia-associated variants may shed a light not only on understanding the pathogenesis of early-onset high myopia but also may provide clues in understanding the molecular mechanism of common myopia.

Table 4.2 Genetic loci and genes for nonsyndromic Mendelian high myopia

Locus	Inheritance	OMIM	Location	Gene	OMIM	Reference	PMID
MYP1	xlHM	310460	Xq28	OPN1LW	300822	Guo (2010); Li (2015)	21060050; 26114493
MYP2	adHM	160700	18p11.31	NA	NA	Young TL et al. (1998)	9634508
MYP3	adHM	603221	12q21-q23	NA	NA	Young TL et al. (1998)	9792869
MYP5	adHM	608474	17q21-q22	NA	NA	Paluru P et al. (2003)	12714612
MYP6	adHM	608908	22q13.33	SCO2	604272	Tran-Viet et al. (2013)	23643385
MYP11	adHM	609994	4q22-q27	NA	NA	Zhang Q et al. (2005)	16052171
MYP12	adHM	609995	2q37.1	NA	NA	Paluru PC et al. (2005)	15980214
MYP13	xlHM	300613	Xq23-q27.2	NA	NA	Zhang et al. (2006)	16648373
MYP15	adHM	612717	10q21.1	NA	NA	Nallasamy S, 2007	17327828
MYP16	adHM	612554	5p15.33-p15.2	NA	NA	Lam CY et al. (2008)	18421076
MYP17	adHM	608367	7p15	NA	NA	Paget et al. (2008)	19122830
MYP18	arHM	255500	14q22.1-q24.2	NA	NA	Yang et al. (2009)	19204786
MYP19	adHM	613969	5p15.1-p13.3	NA	NA	Ma et al. (2010)	21042559
MYP20	adHM	614166	13q12.12	NA	NA	Shi et al. (2011)	21640322
MYP21	adHM	614167	1p22	ZNF644	614159	Shi et al. (2011)	21695231
MYP22	adHM	615420	4q35	CCDC111	615421	Zhao et al. (2013)	23579484
MYP23	arHM	615431	4p16	LRPAP1	104225	Aldahmesh et al. (2013)	23830514
MYP24	adHM	615946	12q13	SLC39A5	608730	Guo et al. (2014)	24891338
MYP25	adHM	617238	5q31	P4HA2	600608	Guo et al. (2015)	25741866
MYP26	xfHM	301010	Xq13	ARR3	301770	Xiao et al. (2016)	27829781
MYP27	adHM	618827	8q24.23	CPSF1	606027	Ouyang et al. (2019)	30689892
MYP?	xlHM	NA	Xp11.4	NYX	300278	Zhang (2007); Yip (2013)	17392683; 23406521
MYP?	arHM	NA	2p13.1	LOXL3	607163	Li et al. (2016)	26957899
MYP?	adHM	NA	19p13.3	BSG	109480	Jin et al. (2017)	28373534
MYP?	adHM?	NA	13q32.1	DZIP1	608671	Lee et al. (2017)	28085539
MYP?	adHM?	NA	16p12.3	XYLT1	608124	Lee et al. (2017)	28085539
MYP?	adHM	NA	2p22.2	NDUFAF7	615898	Wang et al. (2017)	28837730
MYP?	adHM	NA	6p12.3	TNFRSF21	605732	Pan et al. (2019)	31189563

MYP4 is replaced by MYP17 because the previous mapping locus was not proved by themselves. MYP7, MYP8, MYP9, MYP10, and MYP14 are not listed here as they are genetic loci for complex common myopia
The current content listed under OMIM 310460 is controversial. Its old version is reasonable but disappeared
adHM autosomal dominant high myopia, *arHM* autosomal recessive high myopia, *xlHM* X-linked recessive high myopia, *xfHM* X-linked female-limited high myopia, *NA* not available

4.5   Genes for Syndromic Pathologic Myopia

Mendelian high myopia accompanied with ocular or systemic anomalies is usually present early in childhood and is much more likely to present with pathologic myopic changes in the posterior segment of the eyes beside other ocular or systemic signs. Sometimes, such syndromic high myopia may be initially treated as nonsyndromic high myopia since other ocular or systemic signs may not be prominent or well-developed in childhood [73]. Mutations in some genes may cause either nonsyndromic high myopia or syndromic high myopia, such genes as *NYX*, *LOXL3*, *OPN1LW*, etc. So far, high myopia has been reported as a sign in a number of ocular or systemic diseases, in which causative mutations in at least 84 genes have been reported (Tables 4.3 and 4.4) [65, 74–151]. For diseases associated with mutations in the 84 genes, high myopia may be a frequent sign in some genes but

may be rarely mentioned in one or a few families in other genes. Mutations in all these genes are most frequent cause of high myopia seen in early childhood [75, 99]. The proportion of contribution by mutations in these genes may be even higher, about 30%, if probands with high myopia and other ocular or systemic changes are counted. In the following paragraphs, genes responsible for pathologic myopia accompanied with ocular diseases or with systemic diseases will be discussed separately. In rare circumstance, mutations in a gene may cause pathologic myopia either with ocular disease or with systemic disease, such gene as *COL2A1*.

4.5.1   Pathologic Myopia Accompanied with Ocular Diseases

Pathologic myopia or high myopia has been recorded in a number of ocular diseases based on PubMed search and

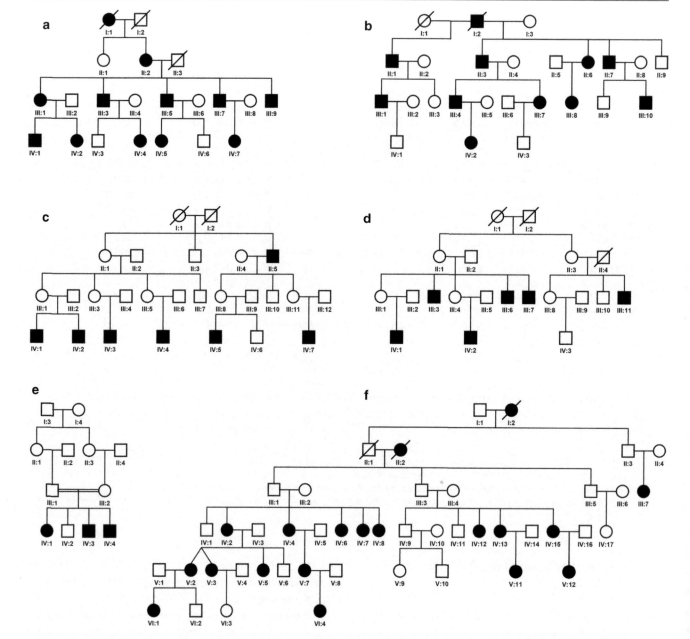

Fig. 4.2 Pedigrees demonstrating patterns of inheritance for pathologic high myopia. (**a**) MYP11, adHM, (**b**) COL2A1, syndromic HM, (**c**) MYP1, OPN1LW, xlHM, (**d**) MYP13, xlHM, (**e**) MYP18, arHM, (**f**) MYP26, ARR3, female-limited xlHM. adHM, autosomal dominant high myopia; xlHM, X-linked recessive high myopia; arHM, autosomal recessive high myopia. X-linked female-limited transmission is a new pattern of inheritance

OMIM search. Clarification of the searched results by checking the original reports has identified 37 genes (Table 4.3), in which high myopia was recorded as a sign in the corresponding ocular diseases caused by mutations in these genes [65, 74–106]. In a few of the 37 genes, mutations in the same gene may cause different diseases due to varied phenotypes, in which high myopia may only present in one or two forms of the related diseases. In these cases, only the most common disease with high myopia is listed in Table 4.3.

Ocular diseases with syndromic pathologic myopia due to mutations in the 37 genes can be subdivided into the following groups: congenital stationary night blindness (*GRM6*, *LRIT3*, *TRPM1*, *CACNA1F*, and *NYX*), retinitis pigmentosa (*PRPF3*, *RP1*, *CYP4V2*, *RBP3*, *TTC8*, *RP2*, and *RPGR*), cone dysfunction or cone-rod dystrophy (*GUCY2D*, *CNGB3*, *KCNV2*, *PDE6C*, *PROM1*, *RAB28*, *TTLL5*, *OPN1LW*, and *OPN1MW*), exudative vitreoretinopathy (*FZD4* and *TSPAN12*), and several other diseases. Syndromic pathologic myopia is more frequently seen in ocular diseases due to mutations in the

Table 4.3 High myopia as a sign in other ocular diseases with known causative genes

Gene	Gene MIM no.	Location	Phenotype	Inheritance	Phenotype MIM no.	Reference	PMID no.
COL2A1	120140	12q13.11	Nonsyndromic ocular Stickler syndrome, type I	AD	609508	Richards et al. (2006)	16752401
FZD4	604579	11q14.2	Exudative vitreoretinopathy 1	AD	133780	Sun et al. (2015)	26747767
GUCY2D	600179	17p13.1	Cone-rod dystrophy 6	AD	601777	Gregory-Evans et al. (2000)	10647719
OPA1	605290	3q29	Optic atrophy 1	AD	165500	Chen et al. (2007)	17188070
PAX6	607108	11p13	Aniridia	AD	106210	Hewitt et al. (2007)	17896318
PRPF3	607301	1q21.2	Retinitis pigmentosa 18	AD	601414	Vaclavik et al. (2010)	20309403
PRPH2	179605	6p21.1	Macular dystrophy, patterned, 1	AD	169150	Sun et al. (2015)	26747767
TSPAN12	613138	7q31.31	Exudative vitreoretinopathy 5	AD	613310	Sun et al. (2015)	26747767
VCAN	118661	5q14.2-q14.3	Wagner syndrome 1	AD	143200	Miyamoto et al. (2005)	16043844
RP1	603937	8q11.2-q12.1	Retinitis pigmentosa 1	AD, AR	180100	Chassine et al. (2015)	25883087
ADAMTS18	607512	16q23.1	Microcornea, myopic chorioretinal atrophy, and telecanthus	AR	615458	Aldahmesh et al. (2013)	23818446
ADAMTSL4	610113	1q21.2	Ectopia lentis et pupillae	AR	225200	Neuhann et al. (2015)	25975359
CNGB3	605080	8q21.3	Achromatopsia 3	AR	262300	Sundin et al. (2000)	10888875
CYP4V2	608614	4q35.1-q35.2	Bietti crystalline corneoretinal dystrophy	AR	210370	Wang et al. (2012)	22693542
GRM6	604096	5q35.3	Night blindness, congenital stationary (complete), 1B, autosomal recessive	AR	257270	Dryja et al. (2005)	15781871
KCNV2	607604	9p24.2	Retinal cone dystrophy 3B	AR	610356	Michaelides et al. (2005)	15722315
LRIT3	615004	4q25	Night blindness, congenital stationary (complete), 1F, autosomal recessive	AR	615058	Zeitz et al. (2013)	23246293
LTBP2	602091	14q24.3	Microspherophakia and/or megalocornea, with ectopia lentis and with or without secondary glaucoma	AR	251750	Desir et al. (2010)	20179738
MYCBP2	610392	13q22.3	High myopia-excavated optic disc anomaly	AR	NA	Bredrup et al. (2015)	25634536
PDE6C	600827	10q23.33	Cone dystrophy 4	AR	613093	Sun et al. (2015)	26747767
P3H2 (LEPREL1)	610341	3q28	High myopia with cataract and vitreoretinal degeneration (MCVD)	AR	614292	Mordechai et al. (2011)	21885030
PROM1	604365	4p15.32	Cone-rod dystrophy 12	AR	612657	Pras E et al. (2009)	19718270
RAB28	612994	4p15.33	Cone-rod dystrophy 18	AR	615374	Roosing et al. (2013)	23746546
RBP3	180290	10q11.22	?Retinitis pigmentosa 66	AR	615233	Arno G et al. (2015)	25766589
SLC38A8	615585	16q23.3	Foveal hypoplasia 2, with or without optic nerve misrouting and/or anterior segment dysgenesis	AR	609218	Perez et al. (2014)	24045842
TBC1D24	613577	16p13.3	DOOR syndrome	AR	220500	James et al. (2007)	17994565
TRPM1	603576	15q13.3	Night blindness, congenital stationary (complete), 1C, autosomal recessive	AR	613216	Li et al. (2009)	19878917
TTC8	608132	14q31.3	?Retinitis pigmentosa 51	AR	613464	Goyal et al. (2016)	26195043
TTLL5	612268	14q24.3	Cone-rod dystrophy 19	AR	615860	Zhou et al. (2018)	29453956

(continued)

Table 4.3 (continued)

Gene	Gene MIM no.	Location	Phenotype	Inheritance	Phenotype MIM no.	Reference	PMID no.
VSX2	142993	14q24.3	Microphthalmia, isolated 2	AR	610093	Khan et al. (2015)	24001013
GPR143	300808	Xp22.2	Ocular albinism, type I, Nettleship-Falls type	XLR	300500	Preising et al. (2001)	11520764
RP2	300757	Xp11.3	Retinitis pigmentosa 2	XLR	312600	Kaplan et al. (1990)	2227956
RPGR	312610	Xp11.4	Retinitis pigmentosa 3	XL	300029	Meindl et al. (1996)	8673101
CACNA1F	300110	Xp11.23	Congenital stationary night blindness type 2A (and other associated phenotypes)	XLR	300071	Strom et al. (1998)	9662399
NYX	300278	Xp11.4	Night blindness, congenital stationary (complete), 1A, X-linked	XLR	310500	Bech-Hansen et al. (2000)	11062471
OPN1LW	300822	Xq28	Bornholm eye disease	XLR	300843	McClements et al. (2013)	23322568
OPN1LW/ OPN1MW	300822, 300821	Xq28	Cone dystrophy 5	XLR	303700	Gardner et al. (2009)	20579627

AR autosomal recessive, *AD* autosomal dominant, *XLR* X-linked recessive, *NA* nonavailable

following genes: *CACNA1F*, *RPGR*, *NYX*, *GUCY2D*, *FZD4*, and *TSPAN12*. In the early stage, high myopia or pathologic myopia might be the only noticeable sign or complaint for those patients with those ocular diseases, such as retinitis pigmentosa, exudative vitreoretinopathy, congenital stationary night blindness, and cone-rod dystrophy. Follow-up visit and more specialized examination (such as scanning laser ophthalmoscopy, electroretinography, fluorescein angiography, optic coherence tomography, etc.) may be of great value in confirming the original diseases if additional signs are suggestive for other diseases other than pathologic myopia alone. Clinical gene testing is of great value in re-recognizing atypical syndromic pathologic myopia.

So far, pathologic myopia accompanied with ocular diseases is the most common form of high myopia with identifiable genetic defects in the 37 genes, several times more than those with mutations in the 16 genes for nonsyndromic high myopia. Most patients with this type of pathologic myopia are diagnosed as the related ocular diseases rather than pathologic myopia alone. Therefore, the proportion of this type of pathologic myopia is less representative in genetic analysis of high myopia although it is the most common form. For example, a significant proportion of juvenile onset retinal detachment in patients with high myopia is actually caused by mutations in genes responsible for familial exudative vitreoretinopathy.

known, including Stickler syndrome, Marfan syndrome, Knobloch syndrome, and Cohen syndrome. It is not uncommon that some of the patients may be treated as nonsyndromic pathologic myopia when their systemic signs are atypical or not well-developed, especially for those systemic diseases rarely seen in the eye clinic (Table 4.4). The association of pathologic myopia with some of these systemic diseases may need further validation since high myopia or pathologic myopia may have been only reported in a few cases for many of these diseases.

The majority of pathologic myopia with systemic diseases is commonly caused by mutations in a few of the 47 genes, such as *COL2A1*, *FBN1*, and *COL11A1*. In clinical gene test for eye diseases, mutations in *COL2A1* are among one of the several top-ranking genes. At the eye clinic, however, mutations in many other genes are rarely seen in patients with pathologic myopia. In total, the number of pathologic myopias caused by the 47 genes is about twice of the number of pathologic myopias caused by the 16 genes responsible for nonsyndromic high myopia. Inclusion of all these genes in the analysis of eye genomics in future studies will not only clarify the frequency of pathologic myopia and other ocular changes associated with these genes but also expand the extent of eye phenotypes associated with these systemic diseases.

4.5.2 Pathologic Myopia Accompanied with Systemic Diseases

Pathologic myopia or high myopia has also been described as a prominent ocular phenotype in at least 47 systemic diseases that are caused by mutations in 47 genes (Table 4.4), respectively [107–151]. Some of these diseases are well-

4.6 Clinical Gene Test for Pathologic Myopia

Clinical gene test (CGT) has becoming very popular in clinical practice worldwide. Patients inquiring for consultation with results from CGT are more and more common in outpatient clinic. Patients with pathologic myopia and their par-

Table 4.4 High myopia as a sign in systemic diseases with known causative genes

Gene	Gene MIM no.	Location	Phenotype	Inheritance	Phenotype MIM no.	Reference	PMID no.
ASXL1	612990	20q11.21	Bohring-Opitz syndrome	AD	605039	Hoischen et al. (2011)	21706002
COL11A1	120280	1p21.1	Stickler syndrome, type II (and Marshall syndrome)	AD	604841	Richards et al. (1996)	8872475
COL2A1	120140	12q13.11	Stickler syndrome, type I (and several other related diseases)	AD	108300	Lee et al. (1989)	2543071
FBN1	134797	15q21.1	Marfan syndrome (and associated phenotypes)	AD	154700	Dietz et al. (1991)	1852208
NIPBL	608667	5p13.2	Cornelia de Lange syndrome 1	AD	122470	Levin et al. (1990)	2348318
PACS1	607492	11q13.1-q13.2	Schuurs-Hoeijmakers syndrome	AD	615009	Schuurs-Hoeijmakers et al. (2016)	26842493
PAX2	167409	10q24.31	Papillorenal syndrome	AD	120330	Sanyanusin et al. (1995)	7795640
PTPN11	176876	12q24.13	Noonan syndrome 1	AD	163950	Marin Lda et al. (2012)	21815719
TCF4	602272	18q21.2	Pitt-Hopkins syndrome	AD	610954	Sweetser et al. (2018)	22934316
ZEB2	605802	2q22.3	Mowat-Wilson syndrome	AD	235730	Gregory-Evans et al. (2004)	15384097
ADAMTS17	607511	15q26.3	Weill-Marchesani-like syndrome	AR	613195	Morales et al. (2009)	19836009
ADAMTS10	608990	19p13.2	Weill-Marchesani syndrome 1, recessive	AR	277600	Dagoneau et al. (2004)	15368195
ATP6V0A2	611716	12q24.31	Cutis laxa, autosomal recessive, type IIA	AR	219200	Van Maldergem et al. (2008)	18716235
B3GALNT2	610194	1q42.3	Muscular dystrophy-dystroglycanopathy (congenital with brain and eye anomalies), type A, 11	AR	615181	Stevens et al. (2013)	23453667
CBS	613381	21q22.3	Homocystinuria, B6-responsive and nonresponsive types	AR	236200	Cruysberg et al. (1996)	8898592
CLDN19	610036	1p34.2	Hypomagnesemia 5, renal, with ocular involvement	AR	248190	Konrad et al. (2006)	17033971
COL18A1	120328	21q22.3	Knobloch syndrome, type 1	AR	267750	Sertie et al. (2000)	10942434
COL9A1	120210	6q13	Stickler syndrome, type IV	AR	614134	Van Camp et al. (2006)	16909383
COL9A2	120260	1p34.2	Stickler syndrome, type V	AR	614284	Baker et al. (2011)	21671392
COL9A3	120270	20q13.33	Stickler syndrome	AR	NA	Faletra et al. (2014)	24273071
CRIPT	604594	2p21	Short stature with microcephaly and distinctive facies	AR	615789	Leduc et al. (2016)	27250922
C8orf37	614477	8q22.1	Cone-rod dystrophy 16	AR	614500	Katagiri et al. (2016)	25113443
DAG1	128239	3p21.31	Muscular dystrophy-dystroglycanopathy (congenital with brain and eye anomalies), type A, 9	AR	616538	Geis et al. (2013)	24052401
ELOVL4	605512	6q14.1	Ichthyosis, spastic quadriplegia, and mental retardation	AR	614457	Aldahmesh et al. (2011)	22100072
ERBB3	190151	12q13.2	Lethal congenital contractural syndrome 2	AR	607598	Narkis et al. (2007)	17701904
FKRP	606596	19q13.32	Muscular dystrophy-dystroglycanopathy (congenital with brain and eye anomalies), type A, 5	AR	613153	Beltran-Valero de Bernabe et al. (2004)	15121789
GZF1	613842	20p11.21	Joint laxity, short stature, and myopia	AR	617662	Patel et al. (2017)	28475863
HTT	613004	4p16.3	Lopes-Maciel-Rodan syndrome	AR	617435	Rodan et al. (2016)	27329733
IRX5	606195	16q12.2	Hamamy syndrome	AR	611174	Hamamy et al. (2007)	17230486

(continued)

Table 4.4 (continued)

Gene	Gene MIM no.	Location	Phenotype	Inheritance	Phenotype MIM no.	Reference	PMID no.
LAMA1	150320	18p11.31	Poretti-Boltshauser syndrome	AR	615960	Aldinger et al. (2014)	25105227
LAMB2	150325	3p21.31	Pierson syndrome	AR	609049	Kagan et al. (2008)	17943323
LOXL3	607163	2p13.1	Stickler syndrome	AR	NA	Alzahrani et al. (2015)	25663169
LRP2	600073	2q31.1	Donnai-Barrow syndrome	AR	222448	Kantarci et al. (2007)	17632512
NBAS	608025	2p24.3	Short stature, optic nerve atrophy, and Pelger-Huet anomaly	AR	614800	Nucci et al. (2019)	30845840
P4HA1	176710	10q22.1	Congenital connective tissue/myopathy overlap disorders	AR	NA	Zhou et al. (2017)	28419360
PLOD1	153454	1p36.22	Ehlers-Danlos syndrome, type VI	AR	225400	Hautala et al. (1993)	8449506
POLR1C	610060	6p21.1	Leukodystrophy, hypomyelinating, 11	AR	616494	Bernard et al. (2012)	22855961
POLR3A	614258	10q22.3	Leukodystrophy, hypomyelinating, 7, with or without oligodontia and/or hypogonadotropic hypogonadism	AR	607694	Bernard et al. (2012)	22855961
POLR3B	614366	12q23.3	Leukodystrophy, hypomyelinating, 8, with or without oligodontia and/or hypogonadotropic hypogonadism	AR	614381	Bernard et al. (2012)	22855961
POMGNT1	606822	1p34.1	Muscular dystrophy-dystroglycanopathy (congenital with brain and eye anomalies), type A, 3	AR	253280	Vervoort et al. (2004)	15236414
PRDM5	614161	4q27	Brittle cornea syndrome 2	AR	614170	Burkitt Wright et al. (2011)	21664999
QARS1	603727	3p21.31	Microcephaly, progressive, seizures, and cerebral and cerebellar atrophy	AR	615760	Leshinsky-Silver et al. (2017)	28620870
ROBO3	608630	11q24.1	Familial horizontal gaze palsy and progressive scoliosis 1	AR	607313	Khna et al. (2008)	19041479
SLITRK6	609681	13q31.1	Deafness and myopia	AR	221200	Tekin et al. (2013)	23543054
VPS13B	607817	8q22.2	Cohen syndrome	AR	216550	Rodrigues et al. (2018)	30473963
ZNF469	612078	16q24.2	Brittle cornea syndrome 1	AR	229200	Burkitt Wright et al. (2013)	23642083
HS6ST2	300545	Xq26.2	Paganini-Miozzo syndrome	XLR	301025	Paganini et al. (2019)	30471091

AR autosomal recessive, *AD* autosomal dominant, *XLR* X-linked recessive, *NA* nonavailable

ents are among the most common population seeking for CGT and genetic counseling in the eye clinic since pathologic myopia is one of the most common causes of legal blindness and is closely associated with genetics, especially for those patients with early-onset high myopia or with early-onset severe complication due to pathologic myopia. Routine CGT for patients suspected with monogenic eye diseases will greatly change our established knowledge of the disease etiology, phenotypes, classification, diagnosis, prevention, as well as treatment strategy for many hereditary eye diseases, including pathologic myopia.

CGT can be performed on a single gene, a group of genes, all causative genes in specialized field, and all genes for Mendelian diseases by using Sanger sequencing, targeted exome sequencing, whole exome sequencing, and/or whole genome sequencing. With the development of sequencing techniques and more efficient analyzing tools, the cost of different analyses will be getting cheaper over time. In a few years, whole genome sequencing will become the most popular choice for CGT due to the following reasons: (1) obtain the most complete information at once for all genetic defects for the whole body that is the most economic way for comprehensive analysis, (2) no need for sequencing again if new genes for a disease will be identified later, and (3) able to detect causative variants in regions without functional genes or in intronic regions. CGT can be carried out by certified hospital-based lab or commercially available companies. It can be recommended by physicians or can be requested by family members or patients. More patients and their relatives suffering from severe monogenic diseases can benefit from

CGT if its cost can be covered by government or insurance company benefits. Ethics regarding the clinical application of CGT results should be well considered.

At present, detection of variants is not a problem. However, interpretation of CGT results is very challenging since two important aspects have to be well characterized further: the criteria for defining a pathogenic mutation in individual gene and phenotypic characteristics of mutations at individual gene level. These two problems have to be treated very carefully as usage of CGT results in clinical practice is completely different from publication of mutation reports in journals. Genetic counseling based on incorrect CGT information may result in significant consequence where we may never have a chance to submit a correction as proofing papers for publication.

Establishment of association of mutations in a gene with a disease, including pathologic myopia, is a key initial step for CGT. Such initial study usually starts with typical manifestation. However, typical manifestation is uncommon for many kinds of hereditary diseases, including pathologic myopia. Occasionally, atypical manifestation is the typical phenotypes for some diseases, like those caused by mutations in genes responsible for familial exudative vitreoretinopathy. Many pathologic myopias, especially those associated with juvenile retinal detachment, are actually atypical or varied types of familial exudative vitreoretinopathy. Development of new techniques has greatly improved upon simple ophthalmoscopy, such as scanning laser ophthalmoscopy, fluorescein angiography, electroretinography, optical coherence tomography, and so on. Genomic medicine may greatly change our view on many eye diseases, rare or common, hereditary or complex. In the near future, pathologic myopia may be further classified based on genome information.

Usually, once mutations in a gene are reported to be responsible for a disease, a number of subsequent studies may be followed. These actually enriched our understanding between the gene and the diseases. At the meantime, some genes and some "mutations" previously reported to be responsible for monogenic diseases are problematic, including pathologic myopia as well as high myopia, especially at the era of next-generation sequencing when detection of variants in genes has become very easy. Mutations in some genes reported to be responsible for high myopia may be wrong due to limited supportive evidence or limited variant in general population. Even for those genes definitely contributing to high myopia when mutated, not all rare variants (even predicted to be pathogenic) are causative. Truncation variants and/or rare damaging missense variants may be pathogenic in some genes, while only certain specific mutations are pathogenic in others. The ACMG recommended "standards and guidelines for the interpretation of sequence variants" is a valuable resource for CGT in general, but it will be difficult in resolving problem at individual gene level

[152]. These problems can be improved through comprehensive analysis of all variants of individual gene together with well-characterized clinical data in individuals with such variants.

4.7 Perspectives

In this chapter, progress in genetic study on pathologic myopia as well as high myopia is briefly introduced. Although such myopia has been studied either as a complex trait or a Mendelian trait, significant and firm advance has been made for monogenic pathologic myopia, both nonsyndromic form and syndromic form, with the latter associated with either ocular diseases or systemic diseases. Pathologic myopia is more frequently seen in patients with early-onset high myopia, which has been shown to be genetically different from late-onset high myopia that is closely related to extensive near work [99, 153]. Clinical application of the genetic information on pathologic myopia should be treated very carefully although clinical gene test is readily available in many countries, both developed and developing. In the near future, a number of additional studies are expected for pathologic myopia: identification of additional genetic defects responsible for monogenic pathologic myopia or complex pathologic myopia, including novel functional genes, noncoding regions inside/nearby functional genes [154–160], chromosome regions without known functional genes [161–165], and genetic modifiers involving oligogenic inheritance [166]; the spectrum of mutations and the extent of phenotypes in individual gene level; contribution of individual gene in pathologic myopia; and the proportion of pathologic myopia originated from early-onset high myopia and late-onset high myopia; investigation of the molecular pathogenesis of pathologic myopia induced by gene defects and its potential role in understanding common myopia; and prevention and treatment of the complication related to pathologic myopia based on individual genes. It is believed that pathologic myopia will have a completely new face in the era of genome medicine in the near future.

Acknowledgment This work was supported by the National Natural Science Foundation of China (81770965, 30725044).

References

1. Ohno-Matsui K. What is the fundamental nature of pathologic myopia? Retina. 2017;37(6):1043–8.
2. Ohno-Matsui K, Lai TY, Lai CC, Cheung CM. Updates of pathologic myopia. Prog Retin Eye Res. 2016;52:156–87.
3. Fredrick DR. Myopia. BMJ. 2002;324(7347):1195–9.
4. Curtin BJ. Physiologic vs pathologic myopia: genetics vs environment. Ophthalmology. 1979;86(5):681–91.

5. Noble KG, Carr RE. Pathologic myopia. Ophthalmology. 1982;89(9):1099–100.

6. Grossniklaus HE, Green WR. Pathologic findings in pathologic myopia. Retina. 1992;12(2):127–33.

7. Miller WW. Degenerative myopia. Am J Ophthalmol. 1973;75(2):334–5.

8. Bedrossian EH. Progressive myopia with glaucoma. Am J Ophthalmol. 1952;35(4):485–9.

9. Blach RK, Jay B, Macfaul P. The concept of degenerative myopia. Proc R Soc Med. 1965;58:109–12.

10. Wong TY, Ferreira A, Hughes R, Carter G, Mitchell P. Epidemiology and disease burden of pathologic myopia and myopic choroidal neovascularization: an evidence-based systematic review. Am J Ophthalmol. 2014;157(1):9–25.e12.

11. Ruiz-Medrano J, Montero JA, Flores-Moreno I, Arias L, Garcia-Layana A, Ruiz-Moreno JM. Myopic maculopathy: current status and proposal for a new classification and grading system (ATN). Prog Retin Eye Res. 2019;69:80–115.

12. Li J, Zhang Q. Insight into the molecular genetics of myopia. Mol Vis. 2017;23:1048–80.

13. Zhang Q. Genetics of refraction and myopia. Prog Mol Biol Transl Sci. 2015;134:269–79.

14. Stambolian D. Genetic susceptibility and mechanisms for refractive error. Clin Genet. 2013;84(2):102–8.

15. Hornbeak DM, Young TL. Myopia genetics: a review of current research and emerging trends. Curr Opin Ophthalmol. 2009;20(5):356–62.

16. Baird PN, Schache M, Dirani M. The GEnes in Myopia (GEM) study in understanding the aetiology of refractive errors. Prog Retin Eye Res. 2010;29(6):520–42.

17. Fan Q, Barathi VA, Cheng CY, Zhou X, Meguro A, Nakata I, et al. Genetic variants on chromosome 1q41 influence ocular axial length and high myopia. PLoS Genet. 2012;8(6):e1002753.

18. Tang WC, Yip SP, Lo KK, Ng PW, Choi PS, Lee SY, et al. Linkage and association of myocilin (MYOC) polymorphisms with high myopia in a Chinese population. Mol Vis. 2007;13:534–44.

19. Khor CC, Miyake M, Chen LJ, Shi Y, Barathi VA, Qiao F, et al. Genome-wide association study identifies ZFHX1B as a susceptibility locus for severe myopia. Hum Mol Genet. 2013;22(25):5288–94.

20. Li Z, Qu J, Xu X, Zhou X, Zou H, Wang N, et al. A genomewide association study reveals association between common variants in an intergenic region of 4q25 and high-grade myopia in the Chinese Han population. Hum Mol Genet. 2011;20(14):2861–8.

21. Lu B, Jiang D, Wang P, Gao Y, Sun W, Xiao X, et al. Replication study supports CTNND2 as a susceptibility gene for high myopia. Invest Ophthalmol Vis Sci. 2011;52(11):8258–61.

22. Li YJ, Goh L, Khor CC, Fan Q, Yu M, Han S, et al. Genomewide association studies reveal genetic variants in CTNND2 for high myopia in Singapore Chinese. Ophthalmology. 2011;118(2):368–75.

23. Shi Y, Gong B, Chen L, Zuo X, Liu X, Tam PO, et al. A genomewide meta-analysis identifies two novel loci associated with high myopia in the Han Chinese population. Hum Mol Genet. 2013;22(11):2325–33.

24. Meng W, Butterworth J, Bradley DT, Hughes AE, Soler V, Calvas P, et al. A genome-wide association study provides evidence for association of chromosome 8p23 (MYP10) and 10q21.1 (MYP15) with high myopia in the French population. Invest Ophthalmol Vis Sci. 2012;53(13):7983–8.

25. Nakanishi H, Yamada R, Gotoh N, Hayashi H, Yamashiro K, Shimada N, et al. A genome-wide association analysis identified a novel susceptible locus for pathological myopia at 11q24.1. PLoS Genet. 2009;5(9):e1000660.

26. Lin HJ, Wan L, Tsai Y, Chen WC, Tsai SW, Tsai FJ. Muscarinic acetylcholine receptor 1 gene polymorphisms associated with high myopia. Mol Vis. 2009;15:1774–80.

27. Jiang B, Yap MK, Leung KH, Ng PW, Fung WY, Lam WW, et al. PAX6 haplotypes are associated with high myopia in Han Chinese. PLoS One. 2011;6(5):e19587.

28. Mak JY, Yap MK, Fung WY, Ng PW, Yip SP. Association of IGF1 gene haplotypes with high myopia in Chinese adults. Arch Ophthalmol. 2012;130(2):209–16.

29. Hawthorne F, Feng S, Metlapally R, Li YJ, Tran-Viet KN, Guggenheim JA, et al. Association mapping of the high-grade myopia MYP3 locus reveals novel candidates UHRF1BP1L, PTPRR, and PPFIA2. Invest Ophthalmol Vis Sci. 2013;54(3):2076–86.

30. Shi Y, Qu J, Zhang D, Zhao P, Zhang Q, Tam POS, et al. Genetic variants at 13q12.12 are associated with high myopia in the Han Chinese population. Am J Hum Genet. 2011;88(6):805–13.

31. Oishi M, Yamashiro K, Miyake M, Akagi-Kurashige Y, Kumagai K, Nakata I, et al. Association between ZIC2, RASGRF1, and SHISA6 genes and high myopia in Japanese subjects. Invest Ophthalmol Vis Sci. 2013;54(12):7492–7.

32. Jiao X, Wang P, Li S, Li A, Guo X, Zhang Q, et al. Association of markers at chromosome 15q14 in Chinese patients with moderate to high myopia. Mol Vis. 2012;18:2633–46.

33. Hayashi H, Yamashiro K, Nakanishi H, Nakata I, Kurashige Y, Tsujikawa A, et al. Association of 15q14 and 15q25 with high myopia in Japanese. Invest Ophthalmol Vis Sci. 2011;52(7):4853–8.

34. Ho DW, Yap MK, Ng PW, Fung WY, Yip SP. Association of high myopia with crystallin beta A4 (CRYBA4) gene polymorphisms in the linkage-identified MYP6 locus. PLoS One. 2012;7(6):e40238.

35. Li J, Gao B, Guan L, Xiao X, Zhang J, Li S, et al. Unique variants in OPN1LW cause both syndromic and nonsyndromic X-linked high myopia mapped to MYP1. Invest Ophthalmol Vis Sci. 2015;56(6):4150–5.

36. Young TL, Ronan SM, Drahozal LA, Wildenberg SC, Alvear AB, Oetting WS, et al. Evidence that a locus for familial high myopia maps to chromosome 18p. Am J Hum Genet. 1998;63(1):109–19.

37. Young TL, Ronan SM, Alvear AB, Wildenberg SC, Oetting WS, Atwood LD, et al. A second locus for familial high myopia maps to chromosome 12q. Am J Hum Genet. 1998;63(5):1419–24.

38. Paluru P, Ronan SM, Heon E, Devoto M, Wildenberg SC, Scavello G, et al. New locus for autosomal dominant high myopia maps to the long arm of chromosome 17. Invest Ophthalmol Vis Sci. 2003;44(5):1830–6.

39. Tran-Viet KN, Powell C, Barathi VA, Klemm T, Maurer-Stroh S, Limviphuvadh V, et al. Mutations in SCO2 are associated with autosomal-dominant high-grade myopia. Am J Hum Genet. 2013;92(5):820–6.

40. Zhang Q, Guo X, Xiao X, Jia X, Li S, Hejtmancik JF. A new locus for autosomal dominant high myopia maps to 4q22-q27 between D4S1578 and D4S1612. Mol Vis. 2005;11:554–60.

41. Paluru PC, Nallasamy S, Devoto M, Rappaport EF, Young TL. Identification of a novel locus on 2q for autosomal dominant high-grade myopia. Invest Ophthalmol Vis Sci. 2005;46(7):2300–7.

42. Zhang Q, Guo X, Xiao X, Jia X, Li S, Hejtmancik JF. Novel locus for X linked recessive high myopia maps to Xq23-q25 but outside MYP1. J Med Genet. 2006;43(5):e20.

43. Nallasamy S, Paluru PC, Devoto M, Wasserman NF, Zhou J, Young TL. Genetic linkage study of high-grade myopia in a Hutterite population from South Dakota. Mol Vis. 2007;13:229–36.

44. Lam CY, Tam PO, Fan DS, Fan BJ, Wang DY, Lee CW, et al. A genome-wide scan maps a novel high myopia locus to 5p15. Invest Ophthalmol Vis Sci. 2008;49(9):3768–78.

45. Paget S, Julia S, Vitezica ZG, Soler V, Malecaze F, Calvas P. Linkage analysis of high myopia susceptibility locus in 26 families. Mol Vis. 2008;14:2566–74.

46. Yang Z, Xiao X, Li S, Zhang Q. Clinical and linkage study on a consanguineous Chinese family with autosomal recessive high myopia. Mol Vis. 2009;15:312–8.

47. Ma JH, Shen SH, Zhang GW, Zhao DS, Xu C, Pan CM, et al. Identification of a locus for autosomal dominant high myopia on chromosome 5p13.3-p15.1 in a Chinese family. Mol Vis. 2010;16:2043–54.

48. Shi Y, Li Y, Zhang D, Zhang H, Li Y, Lu F, et al. Exome sequencing identifies ZNF644 mutations in high myopia. PLoS Genet. 2011;7(6):e1002084.

49. Zhao F, Wu J, Xue A, Su Y, Wang X, Lu X, et al. Exome sequencing reveals CCDC111 mutation associated with high myopia. Hum Genet. 2013;132(8):913–21.

50. Aldahmesh MA, Khan AO, Alkuraya H, Adly N, Anazi S, Al-Saleh AA, et al. Mutations in LRPAP1 are associated with severe myopia in humans. Am J Hum Genet. 2013;93(2):313–20.

51. Guo H, Jin X, Zhu T, Wang T, Tong P, Tian L, et al. SLC39A5 mutations interfering with the BMP/TGF-beta pathway in nonsyndromic high myopia. J Med Genet. 2014;51(8):518–25.

52. Guo H, Tong P, Liu Y, Xia L, Wang T, Tian Q, et al. Mutations of P4HA2 encoding prolyl 4-hydroxylase 2 are associated with nonsyndromic high myopia. Genet Med. 2015;17(4):300–6.

53. Xiao X, Li S, Jia X, Guo X, Zhang Q. X-linked heterozygous mutations in ARR3 cause female-limited early onset high myopia. Mol Vis. 2016;22:1257–66.

54. Zhang Q, Xiao X, Li S, Jia X, Yang Z, Huang S, et al. Mutations in NYX of individuals with high myopia, but without night blindness. Mol Vis. 2007;13:330–6.

55. Li J, Gao B, Xiao X, Li S, Jia X, Sun W, et al. Exome sequencing identified null mutations in LOXL3 associated with early-onset high myopia. Mol Vis. 2016;22:161–7.

56. Jin ZB, Wu J, Huang XF, Feng CY, Cai XB, Mao JY, et al. Trio-based exome sequencing arrests de novo mutations in early-onset high myopia. Proc Natl Acad Sci U S A. 2017;114(16):4219–24.

57. Lee JK, Kim H, Park YM, Kim DH, Lim HT. Mutations in DZIP1 and XYLT1 are associated with nonsyndromic early onset high myopia in the Korean population. Ophthalmic Genet. 2017;38(4):395–7.

58. Wang B, Liu Y, Chen S, Wu Y, Lin S, Duan Y, et al. A novel potentially causative variant of NDUFAF7 revealed by mutation screening in a Chinese family with pathologic myopia. Invest Ophthalmol Vis Sci. 2017;58(10):4182–92.

59. Ouyang J, Sun W, Xiao X, Li S, Jia X, Zhou L, et al. CPSF1 mutations are associated with early-onset high myopia and involved in retinal ganglion cell axon projection. Hum Mol Genet. 2019;28(12):1959–70.

60. Pan H, Wu S, Wang J, Zhu T, Li T, Wan B, et al. TNFRSF21 mutations cause high myopia. J Med Genet. 2019;56(10):671–7.

61. Yip SP, Li CC, Yiu WC, Hung WH, Lam WW, Lai MC, et al. A novel missense mutation in the NYX gene associated with high myopia. Ophthalmic Physiol Opt. 2013;33(3):346–53.

62. Young TL, Atwood LD, Ronan SM, Dewan AT, Alvear AB, Peterson J, et al. Further refinement of the MYP2 locus for autosomal dominant high myopia by linkage disequilibrium analysis. Ophthalmic Genet. 2001;22(2):69–75.

63. Zhang Q, Li S, Xiao X, Jia X, Guo X. Confirmation of a genetic locus for X-linked recessive high myopia outside MYP1. J Hum Genet. 2007;52(5):469–72.

64. Nathans J, Piantanida TP, Eddy RL, Shows TB, Hogness DS. Molecular genetics of inherited variation in human color vision. Science. 1986;232(4747):203–10.

65. McClements M, Davies WI, Michaelides M, Young T, Neitz M, MacLaren RE, et al. Variations in opsin coding sequences cause x-linked cone dysfunction syndrome with myopia and dichromacy. Invest Ophthalmol Vis Sci. 2013;54(2):1361–9.

66. Guo X, Xiao X, Li S, Wang P, Jia X, Zhang Q. Nonsyndromic high myopia in a Chinese family mapped to MYP1: linkage confirmation and phenotypic characterization. Arch Ophthalmol. 2010;128(11):1473–9.

67. Gardner JC, Liew G, Quan YH, Ermetal B, Ueyama H, Davidson AE, et al. Three different cone opsin gene array mutational mechanisms with genotype-phenotype correlation and functional investigation of cone opsin variants. Hum Mutat. 2014;35(11):1354–62.

68. Orosz O, Rajta I, Vajas A, Takacs L, Csutak A, Fodor M, et al. Myopia and late-onset progressive cone dystrophy associate to LVAVA/MVAVA exon 3 interchange haplotypes of opsin genes on chromosome X. Invest Ophthalmol Vis Sci. 2017;58(3):1834–42.

69. Greenwald SH, Kuchenbecker JA, Rowlan JS, Neitz J, Neitz M. Role of a dual splicing and amino acid code in myopia, cone dysfunction and cone dystrophy associated with L/M opsin interchange mutations. Transl Vis Sci Technol. 2017;6(3):2.

70. Patterson EJ, Kalitzeos A, Kasilian M, Gardner JC, Neitz J, Hardcastle AJ, et al. Residual cone structure in patients with X-linked cone opsin mutations. Invest Ophthalmol Vis Sci. 2018;59(10):4238–48.

71. Mountford JK, Davies WIL, Griffiths LR, Yazar S, Mackey DA, Hunt DM. Differential stability of variant OPN1LW gene transcripts in myopic patients. Mol Vis. 2019;25:183–93.

72. Jiang D, Li J, Xiao X, Li S, Jia X, Sun W, et al. Detection of mutations in LRPAP1, CTSH, LEPREL1, ZNF644, SLC39A5, and SCO2 in 298 families with early-onset high myopia by exome sequencing. Invest Ophthalmol Vis Sci. 2014;56(1):339–45.

73. Zhou L, Xiao X, Li S, Jia X, Wang P, Sun W, et al. Phenotypic characterization of patients with early-onset high myopia due to mutations in COL2A1 or COL11A1: why not stickler syndrome? Mol Vis. 2018;24:560–73.

74. Richards AJ, Laidlaw M, Whittaker J, Treacy B, Rai H, Bearcroft P, et al. High efficiency of mutation detection in type 1 stickler syndrome using a two-stage approach: vitreoretinal assessment coupled with exon sequencing for screening COL2A1. Hum Mutat. 2006;27(7):696–704.

75. Sun W, Huang L, Xu Y, Xiao X, Li S, Jia X, et al. Exome sequencing on 298 probands with early-onset high myopia: approximately one-fourth show potential pathogenic mutations in RetNet genes. Invest Ophthalmol Vis Sci. 2015;56(13):8365–72.

76. Gregory-Evans K, Kelsell RE, Gregory-Evans CY, Downes SM, Fitzke FW, Holder GE, et al. Autosomal dominant cone-rod retinal dystrophy (CORD6) from heterozygous mutation of GUCY2D, which encodes retinal guanylate cyclase. Ophthalmology. 2000;107(1):55–61.

77. Chen S, Zhang Y, Wang Y, Li W, Huang S, Chu X, et al. A novel OPA1 mutation responsible for autosomal dominant optic atrophy with high frequency hearing loss in a Chinese family. Am J Ophthalmol. 2007;143(1):186–8.

78. Hewitt AW, Kearns LS, Jamieson RV, Williamson KA, van Heyningen V, Mackey DA. PAX6 mutations may be associated with high myopia. Ophthalmic Genet. 2007;28(3):179–82.

79. Vaclavik V, Gaillard MC, Tiab L, Schorderet DF, Munier FL. Variable phenotypic expressivity in a Swiss family with autosomal dominant retinitis pigmentosa due to a T494M mutation in the PRPF3 gene. Mol Vis. 2010;16:467–75.

80. Miyamoto T, Inoue H, Sakamoto Y, Kudo E, Naito T, Mikawa T, et al. Identification of a novel splice site mutation of the CSPG2 gene in a Japanese family with Wagner syndrome. Invest Ophthalmol Vis Sci. 2005;46(8):2726–35.

81. Chassine T, Bocquet B, Daien V, Avila-Fernandez A, Ayuso C, Collin RW, et al. Autosomal recessive retinitis pigmentosa with RP1 mutations is associated with myopia. Br J Ophthalmol. 2015;99(10):1360–5.

82. Aldahmesh MA, Alshammari MJ, Khan AO, Mohamed JY, Alhabib FA, Alkuraya FS. The syndrome of microcornea, myopic chorioretinal atrophy, and telecanthus (MMCAT) is caused by mutations in ADAMTS18. Hum Mutat. 2013;34(9):1195–9.

83. Neuhann TM, Stegerer A, Riess A, Blair E, Martin T, Wieser S, et al. ADAMTSL4-associated isolated ectopia lentis: further

patients, novel mutations and a detailed phenotype description. Am J Med Genet A. 2015;167A(10):2376–81.

84. Sundin OH, Yang JM, Li Y, Zhu D, Hurd JN, Mitchell TN, et al. Genetic basis of total colourblindness among the Pingelapese islanders. Nat Genet. 2000;25(3):289–93.

85. Wang Y, Guo L, Cai SP, Dai M, Yang Q, Yu W, et al. Exome sequencing identifies compound heterozygous mutations in CYP4V2 in a pedigree with retinitis pigmentosa. PLoS One. 2012;7(5):e33673.

86. Dryja TP, McGee TL, Berson EL, Fishman GA, Sandberg MA, Alexander KR, et al. Night blindness and abnormal cone elec-troretinogram ON responses in patients with mutations in the GRM6 gene encoding mGluR6. Proc Natl Acad Sci U S A. 2005;102(13):4884–9.

87. Michaelides M, Holder GE, Webster AR, Hunt DM, Bird AC, Fitzke FW, et al. A detailed phenotypic study of "cone dystrophy with supernormal rod ERG". Br J Ophthalmol. 2005;89(3):332–9.

88. Zeitz C, Jacobson SG, Hamel CP, Bujakowska K, Neuille M, Orhan E, et al. Whole-exome sequencing identifies LRIT3 muta-tions as a cause of autosomal-recessive complete congenital sta-tionary night blindness. Am J Hum Genet. 2013;92(1):67–75.

89. Desir J, Sznajer Y, Depasse F, Roulez F, Schrooyen M, Meire F, et al. LTBP2 null mutations in an autosomal recessive ocular syndrome with megalocornea, spherophakia, and secondary glau-coma. Eur J Hum Genet. 2010;18(7):761–7.

90. Bredrup C, Johansson S, Bindoff LA, Sztromwasser P, Krakenes J, Mellgren AE, et al. High myopia-excavated optic disc anomaly associated with a frameshift mutation in the MYC-binding protein 2 gene (MYCBP2). Am J Ophthalmol. 2015;159(5):973–9.e2.

91. Mordechai S, Gradstein L, Pasanen A, Ofir R, El Amour K, Levy J, et al. High myopia caused by a mutation in LEPREL1, encoding prolyl 3-hydroxylase 2. Am J Hum Genet. 2011;89(3):438–45.

92. Pras E, Abu A, Rotenstreich Y, Avni I, Reish O, Morad Y, et al. Cone-rod dystrophy and a frameshift mutation in the PROM1 gene. Mol Vis. 2009;15:1709–16.

93. Roosing S, Rohrschneider K, Beryozkin A, Sharon D, Weisschuh N, Staller J, et al. Mutations in RAB28, encoding a farnesylated small GTPase, are associated with autosomal-recessive cone-rod dystrophy. Am J Hum Genet. 2013;93(1):110–7.

94. Arno G, Hull S, Robson AG, Holder GE, Cheetham ME, Webster AR, et al. Lack of interphotoreceptor retinoid binding protein caused by homozygous mutation of RBP3 is associated with high myopia and retinal dystrophy. Invest Ophthalmol Vis Sci. 2015;56(4):2358–65.

95. Perez Y, Gradstein L, Flusser H, Markus B, Cohen I, Langer Y, et al. Isolated foveal hypoplasia with secondary nystagmus and low vision is associated with a homozygous SLC38A8 mutation. Eur J Hum Genet. 2014;22(5):703–6.

96. James AW, Miranda SG, Culver K, Hall BD, Golabi M. DOOR syndrome: clinical report, literature review and discussion of natu-ral history. Am J Med Genet A. 2007;143A(23):2821–31.

97. Li Z, Sergouniotis PI, Michaelides M, Mackay DS, Wright GA, Devery S, et al. Recessive mutations of the gene TRPM1 abrogate ON bipolar cell function and cause complete congenital stationary night blindness in humans. Am J Hum Genet. 2009;85(5):711–9.

98. Goyal S, Jager M, Robinson PN, Vanita V. Confirmation of TTC8 as a disease gene for nonsyndromic autosomal recessive retinitis pigmentosa (RP51). Clin Genet. 2016;89(4):454–60.

99. Zhou L, Xiao X, Li S, Jia X, Zhang Q. Frequent mutations of RetNet genes in eoHM: further confirmation in 325 probands and comparison with late-onset high myopia based on exome sequenc-ing. Exp Eye Res. 2018;171:76–91.

100. Khan AO, Aldahmesh MA, Noor J, Salem A, Alkuraya FS. Lens subluxation and retinal dysfunction in a girl with homozygous VSX2 mutation. Ophthalmic Genet. 2015;36(1):8–13.

101. Preising M, Op de Laak JP, Lorenz B. Deletion in the OA1 gene in a family with congenital X linked nystagmus. Br J Ophthalmol. 2001;85(9):1098–103.

102. Kaplan J, Bonneau D, Frezal J, Munnich A, Dufier JL. Clinical and genetic heterogeneity in retinitis pigmentosa. Hum Genet. 1990;85(6):635–42.

103. Meindl A, Dry K, Herrmann K, Manson F, Ciccodicola A, Edgar A, et al. A gene (RPGR) with homology to the RCC1 guanine nucleotide exchange factor is mutated in X-linked retinitis pig-mentosa (RP3). Nat Genet. 1996;13(1):35–42.

104. Strom TM, Nyakatura G, Apfelstedt-Sylla E, Hellebrand H, Lorenz B, Weber BH, et al. An L-type calcium-channel gene mutated in incomplete X-linked congenital stationary night blind-ness. Nat Genet. 1998;19(3):260–3.

105. Bech-Hansen NT, Naylor MJ, Maybaum TA, Sparkes RL, Koop B, Birch DG, et al. Mutations in NYX, encoding the leucine-rich proteoglycan nyctalopin, cause X-linked complete congenital sta-tionary night blindness. Nat Genet. 2000;26(3):319–23.

106. Gardner JC, Webb TR, Kanuga N, Robson AG, Holder GE, Stockman A, et al. X-linked cone dystrophy caused by muta-tion of the red and green cone opsins. Am J Hum Genet. 2010;87(1):26–39.

107. Hoischen A, van Bon BW, Rodriguez-Santiago B, Gilissen C, Vissers LE, de Vries P, et al. De novo nonsense mutations in ASXL1 cause Bohring-Opitz syndrome. Nat Genet. 2011;43(8):729–31.

108. Richards AJ, Yates JR, Williams R, Payne SJ, Pope FM, Scott JD, et al. A family with Stickler syndrome type 2 has a mutation in the COL11A1 gene resulting in the substitution of glycine 97 by valine in alpha 1 (XI) collagen. Hum Mol Genet. 1996;5(9):1339–43.

109. Lee B, Vissing H, Ramirez F, Rogers D, Rimoin D. Identification of the molecular defect in a family with spondyloepiphyseal dys-plasia. Science. 1989;244(4907):978–80.

110. Dietz HC, Cutting GR, Pyeritz RE, Maslen CL, Sakai LY, Corson GM, et al. Marfan syndrome caused by a recurrent de novo missense mutation in the fibrillin gene. Nature. 1991;352(6333):337–9.

111. Levin AV, Seidman DJ, Nelson LB, Jackson LG. Ophthalmologic findings in the Cornelia de Lange syndrome. J Pediatr Ophthalmol Strabismus. 1990;27(2):94–102.

112. Schuurs-Hoeijmakers JH, Landsverk ML, Foulds N, Kukolich MK, Gavrilova RH, Greville-Heygate S, et al. Clinical delineation of the PACS1-related syndrome--report on 19 patients. Am J Med Genet A. 2016;170(3):670–5.

113. Sanyanusin P, Schimmenti LA, McNoe LA, Ward TA, Pierpont ME, Sullivan MJ, et al. Mutation of the PAX2 gene in a family with optic nerve colobomas, renal anomalies and vesicoureteral reflux. Nat Genet. 1995;9(4):358–64.

114. Marin Lda R, da Silva FT, de Sa LC, Brasil AS, Pereira A, Furquim IM, et al. Ocular manifestations of Noonan syndrome. Ophthalmic Genet. 2012;33(1):1–5.

115. Sweetser DA, Elsharkawi I, Yonker L, Steeves M, Parkin K, Thibert R. Pitt-Hopkins syndrome. In: Adam MP, Ardinger HH, Pagon RA, Wallace SE, Bean LJH, Stephens K, et al., editors. GeneReviews((R)). Seattle: University of Washington; 1993.

116. Gregory-Evans CY, Vieira H, Dalton R, Adams GG, Salt A, Gregory-Evans K. Ocular coloboma and high myopia with Hirschsprung disease associated with a novel ZFHX1B missense mutation and trisomy 21. Am J Med Genet A. 2004;131(1):86–90.

117. Morales J, Al-Sharif L, Khalil DS, Shinwari JM, Bavi P, Al-Mahrouqi RA, et al. Homozygous mutations in ADAMTS10 and ADAMTS17 cause lenticular myopia, ectopia lentis, glau-coma, spherophakia, and short stature. Am J Hum Genet. 2009;85(5):558–68.

118. Dagoneau N, Benoist-Lasselin C, Huber C, Faivre L, Megarbane A, Alswaid A, et al. ADAMTS10 mutations in autosomal recessive Weill-Marchesani syndrome. Am J Hum Genet. 2004;75(5):801–6.

119. Van Maldergem L, Yuksel-Apak M, Kayserili H, Seemanova E, Giurgea S, Basel-Vanagaite L, et al. Cobblestone-like brain dysgenesis and altered glycosylation in congenital cutis laxa, Debre type. Neurology. 2008;71(20):1602–8.

120. Stevens E, Carss KJ, Cirak S, Foley AR, Torelli S, Willer T, et al. Mutations in B3GALNT2 cause congenital muscular dystrophy and hypoglycosylation of alpha-dystroglycan. Am J Hum Genet. 2013;92(3):354–65.

121. Cruysberg JR, Boers GH, Trijbels JM, Deutman AF. Delay in diagnosis of homocystinuria: retrospective study of consecutive patients. BMJ. 1996;313(7064):1037–40.

122. Konrad M, Schaller A, Seelow D, Pandey AV, Waldegger S, Lesslauer A, et al. Mutations in the tight-junction gene claudin 19 (CLDN19) are associated with renal magnesium wasting, renal failure, and severe ocular involvement. Am J Hum Genet. 2006;79(5):949–57.

123. Sertie AL, Sossi V, Camargo AA, Zatz M, Brahe C, Passos-Bueno MR. Collagen XVIII, containing an endogenous inhibitor of angiogenesis and tumor growth, plays a critical role in the maintenance of retinal structure and in neural tube closure (Knobloch syndrome). Hum Mol Genet. 2000;9(13):2051–8.

124. Van Camp G, Snoeckx RL, Hilgert N, van den Ende J, Fukuoka H, Wagatsuma M, et al. A new autosomal recessive form of Stickler syndrome is caused by a mutation in the COL9A1 gene. Am J Hum Genet. 2006;79(3):449–57.

125. Baker S, Booth C, Fillman C, Shapiro M, Blair MP, Hyland JC, et al. A loss of function mutation in the COL9A2 gene causes autosomal recessive Stickler syndrome. Am J Med Genet A. 2011;155A(7):1668–72.

126. Faletra F, D'Adamo AP, Bruno I, Athanasakis E, Biskup S, Esposito L, et al. Autosomal recessive Stickler syndrome due to a loss of function mutation in the COL9A3 gene. Am J Med Genet A. 2014;164A(1):42–7.

127. Leduc MS, Niu Z, Bi W, Zhu W, Miloslavskaya I, Chiang T, et al. CRIPT exonic deletion and a novel missense mutation in a female with short stature, dysmorphic features, microcephaly, and pigmentary abnormalities. Am J Med Genet A. 2016;170(8):2206–11.

128. Katagiri S, Hayashi T, Yoshitake K, Akahori M, Ikeo K, Gekka T, et al. Novel C8orf37 mutations in patients with early-onset retinal dystrophy, macular atrophy, cataracts, and high myopia. Ophthalmic Genet. 2016;37(1):68–75.

129. Geis T, Marquard K, Rodl T, Reihle C, Schirmer S, von Kalle T, et al. Homozygous dystroglycan mutation associated with a novel muscle-eye-brain disease-like phenotype with multicystic leucodystrophy. Neurogenetics. 2013;14(3–4):205–13.

130. Aldahmesh MA, Mohamed JY, Alkuraya HS, Verma IC, Puri RD, Alaiya AA, et al. Recessive mutations in ELOVL4 cause ichthyosis, intellectual disability, and spastic quadriplegia. Am J Hum Genet. 2011;89(6):745–50.

131. Narkis G, Ofir R, Manor E, Landau D, Elbedour K, Birk OS. Lethal congenital contractural syndrome type 2 (LCCS2) is caused by a mutation in ERBB3 (Her3), a modulator of the phosphatidylinositol-3-kinase/Akt pathway. Am J Hum Genet. 2007;81(3):589–95.

132. Beltran-Valero de Bernabe D, Voit T, Longman C, Steinbrecher A, Straub V, Yuva Y, et al. Mutations in the FKRP gene can cause muscle-eye-brain disease and Walker-Warburg syndrome. J Med Genet. 2004;41(5):e61.

133. Patel N, Shamseldin HE, Sakati N, Khan AO, Softa A, Al-Fadhli FM, et al. GZF1 mutations expand the genetic heterogeneity of Larsen syndrome. Am J Hum Genet. 2017;100(5):831–6.

134. Rodan LH, Cohen J, Fatemi A, Gillis T, Lucente D, Gusella J, et al. A novel neurodevelopmental disorder associated with compound heterozygous variants in the huntingtin gene. Eur J Hum Genet. 2016;24(12):1826–7.

135. Hamamy HA, Teebi AS, Oudjhane K, Shegem NN, Ajlouni KM. Severe hypertelorism, midface prominence, prominent/simple ears, severe myopia, borderline intelligence, and bone fragility in two brothers: new syndrome? Am J Med Genet A. 2007;143A(3):229–34.

136. Aldinger KA, Mosca SJ, Tetreault M, Dempsey JC, Ishak GE, Hartley T, et al. Mutations in LAMA1 cause cerebellar dysplasia and cysts with and without retinal dystrophy. Am J Hum Genet. 2014;95(2):227–34.

137. Kagan M, Cohen AH, Matejas V, Vlangos C, Zenker M. A milder variant of Pierson syndrome. Pediatr Nephrol. 2008;23(2):323–7.

138. Alzahrani F, Al Hazzaa SA, Tayeb H, Alkuraya FS. LOXL3, encoding lysyl oxidase-like 3, is mutated in a family with autosomal recessive Stickler syndrome. Hum Genet. 2015;134(4):451–3.

139. Kantarci S, Al-Gazali L, Hill RS, Donnai D, Black GC, Bieth E, et al. Mutations in LRP2, which encodes the multiligand receptor megalin, cause Donnai-Barrow and facio-oculo-acoustico-renal syndromes. Nat Genet. 2007;39(8):957–9.

140. Nucci F, Lembo A, Farronato M, Farronato G, Nucci P, Serafino M. Oculofacial alterations in NBAS-SOPH like mutations: case report. Eur J Ophthalmol. 2020;30(2):NP12–5.

141. Zou Y, Donkervoort S, Salo AM, Foley AR, Barnes AM, Hu Y, et al. P4HA1 mutations cause a unique congenital disorder of connective tissue involving tendon, bone, muscle and the eye. Hum Mol Genet. 2017;26(12):2207–17.

142. Hautala T, Heikkinen J, Kivirikko KI, Myllyla R. A large duplication in the gene for lysyl hydroxylase accounts for the type VI variant of Ehlers-Danlos syndrome in two siblings. Genomics. 1993;15(2):399–404.

143. Bernard G, Vanderver A. POLR3-related leukodystrophy. In: Adam MP, Ardinger HH, Pagon RA, Wallace SE, Bean LJH, Stephens K, et al., editors. GeneReviews((R)). Seattle: University of Washington; 1993.

144. Vervoort VS, Holden KR, Ukadike KC, Collins JS, Saul RA, Srivastava AK. POMGnT1 gene alterations in a family with neurological abnormalities. Ann Neurol. 2004;56(1):143–8.

145. Burkitt Wright EMM, Spencer HL, Daly SB, Manson FDC, Zeef LAH, Urquhart J, et al. Mutations in PRDM5 in brittle cornea syndrome identify a pathway regulating extracellular matrix development and maintenance. Am J Hum Genet. 2011;88(6):767–77.

146. Leshinsky-Silver E, Ling J, Wu J, Vinkler C, Yosovich K, Bahar S, et al. Severe growth deficiency, microcephaly, intellectual disability, and characteristic facial features are due to a homozygous QARS mutation. Neurogenetics. 2017;18(3):141–6.

147. Khan AO, Oystreck DT, Al-Tassan N, Al-Sharif L, Bosley TM. Bilateral synergistic convergence associated with homozygous ROB03 mutation (p.Pro771Leu). Ophthalmology. 2008;115(12):2262–5.

148. Tekin M, Chioza BA, Matsumoto Y, Diaz-Horta O, Cross HE, Duman D, et al. SLITRK6 mutations cause myopia and deafness in humans and mice. J Clin Invest. 2013;123(5):2094–102.

149. Rodrigues JM, Fernandes HD, Caruthers C, Braddock SR, Knutsen AP. Cohen syndrome: review of the literature. Cureus. 2018;10(9):e3330.

150. Burkitt Wright EM, Porter LF, Spencer HL, Clayton-Smith J, Au L, Munier FL, et al. Brittle cornea syndrome: recognition, molecular diagnosis and management. Orphanet J Rare Dis. 2013;8:68.

151. Paganini L, Hadi LA, Chetta M, Rovina D, Fontana L, Colapietro P, et al. A HS6ST2 gene variant associated with X-linked intellectual disability and severe myopia in two male twins. Clin Genet. 2019;95(3):368–74.

152. Richards S, Aziz N, Bale S, Bick D, Das S, Gastier-Foster J, et al. Standards and guidelines for the interpretation of sequence variants: a joint consensus recommendation of the American College of Medical Genetics and Genomics and the Association for Molecular Pathology. Genet Med. 2015;17(5):405–24.

153. Holden BA, Fricke TR, Wilson DA, Jong M, Naidoo KS, Sankaridurg P, et al. Global prevalence of myopia and high myopia and temporal trends from 2000 through 2050. Ophthalmology. 2016;123(5):1036–42.

154. Brandler WM, Antaki D, Gujral M, Kleiber ML, Whitney J, Maile MS, et al. Paternally inherited cis-regulatory structural variants are associated with autism. Science. 2018;360(6386):327–31.

155. Zhou J, Park CY, Theesfeld CL, Wong AK, Yuan Y, Scheckel C, et al. Whole-genome deep-learning analysis identifies contribution of noncoding mutations to autism risk. Nat Genet. 2019;51(6):973–80.

156. An JY, Lin K, Zhu L, Werling DM, Dong S, Brand H, et al. Genome-wide de novo risk score implicates promoter variation in autism spectrum disorder. Science. 2018;362(6420):6576.

157. Cummings BB, Marshall JL, Tukiainen T, Lek M, Donkervoort S, Foley AR, et al. Improving genetic diagnosis in Mendelian disease with transcriptome sequencing. Sci Transl Med. 2017;9(386):5209.

158. Fresard L, Smail C, Ferraro NM, Teran NA, Li X, Smith KS, et al. Identification of rare-disease genes using blood transcriptome sequencing and large control cohorts. Nat Med. 2019;25(6):911–9.

159. Kremer LS, Bader DM, Mertes C, Kopajtich R, Pichler G, Iuso A, et al. Genetic diagnosis of Mendelian disorders via RNA sequencing. Nat Commun. 2017;8:15824.

160. Spielmann M, Mundlos S. Looking beyond the genes: the role of non-coding variants in human disease. Hum Mol Genet. 2016;25(R2):R157–R65.

161. Hnisz D, Day DS, Young RA. Insulated neighborhoods: structural and functional units of mammalian gene control. Cell. 2016;167(5):1188–200.

162. Doan RN, Bae BI, Cubelos B, Chang C, Hossain AA, Al-Saad S, et al. Mutations in human accelerated regions disrupt cognition and social behavior. Cell. 2016;167(2):341–54.e12.

163. Short PJ, McRae JF, Gallone G, Sifrim A, Won H, Geschwind DH, et al. De novo mutations in regulatory elements in neurodevelopmental disorders. Nature. 2018;555(7698):611–6.

164. Guo Y, Xu Q, Canzio D, Shou J, Li J, Gorkin DU, et al. CRISPR inversion of CTCF sites alters genome topology and enhancer/promoter function. Cell. 2015;162(4):900–10.

165. Tang Z, Luo OJ, Li X, Zheng M, Zhu JJ, Szalaj P, et al. CTCF-mediated human 3D genome architecture reveals chromatin topology for transcription. Cell. 2015;163(7):1611–27.

166. Gifford CA, Ranade SS, Samarakoon R, Salunga HT, de Soysa TY, Huang Y, et al. Oligogenic inheritance of a human heart disease involving a genetic modifier. Science. 2019;364(6443):865–70.

Public Health Impact of Pathologic Myopia

Yee Ling Wong, Ryan Eyn Kidd Man, Eva Fenwick,
Seang Mei Saw, Chee Wai Wong,
Chiu Ming Gemmy Cheung, and Ecosse L. Lamoureux

5.1 Epidemiology of Pathologic Myopia (PM)

5.1.1 Overview and Definition of PM

Myopia is reaching epidemic proportions worldwide [1–3], especially in Asian countries [4–6]. This condition is one of the main causes of correctable visual impairment (VI), and the conventional methods used to correct myopic refraction include spectacles, contact lenses, or surgical procedures [7]. The prevalence of myopia among adults ranges between 16.4% and 48.1% worldwide, and that of high myopia (mostly defined as spherical equivalent [SE] ≤ -5 or ≤ -6 diopters [D]) varies between 0.8% and 9.1% [3, 8]. These rates are generally higher in Asian countries [3], with an earlier onset linked to greater myopia severity [9, 10].

The excessive axial elongation of the eye, as a result of severe myopic refractive error, is often associated with pathological changes of the posterior pole [11, 12], including posterior staphyloma, optic disc changes, peripheral retinal tears, rhegmatogenous retinal detachment (RRD), myopic traction maculopathy (MTM), and myopic macular degeneration (MMD) [2, 13–15]. The vision loss attribut- able to this condition, known as pathologic myopia (PM), is largely uncorrectable, unlike myopic refractive error. Different study groups have utilized varying nomenclature for PM, for instance, myopic retinopathy, myopic macu- lopathy, and myopic macular degeneration, with accompa- nying differences in classification systems and definitions. Chorioretinal atrophy, lacquer cracks, myopic choroidal neovascularization (mCNV), Fuchs spot, and posterior staphyloma are the common retinal signs that have been employed in the various PM definitions [16], with a key variable component being the presence or absence of poste- rior staphyloma. Recently, an international photographic classification system (META-PM classification) by Ohno- Matsui (2015) was established [17], with the intent of stan- dardizing PM grading via the presence and severity of MMD on color fundal imaging: non-myopic retinal degen- erative lesion (category 0), tessellated fundus only (cate- gory 1), diffuse chorioretinal atrophy (category 2), patchy chorioretinal atrophy (category 3), and macular atrophy (category 4). "Plus" lesions supplement the META-PM cat- egories, which comprise lacquer cracks, mCNV, and Fuchs spot. PM is considered present if categories 2, 3, 4, or any "plus" lesion are seen [13].

Y. L. Wong
Singapore Eye Research Institute, Singapore National Eye Centre, Singapore, Singapore

Essilor Centre for Innovation and Technologies AMERA, Singapore, Singapore

National University of Singapore, Singapore, Singapore
e-mail: yeeling.wong@essilor.com.sg

R. E. K. Man · E. Fenwick · C. W. Wong · C. M. G. Cheung
Singapore Eye Research Institute, Singapore National Eye Centre, Singapore, Singapore

DUKE-NUS Medical School, Singapore, Singapore
e-mail: man.eyn.kidd.ryan@seri.com.sg;
eva.fenwick@seri.com.sg; wong.chee.wai@singhealth.com.sg;
gemmy.cheung.c.m@snec.com.sg

S. M. Saw
Singapore Eye Research Institute, Singapore National Eye Centre, Singapore, Singapore

National University of Singapore, Singapore, Singapore
e-mail: ephssm@nus.edu.sg

E. L. Lamoureux (✉)
Singapore Eye Research Institute, Singapore National Eye Centre, Singapore, Singapore

Essilor Centre for Innovation and Technologies AMERA, Singapore, Singapore

DUKE-NUS Medical School, Singapore, Singapore

National University of Singapore, Singapore, Singapore
e-mail: ecosse.lamoureux@seri.com.sg

© Springer Nature Switzerland AG 2021
R. F. Spaide et al. (eds.), *Pathologic Myopia*, https://doi.org/10.1007/978-3-030-74334-5_5

5.1.2 Prevalence, Incidence, and Progression of PM

Several population-based studies have reported the prevalence rates of PM, such as the Blue Mountains Eye Study at 1.2% [18], the Handan Eye Study at 0.9% [19], the Beijing Eye Study at 3.1% [20], the Shihpai Eye Study at 3.0% [21], and the Hisayama Study at 1.7% [22]. Recent population-based studies utilizing the META-PM classifications have also supported these findings, namely, the Central India Eye and Medical Study in Rural India at 0.2% [23], the Singapore Epidemiology of Eye Diseases Study in Singapore at 3.8% [24], and the Yangxi Eye Study in rural Southern China at 1.2% [25]. Overall, the prevalence of PM ranges between 0.2% and 3.8%. However, the inconsistent use of PM definitions limits our ability to compare findings, and underscores the need for a standardized and comprehensive definition of PM, that includes the atrophic, tractional, and neovascular components, to be adopted across all PM epidemiological studies [13, 15, 26].

Except for three studies conducted in Asian adult populations [27–29], there are few data on PM incidence [3]. In the Handan Eye Study (2006–2007 to 2012–2013), the 5-year incidence of PM among 2236 myopic eyes of adults in rural China was 0.2% [27]. The Singapore Epidemiology of Eye Diseases Study (2004–2011 to 2010–2017) reported a similarly low 6-year incidence of 1.2% among 3373 myopic eyes of adults in Singapore [28]. In contrast, the Beijing Eye Study reported a 10-year incidence of PM at 19.0% in 79 highly myopic eyes of Chinese adults [29]; however, this study excluded those with low or moderate myopia who are at lower risk of developing PM than those with high myopia, which may have resulted in an overestimation of incidence of PM [24].

In terms of progression, the 5-year progression of PM was reported to be 15.1% in 139 eyes in the Beijing Eye Study [20], 23.9% among 46 eyes in the Blue Mountains Eye Study [18], and 35.3% among 51 eyes in the Handan Eye Study [27]. The 6-year progression of PM was 17.0% among 288 eyes with PM at baseline in Singapore [28], while the 10-year progression was 77.4% among 31 highly myopic eyes with preexisting PM in the Beijing Eye Study [29]. Clinic-based case-series studies of highly myopic Japanese patients with ≥10 years of follow-up demonstrated similarly high PM progression rates (54.7–74.3%) [30, 31].

Of note, the prevalence of PM appears to be increasing over time, as reported in several studies [18, 20, 27–29, 32]. For example, the Japanese PM prevalence rates have more than doubled over a period of a decade as noted in the Hisayama Study, from 1.6% in 2005, 3.0% in 2012, to 3.6% in 2017 (p-trend <0.001) [32]. This increasing trend underscores the importance of research to elicit the risk factors,

public health, and quality of life (QoL) impact and public health strategies to combat this growing problem.

5.1.3 Risk Factors of PM

The risk factors of PM include older age, worse myopic refractive error, and longer axial length [18–22, 24, 30, 31]. According to Hayashi's hypothesis, the presence of fundus tessellation is associated with development of MMD [31]. While not clinically associated with visual acuity, fundus tessellation is associated with a thinner choroid [33–36] which is linked to anatomical changes that increase the risk of chorioretinal atrophy [37, 38]. The problem with fundus tesselation as a diagnostic entity is that it is not universally useful. In Northern Europeans, especially those with blond fundi, choroidal vessels are easily visible independent of the presence of myopia. Eyes with more severe MMD lesions at baseline have higher risk of progression than those with less severe ones [13, 14].

5.2 Public Health Impact of PM

Given the projected doubling of myopia and high myopia prevalence rates from the year 2000 to 2050 [39], those for PM and PM-related VI are expected to increase concurrently [40, 41]. The public health burden of PM is therefore likely to magnify significantly, as outlined in the following sections.

5.2.1 Blindness and VI Associated with PM

PM is one of the leading causes of blindness in countries worldwide [42–45], with the global prevalence of PM-related VI estimated to rise from 0.1% in 2000 to 0.6% in 2050 if there are no changes in current intervention strategies [46]. PM was the cause of VI in 0.2–0.4% of individuals in the Beijing Eye Study [42], the Tajimi Study [43], and the Chinese American Eye Study (Table 5.1) [47]. In contrast to Asian ethnicities, the prevalence of PM-related VI appears to be much lower in Western populations, ranging between 0.05% and 0.1% of individuals as reported in the Rotterdam Study [48], the Copenhagen City Eye Study [49], and the Los Angeles Latino Eye Study [50]. All studies used the World Health Organization (WHO) definition of VI (best-corrected visual acuity between 20/60 and 20/400). Based on these population-based estimates, the prevalence of PM-related VI appears to be at least two- to fourfold higher among Asian (0.2–0.4%), compared to Western and European (<0.1%), countries.

Table 5.1 Prevalence of visual impairment (VI) associated with pathologic myopia in population-based studies worldwide

Study name	Country	Subjects (eyes) in study	VI attributable to PM, %
The Beijing Eye Study	Beijing, China	4409 (8816)	0.4%[a]
The Tajimi Study	Tajimi, Japan	2977 (5934)	0.3%[b]
The Chinese American Eye Study	California	4582	0.2%[b]
The Rotterdam Study	Rotterdam, the Netherlands	6775 (13,550)	0.1%[b]
The Copenhagen City Eye Study	Copenhagen, Denmark	9934	0.1%[a]
The Los Angeles Latino Eye Study	California	6129 (12,258)	0.05%[a]

[a]Refers to subjects
[b]Refers to eyes

5.2.2 The Quality of Life (QoL) Impact of PM

The impact of PM on patient-reported outcomes, including QoL and vision-specific functioning (VSF), has not been well-documented, with only a few clinic-based studies reporting on the association between PM and poor VSF [51, 52]. To address this limitation, our group in Singapore assessed the impact of PM on vision-related QoL domains in population-based analyses using the 11-item Visual Functioning Index (VF-11) [53] and 32-item Impact of Vision Impairment (IVI) questionnaire [24, 28, 54]. We found that the presence of severe PM (Meta-PM categories 3 or 4) was significantly associated with poorer VSF compared to those without the disease, after multivariable adjustment including presenting visual acuity [24]. In particular, individuals with severe PM had significantly greater difficulty in performing 3 of 11 items on the VF-11, including playing games ($P = 0.04$), recognizing friends ($P < 0.001$), and seeing stairs ($P = 0.03$), compared to those without PM.

The presence of severe PM was also significantly associated with decrements in all three domains of the IVI, including reading ($P = 0.04$), mobility ($P = 0.02$), and emotional well-being ($P = 0.04$) [28]. Importantly, these decrements were independent of presenting distance visual acuity, suggesting that factors beyond vision (e.g., contrast sensitivity, depth perception, color vision, concerns, inconveniences, etc.) may play a role in the QoL of patients with PM. Rehabilitation management for PM should therefore include strategies to optimize reading abilities, promote mobility, and improve emotional well-being.

5.3 Public Health Strategies to Manage the Burden of PM

The exact pathogenesis of PM remains unclear, and well-replicated evidence on the genetic determinants of PM is still lacking [55–58]. In the next few sections, we advocate three strategies to combat the detrimental public health impact of PM and some future research directions in evaluating the disease's patient-centered impact.

5.3.1 Strategy 1: Health Promotion Programs

5.3.1.1 Myopia Prevention and Control

Myopia control interventions, such as health behavior interventions, optical aids, and pharmacological solutions, are important in reducing the risk of future incidence and progression of PM. The benefits of health behavior programs, including numerous trials on promoting more outdoor time and less time on near-work activities [59–61], have been highlighted in recent articles from the International Myopia Institute [7]. These trials have demonstrated the protective effect of increased outdoor time on myopia, most assessed using subjective self-reporting (recall bias) rather than objective measurements. However, novel light exposure measurement devices that provide light-related measurements have been recently developed [62], which appear to be viable tools for assessing objective light exposure and may be useful in quantifying the effectiveness of future health behavior intervention programs on preventing or slowing the development of myopia. If there is a need to correct myopic refractive error in children, optical aids with myopia control properties, such as bifocal or multifocal spectacle lenses, contact lenses, and orthokeratology lenses, can be used instead of conventional visual aids [63–66]. Pharmacological solutions, namely, atropine, are also an alternative form of myopia control. Although these interventions are targeted at myopia in general rather than PM specifically, prevention of myopia onset and slowing down myopia progression are key to reducing the risk of PM in later life.

5.3.1.2 Public Health Education Campaigns and Regular Screening

Myopia prevention and control programs and policies, targeted at children at the community or national levels, are employed in numerous countries, such as Taiwan, Singapore, and China [59, 60, 67, 68], through increased outdoor time in class during school. The public health message of spending more time outdoors to combat myopia is generally well-understood, but individuals with myopia are typically unaware that their refractive state may progress to pathological complications that may lead to irreversible vision loss [2, 69]. Therefore, public health education campaigns on the increased risk of irreversible visual complications with greater myopia severity and older age at the community, regional, and national levels are needed to increase awareness, particularly for older myopic adults who are at greater risk. Since older age and higher myopic refractive errors are important PM risk factors, identification of at-risk individuals for targeted monitoring and early intervention may help reduce disease incidence and progression. As such, public education campaigns should also be tailored toward persons with a high PM risk profile to encourage these individuals to undergo regular eye screening examinations with their eye care professional or specialist (such as optometrist, ophthalmologist, or retinal specialist). Increased subsidies for these individuals by government agencies may also aid in the provision of intermediate and long-term care services by affected persons. In addition, eye care professionals, particularly frontline providers such as opticians and optometrists, can inform and educate their patients on the increased risk of PM, as well as set up regular eye checks and examinations for at-risk individuals. Regular screening may facilitate early detection of other myopia-related complications, such as mCNV and MTM, which can be stopped from progressing with efficient treatment and surgical management [70]. Public health education efforts should also be directed toward increasing awareness of the symptoms of these complications in at-risk individuals, so that affected individuals can seek timely medical care.

5.3.2 Strategy 2: Provisions for Treating Complications of PM

Irreversible visual loss may be preventable with early treatment of certain complications of PM. In tandem with public health education efforts, resources should be allocated to the provision of diagnostic equipment and treatment facilities. Training of healthcare professionals to provide these services should be undertaken to meet the increasing demand.

5.3.2.1 Diagnostics

MTM and mCNV, particularly in their early stages where treatment outcomes may be optimal, are often difficult or impossible to diagnose based on clinical examination or fundus photography alone. Optical coherence tomography is often a necessary component of the diagnostic process for mCNV and MTM for the detection of subretinal exudation and foveal detachment, respectively. In areas where there is a lack of access to ophthalmic expertise for the examination of the peripheral retina, ultrawide-field fundus photography may be useful for detecting peripheral retinal tears and reti-

nal detachments. Accurate and precise diagnosis of these conditions is also dependent on the healthcare professionals trained to deliver these services. In low-resource areas, teleophthalmology services, paired with an efficient referral pathway to tertiary treatment centers, may be a cost-effective alternative to having trained healthcare professionals onsite.

5.3.2.2 Treatment

Intravitreal anti-vascular endothelial growth factor (anti-VEGF) is an effective treatment for mCNV if administered early, i.e., within a few weeks of onset. However, facilities and trained personnel for the delivery of anti-VEGF injections may only be available in tertiary healthcare centers. Similarly, patients with MTM may require early surgery by ophthalmic surgeons with advanced surgical techniques and equipment. The delivery of such highly specialized medical services in low-resource areas is a pertinent issue that needs to be addressed, for example, by locating satellite intravitreal injection and surgical facilities strategically in areas where the prevalence of myopia may be high.

5.3.3 Strategy 3: Low Vision Care and Rehabilitation

As vision loss associated with PM is often irreversible, low vision care and rehabilitation are recommended in order to improve individuals' ability to complete visual tasks and optimize their QoL [71–73]. Low vision care and services include clinical treatment, rehabilitation services, and the use of adaptive technologies. Clinical low vision care encompasses a comprehensive examination of the condition of the eyes and vision by an ophthalmologist and/or an optometrist, including an assessment of the patient's remaining visual function. Rehabilitation services include assistance with activities of daily living, counseling, orientation and mobility training, peer support groups, community and social services, advocacy (support groups and organizations) and education, and employment and training [71–73].

5.4 Future Direction and Work: Item Banking and Computerized Adaptive Testing in Myopia

Increasing emphasis has been placed on understanding the QoL impact of PM and effectiveness of treatment therapies from the patient's perspective using patient-reported outcome measures (PROMs) in research and clinical practice, in order to improve clinical care and patient-provider relationship, as well as inform comparative effectiveness research and value-based care models [74]. Indeed, PROMs are now required by regulatory authorities such as the Food and Drug

Administration (FDA) in the USA [75] and the National Institute for Health and Care Excellence (NICE) in Europe [76] to be used in trials involving patients to evaluate the impact of treatment therapies and interventions from the patient's perspective.

PROMs are typically questionnaires utilizing Likert (e.g., *Strongly Agree, Somewhat Agree, Neither Agree nor Disagree, Somewhat disagree, Strongly Disagree*) and/or Likert-type (e.g., *Not at all, A little bit, A moderate amount, A lot, Unable to do*) rating scales that patients have to fill in. Several PROMs have been developed specifically to measure the QoL impact of myopia, such as the National Eye Institute Refractive Quality of Life (NEI-RQL) [77] and the Quality of Life Impact of Refractive Correction (QIRC) [78] questionnaires. However, current myopia PROMs have several major shortcomings. First, they are paper-pencil based and therefore comprise a fixed number of items (i.e., questions) that responders must answer. As the number of items is necessarily limited to reduce participant burden, available myopia-specific questionnaires either *target only specific subsets of the myopic population* (e.g., *persons wearing glasses*) [78] or *focus on only limited aspects of QoL* (e.g., *activity limitation and symptoms*) [79]. Second, modern psychometric techniques (e.g., Rasch analysis) have highlighted several limitations of these questionnaires, including *poor validity, reliability, and targeting* [80]. These shortcomings make comparison of results between studies difficult, and do not allow for a comprehensive and nuanced QoL assessment of patients at the extreme ends of participant ability, particularly individuals suffering from PM, where QoL data are already lacking.

The limitations of paper-pencil PROMs can, however, be overcome by sophisticated psychometric methods of questionnaire development and validation, namely, item banking (IB) and computerized adaptive testing (CAT). An IB is a large pool of items calibrated (or ranked) for difficulty on the same linear scale based on participant response and use of modern psychometric techniques (e.g., Rasch analysis, a form of item response theory [IRT]) [81]. IBs are operationalized using CAT, which is a computer-based "smart" technology that selects the items to be administered based on participants' responses to previous items [82]. By presenting targeted items from a calibrated IB to the respondent, CAT minimizes measurement error and reduces test length without loss of precision and reliability [82]. Preliminary results for RetCAT (a suite of diabetic retinopathy (DR)-specific QoL CATs), developed by our team at the Singapore Eye Research Institute (SERI), showed that ≤7 *items* per CAT are required to obtain precise estimates of patients' QoL [83]. However, IBs and CAT have yet to be developed to comprehensively assess the impact of myopia, in particular PM, and its corrective interventions on QoL. Given the mounting public health burden resulting from this ocular condition in Asia

[42–45], the emergence of treatment therapies such as anti-vascular endothelial growth factor (VEGF) injections [84], and the global push to incorporate PROM data in value-based healthcare systems [85], a comprehensive and culturally valid CAT is needed to assess the impact of this devastating disease and effectiveness of related corrections from the patient's perspective in Singapore and Asia more widely.

5.5 Conclusion

With the rising epidemic of myopia in Asian countries and the increased risk of irreversible vision loss associated with PM, strategies to prevent and reduce the development and progression of this condition should be an important objective for individual patient care and a critical public health goal. The implementation of public health programs by healthcare authorities or tertiary eye centers to raise public awareness of the sight-threatening complications of PM; advancements in medical or surgical treatments; investment in training, technology, and equipment; low vision care and rehabilitation for affected individuals; and importantly myopia control interventions to prevent and/or slow down myopia progression in early life are needed to reduce the risk of PM development and progression and mitigate its impact on patients' QoL. A more comprehensive understanding of the patient-reported impact of PM, obtained using targeted IB and CAT, may also be central to informing individualized PM management plans for better clinical and QoL outcomes. While PM is emerging as a significant public health issue, these challenges can be resolved with the implementation of evidence-based public health interventions.

References

1. Tano Y. Pathologic myopia: where are we now? Am J Ophthalmol. 2002;134(5):645–60.
2. Saw SM, Gazzard G, Shih-Yen EC, Chua WH. Myopia and associated pathological complications. Ophthalmic Physiol Opt. 2005;25(5):381–91.
3. Wong Y-L, Saw S-M. Epidemiology of pathologic myopia in Asia and worldwide. Asia Pac J Ophthalmol. 2016;5(6):394–402.
4. Dolgin E. The myopia boom. Nature. 2015;519(7543):276–8.
5. Wong TY, Loon SC, Saw SM. The epidemiology of age related eye diseases in Asia. Br J Ophthalmol. 2006;90(4):506–11.
6. Verkicharla PK, Ohno-Matsui K, Saw SM. Current and predicted demographics of high myopia and an update of its associated pathological changes. Ophthalmic Physiol Opt. 2015;35(5):465–75.
7. Wildsoet CF, Chia A, Cho P, et al. IMI–interventions for controlling myopia onset and progression report. Invest Ophthalmol Vis Sci. 2019;60(3):M106–M31.
8. Wu P-C, Huang H-M, Yu H-J, Fang P-C, Chen C-T. Epidemiology of myopia. Asia Pac J Ophthalmol. 2016;5(6):386–93.

9. Chua SY, Sabanayagam C, Cheung YB, et al. Age of onset of myopia predicts risk of high myopia in later childhood in myopic Singapore children. Ophthalmic Physiol Opt. 2016;36(4):388–94.

10. Jones D, Luensmann D. The prevalence and impact of high myopia. Eye Contact Lens. 2012;38(3):188–96.

11. D-E S. Pathological refractive errors: system of ophthalmology, ophthalmic optics, and refraction. St Louis: Mosby; 1970.

12. Young TL. Molecular genetics of human myopia: an update. Optom Vis Sci. 2009;86(1):8–22.

13. Ohno-Matsui K, Lai TY, Lai CC, Cheung CM. Updates of pathologic myopia. Prog Retin Eye Res. 2016;52:156–87.

14. Ohno-Matsui K. What is the fundamental nature of pathologic myopia? Retina. 2017;37:1043–8.

15. Ruiz-Medrano J, Montero JA, Flores-Moreno I, Arias L, García-Layana A, Ruiz-Moreno JM. Myopic maculopathy: current status and proposal for a new classification and grading system (ATN). Prog Retin Eye Res. 2018;69:80–115.

16. Spaide RF, Ohno-Matsui K, Yannuzzi LA. Pathologic myopia. New York: Springer; 2014.

17. Ohno-Matsui K, Kawasaki R, Jonas JB, et al. International photographic classification and grading system for myopic maculopathy. Am J Ophthalmol. 2015;159(5):877–83 e7.

18. Vongphanit J, Mitchell P, Wang JJ. Prevalence and progression of myopic retinopathy in an older population. Ophthalmology. 2002;109(4):704–11.

19. Gao LQ, Liu W, Liang YB, et al. Prevalence and characteristics of myopic retinopathy in a rural Chinese adult population: the Handan Eye Study. Arch Ophthalmol. 2011;129(9):1199–204.

20. Liu HH, Xu L, Wang YX, Wang S, You QS, Jonas JB. Prevalence and progression of myopic retinopathy in Chinese adults: the Beijing Eye Study. Ophthalmology. 2010;117(9):1763–8.

21. Chen SJ, Cheng CY, Li AF, et al. Prevalence and associated risk factors of myopic maculopathy in elderly Chinese: the Shihpai Eye Study. Invest Ophthalmol Vis Sci. 2012;53(8):4868–73.

22. Asakuma T, Yasuda M, Ninomiya T, et al. Prevalence and risk factors for myopic retinopathy in a Japanese population: the Hisayama Study. Ophthalmology. 2012;119(9):1760–5.

23. Jonas JB, Nangia V, Gupta R, Bhojwani K, Nangia P, Panda-Jonas S. Prevalence of myopic retinopathy in rural Central India. Acta Ophthalmol. 2016;95:e399–404.

24. Wong Y-L, Sabanayagam C, Ding Y, et al. Prevalence, risk factors, and impact of myopic macular degeneration on visual impairment and functioning among adults in Singapore. Invest Ophthalmol Vis Sci. 2018;59(11):4603–13.

25. Li Z, Liu R, Jin G, et al. Prevalence and risk factors of myopic maculopathy in rural southern China: the Yangxi Eye Study. Br J Ophthalmol. 2019;103:1797–802.

26. Wong TY, Ferreira A, Hughes R, Carter G, Mitchell P. Epidemiology and disease burden of pathologic myopia and myopic choroidal neovascularization: an evidence-based systematic review. Am J Ophthalmol. 2014;157(1):9–25 e12.

27. Lin C, Li SM, Ohno-Matsui K, et al. Five-year incidence and progression of myopic maculopathy in a rural Chinese adult population: the Handan Eye Study. Ophthalmic Physiol Opt. 2018;38(3):337–45.

28. Wong YL, Sabanayagam C, Wong CW, et al. Six-year changes in myopic macular degeneration in adults of the singapore epidemiology of eye diseases study. Invest Ophthalmol Vis Sci. 2019;60(9):6453.

29. Yan YN, Wang YX, Yang Y, et al. Ten-year progression of myopic maculopathy: the Beijing Eye Study 2001–2011. Ophthalmology. 2018;125:1253–63.

30. Fang Y, Yokoi T, Nagaoka N, et al. Progression of myopic maculopathy during 18-year follow-up. Ophthalmology. 2018;125(6):863–77.

31. Hayashi K, Ohno-Matsui K, Shimada N, et al. Long-term pattern of progression of myopic maculopathy: a natural history study. Ophthalmology. 2010;117(8):1595–611, 611 e1–4.

32. Ueda E, Yasuda M, Fujiwara K, et al. Trends in the prevalence of myopia and myopic maculopathy in a Japanese population: the Hisayama Study. Invest Ophthalmol Vis Sci. 2019;60(8):2781–6.

33. Wong Y-L, Ding Y, Sabanayagam C, et al. Longitudinal changes in disc and retinal lesions among highly myopic adolescents in Singapore over a 10-year period. Eye Contact Lens. 2018;44(5):286–91.

34. Yoshihara N, Yamashita T, Ohno-Matsui K, Sakamoto T. Objective analyses of tessellated fundi and significant correlation between degree of tessellation and choroidal thickness in healthy eyes. PLoS One. 2014;9(7):e103586.

35. Yan YN, Wang YX, Yang Y, et al. Long-term progression and risk factors of fundus tessellation in the Beijing Eye Study. Sci Rep. 2018;8(1):10625.

36. Zhou Y, Song M, Zhou M, Liu Y, Wang F, Sun X. Choroidal and retinal thickness of highly myopic eyes with early stage of myopic chorioretinopathy: tessellation. J Ophthalmol. 2018;2018:2181602.

37. Fang Y, Du R, Nagaoka N, et al. Optical coherence tomography-based diagnostic criteria for different stages of myopic maculopathy. Ophthalmology. 2019;126:1018–32.

38. Wong CW, Phua V, Lee SY, Wong TY, Cheung CMG. Is choroidal or scleral thickness related to myopic macular degeneration? Invest Ophthalmol Vis Sci. 2017;58(2):907–13.

39. Holden BA, Fricke TR, Wilson DA, et al. Global prevalence of myopia and high myopia and temporal trends from 2000 through 2050. Ophthalmology. 2016;123(5):1036–42.

40. Holden BA, Jong M, Davis S, Wilson D, Fricke T, Resnikoff S. Nearly 1 billion myopes at risk of myopia-related sight-threatening conditions by 2050 - time to act now. Clin Exp Optom. 2015;98(6):491–3.

41. Holden BA, Wilson DA, Jong M, et al. Myopia: a growing global problem with sight-threatening complications. Community Eye Health/Int Centre Eye Health. 2015;28(90):35.

42. Xu L, Cui T, Yang H, et al. Prevalence of visual impairment among adults in China: the Beijing Eye Study. Am J Ophthalmol. 2006;141(3):591–3.

43. Iwase A, Araie M, Tomidokoro A, et al. Prevalence and causes of low vision and blindness in a Japanese adult population: the Tajimi Study. Ophthalmology. 2006;113(8):1354–62.e1.

44. Hsu W-M, Cheng C-Y, Liu J-H, Tsai S-Y, Chou P. Prevalence and causes of visual impairment in an elderly Chinese population in Taiwan: the Shihpai Eye Study. Ophthalmology. 2004;111(1):62–9.

45. Xu L, Wang Y, Li Y, et al. Causes of blindness and visual impairment in urban and rural areas in Beijing: the Beijing Eye Study. Ophthalmology. 2006;113(7):1134. e1–11.

46. Fricke TR, Jong M, Naidoo KS, et al. Global prevalence of visual impairment associated with myopic macular degeneration and temporal trends from 2000 through 2050: systematic review, meta-analysis and modelling. Br J Ophthalmol. 2018:bjophthalmol-2017-311266.

47. Varma R, Kim JS, Burkemper BS, et al. Prevalence and causes of visual impairment and blindness in Chinese American adults: the Chinese American eye study. JAMA Ophthalmol. 2016;134(7):785–93.

48. Klaver CC, Wolfs RC, Vingerling JR, Hofman A, de Jong PT. Age-specific prevalence and causes of blindness and visual impairment in an older population: the Rotterdam Study. Arch Ophthalmol. 1998;116(5):653–8.

49. Buch H, Vinding T, La Cour M, Appleyard M, Jensen GB, Nielsen NV. Prevalence and causes of visual impairment and blindness among 9980 Scandinavian adults: the Copenhagen City Eye Study. Ophthalmology. 2004;111(1):53–61.

50. Cotter SA, Varma R, Ying-Lai M, Azen SP, Klein R, Los Angeles Latino eye study Group. Causes of low vision and blindness in adult Latinos: the Los Angeles Latino Eye Study. Ophthalmology. 2006;113(9):1574–82.

51. Takashima T, Yokoyama T, Futagami S, et al. The quality of life in patients with pathologic myopia. Jpn J Ophthalmol. 2001;45(1):84–92.

52. Rose K, Harper R, Tromans C, et al. Quality of life in myopia. Br J Ophthalmol. 2000;84(9):1031–4.

53. Lamoureux EL, Pesudovs K, Thumboo J, Saw S-M, Wong TY. An evaluation of the reliability and validity of the visual functioning questionnaire (VF-11) using Rasch analysis in an Asian population. Invest Ophthalmol Vis Sci. 2009;50(6):2607–13.

54. Fenwick EK, Ong PG, Sabanayagam C, et al. Assessment of the psychometric properties of the Chinese Impact of Vision Impairment questionnaire in a population-based study: findings from the Singapore Chinese Eye Study. Qual Life Res. 2016;25(4):871–80.

55. Wong Y-L, Hysi P, Cheung G, et al. Genetic variants linked to myopic macular degeneration in persons with high myopia: CREAM Consortium. PLoS One. 2019;14(8):e0220143.

56. Nakanishi H, Yamada R, Gotoh N, et al. A genome-wide association analysis identified a novel susceptible locus for pathological myopia at 11q24.1. PLoS Genet. 2009;5(9):e1000660.

57. Yu Z, Zhou J, Chen X, Zhou X, Sun X, Chu R. Polymorphisms in the CTNND2 gene and 11q24. 1 genomic region are associated with pathological myopia in a Chinese population. Ophthalmologica. 2012;228(2):123–9.

58. Chen C-D, Yu Z-Q, Chen X-L, et al. Evaluating the association between pathological myopia and SNPs in RASGRF1. ACTC1 and GJD2 genes at chromosome 15q14 and 15q25 in a Chinese population. Ophthalmic Genet. 2015;36(1):1–7.

59. Wu P-C, Chen C-T, Lin K-K, et al. Myopia prevention and outdoor light intensity in a school-based cluster randomized trial. Ophthalmology. 2018;125(8):1239–50.

60. He M, Xiang F, Zeng Y, et al. Effect of time spent outdoors at school on the development of myopia among children in China: a randomized clinical trial. JAMA. 2015;314(11):1142–8.

61. Jin J-X, Hua W-J, Jiang X, et al. Effect of outdoor activity on myopia onset and progression in school-aged children in northeast China: the Sujiatun Eye Care Study. BMC Ophthalmol. 2015;15(1):73.

62. Wang J, He X-G, Xu X. The measurement of time spent outdoors in child myopia research: a systematic review. Int J Ophthalmol. 2018;11(6):1045.

63. Wolffsohn JS, Kollbaum PS, Berntsen DA, et al. IMI–clinical myopia control trials and instrumentation report. Invest Ophthalmol Vis Sci. 2019;60(3):M132–M60.

64. Huang J, Wen D, Wang Q, et al. Efficacy comparison of 16 interventions for myopia control in children: a network meta-analysis. Ophthalmology. 2016;123(4):697–708.

65. Gong Q, Janowski M, Luo M, et al. Efficacy and adverse effects of atropine in childhood myopia: a meta-analysis. JAMA Ophthalmol. 2017;135(6):624–30.

66. Li S-M, Kang M-T, Wu S-S, et al. Efficacy, safety and acceptability of orthokeratology on slowing axial elongation in myopic children by meta-analysis. Curr Eye Res. 2016;41(5):600–8.

67. Wu P-C, Tsai C-L, Wu H-L, Yang Y-H, Kuo H-K. Outdoor activity during class recess reduces myopia onset and progression in school children. Ophthalmology. 2013;120(5):1080–5.

68. Seet B, Wong TY, Tan DT, et al. Myopia in Singapore: taking a public health approach. Br J Ophthalmol. 2001;85(5):521–6.

69. Morgan IG, Ohno-Matsui K, Saw SM. Myopia. Lancet. 2012;379(9827):1739–48.

70. Saw S-M, Matsumura S, Hoang QV. Prevention and management of myopia and myopic pathology. Invest Ophthalmol Vis Sci. 2019;60(2):488–99.

71. Chiang PPC, O'Connor PM, Keeffe JE. Low vision service provision: a global perspective. Expert Rev Ophthalmol. 2007;2(5):861–74.

72. Scott IU, Smiddy WE, Schiffman J, Feuer WJ, Pappas CJ. Quality of life of low-vision patients and the impact of low-vision services. Am J Ophthalmol. 1999;128(1):54–62.

73. Stelmack J. Quality of life of low-vision patients and outcomes of low-vision rehabilitation. Optom Vis Sci. 2001;78(5):335–42.

74. Van Der Wees PJ, Nijhuis-Van Der Sanden MW, Ayanian JZ, Black N, Westert GP, Schneider EC. Integrating the use of patient-reported outcomes for both clinical practice and performance measurement: views of experts from 3 countries. Milbank Q. 2014;92(4):754–75.

75. U.S. Department of Health and Human Services FDA Center for Drug Evaluation and Research, U.S. Department of Health and Human Services FDA Center for Biologics Evaluation and Research, U.S. Department of Health and Human Services FDA Center for Devices and Radiological Health. Guidance for industry: patient-reported outcome measures: use in medical product development to support labeling claims: draft guidance. Health Qual Life Outcomes. 2006;4:79.

76. National Institute for Health and Clinical Excellence. Patient experience in adult NHS services: improving the experience of care for people using adult NHS services. Patients experience in generic terms. London: National Clinical Guideline Centre; 2012.

77. Berry S, Mangione CM, Lindblad AS, McDonnell PJ. Development of the National Eye Institute refractive error correction quality of life questionnaire: focus groups. Ophthalmology. 2003;110(12):2285–91.

78. Pesudovs K, Garamendi E, Elliott DB. The quality of life impact of refractive correction (QIRC) questionnaire: development and validation. Optom Vis Sci. 2004;81(10):769–77.

79. Vitale S, Schein OD, Meinert CL, Steinberg EP. The refractive status and vision profile: a questionnaire to measure vision-related quality of life in persons with refractive error. Ophthalmology. 2000;107(8):1529–39.

80. Kandel H, Khadka J, Goggin M, Pesudovs K. Patient-reported outcomes for assessment of quality of life in refractive error: a systematic review. Optom Vis Sci. 2017;94(12):1102–19.

81. Cella D, Gershon R, Lai JS, Choi S. The future of outcomes measurement: item banking, tailored short-forms, and computerized adaptive assessment. Qual Life Res. 2007;16(Suppl 1):133–41.

82. Gershon RC. Computer adaptive testing. J Appl Meas. 2005;6(1):109–27.

83. Fenwick E, Khadka J, Pesudovs K, Rees G, Lamoureux E. Quality of life item banks for diabetic retinopathy and diabetic macular oedema: development and initial evaluation using computer adaptive testing. Invest Ophthalmol Vis Sci. 2017;58:6379–87.

84. Tan CS, Sadda SR. Anti-vascular endothelial growth factor therapy for the treatment of myopic choroidal neovascularization. Clin Ophthalmol. 2017;11:1741–6.

85. Baumhauer JF, Bozic KJ. Value-based healthcare: patient-reported outcomes in clinical decision making. Clin Orthop Relat Res. 2016;474(6):1375–8.

Animal Models of Experimental Myopia: Limitations and Synergies with Studies on Human Myopia

Ian G. Morgan, Kathryn A. Rose, and Regan S. Ashby

Interest in human myopia has a long history [1], but research into experimental myopia in animal models is much more recent. After some early attempts at experiments in animals [2, 3], the field took off after the publication of two papers – the first a paper on induced myopia in primates in 1977 by Wiesel and Raviola [4] that was an offshoot of the research on visual pathways that later won Hubel and Wiesel the Nobel Prize. This was rapidly followed by a paper by Wallman and colleagues on experimental myopia in chickens [5]. Since then, experimental myopia has been expanded to a much wider range of species, including common laboratory animals such as mice [6, 7] and guinea pigs [8, 9], as well as more exotic species such as tree shrews [10]. While experimental myopia is a biologically interesting problem in its own right [11], we will deal primarily with what experimental myopia can tell us about human myopia. This perspective means that the ideal animal model should reproduce the developmental features of human myopia in the time course of change in the ocular determinants of refraction and also use methods of inducing experimental myopia that mimic those important in human myopia. Departures from this ideal do not, however, doom a model to irrelevance, since, while the timing and regulatory pathways may be different, many of the basic pathways involved in construction of an eye, and in particular the sclera, may be similar.

I. G. Morgan (✉)
Research School of Biology, Australian National University, Canberra, ACT, Australia
e-mail: ian.morgan@anu.edu.au

K. A. Rose
School of Orthoptics, Graduate School of Health, University of Technology Sydney, Ultimo, NSW, Australia
e-mail: kathryn.rose@uts.edu.au

R. S. Ashby
Centre for Research into Therapeutic Solutions, Faculty of Science and Technology, University of Canberra, Bruce, ACT, Australia
e-mail: regan.ashby@canberra.edu.au

6.1 Refractive Development and Incident Myopia in Children

Given these criteria, a brief overview of refractive development in children is necessary. Children are born with a normal (Gaussian) distribution of spherical equivalent refraction (SER), with a mean hyperopic refraction [12]. Rapid changes over the first year or two after birth result in a narrower distribution of SER, often described as leptokurtotic, largely due to a reduction in highly hyperopic refractive errors. Whether early myopic refractive errors are eliminated is less clear. The major biometric changes involve loss of corneal power, loss of lens power and axial elongation. While the mean SER moves from hyperopia towards emmetropia, at the end of this developmental period, the mean SER remains distinctly hyperopic, often with a mean SER of around 1.0–1.5 D [13–15]. From then on, the cornea stabilises, and over the next few years, these characteristic features of the distribution of SER (hyperopic mean SER and narrow distribution) are seen in most populations that have been studied [16]. By the age of 5–6, the distribution of the ratio of AL to CR is also narrow, suggesting that an important part of the changes up to this age involves matching the axial length of the eye to the corneal power, but the underlying distributions of AL and CR remain normal [17]. In general, the prevalence of myopia is low over this period.

After the cornea stabilises around the age of 2, axial elongation can continue for as much as 20 years, at rates which seem to be influenced by the environments in which the children are growing up [18, 19]. This period of development appears to create the marked differences in the prevalence of myopia currently seen around the world [18]. Up to 10–12 years, there are rapid decreases in lens power [20–22], which minimise increases in myopia associated with axial elongation. The rate of loss of lens power decreases after the age of 10–12, and the lens starts to thicken. Mutti and colleagues [23] have reported that, close to the onset of myopia, loss of lens power ceases abruptly, but this phenomenon has not been reported in all studies [24]. After this age, with a slower rate of loss of lens power, axial elongation is translated almost completely into myopic shifts in refraction. It is important to note that it is impossible to understand refractive development in children without taking into account changes in lens power [25], although this is rarely done because of the difficulty in estimating lens power, which cannot be directly measured.

It is important to note that most human myopia (school myopia) appears after the age of 5–6 across a range of ethnic groups [16], although there is a low percentage of early onset myopia (1–2%) in many populations. In children in mainland China, there is little myopia in children attending preschools [26–28], although myopia then develops rapidly over the first few years of primary school [29, 30]. The low prevalence of myopia in preschool and at the beginning of school is also seen in populations of European ancestry [31–33], although the subsequent development of myopia is much slower.

Some deviations from this pattern have been reported. Some studies on preschool-age children have reported quite high (up to 5%) myopia prevalence rates, specifically in those of Asian, African-American and Hispanic origin in the USA [34, 35] and in Chinese in Singapore [36]. Some of these observations may be due to variations in methodology, including the rigour of cycloplegia, since the data show an unusual pattern of higher prevalences in younger children, with a gradual reduction as children get older. There is more compelling evidence that in some Chinese populations, particularly in Singapore [37], Hong Kong [38] and Taiwan [39], there is more myopia when children start school than is seen in mainland China. The factors that account for these differences have not been identified, although differences in early educational pressures are an obvious possibility.

An important feature of human myopia is that, although the term emmetropisation is widely used [40–42] the epidemiological evidence suggests that in natural environments, in which children are not under much educational pressure and spend reasonable amounts of time outdoors, refractions tend to converge on mild hyperopia rather than emmetropia at the age of 6 [16]. For example, in children starting school in such diverse environments as Chinese cities [28–30] and Sydney [17], the mean SER in the first year of primary school, at age 6, is close to +1.3 D – a level at which normal visual acuity can be achieved through accommodation by most people up to the age of about 40 [43]. This "preferred state" is also seen in non-human primates [44, 45].

In populations where the prevalence of myopia is low, this refractive state persists into at least the early adult years, provided that cycloplegia is used [46]. In contrast, in populations which later develop significant myopia, the refractive distribution shifts towards myopia, but emmetropia never becomes the dominant refractive category. Instead, it appears that as some children enter the emmetropic category, others pass from emmetropia to myopia [16]. The loss of control of axial elongation seems to come before children become clinically myopic, and seems to be detectable as an increased rate of myopic shift, comparable to the rate of myopic progression seen after myopia is established, for at least a year before the onset of myopia [22, 47, 48].

In human refractive development, we therefore need to consider several developmental phases defined by changes in refraction and in the biometric components of refraction. At least four phases can be distinguished (Fig. 6.1). The first involves establishment of a tight distribution of refraction

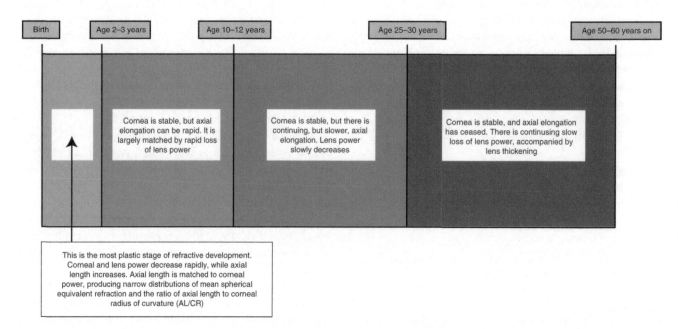

Fig. 6.1 Phases of refractive development in humans. Four phases can be distinguished. A highly plastic neonatal stage lasts 2–3 years, after which the cornea stabilises. Following this, axial elongation can continue for at least 20 years. For some of this time, loss of lens power tends to minimise the myopic refractive shift associated with axial elon-gation, but around the age of 10–12, the rate of loss of lens power decreases but is then maintained at a slow rate for several decades. This results in hyperopic shifts for much of adult life, except where marked increases in lens power associated with cataract lead to marked myopic shifts in the elderly

with a mildly hyperopic peak, generally over the first 2 years after birth. This stage involves increases in axial length and loss of both corneal and lens power. This is followed by a period from the age of 3–6 years in which there are further increases in axial length, but where myopic shifts in refraction are largely neutralised by loss of lens power, where the peak refraction is maintained at around +1 D or slightly higher. In low myopia environments, in which children are not subjected to excessive educational pressures, and they spend adequate amounts of time outdoors, this state can be maintained well into adult life. However, in environments in which axial elongation is accelerated markedly by myopiagenic environments, there are large myopic shifts in refraction which slow and eventually terminate, as the developmental plasticity in axial length decreases with age and terminates.

Thus, in many ways, rather than a process of failed emmetropisation, the process of refractive development and the onset of myopia in children is better described as a process of convergence of refraction towards mild hyperopia by around the age of 5–6 years, with myopiagenic environments, characterised by intense educational pressure and limited time outdoors, able to overwhelm this tendency. This leads to loss of control over refractive development, with subsequent rapid myopic shifts leading to myopia and further myopia progression limited by declining plasticity in axial elongation.

In the final stage, axial elongation has effectively ceased, but slow loss of lens power continues, resulting in slow hyperopic shifts in refraction with increasing age. During this phase, myopic shifts in refraction can also be seen in those individuals who develop cataract later in life. The boundaries between these stages are not tightly defined, particularly that around the age of 6, when in most societies children start attending preschool and school. But they provide an important point of reference for assessing the relevance to human myopia of studies on experimental myopia.

6.2   Experimental Myopia

6.2.1   The Basic Paradigms in Experimental Myopia

The basic methods for research in experimental myopia, and the results obtained, have been extensively reviewed [11]. Wiesel and Raviola [4] carried out their pioneering studies on monkeys with sutured eyelids, an approach with analogies to myopia associated with infantile ptosis [49]. In contrast, Wallman and colleagues placed translucent diffusers over the eyes of chickens to induce myopia [5]. Roughly 10 years later, a different technique for inducing experimental myopia was introduced by Schaeffel, in which negative

lenses were placed over the eyes, and compensatory changes in eye growth were observed [50]. These studies have led to the general use of two paradigms for inducing experimental myopia.

6.2.1.1   Form-Deprivation Myopia (FDM)

This paradigm uses translucent diffusers, fitted over the experimental eye, which allow considerable light through, typically with a reduction of light intensity of less than one log unit. These diffusers, however, markedly reduce spatial contrast, and, in moving animals, the reduced spatial contrast translates automatically into reduced temporal contrast. This kind of manipulation results in rapid development of myopia – for example, in chickens as much as 20 D of myopia is achieved in less than 2 weeks, although the development of myopia is slower in other animals. As in humans, the development of myopia in this paradigm primarily depends on axial elongation and particularly elongation of the vitreous chamber.

6.2.1.2   Lens-Induced Myopia (LIM)

When negative lenses are fitted over the developing eye, the eye responds rapidly with compensatory increased growth, which continues until the imposed defocus has been neutralised [50, 51]. Thus, the experimental eyes move towards emmetropia with the lens in place and develop an intrinsic refractive error which, after the lens is removed, corresponds to the power of the lens fitted. This occurs largely through modulation of vitreous chamber depth. The compensation for imposed defocus achieved in LIM appears to be quite precise.

6.2.1.3   How Different Are FDM and LIM?

These paradigms differ in several ways. Eyes fitted with diffusers have no way of overcoming the reduced spatial and temporal contrast to which they are exposed, for this is not affected by axial elongation. Thus, continued growth does not reduce the level of the stimulation towards growth, and the eyes continue to grow until natural reductions in body growth terminate the process. Accommodation does not seem to be important for the development of FDM [52, 53]. This is therefore an open-loop process, in which there is no feedback to limit growth.

In contrast, in LIM, the eyes are generally fitted with lenses of powers that are within the accommodative capacity of the eyes. It is therefore expected that, for at least part of the time, the animals use accommodation to neutralise the imposed defocus to produce focused images. This accommodative response does not appear to be a crucial factor, since eyes with impaired accommodation seem to develop lens-induced myopia [54, 55]. It is thus generally assumed that the growth responses are stimulated by the magnitude or the sign of defocus, which is detected in some way by the retina, although the mechanisms involved are not understood. Since axial elongation leads to compensation for the imposed hyperopic defocus, as the eye grows, there is a constant reduction in the stimulus to growth, and the process terminates when growth has compensated for the imposed refractive error. In other words, this is a closed-loop system.

Despite the different properties of the paradigms at the level of visual input and feedback, the responses in FDM and LIM are very similar at the cellular and molecular levels [56, 57], suggesting that many of the pathways leading to axial elongation and myopia are shared between the two systems. This is currently a controversial area, and the many similarities do not mean that they are identical. In principle, differences are most likely to be seen in the early stages of the visual processing that leads to changes in eye growth, with commonalities more likely to be seen closer to the changes in scleral composition that underlie increased eye growth.

6.2.1.4 Recovery from Experimental Myopia (REC)

After the introduction of the FDM paradigm, it was discovered that if the diffusers were removed, provided that the animals were still young, the eyes responded by slowing the rate of axial elongation [58]. As a result, the refractive state could return to, or at least towards, emmetropia, due to continued development of the anterior segment of the eye. This process does not appear to be driven by the different shape of the myopic eye but is driven by the defocus, because optical correction of the myopic defocus prevents the changes in eye growth [59, 60]. Unlike the FDM paradigm used to induce the myopia initially, this is therefore also a closed-loop paradigm.

6.2.1.5 Lens-Induced Hyperopia (LIH)

In the same set of experiments that introduced LIM [50, 51], the effects of fitting positive lenses were examined. This should impose myopic defocus on the eye, which cannot be corrected by accommodation, and in this case, the rate of axial elongation slows. Since the anterior segment of the eye continues to develop, associated loss of corneal and lens power can lead to hyperopic shifts in refraction. As with LIM, this is a closed-loop paradigm, and compensation for the imposed lens appears to be quite precise.

6.2.1.6 How Similar Are the REC and LIH Paradigms?

These two paradigms enable investigation of the processes leading to reduced rates of eye growth, which is important for the control of myopia progression. It is generally assumed that the paradigms involve reductions in the rate of axial elongation, but recently evidence has been produced that a proportion of eyes can actually become shorter through active remodelling of the sclera [58]. The REC paradigm

involves an eye and a retina that have been supporting an excessive rate of eye growth, and thus they are in a different state to that seen in a normal eye, at both the retinal and scleral levels. In contrast, the eye and retina in the LIH paradigm are effectively in their control state. Much less work has been done on the cellular and molecular basis of these paradigms, but molecular changes in the sclera appear to be different in the two paradigms [62].

6.2.1.7 What Is the Best Model in Terms of Stimulus Relevance to Human Myopia?

The unfortunate answer to this question is "probably none". With the exception of the very low percentage of myopia associated with congenitally blurred vision, such as with ptosis, congenital cataract or corneal scarring, children do not grow up with the equivalent of translucent plastic goggles over their eyes, and thus the FDM model is generally not regarded as a good model of human myopia. It is often assumed that LIM provides a better model, because the imposed hyperopic defocus generated by fitting negative lenses over the eye can be regarded as analogous to the demands placed on children's eyes by too much near work, although the evidence that near-work demands and myopia are linked has become much weaker, as more quantitative studies have been performed [63, 64]. FDM and human refractive development do share an important characteristic, in that both seem to be influenced by light exposures. The development of FDM is inhibited by bright light exposures [65–67], a protective effect that is mediated by increased dopamine release [66]. This parallels the mechanism involving increased dopamine release by bright light outdoors [68] to explain the protective effect of increased time outdoors against the development of myopia in children [68–70].

Initially, it was believed that the increased accommodation associated with high levels of near work might be the important factor in the development of human myopia. However, studies on animals have shown that experimental myopia can be induced in species without accommodative capacity [52], or with experimental interruptions to accommodation [55], and that atropine can block eye growth in a species (chicken) in which it does not block accommodation [53]. Collectively, this is strong evidence that active accommodation is not a crucial factor in the development of myopia.

In parallel with these developments, while there is a consistent correlation between schooling and educational outcomes and myopia [18], attempts to quantify the association using precise measurement of near-work exposures have produced less than stunning results, and some have concluded that near work may have little role [64]. Emphasis then shifted to the idea that, rather than accommodation itself, it was accommodative lag in periods of near work which was important. However, while accommodation is less accurate in children with myopia than in those with emmetropic refractions [71], there is conflicting evidence on whether this difference precedes or follows the development of myopia [71, 72]. More recently, attention has shifted to the interplay in space and time between hyperopic and myopic defocus on the retina, where myopic defocus appears to be a stronger stimulus [73, 74]. Flitcroft [75, 76] has explored the complex interplay between viewing distance or accommodation and eye shape in indoor and outdoor environments in producing patterns of defocus on the retina, suggesting that this might provide a supplementary explanation of the protective effects of time outdoors to the hypothesis based on bright light exposures and increased dopamine release, despite the strong support from animal experiments for this mechanism. Extrapolating from the animal experiments on myopic defocus to human myopia is problematic, because if myopic defocus plays a major role during development, then myopia should be a self-limiting condition, and it should be dangerous to correct myopic defocus clinically. Neither of these propositions seems to be correct. However, a significant role for myopic defocus is supported by the evidence that imposed myopic defocus seems to be able to control myopia progression [77–79].

It has also been shown that chickens raised on light-dark cycles, in which the light phase consists of dim light (50 lux), slowly become myopic [80], with development of myopia associated with low dopamine release [81]. There has been some interest in this as a model for human myopia, but children becoming myopic are not generally exposed to such extreme conditions, even where time spent outdoors is low and there is an epidemic of myopia. More recently, it has been shown that a similar phenomenon is not observed in non-human primates [82].

Overall, none of the animal models fits well with what we know about human myopia. A simple but powerful illustration of this point is that in both FDM and LIM, brief removal of the optical devices prevents the development of myopia [83–85]. In contrast, it seems almost certain that children are not constantly exposed to risk factors such as near work or low light intensities, and periods without these conditions do not seem to block the development of myopia. Equally, given the strong effect of imposed myopic defocus, there is a paradox, because the ability of myopic defocus to slow axial elongation and the recovery observed in the REC paradigm, if simply applied to human myopia, would suggest that human myopia should be a self-limiting condition, which it clearly is not. Similarly, if myopic defocus was exerting a controlling effect, then it should be deleterious to correct myopic, but again it is not.

Another important difference is that, while compensation appears to be quite precise in the LIM and LIH paradigms, the same precision is not obvious in human refractive development, given that characteristically in 3–5-year-olds, the

mean SER is distinctly hyperopic. Thus, some of the principles that appear to apply to experimental myopia do not seem to apply to human myopia.

Clearly, none of the existing paradigms provides a completely adequate model of human myopia, which means that human epidemiology will continue to play a critical role as the point of reference. But this does not mean that these models are useless. Irrespective of the mechanism by which myopia is induced, these models can be used to study the nature of the changes in ocular components and the corresponding details of changes in gene expression and biochemistry, at a level which is simply impossible in humans.

6.2.1.8 Which Is the Best Species to Study for Relevance to Human Myopia?

At one level, the answer to the question about the most relevant species is almost self-evident – non-human primates or monkeys. Detailed studies of the development of the refractive components of the eye in rhesus monkeys have shown that humans and monkeys share common processes of early loss of corneal power, followed by stabilisation, accompanied by axial elongation and loss of lens power, with a mean SER in the mildly hyperopic rather than the emmetropic range. This is followed by further axial elongation and loss of lens power, with little change in refraction, as discussed previously. They have also shown that the development of myopia in monkeys predominantly depends on increases in axial length, as it does in humans.

But while the pattern of change is similar, the absolute timing is different (Table 6.1). In humans, corneal power (or radius of curvature) stabilises at about 700 days, while in monkeys, it stabilises at around 200 days. This difference is not surprising given the relative differences in maturation and lifespan. It is particularly important to note that most studies on monkeys have been carried out in this early developmental period, typically from 21 days up to around 140 days, corresponding to a developmental period in which there is very little development of myopia in humans.

This difference in developmental stage also applies to the other species that are studied. As a general rule, studies on experimental myopia have overwhelmingly been carried

Table 6.1 Temporal characteristics of refractive development in humans and monkeys (time to reach the midpoint between the measure at birth and the measure at the developmental plateau, assuming non-linear regression) [44]

Ocular component	Human (days)	Monkey (days)
Refraction	276	213
Corneal power	251	75
Axial length	584	196
Anterior chamber depth	384	133
Vitreous chamber depth	815	258

out during developmental periods that correspond most closely to the neonatal period of development in humans, for the simple reason that large and rapid changes can be observed more easily. In humans, this is a period in which significant hyperopia is substantially reduced, and there is loss of corneal power, major loss of lens power and substantial matching of the axial length of the eye to the corneal and lens powers, to produce a tight distribution of refraction. In contrast, during the period in which myopia typically develops in humans, corneal power is stable, and lens power loss decreases and, after the age of 10–12, slows even further.

In the other species that are commonly studied as models of experimental myopia, the developmental patterns deviate more markedly from the human pattern, and guinea pigs [8, 9] and mice [7] show thickening of the crystalline lens, in contrast to humans, although lens power decreases in all three. However, tree shrews show the human pattern of combination of loss of lens power and thinning of the crystalline lens but otherwise have a complicated pattern of development, including a period after eye opening where experimental myopia develops very slowly [96, 97].

Again, this does not mean that the use of models other than non-human primates is irrelevant. Experimentation on monkeys is limited by justified ethical concerns, as well as by logistic and other considerations, and other species have their advantages. Chickens are easy and cheap to obtain, and induction of experimental myopia is extremely rapid. Mice are easy to obtain, but induction and monitoring of myopia is more difficult. The great advantage of mice lies in the existing detailed knowledge of the mouse genome and of their cellular and molecular biochemistry, but this has only rarely been exploited. Guinea pigs provide a diurnal mammalian model, although they probably differ most in terms of the changes in ocular components from the human model. Tree shrews provide a diurnal mammalian model and are close to the primate line, but again their developmental profile does not correspond closely to the human model, and they require specialised breeding facilities.

One important limitation on the use of animal models is that most vertebrates, including birds, have a sclera which consists of two components – a fibrous layer and a cartilaginous layer [86, 87]. In lower vertebrates, the dominant response of the sclera involves expansion of the cartilaginous layer, whereas the fibrous layer appears to become thinner. Mammals, including humans, appear to have at most a vestigial cartilaginous layer, and thus the scleral response consists only of thinning and weakening of the fibrous layer. Thus, chickens are not a good model in which to study changes in the sclera relevant to pathological myopia.

Even with mammalian models, there is another important limitation. In humans, when high myopia first appears, there are few signs of pathological changes that could be described as pathological myopia. These develop in human high myopes over a period of decades, and are thus unlikely to be reproduced in most of the mammalian models, including non-human primates, unless experimental studies are prolonged well beyond the length of the usual experiment. There may, however, be a small place for experimentation on appropriate mammalian models of high myopia, if methods for strengthening the sclera are under consideration.

6.3 Important Features of Experimental Myopia

6.3.1 Local Control and Spatial Localisation

One of the most striking discoveries from experimental myopia is that the control of eye growth primarily occurs within the eye, with little influence from central pathways. In both FDM and LIM, there is minimal impact of sectioning of the optic nerve, cutting off the eye from centrifugal input [55, 88]. Equally, lesions to the ciliary nerve have little effect [55].

This point is further emphasised by the evidence that use of partial diffusers and lenses produces differential growth changes. For example, half diffusers tend to produce excessive growth in roughly half the eye, the half experiencing form deprivation [89], and the same is true of partial lenses [90]. These findings place some important limitations on mechanisms, since global processes such as accommodation would not be expected to operate in this way. It is not clear how precise this spatial localisation is, since most experiments have demonstrated differential control over quite large areas, and it should not be assumed that the spatial localisation is as precise as point-to-point neural pathways can be. Rather, it is probably best to think in terms of circles of influence for any pathway being considered, just as blur of the image turns a point into a blur circle. For example, if the release of dopamine from dopaminergic neurons in the retina is important, as the evidence strongly suggests [91], then this could be controlled by spatially precise modulation of activity within defined pathways linking photoreceptors to ON-bipolar cells to dopaminergic cells. However, once the transmitter has been released, then diffusion of the transmitter, including lateral spread of its effects within the retina and choroid, is likely to produce a circle of influence. How large this circle of influence is will depend on the speed with which the transmitter or messenger diffuses, but this principle is likely to apply at any stage in the growth control pathway where the message is transmitted by soluble, diffusible messengers.

6.3.2   Choroidal Changes

Another important observation from animal experimentation is that, particularly in chicken, there are major changes in the thickness of the choroid, which swells in response to myopic defocus and thins in response to hyperopic defocus [92, 93]. In chickens, the choroid can expand by some hundreds of microns in response to myopic defocus, although thinning is of lesser magnitude. In other species, including non-human primates [94], changes in choroidal thickness are much less marked. This is also true for humans [95, 96].

In chickens, it has been suggested that the swelling of the choroid in response to myopic defocus may act to reduce the level of myopic defocus on a time-scale intermediate between that of accommodation and changes in axial length, by bringing the retina towards the myopic focal plane within minutes to hours of the imposition of myopic defocus. The accuracy of the compensation is still to be determined. Given the smaller magnitude of the responses to hyperopic defocus, less effective compensation would be achieved.

Whatever the reasons for these changes, they may be involved in the transmission of growth control signals from the retina to the sclera, since there is some evidence that choroidal changes are linked to slowing of axial elongation in response to myopic defocus [97–100]. The general role of the choroid has been extensively reviewed [101, 113].

6.3.3   Summary

Despite the many limitations and cautions on the use of animal models of experimental myopia, studies on animal models can investigate issues that cannot be addressed in humans – in particular, animal models of experimental myopia can be used to elucidate details of the molecular and cellular processes involved, which may open up opportunities for pharmacological intervention.

Of the various limitations of studies on experimental myopia, probably the most fundamental is that experimental myopia is generally induced during a different developmental phase to that in which human myopia appears. In addition, the lens models involve a level of precision that does not appear to apply to human myopia. Specifically, the compensation process in LIM (and LIH) appears to be very precise, but, in humans, refractive development appears to be rather imprecise, with refractions in the range from +0.5 to +2.0 D appearing after the first 2–5 years of life. These are maintained into adult life in populations in which the prevalence of myopia is low.

The distinction concerning developmental period may be crucial. Pooled data from four leading laboratories in the field of experimental myopia has shown that in the REC and LIH paradigms, there is evidence that the eyes can actually shrink in chickens, monkeys (both macaques and marmosets) and tree shrews [61], suggesting a more active remodelling process than just the slowing of growth normally assumed. Not all eyes shrink however, and shrinking was more common in tree shrews than in monkeys, which the authors attributed to the earlier developmental age of the tree shrews. All the studies were carried out in the rapid developmental period, and, given the evidence in the paper that this active remodelling becomes less active with age, it is questionable whether anything like this would occur in human myopia, given the differences in developmental stage.

6.4   Synergies Between Genetic Research on Human and Experimental Myopia

We suggest that greater integration of the results from these two streams of research, human myopia and experimental myopia, will increase understanding of the aetiology of myopia and assist in achieving the ultimate goal of controlling human myopia. The interaction is two way – sometimes starting with discoveries in human epidemiology and sometimes with discoveries in experimental myopia. We will discuss some examples that illustrate the synergies that have already occurred and suggest some areas that can be more systematically explored in the future.

One of the most immediate conclusions that could have been drawn from the animal models of myopia is that refractive development could be profoundly altered by changes to visual input – stressing the potential for environmental influences. Unfortunately, there has often been little interchange between the two approaches to myopia research, and conclusions about the tight genetic determination of myopia in humans derived from twin studies [102] were not seriously contrasted with the evidence that refractive development in animals was extremely responsive to environmental manipulation [11]. Instead, these two contrasting conclusions simply coexisted, relatively peacefully.

It took the emergence of an epidemic of myopia in developed parts of East and Southeast Asia to bring the issue to the fore [18, 19]. The realisation of the implications of the rapid increase in the prevalence of myopia in East and Southeast Asia and the development of research in experimental myopia covered much the same period and, in combination, played a major role in the reassessment of the balance between genes and environment in the aetiology of myopia that has taken place over the past decade [103–107].

So far, studies on highly familial, apparently genetic, forms of human myopia have identified a large number of distinct but rare forms of myopia, on the basis of chromosomal localisations or identified genes. While numerous, they account for only a low percentage, perhaps as low as

1–2%, of myopia in most populations. This topic has been extensively reviewed [103–110]. A cluster of mutations associated with scleral constituents [118] has been identified. There may also be a cluster associated with visual processing in the photoreceptor to ON-bipolar cell pathway in the outer retina, of which well-known examples are the myopia-associated rod-cone dystrophies, retinitis pigmentosa and congenital stationary night blindness.

GWAS studies have identified increasing numbers of SNPs associated with myopia. In the most recent analysis with a sample size of over half a million, over 400 genomic regions have been identified as associated with myopia. These contain hundreds to thousands of SNPs, but still account for only a little over 10% (12.1%) of the variation in refraction [105]. A recent analysis has shown that there is considerable overlap between the genes implicated in the GWAS studies and those identified in linkage studies. Mutations of small effect size in regulatory regions are more likely to be found in the GWAS studies, while structural mutations of larger effect size are more likely to be found in linkage studies [108].

Despite these impressive sample sizes, and the plenitude of data, these elegant GWAS studies have so far only confirmed what was largely known from previous work through broad conclusions such as "genome-wide association meta-analysis highlights light-induced signaling as a driver for refractive error" [109]. This has been a basic tenet of animal studies since the earliest evidence that modulation of visual input could induce myopia in experimental models of myopia [11].

So far, these studies have not delivered new insights into pathways that can be translated into pharmacological interventions. The only validated pharmacological intervention to control myopia progression [111, 112], and perhaps onset [113], is the use of atropine eye drops, but cholinergic pathways do not feature prominently in the pathways identified by GWAS. However, whether atropine is acting via cholinergic pathways is under some dispute (see below). Similarly, despite the extensive evidence from animal studies that dopamine plays an important role in the control of ocular growth [91], in particular through pathways that may mediate the ability of light to slow the onset of myopia [114], dopaminergic pathways are not highlighted in GWAS analysis. One of the identified genes with a relatively large effect size, GJD2 [115], encodes for connexin-36, a gap junction protein expressed in both the inner and outer plexiform layers, which plays a role in the coupling and uncoupling of many types of cells within the retina. This involves dopamine-regulated phosphorylation mediated by D1-dopamine receptors, whereas most dopaminergic effects on experimental myopia are mediated by D2-dopamine receptors.

GWAS has now implicated hundreds, if not thousands, of genes as involved in the regulation of eye growth. Further examination of changes in expression of some of these genes

in animal models has the potential to be very illuminating. One limiting factor is that currently identified SNPs only explain a low percentage of the variation in refraction, meaning that practical returns in terms of myopia control may be limited. This limiting factor also means that currently, prospects for the successful prediction of subsequent myopia at an early age based on genetic analysis are not promising [116]. Analysis of what is known as SNP heritability suggests that the most that can be expected from GWAS analysis is an explanation of 25–35% of the variation in refraction [128], which is still too low for useful prediction.

It is clear that to unravel the complexities of the retinal pathways implicated by GWAS analysis, studies in animal models are required. Studies of changes in gene expression in experimental myopia can help to define the site of action of mutant genes identified for human myopia, since they can define, at least in some cases, where relevant changes in the expression of genes and gene products take place. The link between sites of mutations which affect myopia in humans and where changes in gene expression take place in experimental myopia is not likely to be absolute, but substantial overlap would be anticipated. Where genes identified in human myopia studies correspond to those in which changes in expression are reported in experimental myopia, the case will be particularly strong. Studies on animal models have identified a list of candidate genes on the basis of changes in gene expression [117, 118]. These need to be used as candidate genes in studies on human myopia, since the chances of the gene playing a significant role seem likely to be higher if there are large changes in gene expression during the development of myopia. However, so far the list of changes in mRNA expression is relatively short, and they are small in magnitude, but parallel studies are bound to become more systematic in the future.

An interesting approach which is obviously impossible in humans, but highly feasible in experimental animals, is selective breeding. After only two cycles of selective breeding of chickens that show large or small responses to form deprivation, the strains showed marked differences in their responses to FDM, indicating a strong genetic component to the differences [119–121]. Whether this is relevant to human myopia is not clear, since, for these characteristics to segregate in human populations, it would require selective mating on the basis of sensitivity to develop FDM, which seems unlikely. Nevertheless, selectively bred strains could enable elegant dissection of the pathways involved.

GWAS analysis has addressed one of the important controversies concerning the current epidemic of myopia, namely, whether ethnic genetic differences play a role in the high prevalences of myopia characteristically seen in East Asia. Epidemiological evidence suggests that the major differences seen in the prevalence of myopia between ethnic groups are primarily based on different environmental exposures, because the prevalence of myopia reported for an ethnic group can be highly variable depending on location. A striking example comes from the high prevalence of myopia reported for the three major ethnic groups in Singapore. Chinese, Malays and Indians all have very high rates of myopia in Singapore [122, 123], whereas in Malaysia [124] and India [125], the rates are much lower. Recent results from the CREAM study [109] show that the percentage of variation explained by identified myopia-associated SNPs is higher in their Caucasians sample than in their East Asian sample, consistent with a greater role for environmental factors in the population where the epidemic of myopia has appeared.

6.5 Control of the Onset and Progression of Myopia

In the context of pathological myopia, there is now considerable interest in preventing the development of high myopia, because of the higher rate of occurrence of pathological myopia in those with high myopia. This is based on the assumption that lowering the prevalence of high myopia will result in a reduction in the development of pathological myopia. The large CREAM genetic studies have not identified any genes that are specifically associated with pathological myopia, although the SNPs associated with myopia with the largest effect sizes do seem to be associated with pathological myopia [105]. While there are clearly rare genetic forms of high myopia [108, 126], this is consistent with the epidemiological evidence that the recent increases in the prevalence of high myopia are an extension of the epidemic of school myopia, in which those with early onset of school myopia progress towards and achieve high myopia before they complete schooling [108, 126]. There has been considerable progress in this area, with atropine and imposed myopic defocus used to control progression of myopia, while increased time outdoors is used to slow the onset of myopia. Since it has been shown that the rate of myopia progression depends on age rather than the number of years that a child has been myopic [127], and that progression is higher in younger children, delaying the onset of myopia not only reduces the number of years for progression, but eliminates progression at ages where the progression rate is highest. In this area, studies on experimental myopia in animals have helped to increase understanding of the sites and mechanisms of action of the interventions.

6.5.1 Control of Myopia Progression with Atropine

Atropine was introduced to control the progression of myopia, based on the idea that myopia was due to excessive accommodation, and the initial successes seemed to give strong support to the excessive accommodation theory [129].

It is still the best validated technique for preventing myopic progression [111, 112], and it has been extensively used, particularly in Taiwan [130].

When muscarinic agents were first used in experimental myopia, their ability to block axial elongation was taken as strong evidence for an effect on accommodation. However, this assumption was critically explored by McBrien and colleagues, who showed that experimental myopia could be induced in animals with little accommodative capacity, such as grey squirrels [52]. McBrien [63] also pointed out that atropine was effective in chickens, where accommodation was controlled by nicotinic rather than muscarinic acetylcholine receptors. Other studies suggested that experimental myopia developed normally in animals in which accommodation had been experimentally disrupted [55]. A role for accommodation was also difficult to reconcile with the spatial localisation of experimental myopia [89].

Collectively, this evidence shifted attention to alternative sites of action. Studies on chicken chondrocytes and scleral tissue in culture showed that many muscarinic antagonists were able to exert direct effects on these tissues [131]. The other obvious site was the retina itself, given that it has an extensive cholinergic system, with both muscarinic and nicotinic elements. However, evidence on whether retinal sites are involved is ambiguous. Fischer and colleagues used a cholinergic toxin, which had been shown to destroy most cholinergic neurons in the chicken retina [132, 133], to show that eyes in which the cholinergic system had been extensively disrupted could still develop FDM and LIM, which could be blocked with atropine [132]. This evidence tended to favour a non-retinal, perhaps scleral, site of action.

However, other evidence tends to support a retinal site. Specifically, one of the earliest responses detected in response to myopigenic optical devices, which can be detected within 30 min, is decreased expression of the immediate early gene Egr-1 at both the mRNA and protein levels in the glucagon-immunoreactive amacrine cells of the chicken retina [134]. It should be noted that this part of the pathway may be specific to chickens and may not be applicable to the human retina. Atropine reverses this downregulation within 1 h of the fitting of a diffuser or negative lens [135]. It is hard to explain the rapidity of this effect in terms of a primary action of atropine on the sclera, with feedback to the retina. The ultimate test of site of action should come from a full pharmacological analysis of the three processes affected by muscarinic antagonists – block of axial elongation by muscarinic antagonists, block of scleral glycosaminoglycan synthesis and reversal of downregulation of Egr-1 in the retina. Whichever of the latter two replicates the pharmacology of the block of axial elongation is likely to be the site of action, although the subtleties of muscarinic cholinergic pharmacology may make discrimination difficult.

Irrespective of the outcome of this proposed three-way comparison, more detailed analysis of the receptors involved in blocking the development of myopia has been pursued. McBrien and colleagues have shown that the M4 antagonist himbacine blocks experimental myopia [136], and use of snake toxins which have a somewhat greater differential affinity for receptor subtypes has given further support to the idea that M4 receptors are involved [137, 138]. In chicken, which appears to lack Ml receptors, predominantly M4 receptors may be involved. However, in mammals, it appears that both Ml and M4 receptors are involved. This pharmacological characterisation is important because the use of atropine to control myopic progression has been limited because of the associated pupil dilation and block of accommodation which underlie its use as a cycloplegic agent. One approach to this problem is to use lower doses of atropine that avoid some of the side effects [111, 112]. The other is to more precisely define the receptors involved, so that agents with more specific actions can be developed.

Other evidence is accumulating that atropine's effects on axial elongation may be mediated by other types of receptors. The cholinergic pharmacology of block of axial elongation is very inconsistent [139]. Stell and colleagues have further shown that at the concentrations needed to block axial elongation, muscarinic antagonists also block the activation of alphaA2-adrenoceptors [139, 140] and that agonists of those receptors block axial elongation [141]. There are many other inconsistencies in research in this area, and while atropine has become a widely used tool for controlling myopia progression, animal research has so far raised more questions than it has answered in relation to mechanism and site of action.

6.5.2 Optical Control of Myopia Progression

There is considerable evidence that hyperopic defocus stimulates signals that stimulate eye growth, whereas myopic defocus inhibits axial elongation. This area has been extensively reviewed [11]. The kinetics of these signals and their spatial and temporal interactions have been extensively studied. Even short periods of imposed myopic defocus were effective in slowing axial elongation, whereas effective stimulation of axial elongation required essentially constant exposure to hyperopic defocus. Interruptions to FDM by removal of the diffusers of as little as 15 min significantly reduced the development of myopia [83, 84], and the effectiveness of this reduction was markedly increased if the light intensity was increased over this period [65] and decreased if the animals were kept in the dark [142]. In addition, the D2-dopamine antagonist spiperone blocked the inhibitory effects of diffuser removal in the light, and, thus, the inhibitory effect of removal of the diffusers seems to involve light-stimulated release of dopamine [142].

Experiments involving temporal interactions between these signals have also shown that relatively brief periods of

exposure to myopic defocus are able to block the effects of otherwise continuous exposure to hyperopic defocus [73, 74, 143–145]. This is also true when spatial interactions were examined. When only 25% of the field was myopically defocused, the amount of myopia was substantially reduced, and with one third of the field myopically defocused, hyperopic refractions were achieved [146, 147].

Perhaps the most important impact of this work has come from the use of imposed myopic defocus to inhibit the progression of myopia. Both spectacles [77, 79] and contact lenses [78, 148] that incorporate zones of myopic defocus simultaneously with optical correction have been developed. These provide substantial inhibition of myopia progression of at least 60%, for both changes in SER and axial length. These may enable the effective elimination of the increased levels of high myopia that have appeared in recent years, particularly in East and Southeast Asia, with a less invasive intervention than the use of atropine eye drops.

One important question about these effects of defocus is how they are translated into actions at the cellular and biochemical level, since this is necessary for optical interventions to be converted into changes in regulation of gene expression at the scleral level. In this area, there are only a few sign-posts, rather than well-defined pathways at this stage. One of the sign-posts is provided by the rate of release of the retinal transmitter dopamine. The actual rate of release is difficult to measure directly, and it is probably most robustly estimated by the rate of accumulation of the dopamine metabolite DOPAC in the vitreous in the first hours after application of the stimulus [149]. In both the FDM and LIM paradigms, where axial elongation is increased, dopamine release is decreased [149], and there is a parallel decrease in expression of the early intermediate gene Egr-1 [135, 150]. Dopamine appears to be causally involved, since administration of the dopamine agonist ADTN blocks the increase in axial elongation and reverses the decrease in Egr-1 [135]. Preclinical data on the use of levo-DOPA, a precursor of dopamine, indicates that topical application of this agent effectively controls the development of myopia in animal models [151–155]. However, the picture is not simple, because in the LIH paradigm, dopamine release is also decreased [156], but expression of Egr-1 is increased [134], and axial elongation is blocked. This suggests that dopamine release may be regulated by the decline in spatial contrast with blurred vision, or the resulting decline in temporal frequency of stimulation, but how the apparently causal connection between decreased dopamine release, increased expression of Egr-1 and increased axial elongation is reversed is not clear. There are some data implicating regulation of glucagon release as a subsequent step in the pathway [150, 157–160], but if and how these changes lead to the choroidal responses to defocus discussed earlier is not known.

6.5.3   Is Peripheral Defocus Important?

The idea that peripheral defocus might have an important role in the development and control of myopia originated in observations on eye shape in Dutch trainee pilots [161], which suggested that more prolate eyes at baseline (eyes with axial diameter greater than normal relative to equatorial diameter) were more likely to become myopic. Whether this is an accurate reading of the original paper has since been challenged [162], but this report stimulated the general hypothesis that early peripheral hyperopic defocus might promote the development of myopia.

This hypothesis was developed in a series of seminal papers by Smith and colleagues which showed that lesions to the central retina of the monkeys did not prevent the normal process of emmetropisation or prevent the development of FDM [163–165]. This showed that the peripheral retina was able to control central axial elongation, but further experiments were unable to definitively show that peripheral signals could override central signals. This area has now been extensively reviewed [45, 166].

This area has been pursued in two ways. Firstly, since myopic eyes tend to be more prolate than emmetropic eyes, the critical question is whether eyes that become myopic were more prolate than others prior to the onset of myopia. This idea has not fared well, and it appears that the appearance of a prolate eye shape is a consequence of, rather than a cause of, myopia [162, 167–169].

Even if a role for peripheral defocus in the appearance of incident myopia has not stood up, a possible role for peripheral hyperopic defocus as a continuing drive to myopic progression could still be valid. These questions have been addressed through the design of spectacles or contact lenses which reduce the level of peripheral hyperopia [170, 171]. In these clinical trials, the spectacles showed no significant protection from progression in the whole sample, but a significant effect in the subsample with myopic parents. These results underpinned the Zeiss MyoVision spectacles, but recently, these have been reported to have clinically insignificant effects in a Japanese trial [172].

6.5.4   Protective Effects of Time Outdoors

One of the observations that has excited considerable recent interest is that children who spend more time outdoors are less likely to be, or become, myopic [68, 69]. After considering a range of possibilities, we [68, 114] suggested that the most plausible explanation of this effect was that bright light outdoors stimulated the release of dopamine from the retina, which then acted as an inhibitor of axial elongation. This suggestion was based on considerable prior research on experimental myopia, both FDM and LIM, which suggested that one of the early steps in the development of experimental myopia was the suppression of dopamine release, with dopamine agonists able to inhibit axial elongation, as discussed previously.

This hypothesis was immediately translated into experimental situations, and it was shown that raising animals in lights brighter than those normally used in animal houses, from 15,000 to 30,000 lux as compared to normal experimental conditions of 100–500 lux, could substantially inhibit the development of FDM in chickens [68] and primates [173] and slow the development of LIM in chickens [69] and marginally in primates [174, 175]. It was also shown that the ability of bright light to block FDM was itself blocked by a D2-dopamine receptor antagonist, spiperone [69].

These very promising results need to be put into perspective in two ways. Firstly, the ranges of light intensity involved in the protective effects are commonly encountered in human environments. Indoor light intensities are generally in the range from 200 up to 1000 lux, with light intensities in animal houses at the lower end. Outdoor light intensities can range during the day and even in the shade on cloudy days, from several thousand lux up to 150,000 to 200,000 lux on bright sunny days. These, of course, can vary quite significantly by latitude and season, both in intensity and duration. More recent epidemiological results suggest that lower light intensities, of the order of 3–5000 lux, may be protective [176]. The lower light intensities apparently effective on humans may be due to limitations in the animal models, which require fitting of a diffuser or lens over the eye, and the need for constant stimulation to produce myopia. In contrast, the stimulus that drives myopia in humans does not involve obstructing vision and may be more intermittent.

Secondly, the protective effects seem to be quite substantial in the experimental studies discussed above and in epidemiological studies. Longitudinal data from the CLEERE study suggested that more than 14 hours a week of outdoor activity could overcome the higher prevalence of myopia seen in children with myopia parents [69], whereas data from the Sydney Myopia Study indicated that around 3 hours a day outdoors protected children from increased amounts of near work [68, 70]. The ability of increased time outdoors at school to slow the development of myopia in children has been confirmed in intervention trials [29, 176–178], and as a national school-based intervention in Taiwan [179].

The postulated mechanism for the protective effect from the development of myopia of more time outdoors, namely, increased exposure to brighter light outdoors, leading to greater dopamine release from the retina, and greater inhibition of axial elongation, has been confirmed in animal models including non-human primate models and is thus likely to play a major role in the prevention of the onset of myopia.

Using the FDM model of experimental myopia, complete prevention of the development of myopia can be achieved [173]. It is not obvious how this hypothesis could be further tested in humans.

An alternative to this model, based on a role for increased vitamin D production in children who spend more time outdoors, seems to be excluded by detailed longitudinal [180] and Mendelian randomisation [181] analysis. As noted previously, Flitcroft has postulated that the different patterns of defocus experienced indoors versus outdoors may also play a role [75]. This hypothesis is consistent with the numerous studies on the impact of imposed defocus on experimental myopia, but it has not otherwise been tested experimentally or as an intervention. More recently, he has postulated that the different spatial frequency components of indoor and outdoor environments, as well as of rural and urban environments, may play a role [76]. Again, while consistent with animal experimentation, this hypothesis has not been tested as an intervention. How much these mechanisms contribute to the protective effect of time outdoors, if at all, remains to be determined.

6.5.5 Changes in Scleral Metabolism

The sclera is the endpoint tissue in both human and experimental myopia, because changes in the sclera ultimately determine the axial length of the eye. During the development of human myopia, there are marked changes in scleral metabolism which result in thinning of the fibrous layer, which constitutes the bulk of the human sclera. As a result, it is also the site of the development of staphyloma, one of the most destructive pathological features of high myopia. Studies on human myopia have shown that the sclera from myopic eyes is thinner than normal and that marked reductions in the content and structure of collagens, as well as scleral glycosaminoglycans, have taken place. This area has been extensively reviewed [86, 87, 182], but there has been little progress in the past few years. This is surprising, because interventions to prevent changes in the sclera may be feasible.

Studies on human sclera are obviously limited to single-point determinations, except when culture systems, such as human scleral fibroblasts and retinal pigment epithelium cells. The HSF culture system has been used to document regulation of synthesis of brain morphogenetic proteins (BMPs) and matrix metalloproteases (MMPs) by retinoic acid, which have been implicated in the development of experimental myopia. More systematic use of this approach to examining changes in scleral metabolism looks promising.

One of the early events in the development of myopia at the scleral level appears to be upregulation of matrix metalloproteinase (MMP) activity [183].

Further work has implicated myofibroblasts in controlling the properties of the sclera [184, 185]. Myofibroblasts differentiate from fibroblasts and are highly contractile cells which express the smooth muscle protein alpha-smooth muscle actin. The differentiation of these cells can occur in response to local stresses, a process involving regulation of the synthesis of extracellular matrix constituents. They could therefore play a role in enabling the sclera to adjust for fluctuating intraocular pressure and other stresses. Cell adhesion molecules such as integrins play a key role in mediating cell-matrix interactions, and again McBrien and colleagues have shown rapid downregulation of the expression of alpha and alpha2 integrin subunits [186]. The expression of these two subunits seems to be differentially regulated during the development of myopia.

McBrien has proposed that transforming growth factor-beta (TGF-beta) is a key regulator in the sclera [182]. The three mammalian isoforms of TGF-beta change rapidly in response to stimuli that induce experimental myopia and regulate collagen and glycosaminoglycan production, as well as sclera, but it is only in the sclera that regulation occurs in relation to myopigenic stimuli.

It is important to note that mutations in many genes involved in this complex integrated response have been identified in human genetic studies as candidate genes, along with a number other scleral constituents [107, 109]. This suggests that the sclera in myopia can be both the direct site of action of mutations that affect extracellular matrix metabolism and cause a weaker sclera and the site of modulation of scleral metabolism in response to upstream mutations.

6.5.6 A Heuristic Model of Growth Control

Based on the evidence we have reviewed in this chapter, we propose a model that we believe will be useful for orienting future studies on both human and experimental myopia (Fig. 6.2). Key players are the transmitter dopamine and the dopaminergic amacrine cells. These may be involved in a number of human conditions in which myopia is a feature, including rod-cone dystrophies, retinitis pigmentosa and congenital stationary night blindness. The mutations involved, which primarily affect visual processing at the photoreceptor and ON-bipolar cell level, may also affect the functioning of the downstream dopaminergic amacrine cells, and when this results in reduced dopamine release, then, based on the findings in animal models, myopia might be expected to develop, although the possibility that dopaminergic function has been perturbed in these conditions has not yet been tested.

Dopamine release is also controlled by environmental conditions. Simulation with low contrast and low spatial frequency patterns, such as are experienced in experimental

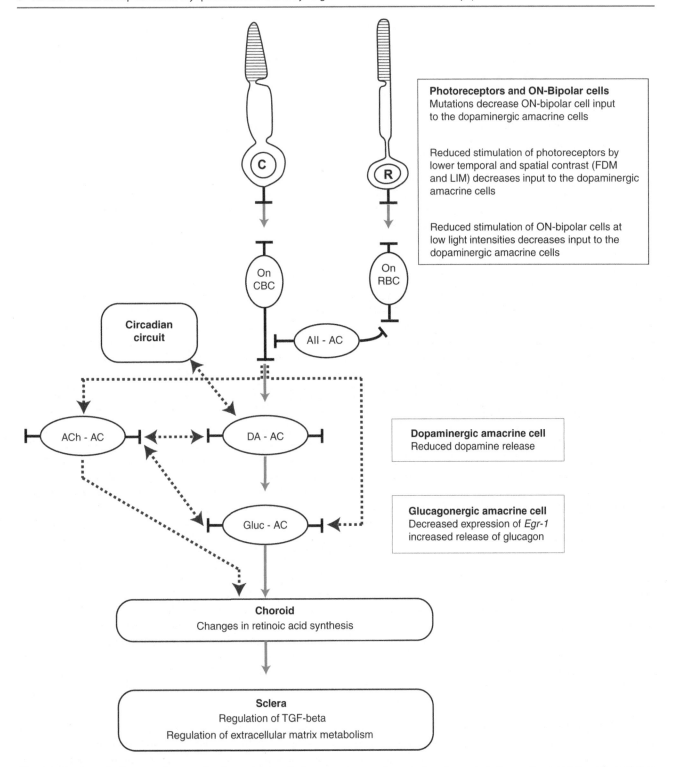

Photoreceptors and ON-Bipolar cells
Mutations decrease ON-bipolar cell input
to the dopaminergic amacrine cells

Reduced stimulation of photoreceptors by
lower temporal and spatial contrast (FDM
and LIM) decreases input to the dopaminergic
amacrine cells

Reduced stimulation of ON-bipolar cells at
low light intensities decreases input to the
dopaminergic amacrine cells

Dopaminergic amacrine cell
Reduced dopamine release

Glucagonergic amacrine cell
Decreased expression of *Egr-1*
increased release of glucagon

Fig. 6.2 A schematic diagram of a general pathway that may be important in the control of eye growth. A key element is the link from photoreceptors though ON-bipolar cells and dopaminergic amacrine cells into the inner retina, where the first stages of growth signal cascades, which ultimately control scleral metabolism and growth, are generated. Animal studies strongly support a role for dopaminergic amacrine cells in growth control, and recent studies on the protective effect of time outdoors in children also suggest that dopamine may be involved in human myopia. Key: C Cone photoreceptor, R Rod photoreceptor, On CBC On-cone bipolar cell, On RBC On-rod bipolar cell, All-AC All amacrine cell, Ach-AC Acetylcholine amacrine cell, DA-AC Dopaminergic amacrine cell, Gluc-AC Glucagonergic amacrine cell

FDM, leads to myopia associated with low dopamine release from the retina. Based on the involvement of dopamine in these animal models, it was postulated that the protective effects of bright light outdoors on the development of myopia in children might be mediated by increased release of dopamine, and subsequent reduction in axial elongation – a further hypothesis based on animal experimentation. It is difficult to imagine how this hypothesis could be tested on humans, but it has been tested in animal models of myopia, where increased light intensity has been shown to reduce the development of experimental myopia, and particularly of FDM. The protective effect of exposure to bright light was blocked by administration of a dopaminergic antagonist, providing further support for the hypothesis.

Within the inner retina, a key event in animal models that correlates with the development of myopia is decreased dopamine release and the downregulation of the expression of the early immediate gene Egr-1. Dopamine agonists and muscarinic antagonists, which block experimental myopia, reverse this downregulation, resulting in enhanced levels of expression of Egr-1. Similar effects are observed after removal of the diffuser or negative lens. Most of the experiments have been carried on chickens, but there is limited evidence that similar regulatory events also occur in mammalian retinas. This nexus of changes provides a good basis for screening for myopia control agents, since so far, all agents that block the development of experimental myopia reverse the downregulation of Egr-1 expression seen in the FDM and LIM paradigms.

An obvious question is what further pathways are regulated by Egr-1. Glucagon amacrine cells have been implicated, but so far little detailed work has been done. Later steps in the process, such as changes in the choroid, have hardly been studied, and these changes in the retina and choroid have not yet been clearly linked to the metabolic and structural changes in the sclera that directly underpin the development of myopia.

6.6   Conclusions

A range of paradigms in which changes in myopia, or more generally in eye growth, can be induced experimentally have been developed. None of them precisely matches the characteristic patterns of development of human myopia, with particular problems associated with the methods used to induce myopia and the developmental stage at which myopia is induced. Non-human primates provide the animal model that best matches human myopia, but there are considerable commonalities between the models at a molecular level. It is important to note that some of the implications drawn from animal models, such as the idea that myopia should be self-limiting because myopic defocus prevents axial elongation, and that correction of myopia is dangerous since it would promote progression, are erroneous. Thus, considerable caution needs to be exercised in extrapolating from animal models to human myopia.

Arguably, despite these cautions, the most important contribution made by animal experimentation is the evidence that defocus can influence axial elongation. In particular, the evidence that imposed myopia defocus can inhibit axial elongation has led directly to the development of both spectacle and contact lenses that can control myopia progression, which have an important role to play in limiting the development of high myopia and ultimately pathological myopia.

Animal models have also played a key role in confirming that the protective effects of time outdoors are mediated, at least in part, by exposure to bright light, increases in the release of dopamine from the retina and inhibition of axial elongation. The information flow in this case was from human epidemiology to an experimental hypothesis, which was then tested with animal models, since testing it directly in humans would be impossible. Early experiments with the animal models did look at variations in light exposures, but not in a way that led to the hypothesis that light exposure could inhibit myopia.

Animal models have played a more confusing role in relation to atropine. The simple idea that atropine acts on muscarinic receptors in the retina to control axial elongation is not consistent with the evidence from animal experiments, but so far a definite mechanism and site of action have not been determined, and most of the information we have on the site an action of atropine, now widely used to control myopia progression in children, comes from animal studies. At this stage, however, it has to be said that neither site nor mechanism of action has been determined.

These examples show how there can be powerful synergy between animal studies and human studies, resulting in interventions to control human myopia. With the vast increase in recent years in our understanding of the aetiology and environmental risk factors for human myopia and of biological pathways that control eye growth, further advances seem likely to occur. Unfortunately, the prospects for developing an animal model of pathological myopia are not promising, because the epidemiology of human pathological myopia suggests that it requires the development of high myopia, and a substantial time for significant pathology to appear. But, more optimistically, the development of methods for the control of the onset and progression of myopia, where animal models have made substantial contributions, should enable substantial reductions in the burden of high myopia and pathological myopia in the future.

References

1. Curtin BJ. The myopias. New York: Harper and Row; 1985.
2. Levinsohn G. Reply to criticisms of my theory on the genesis of myopia. Arch Ophthalmol. 1936;15:84.
3. Young FA. The development and retention of myopia by monkeys. Am J Optom Arch Am Acad Optom. 1961;38:545–55. Epub 1961/10/01.
4. Wiesel TN, Raviola E. Myopia and eye enlargement after neonatal lid fusion in monkeys. Nature. 1977;266(5597):66–8. Epub 1977/03/03.
5. Wallman J, Turkel J, Trachtman J. Extreme myopia produced by modest change in early visual experience. Science. 1978;201(4362):1249–51. Epub 1978/09/29.
6. Tejedor J, de la Villa P. Refractive changes induced by form deprivation in the mouse eye. Invest Ophthalmol Vis Sci. 2003;44(1):32–6. Epub 2002/12/31.
7. Barathi VA, Boopathi VG, Yap EP, Beuerman RW. Two models of experimental myopia in the mouse. Vis Res. 2008;48(7):904–16. Epub 2008/02/22.
8. Howlett MH, McFadden SA. Spectacle lens compensation in the pigmented guinea pig. Vis Res. 2009;49(2):219–27. Epub 2008/11/11.
9. Howlett MH, McFadden SA. Form-deprivation myopia in the guinea pig (Cavia porcellus). Vis Res. 2006;46(1–2):267–83. Epub 2005/09/06.
10. Sherman SM, Norton TT, Casagrande VA. Myopia in the lid-sutured tree shrew (Tupaia glis). Brain Res. 1977;124(1):154–7. Epub 1977/03/18.
11. Wallman J, Winawer J. Homeostasis of eye growth and the question of myopia. Neuron. 2004;43(4):447–68. Epub 2004/08/18.
12. Cook RC, Glasscock RE. Refractive and ocular findings in the newborn. Am J Ophthalmol. 1951;34(10):1407–13. Epub 1951/10/01.
13. Mayer DL, Hansen RM, Moore BD, Kim S, Fulton AB. Cycloplegic refractions in healthy children aged 1 through 48 months. Arch Ophthalmol. 2001;119(11):1625–8. Epub 2001/11/16.
14. Mutti DO, Mitchell GL, Jones LA, Friedman NE, Frane SL, Lin WK, et al. Axial growth and changes in lenticular and corneal power during emmetropization in infants. Invest Ophthalmol Vis Sci. 2005;46(9):3074–80. Epub 2005/08/27.
15. Pennie FC, Wood IC, Olsen C, White S, Charman WN. A longitudinal study of the biometric and refractive changes in full-term infants during the first year of life. Vis Res. 2001;41(21):2799–810. Epub 2001/10/06.
16. Morgan IG, Rose KA, Ellwein LB. Is emmetropia the natural end-point for human refractive development? An analysis of population-based data from the refractive error study in children (RESC). Acta Ophthalmol. 2010;88(8):877–84. Epub 2009/12/05.
17. Ojaimi E, Rose KA, Morgan IG, Smith W, Martin FJ, Kifley A, et al. Distribution of ocular biometric parameters and refraction in a population-based study of Australian children. Invest Ophthalmol Vis Sci. 2005;46(8):2748–54. Epub 2005/07/27.
18. Morgan IG, French AN, Ashby RS, et al. The epidemics of myopia: Aetiology and prevention. Prog Retin Eye Res. 2018;62:134–49.
19. Morgan IG, He M, Rose KA. EPIDEMIC OF PATHOLOGIC MYOPIA: what can laboratory studies and epidemiology tell us? Retina. 2017;37:989–97.
20. Iribarren R, Morgan IG, Chan YH, Lin X, Saw SM. Changes in lens power in Singapore Chinese children during refractive development. Invest Ophthalmol Vis Sci. 2012;53:5124–30.
21. Jones LA, Mitchell GL, Mutti DO, Hayes JR, Moeschberger ML, Zadnik K. Comparison of ocular component growth curves among refractive error groups in children. Invest Ophthalmol Vis Sci. 2005;46(7):2317–27. Epub 2005/06/28.
22. Wong HB, Machin D, Tan SB, Wong TY, Saw SM. Ocular component growth curves among Singaporean children with different refractive error status. Invest Ophthalmol Vis Sci. 2010;51(3):1341–7. Epub 2009/10/31.
23. Mutti DO, Mitchell GL, Sinnott LT, Jones-Jordan LA, Moeschberger ML, Cotter SA, et al. Corneal and crystalline lens dimensions before and after myopia onset. Optom Vis Sci. 2012;89(3):251–62. Epub 2012/01/10.
24. Xiang F, He M, Morgan IG. Annual changes in refractive errors and ocular components before and after the onset of myopia in Chinese children. Ophthalmology. 2012;119(7):1478–84. Epub 2012/05/15.
25. Iribarren R. Crystalline lens and refractive development. Prog Retin Eye Res. 2015;47:86–106.
26. Guo X, Fu M, Ding X, Morgan IG, Zeng Y, He M. Significant axial elongation with minimal change in refraction in 3- to 6-year-old Chinese preschoolers: the Shenzhen Kindergarten eye study. Ophthalmology. 2017;
27. Lan W, Zhao F, Lin L, et al. Refractive errors in 3-6 year-old Chinese children: a very low prevalence of myopia? PLoS One. 2013;8:e78003.
28. Ma Y, Qu X, Zhu X, et al. Age-specific prevalence of visual impairment and refractive error in children aged 3-10 years in Shanghai, China. Invest Ophthalmol Vis Sci. 2016;57:6188–96.
29. He M, Xiang F, Zeng Y, et al. Effect of time spent outdoors at school on the development of myopia among children in China: a randomized clinical trial. JAMA. 2015;314:1142–8.
30. Wu JF, Bi HS, Wang SM, et al. Refractive error, visual acuity and causes of vision loss in children in Shandong, China. The Shandong children eye study. PLoS One. 2013;8:e82763.
31. Giordano L, Friedman DS, Repka MX, Katz J, Ibironke J, Hawes P, et al. Prevalence of refractive error among preschool children in an urban population: the Baltimore Pediatric Eye Disease Study. Ophthalmology. 2009;116(4):739–46, 46 e1–4. Epub 2009/02/27.
32. O'Donoghue L, McClelland JF, Logan NS, Rudnicka AR, Owen CG, Saunders KJ. Refractive error and visual impairment in school children in Northern Ireland. Br J Ophthalmol. 2010;94:1155–9.
33. Twelker JD, Mitchell GL, Messer DH, et al. Children's ocular components and age, gender, and ethnicity. Optom Vis Sci. 2009;86:918–35.
34. Wen G, Tarczy-Hornoch K, McKean-Cowdin R, et al. Prevalence of myopia, hyperopia, and astigmatism in non-Hispanic white and Asian children: multi-ethnic pediatric eye disease study. Ophthalmology. 2013;120:2109–16.
35. Multi-Ethnic Pediatric Eye Disease Study Group. Prevalence of myopia and hyperopia in 6- to 72-month-old African American and Hispanic children: the multi-ethnic pediatric eye disease study. Ophthalmology. 2010;117(1):140–7.e3. Epub 2009/11/21.
36. Dirani M, Chan YH, Gazzard G, Hornbeak DM, Leo SW, Selvaraj P, et al. Prevalence of refractive error in Singaporean Chinese children: the strabismus, amblyopia, and refractive error in young Singaporean children (STARS) study. Invest Ophthalmol Vis Sci. 2010;51(3):1348–55. Epub 2009/11/26.
37. Saw SM, Carkeet A, Chia KS, Stone RA, Tan DT. Component dependent risk factors for ocular parameters in Singapore Chinese children. Ophthalmology. 2002;109:2065–71.
38. Yam JC, Tang SM, Kam KW, et al. High prevalence of myopia in children and their parents in Hong Kong Chinese Population: the Hong Kong children eye study. Acta Ophthalmol. 2020; in press
39. Lin LL, Shih YF, Hsiao CK, CJ. Prevalence of myopia in Taiwanese schoolchildren: 1983 to 2000. Ann Acad Med Singapore. 2004;33:27–33.
40. Flitcroft DI. Is myopia a failure of homeostasis? Exp Eye Res. 2013;114:16–24.

41. Flitcroft DI. Emmetropisation and the aetiology of refractive errors. Eye (Lond). 2014;28:169–79.

42. Wildsoet CF. Active emmetropization–evidence for its existence and ramifications for clinical practice. Ophthalmic Physiol Opt. 1997;17(4):279–90. Epub 1997/07/01.

43. Anderson HA, Glasser A, Manny RE, Stuebing KK. Age-related changes in accommodative dynamics from preschool to adulthood. Invest Ophthalmol Vis Sci. 2010;51(1):614–22. Epub 2009/08/18.

44. Qiao-Grider Y, Hung LF, Kee CS, Ramamirtham R. Smith 3rd EL. Normal ocular development in young rhesus monkeys (Macaca mulatta). Vis Res. 2007;47(11):1424–44. Epub 2007/04/10.

45. Smith EL 3rd. Prentice award lecture 2010: a case for peripheral optical treatment strategies for myopia. Optom Vis Sci. 2011;88(9):1029–44. Epub 2011/07/13.

46. Sorsby A, Sheridan M, Leary GA, Benjamin B. Vision, visual acuity, and ocular refraction of young men: findings in a sample of 1,033 subjects. Br Med J. 1960;1(5183):1394–8. Epub 1960/05/07.

47. Mutti DO, Sinnott LT, Mitchell GL, et al. Relative peripheral refractive error and the risk of onset and progression of myopia in children. Invest Ophthalmol Vis Sci. 2011;52:199–205.

48. Thorn F, Gwiazda J, Held R. Myopia progression is specified by a double exponential growth function. Optom Vis Sci. 2005;82:286–97.

49. Hoyt CS, Stone RD, Fromer C, Billson FA. Monocular axial myopia associated with neonatal eyelid closure in human infants. Am J Ophthalmol. 1981;91(2):197–200. Epub 1981/02/01.

50. Schaeffel F, Glasser A, Howland HC. Accommodation, refractive error and eye growth in chickens. Vis Res. 1988;28(5):639–57. Epub 1988/01/01.

51. Irving EL, Callender MG, Sivak JG. Inducing myopia, hyperopia, and astigmatism in chicks. Optom Vis Sci. 1991;68(5):364–8. Epub 1991/05/01.

52. McBrien NA, Moghaddam HO, New R, Williams LR. Experimental myopia in a diurnal mammal (Sciurus carolinensis) with no accommodative ability. J Physiol. 1993;469:427–41. Epub 1993/09/01.

53. McBrien NA, Moghaddam HO, Reeder AP. Atropine reduces experimental myopia and eye enlargement via a nonaccommodative mechanism. Invest Ophthalmol Vis Sci. 1993;34(1):205–15. Epub 1993/01/01.

54. Schaeffel F, Troilo D, Wallman J, Howland HC. Developing eyes that lack accommodation grow to compensate for imposed defocus. Vis Neurosci. 1990;4(2):177–83. Epub 1990/02/01.

55. Wildsoet C. Neural pathways subserving negative lens-induced emmetropization in chicks–insights from selective lesions of the optic nerve and ciliary nerve. Curr Eye Res. 2003;27(6):371–85. Epub 2004/01/06.

56. Guo L, Frost MR, He L, Siegwart JT Jr, Norton TT. Gene expression signatures in tree shrew sclera in response to three myopiagenic conditions. Invest Ophthalmol Vis Sci. 2013;54:6806–19.

57. Morgan IG, Ashby RS, Nickla DL. Form deprivation and lens-induced myopia: are they different? Ophthalmic Physiol Opt. 2013;33:355–61.

58. Wallman J, Adams JI. Developmental aspects of experimental myopia in chicks: susceptibility, recovery and relation to emmetropization. Vis Res. 1987;27(7):1139–63. Epub 1987/01/01.

59. McBrien NA, Gentle A, Cottriall C. Optical correction of induced axial myopia in the tree shrew: implications for emmetropization. Optom Vis Sci. 1999;76(6):419–27. Epub 1999/07/23.

60. Wildsoet CF, Schmid KL. Optical correction of form deprivation myopia inhibits refractive recovery in chick eyes with intact or sectioned optic nerves. Vis Res. 2000;40(23):3273–82. Epub 2000/09/29. .PubMed

61. Zhu X, McBrien NA, Smith EL 3rd, Troilo D, Wallman J. Eyes in various species can shorten to compensate for myopic defocus. Invest Ophthalmol Vis Sci. 2013;54:2634–44.

62. Guo L, Frost MR, Siegwart JT Jr, Norton TT. Gene expression signatures in tree shrew sclera during recovery from minus-lens wear and during plus-lens wear. Mol Vis. 2019;25:311–28.

63. Huang HM, Chang DS, Wu PC. The Association between near work activities and myopia in children-a systematic review and meta-analysis. PLoS One. 2015;10:e0140419.

64. Mutti DO, Zadnik K. Has near work's star fallen? Optom Vis Sci. 2009;86(2):76–8. Epub 2009/01/22.

65. Ashby R, Ohlendorf A, Schaeffel F. The effect of ambient illuminance on the development of deprivation myopia in chicks. Invest Ophthalmol Vis Sci. 2009;50(11):5348–54. Epub 2009/06/12.

66. Ashby RS, Schaeffel F. The effect of bright light on lens compensation in chicks. Invest Ophthalmol Vis Sci. 2010;51(10):5247–53. Epub 2010/05/07.

67. Smith EL 3rd, Hung LF, Huang J. Protective effects of high ambient lighting on the development of form-deprivation myopia in rhesus monkeys. Invest Ophthalmol Vis Sci. 2012;53(1):421–8. Epub 2011/12/16.

68. Rose KA, Morgan IG, Ip J, Kifley A, Huynh S, Smith W, et al. Outdoor activity reduces the prevalence of myopia in children. Ophthalmology. 2008;115(8):1279–85. Epub 2008/02/26.

69. Jones LA, Sinnott LT, Mutti DO, Mitchell GL, Moeschberger ML, Zadnik K. Parental history of myopia, sports and outdoor activities, and future myopia. Invest Ophthalmol Vis Sci. 2007;48(8):3524–32. Epub 2007/07/27.

70. Rose KA, Morgan IG, Smith W, Burlutsky G, Mitchell P, Saw SM. Myopia, lifestyle, and schooling in students of Chinese ethnicity in Singapore and Sydney. Arch Ophthalmol. 2008;126(4):527–30. Epub 2008/04/17.

71. Gwiazda J, Thorn F, Held R. Accommodation, accommodative convergence, and response AC/A ratios before and at the onset of myopia in children. Optom Vis Sci. 2005;82(4):273–8. Epub 2005/04/15.

72. Mutti DO, Mitchell GL, Hayes JR, Jones LA, Moeschberger ML, Cotter SA, et al. Accommodative lag before and after the onset of myopia. Invest Ophthalmol Vis Sci. 2006;47(3):837–46. Epub 2006/03/01.

73. Zhu X, Park TW, Winawer J, Wallman J. In a matter of minutes, the eye can know which way to grow. Invest Ophthalmol Vis Sci. 2005;46(7):2238–41. Epub 2005/06/28.

74. Zhu X, Winawer JA, Wallman J. Potency of myopic defocus in spectacle lens compensation. Invest Ophthalmol Vis Sci. 2003;44:2818–27.

75. Flitcroft DI. The complex interactions of retinal, optical and environmental factors in myopia aetiology. Prog Retin Eye Res. 2012;31(6):622–60. Epub 2012/07/10.

76. Flitcroft DI, Harb EN, Wildsoet CF. The spatial frequency content of urban and indoor environments as a potential risk factor for myopia development. Invest Ophthalmol Vis Sci. 2020;61:42.

77. Bao J, Yang A, Huang Y, et al. One-year myopia control efficacy of spectacle lenses with aspherical lenslets. Br J Ophthalmol. 2021;

78. Chamberlain P, Peixoto-de-Matos SC, Logan NS, Ngo C, Jones D, Young G. A 3-year randomized clinical trial of MiSight lenses for myopia control. Optom Vis Sci. 2019;96:556–67.

79. Lam CSY, Tang WC, Tse DY, et al. Defocus Incorporated Multiple Segments (DIMS) spectacle lenses slow myopia progression: a 2-year randomised clinical trial. Br J Ophthalmol. 2020;104:363–8.

80. Cohen Y, Belkin M, Yehezkel O, Solomon AS, Polat U. Dependency between light intensity and refractive develop-

ment under light–dark cycles. Exp Eye Res. 2011;92(1):40–6. Epub 2010/11/09.

81. Cohen Y, Peleg E, Belkin M, Polat U, Solomon AS. Ambient illuminance, retinal dopamine release and refractive development in chicks. Exp Eye Res. 2012;103:33–40. Epub 2012/09/11.

82. She Z, Hung LF, Arumugam B, Beach KM, Smith EL 3rd. Effects of low intensity ambient lighting on refractive development in infant rhesus monkeys (Macaca mulatta). Vision Res. 2020;176:48–59.

83. Napper GA, Brennan NA, Barrington M, Squires MA, Vessey GA, Vingrys AJ. The duration of normal visual exposure necessary to prevent form deprivation myopia in chicks. Vis Res. 1995;35(9):1337–44. Epub 1995/05/01.

84. Napper GA, Brennan NA, Barrington M, Squires MA, Vessey GA, Vingrys AJ. The effect of an interrupted daily period of normal visual stimulation on form deprivation myopia in chicks. Vis Res. 1997;37(12):1557–64. Epub 1997/06/01.

85. Schmid KL, Wildsoet CF. Effects on the compensatory responses to positive and negative lenses of intermittent lens wear and ciliary nerve section in chicks. Vision Res. 1996;36:1023–36.

86. McBrien NA, Gentle A. Role of the sclera in the development and pathological complications of myopia. Prog Retin Eye Res. 2003;22(3):307–38. Epub 2003/07/11.

87. Rada JA, Shelton S, Norton TT. The sclera and myopia. Exp Eye Res. 2006;82(2):185–200. Epub 2005/10/06.

88. Troilo D, Gottlieb MD, Wallman J. Visual deprivation causes myopia in chicks with optic nerve section. Curr Eye Res. 1987;6(8):993–9. Epub 1987/08/01.

89. Wallman J, Gottlieb MD, Rajaram V, Fugate-Wentzek LA. Local retinal regions control local eye growth and myopia. Science. 1987;237(4810):73–7. Epub 1987/07/03.

90. Diether S, Schaeffel F. Local changes in eye growth induced by imposed local refractive error despite active accommodation. Vis Res. 1997;37(6):659–68. Epub 1997/03/01.

91. Feldkaemper M, Schaeffel F. An updated view on the role of dopamine in myopia. Exp Eye Res. 2013;114:106–19.

92. Wallman J, Wildsoet C, Xu A, Gottlieb MD, Nickla DL, Marran L, et al. Moving the retina: choroidal modulation of refractive state. Vis Res. 1995;35(1):37–50. Epub 1995/01/01.

93. Wildsoet C, Wallman J. Choroidal and scleral mechanisms of compensation for spectacle lenses in chicks. Vis Res. 1995;35(9):1175–94. Epub 1995/05/01.

94. Troilo D, Nickla DL, Wildsoet CF. Choroidal thickness changes during altered eye growth and refractive state in a primate. Invest Ophthalmol Vis Sci. 2000;41(6):1249–58. Epub 2000/05/08.

95. Chakraborty R, Read SA, Collins MJ. Monocular myopic defocus and daily changes in axial length and choroidal thickness of human eyes. Exp Eye Res. 2012;103:47–54. Epub 2012/09/14.

96. Chakraborty R, Read SA, Collins MJ. Diurnal variations in axial length, choroidal thickness, intraocular pressure, and ocular biometrics. Invest Ophthalmol Vis Sci. 2011;52(8):5121–9. Epub 2011/05/17.

97. Nickla DL, Damyanova P, Lytle G. Inhibiting the neuronal isoform of nitric oxide synthase has similar effects on the compensatory choroidal and axial responses to myopic defocus in chicks as does the non-specific inhibitor L-NAME. Exp Eye Res. 2009;88(6):1092–9. Epub 2009/05/20.

98. Nickla DL, Totonelly K. Choroidal thickness predicts ocular growth in normal chicks but not in eyes with experimentally altered growth. Clin Exp Optom. 2015;98:564–70.

99. Nickla DL, Totonelly K. Dopamine antagonists and brief vision distinguish lens-induced- and form-deprivation-induced myopia. Exp Eye Res. 2011;93(5):782–5. Epub 2011/08/30.

100. Nickla DL, Wilken E, Lytle G, Yom S, Mertz J. Inhibiting the transient choroidal thickening response using the nitric oxide synthase inhibitor l-NAME prevents the ameliorative effects of visual expe-

rience on ocular growth in two different visual paradigms. Exp Eye Res. 2006;83(2):456–64. Epub 2006/04/26.

101. Nickla DL, Wallman J. The multifunctional choroid. Prog Retin Eye Res. 2010;29(2):144–68. Epub 2010/01/02.

102. Sorsby A, Sheridan M, Leary GA. Refraction and its components in twins. Memo Med Res Counc. 1961;301(Special):1–43.

103. Morgan I, Rose K. How genetic is school myopia? Prog Retin Eye Res. 2005;24(1):1–38. Epub 2004/11/24.

104. Morgan IG, Rose KA. Myopia: is the nature-nurture debate finally over? Clin Exp Optom. 2019;102:3–17.

105. Hysi PG, Choquet H, Khawaja AP, et al. Meta-analysis of 542,934 subjects of European ancestry identifies new genes and mechanisms predisposing to refractive error and myopia. Nat Genet. 2020;52:401–7.

106. Morgan IG, Ohno-Matsui K, Saw SM. Myopia. Lancet. 2012;379:1739–48.

107. Wojciechowski R. Nature and nurture: the complex genetics of myopia and refractive error. Clin Genet. 2011;79(4):301–20. Epub 2010/12/16.

108. Flitcroft DI, Loughman J, Wildsoet CF, Williams C, Guggenheim JA, Consortium C. Novel myopia genes and pathways identified from syndromic forms of myopia. Invest Ophthalmol Vis Sci. 2018;59:338–48.

109. Tedja MS, Wojciechowski R, Hysi PG, et al. Genome-wide association meta-analysis highlights light-induced signaling as a driver for refractive error. Nat Genet. 2018;50:834–48.

110. Wojciechowski R, Hysi PG. Focusing in on the complex genetics of myopia. PLoS Genet. 2013;9:e1003442.

111. Chia A, Chua WH, Cheung YB, Wong WL, Lingham A, Fong A, et al. Atropine for the treatment of childhood myopia: safety and efficacy of 0.5%, 0.1%, and 0.01% doses (atropine for the treatment of myopia 2). Ophthalmology. 2012;119(2): 347–54.

112. Yam JC, Jiang Y, Tang SM, et al. Low-Concentration Atropine for Myopia Progression (LAMP) study: a randomized, double-blinded, placebo-controlled trial of 0.05%, 0.025%, and 0.01% atropine eye drops in myopia control. Ophthalmology. 2019;126:113–24.

113. Fang YT, Chou YJ, Pu C, Lin PJ, Liu TL, Huang N, et al. Prescription of atropine eye drops among children diagnosed with myopia in Taiwan from 2000 to 2007: a nationwide study. Eye (Lond). 2013;27(3):418–24. Epub 2013/01/05.

114. French AN, Ashby RS, Morgan IG, Rose KA. Time outdoors and the prevention of myopia. Exp Eye Res. 2013;114:58–68.

115. Solouki AM, Verhoeven VJ, van Duijn CM, Verkerk AJ, Ikram MK, Hysi PG, et al. A genome-wide association study identifies a susceptibility locus for refractive errors and myopia at 15q14. Nat Genet. 2010;42(10):897–901. Epub 2010/09/14.

116. Guggenheim JA, Ghorbani Mojarrad N, Williams C, Flitcroft DI. Genetic prediction of myopia: prospects and challenges. Ophthalmic Physiol Opt. 2017;37:549–56.

117. Stone RA, Khurana TS. Gene profiling in experimental models of eye growth: clues to myopia pathogenesis. Vis Res. 2010;50(23):2322–33. Epub 2010/04/07.

118. Stone RA, Pardue MT, Iuvone PM, Khurana TS. Pharmacology of myopia and potential role for intrinsic retinal circadian rhythms. Exp Eye Res. 2013;114:35–47.

119. Chen YP, Hocking PM, Wang L, Povazay B, Prashar A, To CH, et al. Selective breeding for susceptibility to myopia reveals a gene-environment interaction. Invest Ophthalmol Vis Sci. 2011;52(7):4003–11. Epub 2011/03/26.

120. Chen YP, Prashar A, Erichsen JT, To CH, Hocking PM, Guggenheim JA. Heritability of ocular component dimensions in chickens: genetic variants controlling susceptibility to experimentally induced myopia and pretreatment eye size are distinct. Invest Ophthalmol Vis Sci. 2011;52(7):4012–20. Epub 2011/03/26.

121. Chen YP, Prashar A, Hocking PM, Erichsen JT, To CH, Schaeffel F, et al. Sex, eye size, and the rate of myopic eye growth due to form deprivation in outbred white leghorn chickens. Invest Ophthalmol Vis Sci. 2010;51(2):651–7. Epub 2009/09/10.

122. Au Eong KG, Tay TH, Lim MK. Race, culture and Myopia in 110,236 young Singaporean males. Singapore Med J. 1993;34:29–32.

123. Koh V, Yang A, Saw SM, et al. Differences in prevalence of refractive errors in young Asian males in Singapore between 1996-1997 and 2009-2010. Ophthalmic Epidemiol. 2014;21:247–55.

124. Goh PP, Abqariyah Y, Pokharel GP, Ellwein LB. Refractive error and visual impairment in school-age children in Gombak District, Malaysia. Ophthalmology. 2005;112:678–85.

125. Saxena R, Vashist P, Tandon R, et al. Prevalence of myopia and its risk factors in urban school children in Delhi: the North India Myopia Study (NIM Study). PLoS One. 2015;10:e0117349.

126. Hawthorne FA, Young TL. Genetic contributions to myopic refractive error: insights from human studies and supporting evidence from animal models. Exp Eye Res. 2013;114:141–9.

127. Chua SY, Sabanayagam C, Cheung YB, et al. Age of onset of myopia predicts risk of high myopia in later childhood in myopic Singapore children. Ophthalmic Physiol Opt. 2016;36:388–94.

128. Sankaridurg PR, Holden BA. Practical applications to modify and control the development of ametropia. Eye (Lond). 2014;28:134–41.

129. Bedrossian RH. The effect of atropine on myopia. Ophthalmology. 1979;86(5):713–9. Epub 1979/05/01.

130. Fang YT, Chou YJ, Pu C, et al. Prescription of atropine eye drops among children diagnosed with myopia in Taiwan from 2000 to 2007: a nationwide study. Eye (Lond). 2013;27:418–24.

131. Lind GJ, Chew SJ, Marzani D, Wallman J. Muscarinic acetylcholine receptor antagonists inhibit chick scleral chondrocytes. Invest Ophthalmol Vis Sci. 1998;39(12):2217–31. Epub 1998/11/06.

132. Fischer AJ, Miethke P, Morgan IG, Stell WK. Cholinergic amacrine cells are not required for the progression and atropine-mediated suppression of form-deprivation myopia. Brain Res. 1998;794:48–60.

133. Millar TJ, Ishimoto I, Boelen M, Epstein ML, Johnson CD, Morgan IG. The toxic effects of ethylcholine mustard aziridinium ion on cholinergic cells in the chicken retina. J Neurosci. 1987;7:343–56.

134. Fischer AJ, McGuire JJ, Schaeffel F, Stell WK. Light- and focus-dependent expression of the transcription factor ZENK in the chick retina. Nat Neurosci. 1999;2(8):706–12. Epub 1999/07/21.

135. Ashby R, McCarthy CS, Maleszka R, Megaw P, Morgan IG. A muscarinic cholinergic antagonist and a dopamine agonist rapidly increase ZENK mRNA expression in the form-deprived chicken retina. Exp Eye Res. 2007;85(1):15–22. Epub 2007/05/15.

136. Cottriall CL, Truong HT, McBrien NA. Inhibition of myopia development in chicks using himbacine: a role for M(4) receptors? Neuroreport. 2001;12(11):2453–6. Epub 2001/08/10.

137. McBrien NA, Arumugam B, Gentle A, Chow A, Sahebjada S. The M4 muscarinic antagonist MT-3 inhibits myopia in chick: evidence for site of action. Ophthalmic Physiol Opt. 2011;31:529–39.

138. Arumugam B, McBrien NA. Muscarinic antagonist control of myopia: evidence for M4 and M1 receptor-based pathways in the inhibition of experimentally-induced axial myopia in the tree shrew. Invest Ophthalmol Vis Sci. 2012;53(9):5827–37. Epub 2012/07/28

139. Luft WA, Ming Y, Stell WK. Variable effects of previously untested muscarinic receptor antagonists on experimental myopia. Invest Ophthalmol Vis Sci. 2003;44:1330–8.

140. Carr BJ, Mihara K, Ramachandran R, et al. Myopia-inhibiting concentrations of Muscarinic receptor antagonists block activation of Alpha2A-Adrenoceptors In Vitro. Invest Ophthalmol Vis Sci. 2018;59:2778–91.

141. Carr BJ, Nguyen CT, Stell WK. Alpha2 -adrenoceptor agonists inhibit form-deprivation myopia in the chick. Clin Exp Optom. 2019;102:418–25.

142. McCarthy CS, Megaw P, Devadas M, Morgan IG. Dopaminergic agents affect the ability of brief periods of normal vision to prevent form-deprivation myopia. Exp Eye Res. 2007;84(1):100–7. Epub 2006/11/11

143. Winawer J, Wallman J. Temporal constraints on lens compensation in chicks. Vision Res. 2002;42:2651–68.

144. Winawer J, Zhu X, Choi J, Wallman J. Ocular compensation for alternating myopic and hyperopic defocus. Vision Res. 2005;45:1667–77.

145. Zhu X, Winawer JA, Wallman J. Potency of myopic defocus in spectacle lens compensation. Invest Ophthalmol Vis Sci. 2003;44(7):2818–27. Epub 2003/06/26.

146. Tse DY, Lam CS, Guggenheim JA, Lam C, Li KK, Liu Q, et al. Simultaneous defocus integration during refractive development. Invest Ophthalmol Vis Sci. 2007;48(12):5352–9. Epub 2007/12/07.

147. Tse DY, To CH. Graded competing regional myopic and hyperopic defocus produces summated emmetropization set points in chick. Invest Ophthalmol Vis Sci. 2011;52:8056–62.

148. Lam CS, Tang WC, Tse DY, Tang YY, To CH. Defocus Incorporated Soft Contact (DISC) lens slows myopia progression in Hong Kong Chinese schoolchildren: a 2-year randomised clinical trial. Br J Ophthalmol. 2014;98:40–5.

149. Megaw P, Morgan I, Boelen M. Vitreal dihydroxyphenylacetic acid (DOPAC) as an index of retinal dopamine release. J Neurochem. 2001;76(6):1636–44. Epub 2001/03/22.

150. Ashby R, Kozulin P, Megaw PL, Morgan IG. Alterations in ZENK and glucagon RNA transcript expression during increased ocular growth in chickens. Mol Vis. 2010;16:639–49. Epub 2010/04/21.

151. Thomson K, Karouta C, Ashby R. Form-deprivation and lens-induced myopia are similarly affected by pharmacological manipulation of the dopaminergic system in chicks. Invest Ophthalmol Vis Sci. 2020;61:4.

152. Thomson K, Karouta C, Ashby R. Topical application of dopaminergic compounds can inhibit deprivation myopia in chicks. Exp Eye Res. 2020;200:108233.

153. Thomson K, Karouta C, Morgan I, Kelly T, Ashby R. Effectiveness and safety of topical levodopa in a chick model of myopia. Sci Rep. 2019;9:18345.

154. Thomson K, Morgan I, Karouta C, Ashby R. Levodopa inhibits the development of lens-induced myopia in chicks. Sci Rep. 2020;10:13242.

155. Thomson K, Morgan I, Kelly T, Karouta C, Ashby R. Coadministration With carbidopa enhances the antimyopic effects of levodopa in chickens. Invest Ophthalmol Vis Sci. 2021;62:25.

156. Nickla DL, Sarfare S, McGeehan B, et al. Visual conditions affecting eye growth alter diurnal levels of vitreous DOPAC. Exp Eye Res. 2020;200:108226.

157. Feldkaemper M, Schaeffel F. An updated view on the role of dopamine in myopia. Exp Eye Res. 2013;114:106–19.

158. Mathis U, Schaeffel F. Glucagon-related peptides in the mouse retina and the effects of deprivation of form vision. Graefes Arch Clin Exp Ophthalmol. 2007;245:267–75.

159. Vessey KA, Lencses KA, Rushforth DA, Hruby VJ, Stell WK. Glucagon receptor agonists and antagonists affect the growth of the chick eye: a role for glucagonergic regulation of emmetropization? Invest Ophthalmol Vis Sci. 2005;46:3922–31.

160. Vessey KA, Rushforth DA, Stell WK. Glucagon- and secretin-related peptides differentially alter ocular growth and the development of form-deprivation myopia in chicks. Invest Ophthalmol Vis Sci. 2005;46:3932–42.

161. Hoogerheide J, Rempt F, Hoogenboom WP. Acquired myopia in young pilots. Ophthalmologica. 1971;163(4):209–15. Epub 1971/01/01.

162. Atchison DA, Rosen R. The possible role of peripheral refraction in development of myopia. Optom Vis Sci. 2016;93:1042–4.

163. Smith EL 3rd, Hung LF, Huang J. Relative peripheral hyperopic defocus alters central refractive development in infant monkeys. Vision Res. 2009;49:2386–92.

164. Smith EL 3rd, Hung LF, Huang J, Blasdel TL, Humbird TL, Bockhorst KH. Effects of optical defocus on refractive development in monkeys: evidence for local, regionally selective mechanisms. Invest Ophthalmol Vis Sci. 2010;51(8):3864–73. Epub 2010/03/12.

165. Smith EL 3rd, Ramamirtham R, Qiao-Grider Y, et al. Effects of foveal ablation on emmetropization and form-deprivation myopia. Invest Ophthalmol Vis Sci. 2007;48:3914–22.

166. Troilo D, Smith EL 3rd, Nickla DL, et al. IMI - report on experimental Models of emmetropization and myopia. Invest Ophthalmol Vis Sci. 2019;60:M31–88.

167. Sng CC, Lin XY, Gazzard G, Chang B, Dirani M, Chia A, et al. Peripheral refraction and refractive error in Singapore Chinese children. Invest Ophthalmol Vis Sci. 2011;52(2):1181–90. Epub 2010/10/12.

168. Sng CC, Lin XY, Gazzard G, Chang B, Dirani M, Lim L, et al. Change in peripheral refraction over time in Singapore Chinese children. Invest Ophthalmol Vis Sci. 2011;52(11):7880–7. Epub 2011/08/30.

169. Atchison DA, Li SM, Li H, et al. Relative peripheral hyperopia does not predict development and progression of myopia in children. Invest Ophthalmol Vis Sci. 2015;56:6162–70.

170. Sankaridurg P, Donovan L, Varnas S, Ho A, Chen X, Martinez A, et al. Spectacle lenses designed to reduce progression of myopia: 12-month results. Optom Vis Sci. 2010;87(9):631–41. Epub 2010/07/14.

171. Sankaridurg P, Holden B, Smith E 3rd, Naduvilath T, Chen X, de la Jara PL, et al. Decrease in rate of myopia progression with a contact lens designed to reduce relative peripheral hyperopia: one-year results. Invest Ophthalmol Vis Sci. 2011;52(13):9362–7. Epub 2011/11/01.

172. Kanda H, Oshika T, Hiraoka T, et al. Effect of spectacle lenses designed to reduce relative peripheral hyperopia on myopia progression in Japanese children: a 2-year multicenter randomized controlled trial. Jpn J Ophthalmol. 2018;62:537–43.

173. Karouta C, Ashby RS. Correlation between light levels and the development of deprivation myopia. Invest Ophthalmol Vis Sci. 2015;56:299–309.

174. Norton TT, Siegwart JT Jr. Light levels, refractive development, and myopiaDOUBLEHYPHENa speculative review. Exp Eye Res. 2013;114:48–57.

175. Smith EL 3rd, Hung LF, Arumugam B, Huang J. Negative lens-induced myopia in infant monkeys: effects of high ambient lighting. Invest Ophthalmol Vis Sci. 2013;54:2959–69.

176. Wu PC, Chen CT, Lin KK, et al. Myopia prevention and outdoor light intensity in a school-based cluster randomized trial. Ophthalmology. 2018;125:1239–50.

177. Jin JX, Hua WJ, Jiang X, et al. Effect of outdoor activity on myopia onset and progression in school-aged children in northeast China: the Sujiatun Eye Care Study. BMC Ophthalmol. 2015;15:73.

178. Wu PC, Tsai CL, Wu HL, Yang YH, Kuo HK. Outdoor activity during class recess reduces myopia onset and progression in school children. Ophthalmology. 2013;120:1080–5.

179. Wu PC, Chen CT, Chang LC, et al. Increased time outdoors is followed by reversal of the long-term trend to reduced visual acuity in Taiwan primary school students. Ophthalmology. 2020;127:1462.

180. Guggenheim JA, Williams C, Northstone K, et al. Does vitamin D mediate the protective effects of time outdoors on myopia? Findings from a prospective birth cohort. Invest Ophthalmol Vis Sci. 2014;55:8550–8.

181. Cuellar-Partida G, Williams KM, Yazar S, et al. Genetically low vitamin D concentrations and myopic refractive error: a Mendelian randomization study. Int J Epidemiol. 2017;46:1882–90.

182. McBrien NA. Regulation of scleral metabolism in myopia and the role of transforming growth factor-beta. Exp Eye Res. 2013;114:128–40.

183. Guggenheim JA, McBrien NA. Form-deprivation myopia induces activation of scleral matrix metalloproteinase-2 in tree shrew. Invest Ophthalmol Vis Sci. 1996;37(7):1380–95. Epub 1996/06/01.

184. Jobling AI, Gentle A, Metlapally R, McGowan BJ, McBrien NA. Regulation of scleral cell contraction by transforming growth factor-beta and stress: competing roles in myopic eye growth. J Biol Chem. 2009;284(4):2072–9. Epub 2008/11/18.

185. McBrien NA, Jobling AI, Gentle A. Biomechanics of the sclera in myopia: extracellular and cellular factors. Optom Vis Sci. 2009;86(1):E23–30. Epub 2008/12/24.

186. Metlapally R, Jobling AI, Gentle A, McBrien NA. Characterization of the integrin receptor subunit profile in the mammalian sclera. Mol Vis. 2006;12:725–34. Epub 2006/07/25.

The Sclera and Its Role in Regulation of the Refractive State

7

Jody A. Summers

7.1 Introduction

The sclera is a dense, fibrous, viscoelastic connective tissue that defines the shape of the eye. Moreover, the sclera provides a strong framework that supports the visual apparatus of the inner eye, withstands the expansive force generated by intraocular pressure, and protects the eye contents from external trauma. However, the role of the sclera is much more than that of a static container. Strong evidence from clinical and experimental studies indicates that the biochemical and biomechanical properties of the sclera are actively modulated in response to visual stimuli to adjust the axial length of the globe to minimize refractive error. As we will discuss below, the sclera is now known to undergo constant remodeling throughout life, and this remodeling is highly dependent on scleral fibroblast phenotype and extracellular matrix composition. Moreover, results from research over the last 30 years have established that scleral remodeling is regulated by genetic as well as environmental influences that can have profound effects on ocular size and the refractive state.

7.2 Development

The human sclera differentiates from neural crest and mesoderm in the sixth week of human embryonic development. The majority of the sclera differentiates from neural crest that surrounds the optic cup of neuroectoderm; however, a small temporal portion of the sclera differentiates from mesoderm which also contributes to the striated extraocular muscles and vascular endothelia [1, 2]. The human sclera differentiates from anterior to posterior and from inside to outside [3–5]. Electron microscopic studies of human embryos and fetuses show that the developmental process has already started in the region destined to become the limbus by the sixth week, and progresses backward to the equator by the eighth week, and to the posterior pole by the twelfth week [5, 6]. By the fourth month, the scleral spur appears as circularly oriented fibers, and by the fifth month, scleral fibers around the axons of the optic nerve form the lamina cribrosa [5]. Immature collagen can be detected in the sixth week as patches of small fibrils, and elastin deposits appear in the ninth week of development and increase in amount through week 24 [7]. Defects in the synthesis of extracellular matrix (ECM) components during scleral development may account for the scleral involvement in Marfan syndrome (elastin defect), osteogenesis imperfecta (collagen type I defect), and Ehlers-Danlos syndrome (lysyl-protocollagen hydroxylase) [8, 9].

7.3 The Structure of the Sclera

The human sclera has a radius of curvature of approximately 12 mm. The sclera is the thinnest (0.3 mm) under the insertion of the muscle tendons and is the thickest (1.0 mm) at the posterior pole near the optic nerve head. The sclera is divided into three layers: the episclera, the stroma, and the lamina fusca. The scleral stroma constitutes 90% of the scleral thickness and is largely responsible for its biomechanical properties [10].

The sclera has regional specializations for the positioning of the cornea, for the entry and exit of important nerves and blood vessels, as well as for the attachment of extraocular muscles. Despite these regional variations in structure, the sclera must be able to control eye shape during significant events that promote deformation of the globe, such as eye movements, accommodation, and intraocular pressure fluctuations. In doing so, the sclera is able to ensure stable refrac-

Supported by National Eye Institute Grant R01 EY09391 (JAS)

J. A. Summers (✉)
Department of Cell Biology, Oklahoma Center of Neuroscience,
University of Oklahoma Health Science Center,
Oklahoma City, OK, USA
e-mail: jody-summers@ouhsc.edu

tion and prevent rupture of the ocular globe. The sclera meets these requirements through a specialized dense irregular connective tissue stroma.

The scleral stroma is composed of collagen fibrils embedded in a matrix of proteoglycans and non-collagenous glycoproteins. The collagen fibrils are variable in diameter, ranging in size from 25 to 230 nm [11], and are organized into a complex arrangement of interwoven layers, or lamellae (Fig. 7.1). This arrangement of collagen fibrils gives the sclera its strength and rigidity despite its constant movement and pull from the extraocular muscles.

Located between the collagenous lamellae are the scleral fibroblasts, which are responsible for the synthesis and remodeling of the scleral stroma (Fig. 7.1).

It is the biochemical composition of the scleral ECM that is key to the maintenance of its characteristic rigidity, strength, and elasticity. The sclera of most vertebrates con-

sists of two layers: an inner layer of cartilage and an outer fibrous layer. Eutherian mammals, as well as snakes and salamanders, have lost the cartilage layer, although ECM molecules previously believed unique to cartilage, such as aggrecan, proline-arginine-rich and leucine-rich repeat protein (PRELP), and cartilage olimeric matrix protein (COMP), have been identified in the human sclera [12] suggesting that cartilaginous components have been retained in the sclera through evolution and serve important biochemical and biomechanical functions [13–15]. Moreover, the presence of cartilaginous molecules in the sclera may account for the association of scleritis with various rheumatic diseases such as rheumatoid arthritis and polychondritis [16–18].

Collagen In mammals, the sclera tissue contains approximately 30% collagen by wet weight, consisting predominantly of type I collagen [19, 20]. As discussed above, the formation

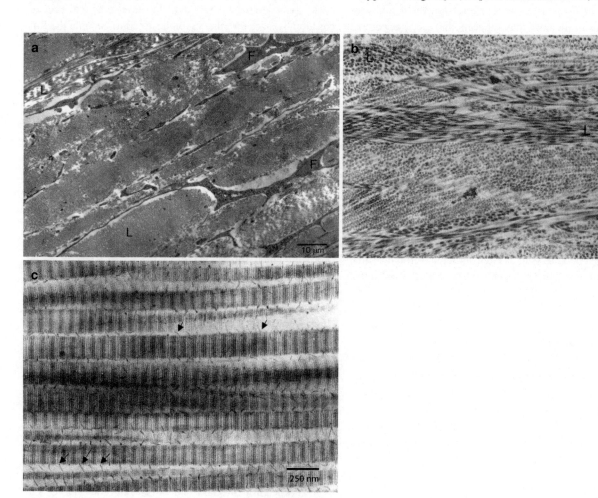

Fig. 7.1 Lamellar organization of collagen of the human sclera. (**a**) Transmission electron microscopic (TEM) image demonstrating the arrangement of scleral fibroblasts (F) located between irregularly arranged collagenous lamellae (L). Within each lamella, collagen fibrils are oriented in the same general direction. (**b**) Higher magnification of anterior human sclera in which collagenous lamellae are interwoven in some areas. (**c**) Higher magnification of scleral collagen fibrils follow-ing staining of anionic glycosaminoglycans on proteoglycans with the cationic dye cuprolinic blue. Proteoglycans can be visualized as fine filaments (arrows) associated with collagen fibrils in longitudinal section. (**a**) Bar = 10 μm; (**b**) Bar = 2 μm; (**c**) Bar = 250 nm. (Panel (**c**) is reproduced from Watson and Young [175]. Reproduced with permission © Elsevier)

of the collagenous matrix of the human sclera can be observed in the sixth week of development, as aggregates of thin-diameter collagen fibrils. As development continues, collagen is deposited in an anterior to posterior manner such that the most immature collagen fibrils are located in the posterior sclera. Due to this spatial pattern of development, the posterior region of the sclera contains a population of smaller diameter collagen fibrils as compared with the anterior region of the sclera throughout early fetal development up to week 16, when differences between the anterior and posterior regions become undetectable [7]. By week 24 of scleral development, the diameter of the collagen fibrils has reached the diameter of adult collagen fibrils with an average range of 94–102 nm and an overall range of 25–250 nm. Because the scleral collagen fibrils exhibit such a wide range in diameter, fibrillar spacing within the ECM of the sclera is found to be irregular as compared to the regular fibril spacing of the cornea.

In addition to type I collagen, the human sclera has been shown to contain collagen types III, IV, V, VI, VIII, XII, and XIII [21–23]. Collagen type I is the major collagen present in the human sclera, accounting for approximately 95% of the total collagen present. Interestingly, high congenital myopia is pathognomonic for Stickler's syndrome, a genetic disorder most commonly involving mutations in the collagen type II (COL2A1) gene, suggesting a major role for collage type II in scleral development and structure [24]. However, although collagen type II has been identified in the sclera of embryonic mice [25], and is a major fibrillar collagen of the largely cartilaginous avian sclera, collagen type II expression has not been detected in human sclera [12, 26].

Immunohistochemical analysis of both fetal and adult human specimens has shown that collagens type I and VI steadily increase with age, while collagens type IV, V, and VIII decrease with age. The presence of collagen III appears to remain fairly constant throughout fetal and adult life. Using atomic force microscopy [27], scleral collagen fibers can be visualized in close association with discrete cross-bridge structures between adjacent fibrils, which occur at regular intervals, one every 67 nm along the collagen fibril. It is speculated that these cross-bridges consist of aggregated proteoglycans associated with type VI collagen [28, 29].

Collagen fibrils within the sclera are organized into irregularly arranged and somewhat interwoven lamellae (Fig. 7.1). This lamellar organization is similar to the collagen arrangement of the cornea, but scleral collagen fibrils are highly variable in their diameter, lamellae vary in thickness, and the orientation of each lamella is irregular with respect to neighboring lamella. Based on studies in the cornea [29], it is likely that the outer edges of each lamella, which are adjacent to the scleral fibroblasts, contain the most immature collagen fibrils relative to those in the centers of each collagenous lamella.

Proteoglycans Collagen fibrillogenesis, fibril orientation, size, and arrangement are influenced by a number of noncollagenous ECM components [30–32]. Specifically, proteoglycans are known modulators of collagen fibril assembly and arrangement and are found in abundance throughout the ECM of the sclera. Proteoglycans consist of a core protein with at least one attached glycosaminoglycan (GAG) side chain made up of repeating sulfated disaccharide units. Due to the presence of negative charges on sulfate residues of GAGs, proteoglycans can be visualized in tissues by staining with cationic dyes such as cuprolinic blue (Fig. 7.1c) [33]. GAGs are categorized into four main groups: (1) hyaluronan, (2) chondroitin sulfate and dermatan sulfate, (3) heparan sulfate and heparin, and (4) keratan sulfate. Glycosaminoglycans are present in scleral development as early as the 13th week. Analysis of scleral tissue shows moderate staining for dermatan sulfate and intense staining for chondroitin sulfate (CS) throughout fetal development. Hyaluronic acid (HA) is present in the sclera at 13 weeks of development and then decreases with the progression of development. Small amounts of heparan sulfate are found in both fetal and adult scleras [21]. The GAGs of the adult sclera are dispersed in a heterogeneous manner throughout the ECM. A higher percentage of chondroitin sulfate and uronic acid has been observed in the posterior pole of the sclera as compared to the anterior and equatorial regions [14]. Staining for hyaluronic acid, on the other hand, is found to be more concentrated in the equatorial region of the sclera than in the posterior sclera [34].

Proteoglycans comprise approximately 0.7–0.9% of the total dry weight of the sclera of which dermatan and chondroitin sulfate proteoglycans are the most abundant. The major sulfated proteoglycans of the sclera include aggrecan, decorin, and biglycan [14]. Aggrecan, the cartilage proteoglycan, consists of a core protein covalently linked to over 100 chondroitin sulfate side chains. The negative charge associated with the GAG chains of aggrecan acts to sequester water molecules within the scleral ECM which is key to proper tissue hydration and elasticity. In contrast to the small proteoglycans which are evenly dispersed throughout all regions of the sclera, aggrecan has been found in highest concentration in the posterior sclera, where it may be responsible for maintaining the pliancy observed in the posterior regions of the sclera [35]. In the ECM of the cartilage, aggrecan associates with hyaluronan via linker proteins to form large hydrated macromolecules [36]; however, this has yet to be demonstrated for sclera.

The human sclera also contains the core proteins of several members of a family of related proteins termed the "small leucine-rich proteoglycans" (SLRPs) [15]. Decorin and biglycan, mentioned above, are the best known and most studied members of the SLRP family [37, 38], and these proteoglycans have been shown to exist in the human sclera as proteoglycans, containing one or two chondroitin/dermatan sulfate side chains, respectively [14]. Additionally, the human sclera contains the SLRP core proteins: lumican, PRELP (proline-arginine-rich and leucine-rich repeat protein), keratocan, fibromodulin, DSPG-3 (dermatan sulfate proteoglycan 3; also known as PG-Lb, epiphycan), chondroadherin, and osteoglycin [15]. All SLRPs contain a common central domain, consisting of ≈ 10 leucine-rich repeats, which have been shown to be involved in strong protein/protein interactions [39]. With the exception of decorin and biglycan, the SLRPs exist in the sclera with short unsulfated or low sulfated GAG side chains. Several members of the SLRP family, including decorin, fibromodulin, lumican, and biglycan, have been shown to bind a variety of ECM components via their core proteins, including type I collagen, where they are thought to guide matrix assembly and organization [30, 31, 40, 41].

Elastic Elastic fibers are synthesized by scleral fibroblasts and are an important component of the scleral extracellular matrix [42]. Elastic fibers in the mature state consist of an amorphous elastin core surrounded by longitudinally aligned microfibrils, composed of a number of glycoproteins, including fibrillin, which forms a scaffold for elastin. Staining for elastin molecules is first evident in the developing sclera around week 9 and increases over time [7]. The distribution of elastin is typically homogenous throughout the fetal stroma and maintains its homogeneity throughout development and into adulthood where elastin concentration is low (approximately 2% of the dry weight). The importance of elastic fibers in the sclera is evidenced by the scleral pathology and high myopia associated with Marfan syndrome, an autosomal dominant disorder due to mutations in the fibrillin gene [43, 44].

Other Glycoproteins Several non-collagenous glycoproteins have been characterized in the in-ground substance of the sclera and generally function to facilitate cell attachment to the extracellular matrix. Immunostaining for fibronectin, vitronectin, and laminin in the fetal sclera indicates that these three glycoproteins appear during the 13th week of fetal development and then diminish as development progresses [7]. In the adult sclera, fibronectin is present diffusely throughout the lamina cribrosa, while vitronectin is distributed as a fine fibrillar staining pattern in the lamina cribrosa, and to a lesser extent in the sclera [45, 46]. Laminin is a trimeric protein that contains an α-chain, a β-chain, and a γ-chain. There are a number of variants of each chain, resulting in 15 different laminins in vivo [47]. Laminin is present throughout the sclera in association with basement membranes of blood vessels, the trabecular meshwork, and Schlemm's canal [48]. Additionally, laminin has been localized to the surface of cribriform plates of the lamina cribrosa of human sclera [49] but is absent in the remaining nonvascular tissue. Interestingly, the alph2a chain of laminin has been identified as a genetic locus associated with myopia development in humans [50] (see below).

Matrix Metalloproteinases Scleral remodeling, as with any tissue, is a dynamic process that involves continual synthesis and degradation of extracellular matrix. Matrix metalloproteinases (MMPs) are a family of neutral proteinases that can initiate the degradation of collagens and other extracellular matrix components [51]. These proteins share significant amino acid homology, are active at neutral pH, require zinc and calcium ions, and are inhibited by tissue inhibitors of metalloproteinases (TIMPs). Human scleral fibroblasts have been shown to express MMP-1 (interstitial collagenase), MMP-2 (gelatinase A), MMP-3 (stromelysin) [52–54], and MMP-9 (gelatinase B) [55] as well as the MMP inhibitor, TIMP-1 [55, 56].

Scleral Fibroblasts Although the composition of the scleral extracellular matrix plays a major role in determining the biomechanical properties of the sclera, several studies provide evidence that scleral cells respond to local biochemical signals originating in the retina and/or choroid by altering their phenotype and their interactions with the scleral matrix to affect changes in scleral remodeling during eye growth. Phillips and McBrien [57] demonstrated that the tree shrew sclera has an initial increase in axial length as a response to increases in IOP, but then axial length progressively decreased over the next hour, resulting in no significant difference in axial length following 60 minutes of elevated pressure as compared with the pre-pressure length measurement. This reduction in axial length was attributed to the presence of α-smooth muscle actin (SMA)-containing myofibroblasts in the scleral stroma. Studies in human, monkey, and guinea pig sclera suggest that myofibroblasts comprise a subset of scleral cells, whose population may increase with age [58, 59]. As has been demonstrated with myofibroblasts from the cornea [60] and skin [61], scleral myofibroblasts can differentiate from noncontractile scleral fibroblasts by imposing mechanical stress on the scleral matrix or through stimulation with cell signaling factors such as transforming growth factor-beta (TGF-B) [62].

Scleral fibroblasts have also been shown to synthesize and secrete relatively large amounts of a protein, transforming growth factor beta-induced, 68kD (TGFB1p) that has the potential to modulate interactions of the scleral fibroblast with the matrix [63]. TGFB1p binds to the cell surface of scleral fibroblasts via the integrin receptors αvβ3 and αvβ5 and inhibits scleral cell attachment to collagen type I in vitro. The anti-adhesive effect of TGFB1p appears to be specific for scleral fibroblasts since TGFB1p does not inhibit attachment of human corneal fibroblasts or human foreskin fibroblasts [63]. Interestingly, *Tgfb1* mRNA levels were shown to be increased in the scleras of tree shrew eyes undergoing minus-lens compensation [64] as well as in the choroids of marmosets [65] and tree shrews [66] during the development of myopia. Based on the in vitro results, suggesting an antiadhesive effect of TGFB1p on scleral fibroblast attachment to collagen, we speculate that changes in scleral levels of TGFB1 may act to disrupt fibroblast-matrix interactions to facilitate slippage of scleral lamellae to facilitate ocular elongation during myopia development. Similarly, myopia development is associated with a reduced production of the collagen binding integrin subunits α1, β1, and α2 by scleral fibroblasts [67] further indicating that reduced fibroblast-matrix interactions within the sclera are necessary for ocular elongation.

7.4 Age-Related Changes in the Sclera

Although the eye nearly reaches adult size by age 10 [68–72], scleral extracellular matrix components are continually being synthesized and accumulated throughout adolescence and young adulthood. The concentration of scleral proteoglycans increases steadily in the human sclera from childhood through the fourth decade of life [35]. Beyond the fourth decade, the scleral population of small proteoglycans (biglycan and decorin) decreases in concentration in all scleral regions. The loss of proteoglycans from the anterior sclera is associated with a coincident decrease in tissue hydration in the aging human sclera [35, 73]. The pattern of accumulation of small proteoglycans in the aging sclera is remarkably similar to the age-related proteoglycan changes observed for human articular cartilage using a competitive radioimmunoassay for decorin (DSPG-2) [74] (Fig. 7.2).

In contrast, the age-related loss of small proteoglycans that occurs with increasing age, the large proteoglycan, aggrecan, remains constant over all ages and is concentrated in the posterior sclera. The retention of aggrecan in the posterior sclera of aging eyes may be related to the observation that the posterior sclera is less rigid than the anterior sclera. Due to its numerous chondroitin sulfate and keratan sulfate glycosaminoglycan side chains, aggrecan binds large amounts of water and contributes to tissue resiliency of cartilage and its ability to withstand compressive forces. If aggrecan has a similar function in the sclera, its presence may allow the posterior sclera to remain pliable, thereby sparing the circulation to the choroid and retina through the posterior ciliary blood vessels. Decreases in aggrecan concentration would significantly reduce the glycosaminoglycan concentration in the posterior sclera and may lead to increased scleral rigidity, which has been associated with hyperopia and high myopia [75].

Additionally, with increasing age, the sclera increases in stiffness, due to the accumulation of nonenzymatic glycation-type cross-links of collagen fibrils with age [76, 77]. This age-related increase in stiffness is greatest in the anterior sclera, followed by the equatorial and then posterior sclera [78].

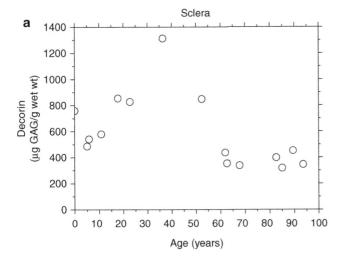

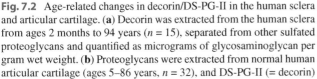

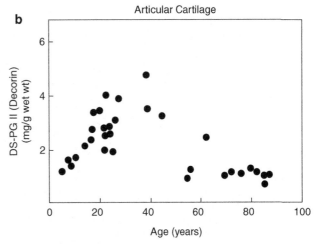

Fig. 7.2 Age-related changes in decorin/DS-PG-II in the human sclera and articular cartilage. (**a**) Decorin was extracted from the human sclera from ages 2 months to 94 years (*n* = 15), separated from other sulfated proteoglycans and quantified as micrograms of glycosaminoglycan per gram wet weight. (**b**) Proteoglycans were extracted from normal human articular cartilage (ages 5–86 years, *n* = 32), and DS-PG-II (= decorin) was determined using a competitive radioimmunoassay. Note the striking similarity in the relative concentrations of decorin/DS-PG-II in the sclera and articular cartilage with increasing age. (From Rada et al. [35]. Reproduced with permission © Association for Research in Vision and Ophthalmology and Sampaio et al. [74]. Reproduced with permission © the Biochemical Society)

7.5   Scleral Changes During Myopia Development

Myopia is the leading cause of visual impairment in the world [79]. Most myopia develops in children between the ages of 8 and 14 [72] and is produced by excessive lengthening of the vitreous chamber of the ocular globe [80, 81] so that the retina comes to lie behind the focal plane of the eye. In animal models of myopia [82, 83] and in humans [84], myopia is accompanied by progressive thinning of the sclera at the posterior pole of the eye, as the ocular globe gradually expands under the force of intraocular pressure. In severe cases of high myopia, scleral thickness can be reduced to as much as 31% of a normal sclera [85]. Severe scleral thinning in high myopia can lead to the formation of posterior scleral staphyloma.

Ultrastructural evaluation of the scleral stroma of highly myopic human eyes shows a more layered, lamellar structure, similar to that of the cornea [82, 86, 87]. Additionally, the sclera of highly myopic eyes is characterized by a pre-ponderance of unusually small diameter collagen fibrils averaging below 60–70 nm in the scleral matrix, a thinning of collagen fiber bundles, and slightly fewer collagen fiber bundles across the entire scleral thickness [82, 86, 88]. Additionally, abnormal fibrils associated with amorphous cementing substance and the presence of fissured or star-shaped fibrils have been observed [80, 86, 88] (Fig. 7.3). These ultramicroscopic alterations seen in myopic sclera suggest a derangement of the growth and organization of the collagen fibrils – either due to abnormal fibril formation or due to the presence of accentuated breakdown or catabolism of the sclera. It is very important to note that the scleral changes described in human myopes, and humans with high myopia, have been found in donor eyes after death, many years after myopia developed. However, studies using mammalian models of myopia have confirmed that the sclera thins during experimental myopia, as a result of active loss of scleral collagen and proteoglycans. Scleral tissue loss during myopia development has been shown to involve both accelerated sclera matrix degradation and slowed production of

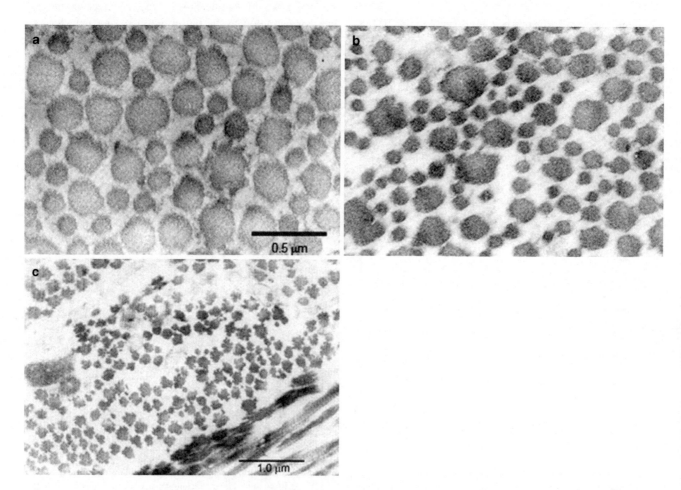

Fig. 7.3 Collagen fibrils in the sclera of normal and highly myopic human eyes. In contrast to the normal human sclera, the highly myopic human sclera shows greater variability in collagen fibril diameters and contains an increased number of smaller diameter collagen fibrils (**a, b**). Additionally, an increase in unusual star-shaped fibrils and fibrils associated with amorphous cementing substance was observed on cross section (**c**). (**a, b**) Bar = 0.5 μm; (**c**) Bar = 1 μm. (Adapted from Curtin [80])

new extracellular matrix, in a complex remodeling process [89, 90].

Few studies have characterized the extracellular matrix in the myopic human sclera. Considering the steady increase in proteoglycan synthesis and accumulation in the sclera through childhood and young adulthood [35], interruption of scleral proteoglycan accumulation in childhood and adolescent years, through genetic or environmental influences, could be expected to lead to disruption of the normal scleral extracellular matrix and result in abnormalities in ocular globe size and refraction. Decreases in glycosaminoglycan and collagen concentration have been identified in the posterior sclera of eyes from highly myopic human donors by some researchers [84] but not by others [91]. However, these studies also examined the sclera of eyes from aged human donors that had been myopic for many years.

Genetics, Scleral Remodeling, and Myopia Evidence supports a genetic component in the determination of axial length and myopia. Children with myopic parents have a higher chance of being affected and have longer axial lengths than those without myopic parents [92]. Twin studies also suggest that myopia is highly heritable and genetic effects can explain up to 88% of the heritability [93, 94]. However, it is likely that common environmental factors shared between parents and siblings contribute to their refractive development as well, thereby confounding the role of heredity in myopia development.

Because the axial length of the eye is a major component in determining the ocular refraction, alterations in any scleral extracellular matrix component are likely to lead to change in scleral shape, which in turn could dramatically affect vision. Genes responsible for myopia in association with other genetic syndromes have been identified: collagen 2A1 and 11A1 for Stickler syndromes type I and II, respectively [24, 95], lysyl-protocollagen hydroxylase for type VI Ehlers-Danlos syndrome [96], collagen 18/A1 for Knobloch syndrome [97], and fibrillin for Marfan syndrome [98]. Each of these genes is expressed in the sclera and serves as a model for possible candidate genes for nonsyndromic high myopia.

Based on results of linkage analysis, it was suggested that certain forms of inherited high myopia are the result of defects in scleral extracellular matrix components that localize at the chromosomal loci 17q [99], 18p (MYP2) [50], and 12q21-23 (MYP3) [100]. Located within these loci are several extracellular matrix genes known to be present in the sclera: collagen 1A1 and chondroadherin (17q), the alpha subunit of laminin (18p), and lumican, decorin, and dermatan sulfate proteoglycan (DSPG-3) (12q). Subsequent linkage analyses indicated that the 12q locus could be responsible for high myopia in approxi-

mately 25% of the UK families [101]. Several large genome-wide studies have been carried out to identify genes associated with myopia development in a number of populations [102–107]. From these studies, a number of candidate genes have been identified in virtually all cell types in the retina, RPE, choroid, and sclera, with a variety of functions, including neurotransmission, ion transport, retinoic acid metabolism, and extracellular matrix remodeling (Fig. 7.4). Taken together, these results suggest that mutations or polymorphisms in a variety of genes may directly result in myopia development, or more likely would predispose a subset of individuals to myopia development in association with environmental factors (discussed below).

Visual Regulation of Scleral Remodeling Animal models of myopia have provided considerable insight into the mechanisms regulating eye size, refraction, and the development of myopia. In the 1970s, it was accidentally discovered that myopia could be induced in monkeys, chicks, tree shrews, and children by depriving the retina of form vision [108–111]. More recently, the same treatment has been shown to produce myopia in mice [112, 113] and guinea pigs [114]. Form vision deprivation is an "open-loop" system, in which the eye will continue to elongate at an accelerated rate for the duration of the deprivation, potentially producing eyes so enormous they bulge out of the eye socket. In contrast, Schaeffel et al. [115] demonstrated through the use of positive and negative lenses of specific refractive powers that chicks could accurately compensate for imposed myopic or hyperopic defocus by modulating the axial length of the eye. Lens compensation was subsequently demonstrated in tree shrews [116], monkeys [117], guinea pigs [118], and mice [113]. The results of these animal studies clearly demonstrate the presence of a vision-dependent "emmetropization" mechanism that acts to minimize refractive error by controlling the axial length of infant and juvenile eyes so that the retina comes to lie at the focal plane and images are focused on the photoreceptors. Interruption of the emmetropization mechanism by obscuring the visual image in children as occurs with congenital cataract, ptosis, or vitreous hemorrhage or with visual form deprivation in animals leads to rapid and significant myopia.

Remarkably, studies using animal models have demonstrated that young eyes can recover from induced myopia following removal of the diffuser or negative lens [119, 120]. This recovery also is considered a manifestation of the emmetropization process by which eyes actively minimize the imposed myopic defocus, brought about through excessive axial elongation. However, in addition to a visual basis for modulating eye growth in recovery, there also exists a homeostatic mechanism to restore the enlarged eye to its natural shape [121].

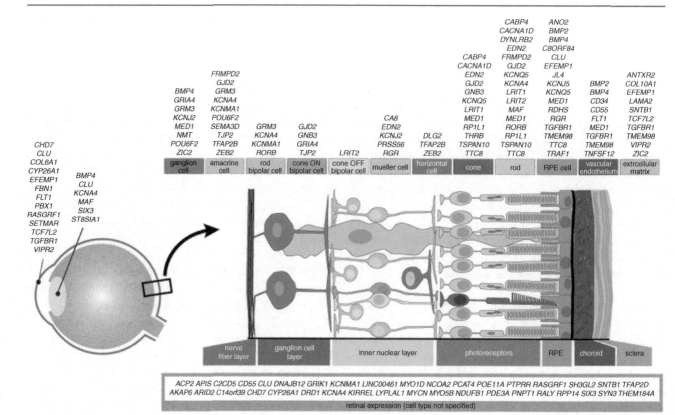

Fig. 7.4 Candidate genes for myopia and their functional sites identified by a genome-wide association study (GWAS). Genes identified on loci associated with refractive error in over 255,000 human subjects were assessed for their gene expression sites and/or functional target cells in the eye. The genes appear to be distributed across all cell types in the neural retina, RPE, vascular endothelium, and extracellular matrix. (From Tedja et al. [107]. Reproduced with permission © Springer Nature)

The key to this recovery is that the young eyes are still elongating as part of their postnatal (or post-hatching) development. When the diffuser or negative lens is removed, the elongated, myopic eye stops elongating. The optics of the eye continue to mature (through continued remodeling of the cornea and lens) so the focal plane gradually moves posteriorly, reducing the myopia.

The location of the retina is generally controlled by the location of the scleral shell, with additional adjustment made by the thickness of the choroid [122]. Thus, it is not at all surprising that significant changes in scleral extracellular matrix synthesis, accumulation, and turnover are associated with the development of induced myopia and recovery [89, 90, 123]. As mentioned above, there are species differences in scleral structure between eutherian mammals (including humans, other primates such as marmoset and macaque monkey, and tree shrews) on the one hand and most other vertebrates, including chicks [124]. The primary difference is that in most vertebrates, the sclera is comprised of an inner layer of the cartilage and an outer fibrous layer that is similar in its composition to the human sclera described in previous sections. In eutherian mammals, the inner layer of the cartilage is absent, so the entire sclera consists of the fibrous, type

I collagen-dominated extracellular matrix. Despite this difference in scleral anatomy, the fibrous sclera of mammals and the fibrous layer of the avian sclera appear to grow similarly. When ocular elongation accelerates, the fibrous sclera thins and loses material both in mammals [89, 90] and birds [83, 125]. The cartilaginous layer of the sclera of birds, however, demonstrates increased growth as the eye elongates, and this is accompanied by an increase in synthesis and accumulation of proteoglycans and an increased dry weight [123, 126]. At some level, all vertebrates probably use similar signaling mechanisms to control the sclera, but do so by controlling growth in the cartilage, where it is present, and by controlling remodeling in the fibrous sclera.

Biomechanical Changes Associated with Myopia The significant scleral thinning and scleral extracellular matrix changes associated with high myopia lead to changes in the biomechanical properties of the sclera. The sclera of myopic human eyes showed lower stiffness values compared to emmetropic eyes, indicating that the sclera in myopic eyes may be more extensible under normal intraocular pressure [127]. In tree shrews, the viscoelasticity in the sclera, as measured as the "creep rate" (continued elongation under a

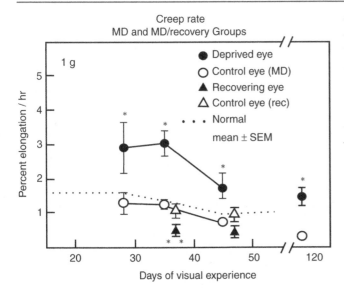

Fig. 7.5 Creep rate of tree shrew scleral strips from deprived (filled circles) and control (open circles) eyes and eyes recovering from form-deprivation myopia (filled triangles) and controls (open triangles) under 1 gram of tension. The data are plotted at the day of treatment when the creep rate was measured (visual experience). The dashed lines are the average creep rate of normal, untreated tree shrew sclera. Single asterisks indicate significant differences ($p < 0.05$) between the treated and control eye values. Double asterisks indicate significant differences between recovering and control eyes ($p < 0.05$). (From Siegwart Jr and Norton [128]. Reproduced with permission © Elsevier)

constant tension similar to that produced by intraocular pressure), was shown to increase significantly during experimentally induced myopia [128] (Fig. 7.5). Within 2 days after a negative lens or a diffuser is put in place and begins to induce myopia, scleral creep rate increased. This increase in viscoelasticity is expected to render the sclera more extensible, so that normal intraocular pressure produces excessive enlargement of the vitreous chamber. Remarkably, when unrestricted vision was restored (recovery), the scleral creep rate decreased significantly below control levels within 2 days by removal of the diffuser, contributing to a recovery from myopia (Fig. 7.5).

The changes in scleral distensibility are thought to be not only due to the reduced proteoglycan and collagen content within the myopic sclera but also due to altered collagen cross-linking. When scleral collagen cross-linking is inhibited by systemic administration of lathyritic agents, the degree of experimental myopia that develops is significantly increased [129]. Interestingly, no changes in ocular elongation were detected in the contralateral control eyes of lathyrogen-treated animals, suggesting that reduced collagen cross-linking in association with other visually induced scleral ECM changes results in exaggerated ocular elongation. More recently, Levy et al. [130] demonstrated that the sclera of myopic tree shrew eyes underwent an increased softening response to cyclic physiological load, compared to

contralateral control eyes. This softening was reversed by exogenous cross-linking of the myopic sclera with genipin. These results exemplify the dynamic nature of the sclera and compel investigation into the molecular basis of the visually driven changes in scleral biomechanics.

Biochemical Changes in the Myopic Sclera: Results from Animal Studies Similar to the posterior sclera of the highly myopic human eye, myopia development in mammalian models of myopia is associated with scleral thinning and significant reduction in scleral collagen fibril diameter [82, 131]. DNA synthesis has been found to be reduced [132], but DNA content in the sclera remains unchanged [131]. There is a net loss of matrix, measured as a reduction in dry weight [82] and a reduction in the amount of type I collagen [89, 133]. The level of sulfated and unsulfated GAGs decreases [89], with hyaluronan levels declining within 24 hours after a negative lens is applied in tree shrews [134]. Similarly, in the common marmoset, the rate of proteoglycan synthesis in the posterior sclera is negatively correlated with the rate of vitreous chamber elongation in eyes developing myopia (accelerated elongation), hyperopia (decelerated elongation), or growing normally [90]. Direct evidence supporting the importance of proteoglycans in maintaining scleral structure and eye shape has come from studies in mice in which mice made deficient in lumican [135] or double knockout mice deficient in both lumican and fibromodulin [136] exhibited abnormalities in scleral collagen fibril diameters and organization, scleral thinning, and an increase in axial elongation, suggesting that these extracellular matrix components are important in maintaining the biomechanical properties of the sclera.

Interestingly, not all matrix proteins are reduced; type III and type V collagens are relatively unaffected [133]. Thus, it appears that there is not a modulation of growth in the fibrous sclera, but rather a remodeling that results in a loss of extracellular matrix. Further, these changes appear to start before, or at least at the same time, as the biomechanical change (increase in creep rate). They likely are modulated, at least in part, by an elevation in both latent and active MMP-2 (gelatinase A) [137]. The tree shrew sclera as well as the outer fibrous layer of the chick sclera undergoes remodeling during the development of myopia, as evidenced by an increased expression of MMP-2 [137, 138]; decreased expression of tissue inhibitor of metalloproteinase (TIMP)-2, an endogenous inhibitor of gelatinase A, [139–141]; decreased rate of proteoglycan synthesis [142]; and overall thinning [83]. Most likely, the scleral remodeling events described for the fibrous scleral layer of chicks and in the mammalian sclera during experimentally induced myopia (i.e., by minus lens wear or form vision deprivation) are similar to those that occur during the development and progression of myopia in humans.

In contrast to the fibrous layer of chick sclera, the cartilaginous scleral layer in chicks demonstrates increased synthesis and accumulation of DNA and of proteoglycans, particularly of aggrecan, and overall thickening during the development of myopia [123, 126, 143]. In chicks, significant increases in proteoglycan synthesis occur within 1 day of the start of form deprivation, presumably associated with cartilage growth, and these changes occur prior to changes in vitreous chamber elongation [144]. Systemic inhibition of proteoglycan synthesis in chicks with β-xyloside significantly reduces the rate of ocular elongation in both form-deprived and contralateral control eyes [145], suggesting that increases in scleral proteoglycan synthesis and accumulation are responsible for ocular elongation during conditions of induced myopia as well as in normal post-hatch ocular growth. In all species examined, the changes in scleral extracellular matrix synthesis and degradation occur more strongly at the posterior pole of the globe [89, 90, 142], suggesting that these animal models of myopia accurately model the scleral changes associated with high myopia in humans. The localized response in the posterior sclera may be related to regional differences in the growth states of the scleral fibroblasts in this region or may be a reflection of a concentration of deprivation-induced changes in the retina, choroid, and sclera along the visual axis. However, this may reflect the organization of the sclera itself because in some of these species (tree shrew, chick), the retinal region with the highest acuity (the analog of the human fovea) is not located at the posterior pole, but is found temporally.

In chicks, tree shrews, and marmosets, scleral changes during the recovery from induced myopia are essentially a reversal of scleral remodeling events associated with form-deprivation or negative-lens-induced myopia. The slowed vitreous chamber elongation in the recovering eyes is associated with decreases in MMP-2 activity, increases in TIMP-2 activity, and increased proteoglycan synthesis in the fibrous sclera of marmosets and tree shrews [146]. GAG levels, which are reduced during myopia development by negative lenses, return to normal [134]. In the posterior cartilaginous sclera of chicks, there is a rapid decrease in proteoglycan synthesis within hours following removal of the occluder and restoration of unrestricted vision [147]. In both chicks and tree shrews, changes in scleral glycosaminoglycan synthesis and levels during recovery occur prior to, or at least as early as, the most rapid deceleration in vitreous chamber elongation [134, 147], suggesting that changes in scleral extracellular matrix remodeling are responsible for changes in ocular elongation.

The multifunctional cytokine, transforming growth factor-beta (TGF-β) has been implicated in regulating scleral extracellular matrix changes associated with the development of myopia. Gene expression of three isoforms of TGF-β (TGF-β1, TGF-β2, and TGF-β3) has been shown to rapidly decrease in the sclera of tree shrew eyes in response to form deprivation [148]. Moreover, comparisons of primary cultures of scleral fibroblasts grown in the presence of TGF-β isoforms at concentrations comparable to that observed in normal and myopic sclera in vivo indicate that the decrease in TGF-β isoforms results in decreases in collagen and proteoglycan synthesis similar to that observed in the sclera of myopic tree shrew eyes [149]. In addition to mediating scleral extracellular matrix changes, changes in local concentration of TGF-β isoforms may modulate α-smooth muscle actin expression in the scleral fibroblasts and thereby regulate scleral fibroblast to myofibroblast differentiation (as discussed above).

Two studies have evaluated global protein expression profiles in the mammalian sclera during the development of myopia. Zhou et al. [150] compared scleral proteins in guinea pig eyes following 7 weeks of form deprivation and following 4 days of recovery from form deprivation and normal eyes using two-dimensional gel electrophoresis. They found 18 scleral proteins that exhibited at least a threefold change in expression in form-deprived eyes as compared with normal eyes, and they found 16 scleral proteins that differed from normal during recovery. Among the highest upregulated proteins were beta A4-crystallin and Ca^{2+}-dependent activator protein for secretion 2 isoform b. Among the most downregulated proteins were peroxiredoxin 4, G12v mutant of human placental Cdc42 GTPase in the GDP form chain B, and putative alpha-tubulin. During recovery, tubulin alpha-6, actin cytoskeletal protein 2, and several crystalline genes were downregulated, including beta A4-crystallin. In a recent study, Frost and Norton [151] compared protein expression in the sclera of tree shrews undergoing lens-induced myopia (LIM) with recovery from LIM and normal sclera using a highly sensitive proteomics approach (DIGE). Using this technique, 79 proteins were shown to be altered in abundance during myopia development and recovery from induced myopia. Lens-induced myopia was associated with a downregulation of structural proteins such as collagen I α 2 as well as proteins involved in cell-matrix interactions (thrombospondin, keratocan) and cytoskeleton remodeling (fortilin, gelsolin). The LIM-induced protein changes might be expected to alter scleral ECM and cell-ECM interactions to facilitate the slippage between scleral lamellae, thereby raising the creep rate of the myopic sclera. During recovery, proteins whose expression had decreased during LIM (e.g., collage I α 2) returned to control levels or slightly above. It is predicated that these changes would stabilize the interlamellar regions, thereby reducing the viscoelasticity of the sclera to normal levels. The lack of similarities in the results of the Zhou et al. [152] and Frost and Norton [151] studies may be attributed to species differences, differences in the method of protein analyses, and/or differences in the experimental paradigms employed.

7.6   Regulation of Scleral Growth and/or Remodeling

Local Control Many aspects of scleral extracellular matrix remodeling are speculated to be under the control of specific growth factors. The finding that age-related changes in scleral proteoglycan synthesis rates in humans are nearly identical to that observed in articular cartilage (Fig. 7.2), peaking in the fourth decade of life [35], suggests that postnatal scleral growth, like that of other connective tissues, is under the control of systemic growth hormone or its downstream effectors, the insulin-like growth factors (IGF-I and IGF-II) [153]. However, one of the most intriguing discoveries in the past 25 years is that the scleral changes associated with visually guided postnatal ocular growth are controlled by a cascade of locally generated chemical events that are initiated in the retina and ultimately cause changes in scleral extracellular matrix (ECM) remodeling [154]. If the optic nerve is severed or action potentials are blocked with tetrodotoxin (TTX), myopia can still be induced by visual deprivation or minus lenses [155, 156]. Furthermore, if occluders or negative lenses are fashioned to affect only a portion of the visual field, only that part of the ocular globe, corresponding the deprived or defocused portion of the retina, will enlarge and become myopic [154]. Recovery from deprivation-induced myopia also occurs in optic nerve-sectioned eyes, although eyes tend to overshoot and become hyperopic in the absence of an intact optic nerve [156]. The notion that postnatal ocular growth is regulated by an intraocular mechanism has stimulated much research on the identification of scleral growth regulators synthesized by neighboring ocular tissues.

The Choroid as a Scleral Growth Regulator As a highly vascular tissue, the choroid is responsible for the synthesis of a number of growth factors that are necessary for the development, growth, and maintenance of its elaborate vasculature. For example, choroidal endothelial and stromal cells have been shown to synthesize vascular endothelial growth factor (VEGF) [157], basic fibroblast growth factor (bFGF or FGF-2) [158, 159], and hepatocyte growth factor (HGF) [160]. These growth factors are necessary to promote and/or inhibit endothelial cell differentiation, proliferation, and migration, as well as vascular maturation, stabilization, maintenance, and permeability. Additionally, the choroid has also been shown to synthesize the matrix metalloproteinases MMP-1, MMP-2, and MMP-3, in association with choroidal capillaries and in the choroidal stroma [161]. The aforementioned growth factors, MMPs and TIMPs, are secreted proteins and exert their effects through receptor-mediated interactions with neighboring cells. Therefore, in addition to their role in maintaining the choroidal vasculature, it is conceivable that these proteins could have effects on cells and tissues outside of the choroid.

Marzani and Wallman [125] were the first to demonstrate that the secreted molecules from the choroid can inhibit scleral proteoglycan synthesis and thereby have the potential to regulate the rate of ocular elongation. This study demonstrated that co-culture of sclera with choroids from untreated eyes inhibited proteoglycan synthesis in the cartilaginous layer of the chick sclera. Moreover, scleral proteoglycan synthesis was more greatly inhibited by choroids isolated from recovering eyes. Conversely, sclera co-cultured with choroids isolated from myopic (form-deprived) eyes demonstrated an increased rate of proteoglycan synthesis relative to that of sclera co-cultured with untreated choroids. Additionally, suprachoroidal fluid removed from recovering choroids inhibits scleral proteoglycan synthesis in vitro as compared with that of fluid isolated from control choroids [162, 163]. Since the changes in scleral proteoglycan synthesis induced by co-culture with choroids or suprachoroidal fluid under different growth conditions mimicked those changes observed in sclera under the same visual conditions in vivo [144], these studies provided the first evidence that the choroid could be the source of scleral growth regulators involved in visually guided ocular elongation.

Retinoic Acid Retinoic acid has been implicated in the signaling cascade between the retina and the sclera that modulates eye growth [164]. The chick choroid synthesizes relatively high levels of all-*trans* retinoic acid (atRA) as compared with the retina or liver, and the rate of atRA synthesis is dramatically affected by the refractive state of the eye. Choroidal synthesis of atRA was shown to be increased in chick eyes during recovery from induced myopia and during compensation for imposed myopic defocus (using plus lenses), and atRA was shown to be decreased in eyes undergoing form-deprivation myopia and compensation for hyperopic defocus (using minus lenses). Interestingly, the time course of the increase in choroidal atRA synthesis [164] was remarkably similar to that of the decrease in rate of sclera proteoglycan synthesis observed in the early phase of recovery from induced myopia [147] (Fig. 7.6a, b) suggesting a causal relationship between choroidal atRA synthesis and scleral proteoglycan synthesis.

Using an ultrasensitive method of quantification [LC (liquid chromatography)/MS/MS], endogenous and newly synthesized atRA were measured in choroids in organ culture [165]. In agreement with Mertz and Wallman [164], atRA concentration was significantly higher in cultures of choroids from eyes recovering for 24 hours–15 days than in cultures of paired controls. Endogenous concentrations of atRA in control and recovering choroid organ cultures were determined to be approximately 5×10^{-9} M and 4×10^{-8} M, respectively (Fig. 7.6c). Moreover, the concentrations of atRA generated by choroids in vitro were within the range to produce significant inhibition of scleral proteoglycan synthe-

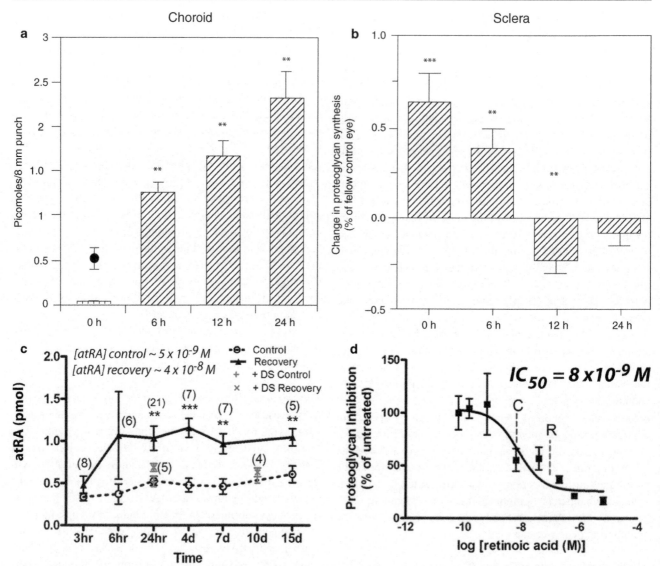

Fig. 7.6 Choroidal retinoic acid synthesis and scleral proteoglycan synthesis during recovery from induced myopia. (**a**) Time course of increase in choroidal all-trans retinoic acid (atRA) synthesis in eyes recovering from form-deprivation myopia. (**b**) Time course of decrease scleral proteoglycan synthesis in eyes recovering from form-deprivation myopia. (**c**) Chick choroids (8-mm punches) from control and recovering eyes were cultured for 3 hours in N2 medium at 37 °C. atRA was quantified in tissue punches, together with culture medium by LC/MS/MS. The atRA synthesis inhibitor, disulfiram (DS, 100 μM), was added to cultures of control and recovering choroids before incubation and subsequent atRA quantification. (**d**) Effect of atRA on scleral proteoglycan synthesis in vitro. Scleral punches were isolated from untreated eyes and incubated in atRA (10^{-10} M to 10^{-5} M) for 24 hours. After incubation with atRA, proteoglycan synthesis was estimated by the amount of $^{35}SO_4$ incorporation into glycosaminoglycans. (Figure (**a**) from Mertz and Wallman [164]. Reproduced with permission © Elsevier. Figure (**b**) adapted from Summers Rada and Hollaway [147]. Reproduced with permission © Elsevier. Figure (**c, d**) from Summers Rada et al. [165]. Reproduced with permission © Association for Research in Vision and Ophthalmology)

sis based on the IC_{50} for atRA on inhibition of scleral proteoglycan synthesis in vitro ($IC_{50} = 8 \times 10^{-9}$ M) [165] (Fig. 7.6d). Taken together, these studies suggest that choroidal synthesis of atRA in response to visual stimuli may modulate scleral proteoglycan synthesis.

In guinea pigs and primates, atRA synthesis is increased in the choroid/sclera [166] and RPE/choroid [167], respectively, during the development of myopia, a condition that is also associated with decreased scleral proteoglycan synthesis. However, in contrast to chicks, decreased proteoglycan synthesis in the mammalian sclera is associated with increased axial elongation [89, 90]. Similar to chicks, atRA has been demonstrated to inhibit proteoglycan synthesis in the primate sclera [167]. Therefore, in both chicks and primates, the visually induced changes in choroidal atRA synthesis and concentration are consistent with the known changes in scleral proteoglycan synthesis that occur during visually guided ocular growth and may represent an evolutionarily conserved mechanism for visually guided ocular growth regulation. How the same visual stimuli (such as hyperopic defocus) can cause opposite changes in choroidal atRA synthesis in chicks and primates is unknown, but suggests the presence of additional regulatory proteins in the cascade between the retina and choroid that differ between primates and chicks.

Tissue concentrations of atRA are tightly controlled by synthesizing and catabolizing enzymes and binding proteins and nuclear receptors [168]. Several studies have documented gene and protein expression of retinoic acid binding proteins, retinoic acid receptors (RARs), and retinaldehyde dehydrogenases (RALDHs) in the retinas, choroids, and sclera of chick eyes under normal and visually induced ocular growth states [165, 169–171]. Several studies have identified significant increases in choroidal RALDH2 mRNA expression during recovery from induced myopia and during compensation for lens-induced myopia (+7D lens) [165, 171, 172], suggesting that increased synthesis of atRA in choroids of recovering eyes is due to increased RALDH2

enzyme activity. Moreover, using a combination of enzymatic assays, Western blotting, and immunohistochemistry, RALDH2 was identified as the major RALDH isoform in the chick choroid and was solely responsible for the increased retinoic acid synthesis seen during recovery from myopia [172]. Within the choroid, RALDH2-positive cells are concentrated in the proximal choroid (near the RPE) and appear as ovoid- and spindle-shaped cells located in the stroma between larger blood and lymphatic vessels as well as some in close association with blood vessels [165, 169, 172] (Fig. 7.7a–d). The number of RALDH2 immunopositive cells in the choroid increases following 1–15 days of recovery [172] (Fig. 7.7e), either as a result of proliferation of RALDH2+ cells, increased RALDH2 protein expression, migration of RALDH2+ cells into the choroid, or a combination of these events. RALDH2+ cells of a similar phenotype to those described in the chick choroid have also been identified in the human choroid [173, 174]. The identification of

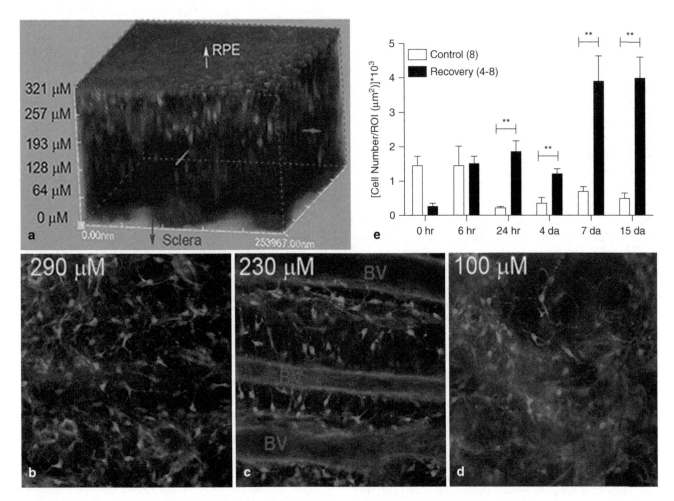

Fig. 7.7 RALDH2-positive (+) cells in the recovering chick choroid. RALDH2+ cells are identified by multiphoton imaging following whole mount immunolabeling of a 4-day recovering choroid with anti-chick RALDH2. RALDH2+ cells (green) are concentrated in the proximal choroid (near the RPE), but also located in the choroidal stroma, some in close association with blood vessels (BV). (a) 3D reconstruction of a region of interest within a recovering choroid from which

RALDH2+ cells were quantified. (b–d) Individual slices (1 μm thick) of the choroid shown in (A), taken throughout the choroidal thickness. Numbers at the top of each image (290 μm, 230 μm, and 100 μm) indicate the location of the choroidal slice, as distance from the sclera. (e). Total RALDH2+ cell number in control and recovering choroids. (Figure (e) from Harper et al. [172]. Reproduced with permission © Association for Research in Vision and Ophthalmology)

atRA and its synthesizing enzyme, RALDH2, as possible mediators of visually induced changes in scleral remodeling and eye size has provided new potential molecular targets for the control of myopia development.

7.7   Conclusions

Research highlighted in this review clearly demonstrates that the sclera is a dynamic tissue, capable of responding rapidly to changes in the visual environment to affect changes in ocular size and refraction. Research over the last decade has identified several genes in the sclera of several animal species, including humans, that are associated with the development of myopia. Therapies designed to slow the loss of extracellular matrix in the human sclera, through inhibition of MMP activity, stimulation of proteoglycan and collagen synthesis, or increase in collagen cross-linking, would be logical approaches to slow the progression of myopia.

Results of many large population-based studies indicate that myopia is a complex trait, affected by multiple genes and environmental factors. Of much interest is the mechanism by which visual environment can be translated to the sclera to initiate cellular and extracellular matrix remodeling events that lead to significant changes in the biomechanical properties of the sclera. The discovery that visually induced changes in eye size are regulated locally, within the eye, has stimulated much research on tissue interactions between the retina, choroid, and sclera in attempts to identify the molecular nature of the retina-to-sclera signaling cascade. The identification of a locally generated chemical signal that acts to regulate scleral extracellular matrix remodeling in vivo will not only elucidate the retinal-scleral signaling cascade involved in emmetropization, but will provide potential therapies aimed at slowing the progression of myopia in children.

Acknowledgments I would like to acknowledge Dr. Josh Wallman who is responsible for most of the significant scientific advances made toward the understanding of emmetropization and myopia development. Josh was my mentor, colleague, and friend for over 25 years and he will be truly missed. The majority of data presented in this review came from projects funded by the National Eye Institute at the National Institutes of Health.

References

1. Ozanics V, Jakobiec FA. Prenatal development of the eye and its anexa. In: Tasman W, Jaeger EA, editors. Duane's foundations of clinical ophthalmology. Philadelphia: Lippincott; 1982. p. 1–93.
2. Johnston MC, Noden DM, Hazelton RD, Coulombre JL, Coulombre AJ. Origins of avian ocular and periocular tissues. Exp Eye Res. 1979;29(1):27–43.
3. Duke-Elder S, Cook CH. Normal and abnormal development. In: Duke-Elder S, editor. System of ophthalmology. St. Louis: CV Mosby; 1966. p. 1–77.
4. Weale RA. A biography of the eye. London: Lewis; 1982.
5. Sellheyer K, Spitznas M. Development of the human sclera. A morphological study. Graefes Arch Clin Exp Ophthalmol. 1988;226(1):89–100.
6. Snell RS, Lemp MA. Clinical anatomy of the eye. Boston: Blackwell Scientific Publications; 1989.
7. Foster CS, Sainz de la Maza M. The sclera. New York: Springer-Verlag; 1994.
8. Wang Q, Forlino A, Marini JC. Alternative splicing in COL1A1 mRNA leads to a partial null allele and two in-frame forms with structural defects in non-lethal osteogenesis imperfecta. J Biol Chem. 1996;271(45):28617–23.
9. Benusiene E, Kucinskas V. COL1A1 mutation analysis in Lithuanian patients with osteogenesis imperfecta. J Appl Genet. 2003;44(1):95–102.
10. Grant CA, Thomson NH, Savage MD, Woon HW, Greig D. Surface characterisation and biomechanical analysis of the sclera by atomic force microscopy. J Mech Behav Biomed Mater. 2011;4(4):535–40.
11. Komai Y, Ushiki T. The three-dimensional organization of collagen fibrils in the human cornea and sclera. Invest Ophthalmol Vis Sci. 1991;32(8):2244–58.
12. Young TL, Scavello GS, Paluru PC, Choi JD, Rappaport EF, Rada JA. Microarray analysis of gene expression in human donor sclera. Mol Vis. 2004;10:163–76.
13. Coster L, Rosenberg LC, van der Rest M, Poole AR. The dermatan sulfate proteoglycans of bovine sclera and their relationship to those of articular cartilage. An immunological and biochemical study. J Biol Chem. 1987;262(8):3809–12.
14. Rada JA, Achen VR, Perry CA, Fox PW. Proteoglycans in the human sclera. Evidence for the presence of aggrecan. Invest Ophthalmol Vis Sci. 1997;38(9):1740–51.
15. Johnson JM, Young TL, Rada JA. Small leucine rich repeat proteoglycans (SLRPs) in the human sclera: identification of abundant levels of PRELP. Mol Vis. 2006;12:1057–66.
16. Sainz de la Maza M, Foster CS, Jabbur NS. Scleritis associated with rheumatoid arthritis and with other systemic immune-mediated diseases. Ophthalmology. 1994;101(7):1281–6; discussion 1287–1288.
17. Isaak BL, Liesegang TJ, Michet CJ Jr. Ocular and systemic findings in relapsing polychondritis. Ophthalmology. 1986;93(5):681–9.
18. Hakin KN, Watson PG. Systemic associations of scleritis. Int Ophthalmol Clin. 1991;31(3):111–29.
19. Keeley FW, Morrin J, Vesely S. Characterization of collagen from normal human sclera. Exp Eye Res. 1984;39(5):533–42.
20. Meek KM. The cornea and sclera. In: Franzl P, editor. Collagen: structure and mechanics. New York: Springer; 2008. p. 359–96.
21. Rada JA, Johnson JM. Sclera. In: Krachmer J, Mannis M, Holland E, editors. Cornea. St. Louis: Mosby; 2004.
22. Wessel H, Anderson S, Fitae D, Halvas E, Hempel J, SundarRaj N. Type XII collagen contributes to diversities in human corneal and limbal extracellular matrices. Invest Ophthalmol Vis Sci. 1997;38:2408–22.
23. Sandberg-Lall M, Hagg PO, Wahlstrom I, Pihlajaniemi T. Type XIII collagen is widely expressed in the adult and developing human eye and accentuated in the ciliary muscle, the optic nerve and the neural retina. Exp Eye Res. 2000;70:775–87.
24. Liberfarb RM, Levy HP, Rose PS, Wilkin DJ, Davis J, Balog JZ, Griffith AJ, Szymko-Bennett YM, Johnston JJ, Francomano CA, et al. The Stickler syndrome: genotype/phenotype correlation in 10 families with Stickler syndrome resulting from seven mutations in the type II collagen gene locus COL2A1. Genet Med. 2003;5(1):21–7.
25. Savontaus M, Ihanamaki T, Metsaranta M, Vuorio E, Sandberg-Lall M. Localization of type II collagen mRNA isoforms in the developing eyes of normal and transgenic mice with a mutation in type II collagen gene. Invest Ophthalmol Vis Sci. 1997;38:930–42.

26. Young TL, Guo XD, King RA, Johnson JM, Rada JA. Identification of genes expressed in a human scleral cDNA library. Mol Vis. 2003;9:508–14.

27. Fullwood NJ, Hammiche A, Pollock HM, et al. Atomic force microscopy of the cornea and sclera. Curr Eye Res. 1995;14:529–35.

28. Meek KM, Fullwood NJ. Corneal and scleral collagens- a microscopist's perspective. Micron. 2001;32:261–72.

29. Birk DE, Trelstad RL. Extracellular compartments in matrix morphogenesis: collagen fibril, bundle, and lamellar formation by corneal fibroblasts. J Cell Biol. 1984;99:2024–33.

30. Rada JA, Cornuet PK, Hassell JR. Regulation of corneal collagen fibrillogenesis in vitro by corneal proteoglycan (Lumican and Decorin) core proteins. Exp Eye Res. 1993;56:635–48.

31. Vogel KG, Paulsson M, Heinegard D. Specific inhibition of type I and type II collagen fibrillogenesis by the small proteoglycan of tendon. Biochem J. 1984;223:587–97.

32. Birk DE, Lande MA. Corneal and scleral collagen fiber formation in vitro. Biochim Biophys Acta. 1981;670:362–9.

33. Young RD. The ultrastructural organization of proteoglycans and collagen in human and rabbit scleral matrix. J Cell Sci. 1985;74:95–104.

34. Trier K, Olsen EB, Ammitzboll T. Regional glycosaminoglycan composition of the human sclera. Acta Ophthalmol. 1990;68:304–6.

35. Rada JA, Achen VR, Penugonda S, et al. Proteoglycan composition in the human sclera during growth and aging. Invest Ophthalmol Vis Sci. 2000;41:1639–48.

36. Muir H. Proteoglycans as organizers of the intercellular matrix. Biochem Soc Trans. 1982;11:613–22.

37. Hocking AM, Shinomura T, McQuillan DJ. Leucine-rich repeat glycoproteins of the extracellular matrix. Matrix Biol. 1998;17:1–19.

38. Iozzo RV. The biology of the small leucine-rich proteoglycans. J Biol Chem. 1999;274:18843–6.

39. Iozzo RV. The family of the small leucine-rich proteoglycans: key regulators of matrix assembly and cellular growth. Crit Rev Biochem Mol Biol. 1997;32:141–74.

40. Hedbom H, Heinegard D. Binding of fibromodulin and decorin to separate sites on fibrillar collagens. J Biol Chem. 1993;268:27307–12.

41. Schonherr E, Witsch-Prehm P, Harrach B, et al. Interaction of biglycan with type I collagen. J Biol Chem. 1995;270:2776–83.

42. Marshall GE. Human scleral elastic system: an immunoelectron microscopic study. Br J Ophthalmol. 1995;79(1):57–64.

43. Maumenee IH. The eye in the Marfan syndrome. Trans Am Ophthalmol Soc. 1981;79:684–733.

44. Robinson PN, Booms P. The molecular pathogenesis of the Marfan syndrome. Cell Mol Life Sci. 2001;58(11):1698–707.

45. Fukuchi T, Ueda J, Abe H, Sawaguchi S. Cell adhesion glycoproteins in the human lamina cribrosa. Jpn J Ophthalmol. 2001;45(4):363–7.

46. Chapman SA, Ayad S, O'Donoghue E, Bonshek RE. Glycoproteins of trabecular meshwork, cornea and sclera. Eye (Lond). 1998;12(Pt 3a):440–8.

47. Yurchenco PD, Patton BL. Developmental and pathogenic mechanisms of basement membrane assembly. Curr Pharm Des. 2009;15(12):1277–94.

48. Dietlein TS, Jacobi PC, Paulsson M, Smyth N, Krieglstein GK. Laminin heterogeneity around Schlemm's canal in normal humans and glaucoma patients. Ophthalmic Res. 1998;30(6):380–7.

49. Hernandez MR, Luo XX, Igoe F, Neufeld AH. Extracellular matrix of the human lamina cribrosa. Am J Ophthalmol. 1987;104(6):567–76.

50. Young TL, Ronan SM, Drahozal LA, Wildenberg SC, Alvear AB, Oetting WS, Atwood LD, Wilkin DJ, King RA. Evidence that a locus for familial high myopia maps to chromosome 18p. Am J Hum Genet. 1998;63(1):109–19.

51. Woessner JF Jr. The family of matrix metalloproteinases. Ann N Y Acad Sci. 1994;732:11–21.

52. Lauhio A, Konttinen YT, Salo T, Tschesche H, Lahdevirta J, Woessner F Jr, Golub LM, Sorsa T. Placebo-controlled study of the effects of three-month lymecycline treatment on serum matrix metalloproteinases in reactive arthritis. Ann N Y Acad Sci. 1994;732:424–6.

53. Gaton DD, Sagara T, Lindsey JD, Weinreb RN. Matrix metalloproteinase-1 localization in the normal human uveoscleral outflow pathway. Invest Ophthalmol Vis Sci. 1999;40(2):363–9.

54. Gaton DD, Sagara T, Lindsey JD, Gabelt BT, Kaufman PL, Weinreb RN. Increased matrix metalloproteinases 1, 2, and 3 in the monkey uveoscleral outflow pathway after topical prostaglandin F(2 alpha)-isopropyl ester treatment. Arch Ophthalmol. 2001;119(8):1165–70.

55. Di Girolamo N, Lloyd A, McCluskey P, Filipic M, Wakefield D. Increased expression of matrix metalloproteinases in vivo in scleritis tissue and in vitro in cultured human scleral fibroblasts. Am J Pathol. 1997;150(2):653–66.

56. Yamaoka A, Matsuo T, Shiraga F, Ohtsuki H. TIMP-1 production by human scleral fibroblast decreases in response to cyclic mechanical stretching. Ophthalmic Res. 2001;33(2):98–101.

57. Phillips JR, McBrien NA. Pressure-induced changes in axial eye length of chick and tree shrew: significance of myofibroblasts in the sclera. Invest Ophthalmol Vis Sci. 2004;45(3):758–63.

58. Poukens V, Glasgow BJ, Demer JL. Nonvascular contractile cells in sclera and choroid of humans and monkeys. Invest Ophthalmol Vis Sci. 1998;39(10):1765–74.

59. Backhouse S. The impact of induced myopia on scleral properties in the guinea pig. In: McBrien NA, Morgan I, editors. Myopia: proceedings of the 12th international conference. Optom Vis Sci; 2009. p. 67–72.

60. Masur SK, Dewal HS, Dinh TT, Erenburg I, Petridou S. Myofibroblasts differentiate from fibroblasts when plated at low density. Proc Natl Acad Sci U S A. 1996;93(9):4219–23.

61. Tomasek JJ, Haaksma CJ, Eddy RJ, Vaughan MB. Fibroblast contraction occurs on release of tension in attached collagen lattices: dependency on an organized actin cytoskeleton and serum. Anat Rec. 1992;232(3):359–68.

62. McBrien NA, Jobling AI, Gentle A. Biomechanics of the sclera in myopia: extracellular and cellular factors. Optom Vis Sci. 2009;86(1):E23–30.

63. Shelton L, Rada JA. Inhibition of human scleral fibroblast cell attachment to collagen type I by TGFBIp. Invest Ophthalmol Vis Sci. 2009;50(8):3542–52.

64. Gao H, Frost MR, Siegwart JT Jr, Norton TT. Patterns of mRNA and protein expression during minus-lens compensation and recovery in tree shrew sclera. Mol Vis. 2011;17:903–19.

65. Shelton L, Troilo D, Lerner MR, Gusev Y, Brackett DJ, Rada JS. Microarray analysis of choroid/RPE gene expression in marmoset eyes undergoing changes in ocular growth and refraction. Mol Vis. 2008;14:1465–79.

66. He L, Frost MR, Siegwart JT, Norton TT. Gene expression signatures in tree shrew choroid during lens-induced myopia and recovery. Exp Eye Res. 2014;123:56–71.

67. McBrien NA, Metlapally R, Jobling AI, Gentle A. Expression of collagen-binding integrin receptors in the mammalian sclera and their regulation during the development of myopia. Invest Ophthalmol Vis Sci. 2006;47(11):4674–82.

68. Larsen JS. The sagittal growth of the eye. IV. Ultrasonic measurement of the axial length of the eye from birth to puberty. Acta Ophthalmol. 1971;49(6):873–86.

69. Larsen JS. The sagittal growth of the eye. 3. Ultrasonic measurement of the posterior segment (axial length of the vitreous) from birth to puberty. Acta Ophthalmol. 1971;49(3):441–53.

70. Larsen JS. The sagittal growth of the eye. II. Ultrasonic measurement of the axial diameter of the lens and the anterior segment from birth to puberty. Acta Ophthalmol. 1971;49(3):427–40.

71. Larsen JS. The sagittal growth of the eye. 1. Ultrasonic measurement of the depth of the anterior chamber from birth to puberty. Acta Ophthalmol. 1971;49(2):239–62.

72. Zadnik K, Satariano WA, Mutti DO, Sholtz RI, Adams AJ. The effect of parental history of myopia on children's eye size. JAMA. 1994;271(17):1323–7.

73. Brown CT, Vural M, Johnson M, Trinkaus-Randall V. Age-related changes of scleral hydration and sulfated glycosaminoglycans. Mech Ageing Dev. 1994;77(2):97–107.

74. Sampaio Lde O, Bayliss MT, Hardingham TE, Muir H. Dermatan sulphate proteoglycan from human articular cartilage. Variation in its content with age and its structural comparison with a small chondroitin sulphate proteoglycan from pig laryngeal cartilage. Biochem J. 1988;254(3):757–64.

75. Friedman E. Aging changes of the sclera. In: Albert DM, Jakobiec FA, editors. Principles and practice of ophthalmology: basic sciences. Philadelphia: WB Saunders; 1994. p. 726–8.

76. Coudrillier B, Tian J, Alexander S, Myers KM, Quigley HA, Nguyen TD. Biomechanics of the human posterior sclera: age- and glaucoma-related changes measured using inflation testing. Invest Ophthalmol Vis Sci. 2012;53(4):1714–28.

77. Schultz DS, Lotz JC, Lee SM, Trinidad ML, Stewart JM. Structural factors that mediate scleral stiffness. Invest Ophthalmol Vis Sci. 2008;49(10):4232–6.

78. Geraghty B, Jones SW, Rama P, Akhtar R, Elsheikh A. Age-related variations in the biomechanical properties of human sclera. J Mech Behav Biomed Mater. 2012;16:181–91.

79. Wojciechowski R. Nature and nurture: the complex genetics of myopia and refractive error. Clin Genet. 2011;79(4):301–20.

80. Curtin BJ. The myopias: basic science and clinical management. Philadelphia: Harper & Row; 1985. p. 256–8.

81. Tong L, Wong EH, Chan YH, Balakrishnan V. A multiple regression approach to study optical components of myopia in Singapore school children. Ophthalmic Physiol Opt. 2002;22(1):32–7.

82. McBrien NA, Cornell LM, Gentle A. Structural and ultrastructural changes to the sclera in a mammalian model of high myopia. Invest Ophthalmol Vis Sci. 2001;42(10):2179–87.

83. Gottlieb MD, Joshi HB, Nickla DL. Scleral changes in chicks with form-deprivation myopia. Curr Eye Res. 1990;9(12):1157–65.

84. Avetisov ES, Savitskaya NF, Vinetskaya MI, Iomdina EN. A study of biochemical and biomechanical qualities of normal and myopic eye sclera in humans of different age groups. Metab Pediatr Syst Ophthalmol. 1983;7(4):183–8.

85. Cheng HM, Singh OS, Kwong KK, Xiong J, Woods BT, Brady TJ. Shape of the myopic eye as seen with high-resolution magnetic resonance imaging. Optom Vis Sci. 1992;69(9):698–701.

86. Curtin BJ, Teng CC. Scleral changes in pathological myopia. Trans Am Acad Ophthalmol Otolaryngol. 1958;62(6):777–88; discussion 88–90.

87. Funata M, Tokoro T. Scleral change in experimentally myopic monkeys. Graefes Arch Clin Exp Ophthalmol. 1990;228(2):174–9.

88. Curtin BJ, Iwamoto T, Renaldo DP. Normal and staphylomatous sclera of high myopia. An electron microscopic study. Arch Ophthalmol. 1979;97(5):912–5.

89. Norton TT, Rada JA. Reduced extracellular matrix in mammalian sclera with induced myopia. Vis Res. 1995;35(9):1271–81.

90. Rada JA, Nickla DL, Troilo D. Decreased proteoglycan synthesis associated with form deprivation myopia in mature primate eyes. Invest Ophthalmol Vis Sci. 2000;41(8):2050–8.

91. Blach RK, Jay B, Macfaul P. The concept of degenerative myopia. Proc R Soc Med. 1965;58:109–12.

92. Kurtz D, Hyman L, Gwiazda JE, Manny R, Dong LM, Wang Y, Scheiman M. Role of parental myopia in the progression of myopia and its interaction with treatment in COMET children. Invest Ophthalmol Vis Sci. 2007;48(2):562–70.

93. He M, Hur YM, Zhang J, Ding X, Huang W, Wang D. Shared genetic determinant of axial length, anterior chamber depth, and angle opening distance: the Guangzhou Twin Eye Study. Invest Ophthalmol Vis Sci. 2008;49(11):4790–4.

94. Lopes MC, Andrew T, Carbonaro F, Spector TD, Hammond CJ. Estimating heritability and shared environmental effects for refractive error in twin and family studies. Invest Ophthalmol Vis Sci. 2009;50(1):126–31.

95. Annunen S, Korkko J, Czarny M, Warman ML, Brunner HG, Kaariainen H, Mulliken JB, Tranebjaerg L, Brooks DG, Cox GF, et al. Splicing mutations of 54-bp exons in the COL11A1 gene cause Marshall syndrome, but other mutations cause overlapping Marshall/stickler phenotypes. Am J Hum Genet. 1999;65(4):974–83.

96. Heikkinen J, Toppinen T, Yeowell H, Krieg T, Steinmann B, Kivirikko KI, Myllyla R. Duplication of seven exons in the lysyl hydroxylase gene is associated with longer forms of a repetitive sequence within the gene and is a common cause for the type VI variant of Ehlers-Danlos syndrome. Am J Hum Genet. 1997;60(1):48–56.

97. Mahajan VB, Olney AH, Garrett P, Chary A, Dragan E, Lerner G, Murray J, Bassuk AG. Collagen XVIII mutation in Knobloch syndrome with acute lymphoblastic leukemia. Am J Med Genet A. 2010;152A(11):2875–9.

98. Kainulainen K, Karttunen L, Puhakka L, Sakai L, Peltonen L. Mutations in the fibrillin gene responsible for dominant ectopia lentis and neonatal Marfan syndrome. Nat Genet. 1994;6(1):64–9.

99. Paluru P, Ronan SM, Heon E, Devoto M, Wildenberg SC, Scavello G, Holleschau A, Makitie O, Cole WG, King RA, et al. New locus for autosomal dominant high myopia maps to the long arm of chromosome 17. Invest Ophthalmol Vis Sci. 2003;44(5):1830–6.

100. Young TL, Ronan SM, Alvear AB, Wildenberg SC, Oetting WS, Atwood LD, Wilkin DJ, King RA. A second locus for familial high myopia maps to chromosome 12q. Am J Hum Genet. 1998;63(5):1419–24.

101. Farbrother JE, Kirov G, Owen MJ, Pong-Wong R, Haley CS, Guggenheim JA. Linkage analysis of the genetic loci for high myopia on 18p, 12q, and 17q in 51 U.K. families. Invest Ophthalmol Vis Sci. 2004;45(9):2879–85.

102. Solouki AM, Verhoeven VJ, van Duijn CM, Verkerk AJ, Ikram MK, Hysi PG, Despriet DD, van Koolwijk LM, Ho L, Ramdas WD, et al. A genome-wide association study identifies a susceptibility locus for refractive errors and myopia at 15q14. Nat Genet. 2010;42(10):897–901.

103. Shi Y, Qu J, Zhang D, Zhao P, Zhang Q, Tam PO, Sun L, Zuo X, Zhou X, Xiao X, et al. Genetic variants at 13q12.12 are associated with high myopia in the Han Chinese population. Am J Hum Genet. 2011;88(6):805–13.

104. Li Z, Qu J, Xu X, Zhou X, Zou H, Wang N, Li T, Hu X, Zhao Q, Chen P, et al. A genome-wide association study reveals association between common variants in an intergenic region of 4q25 and high-grade myopia in the Chinese Han population. Hum Mol Genet. 2011;20(14):2861–8.

105. Hysi PG, Young TL, Mackey DA, Andrew T, Fernandez-Medarde A, Solouki AM, Hewitt AW, Macgregor S, Vingerling JR, Li YJ, et al. A genome-wide association study for myopia and refractive error identifies a susceptibility locus at 15q25. Nat Genet. 2010;42(10):902–5.

106. Verhoeven VJ, Hysi PG, Wojciechowski R, Fan Q, Guggenheim JA, Hohn R, Macgregor S, Hewitt AW, Nag A, Cheng CY, et al. Genome-wide meta-analyses of multiancestry cohorts identify multiple new susceptibility loci for refractive error and myopia. Nat Genet. 2013;45(3):314–8.

107. Tedja MS, Wojciechowski R, Hysi PG, Eriksson N, Furlotte NA, Verhoeven VJM, Iglesias AI, Meester-Smoor MA, Tompson SW, Fan Q, et al. Genome-wide association meta-analysis highlights light-induced signaling as a driver for refractive error. Nat Genet. 2018;50(6):834–48.

108. Sherman SM, Norton TT, Casagrande VA. Myopia in the lid-sutured tree shrew (Tupaia glis). Brain Res. 1977;124(1):154–7.

109. Wiesel TN, Raviola E. Myopia and eye enlargement after neonatal lid fusion in monkeys. Nature. 1977;266(5597):66–8.

110. Wallman J, Turkel J, Trachtman J. Extreme myopia produced by modest change in early visual experience. Science. 1978;201(4362):1249–51.

111. O'Leary DJ, Millodot M. Eyelid closure causes myopia in humans. Experientia. 1979;35(11):1478–9.

112. Barathi VA, Boopathi VG, Yap EP, Beuerman RW. Two models of experimental myopia in the mouse. Vis Res. 2008;48(7):904–16.

113. Tkatchenko TV, Shen Y, Tkatchenko AV. Mouse experimental myopia has features of primate myopia. Invest Ophthalmol Vis Sci. 2010;51(3):1297–303.

114. Howlett MH, McFadden SA. Form-deprivation myopia in the guinea pig (Cavia porcellus). Vis Res. 2006;46(1–2):267–83.

115. Schaeffel F, Glasser A, Howland HC. Accommodation, refractive error and eye growth in chickens. Vis Res. 1988;28(5):639–57.

116. Norton TT, Amedo AO, Siegwart JT Jr. The effect of age on compensation for a negative lens and recovery from lens-induced myopia in tree shrews (Tupaia glis belangeri). Vis Res. 2010;50(6):564–76.

117. Smith EL 3rd, Hung LF, Huang J, Blasdel TL, Humbird TL, Bockhorst KH. Effects of optical defocus on refractive development in monkeys: evidence for local, regionally selective mechanisms. Invest Ophthalmol Vis Sci. 2010;51(8):3864–73.

118. Howlett MH, McFadden SA. Spectacle lens compensation in the pigmented guinea pig. Vis Res. 2009;49(2):219–27.

119. Siegwart JT Jr, Norton TT. The susceptible period for deprivation-induced myopia in tree shrew. Vis Res. 1998;38(22):3505–15.

120. Wallman J, Adams JI. Developmental aspects of experimental myopia in chicks: susceptibility, recovery and relation to emmetropization. Vis Res. 1987;27(7):1139–63.

121. Wallman J, Winawer J. Homeostasis of eye growth and the question of myopia. Neuron. 2004;43(4):447–68.

122. Wallman J, Wildsoet C, Xu A, Gottlieb MD, Nickla DL, Marran L, Krebs W, Christensen AM. Moving the retina: choroidal modulation of refractive state. Vis Res. 1995;35(1):37–50.

123. Rada JA, Thoft RA, Hassell JR. Increased aggrecan (cartilage proteoglycan) production in the sclera of myopic chicks. Dev Biol. 1991;147(2):303–12.

124. Walls G. The vertebrate eye and its adaptive radiations. Bloomfield Hills: The Cranbrook Press; 1942.

125. Marzani D, Wallman J. Growth of the two layers of the chick sclera is modulated reciprocally by visual conditions. Invest Ophthalmol Vis Sci. 1997;38(9):1726–39.

126. Christensen AM, Wallman J. Evidence that increased scleral growth underlies visual deprivation myopia in chicks. Invest Ophthalmol Vis Sci. 1991;32(7):2143–50.

127. Curtin BJ. Physiopathologic aspects of scleral stress-strain. Trans Am Ophthalmol Soc. 1969;67:417–61.

128. Siegwart JT Jr, Norton TT. Regulation of the mechanical properties of tree shrew sclera by the visual environment. Vis Res. 1999;39(2):387–407.

129. McBrien NA, Norton TT. Prevention of collagen crosslinking increases form-deprivation myopia in tree shrew. Exp Eye Res. 1994;59(4):475–86.

130. Levy AM, Fazio MA, Grytz R. Experimental myopia increases and scleral crosslinking using genipin inhibits cyclic softening in the tree shrew sclera. Ophthalmic Physiol Opt. 2018;38(3):246–56.

131. Phillips JR, Khalaj M, McBrien NA. Induced myopia associated with increased scleral creep in chick and tree shrew eyes. Invest Ophthalmol Vis Sci. 2000;41:2028–34.

132. Gentle A, McBrien NA. Modulation of scleral DNA synthesis in development of and recovery from induced axial myopia in the tree shrew. Exp Eye Res. 1999;68(2):155–63.

133. Gentle A, Liu Y, Martin JE, Conti GL, McBrien NA. Collagen gene expression and the altered accumulation of scleral collagen during the development of high myopia. J Biol Chem. 2003;278(19):16587–94.

134. Moring AG, Baker JR, Norton TT. Modulation of glycosaminoglycan levels in tree shrew sclera during lens-induced myopia development and recovery. Invest Ophthalmol Vis Sci. 2007;48(7):2947–56.

135. Austin BA, Coulon C, Liu CY, Kao WW, Rada JA. Altered collagen fibril formation in the sclera of lumican-deficient mice. Invest Ophthalmol Vis Sci. 2002;43(6):1695–701.

136. Chakravarti S, Paul J, Roberts L, Chervoneva I, Oldberg A, Birk DE. Ocular and scleral alterations in gene-targeted lumican-fibromodulin double-null mice. Invest Ophthalmol Vis Sci. 2003;44(6):2422–32.

137. Guggenheim JA, McBrien NA. Form-deprivation myopia induces activation of scleral matrix metalloproteinase-2 in tree shrew. Invest Ophthalmol Vis Sci. 1996;37(7):1380–95.

138. Siegwart JT Jr, Norton TT. Selective regulation of MMP and TIMP mRNA levels in tree shrew sclera during minus lens compensation and recovery. Invest Ophthalmol Vis Sci. 2005;46(10):3484–92.

139. Liu HH, Kenning MS, Jobling AI, McBrien NA, Gentle A. Reduced scleral TIMP-2 expression is associated with myopia development: TIMP-2 supplementation stabilizes scleral biomarkers of myopia and limits myopia development. Invest Ophthalmol Vis Sci. 2017;58(4):1971–81.

140. Rada JA, Perry CA, Slover ML, Achen VR. Gelatinase A and TIMP-2 expression in the fibrous sclera of myopic and recovering chick eyes. Invest Ophthalmol Vis Sci. 1999;40(13):3091–9.

141. Rada JA, Brenza HL. Increased latent gelatinase activity in the sclera of visually deprived chicks. Invest Ophthalmol Vis Sci. 1995;36(8):1555–65.

142. Rada JA, Matthews AL, Brenza H. Regional proteoglycan synthesis in the sclera of experimentally myopic chicks. Exp Eye Res. 1994;59(6):747–60.

143. Rada JA, Matthews AL. Visual deprivation upregulates extracellular matrix synthesis by chick scleral chondrocytes. Invest Ophthalmol Vis Sci. 1994;35(5):2436–47.

144. Rada JA, McFarland AL, Cornuet PK, Hassell JR. Proteoglycan synthesis by scleral chondrocytes is modulated by a vision dependent mechanism. Curr Eye Res. 1992;11(8):767–82.

145. Rada JA, Johnson JM, Achen VR, Rada KG. Inhibition of scleral proteoglycan synthesis blocks deprivation-induced axial elongation in chicks. Exp Eye Res. 2002;74(2):205–15.

146. McBrien NA, Gentle A. Role of the sclera in the development and pathological complications of myopia. Prog Retin Eye Res. 2003;22(3):307–38.

147. Summers Rada JA, Hollaway LR. Regulation of the biphasic decline in scleral proteoglycan synthesis during the recovery from induced myopia. Exp Eye Res. 2011;92(5):394–400.

148. Jobling AI, Nguyen M, Gentle A, McBrien NA. Isoform-specific changes in scleral transforming growth factor-beta expression and the regulation of collagen synthesis during myopia progression. J Biol Chem. 2004;279(18):18121–6.

149. McBrien NA. Regulation of scleral metabolism in myopia and the role of transforming growth factor-beta. Exp Eye Res. 2013;114:128–40.

150. Zhou X, Ye J, Willcox MD, Xie R, Jiang L, Lu R, Shi J, Bai Y, Qu J. Changes in protein profiles of guinea pig sclera during development of form deprivation myopia and recovery. Mol Vis. 2010;16:2163–74.

151. Frost MR, Norton TT. Alterations in protein expression in tree shrew sclera during development of lens-induced myopia and recovery. Invest Ophthalmol Vis Sci. 2012;53(1):322–36.

152. Zhou X, Shen M, Xie J, Wang J, Jiang L, Pan M, Qu J, Lu F. The development of the refractive status and ocular growth in C57BL/6 mice. Invest Ophthalmol Vis Sci. 2008;49(12):5208–14.

153. Van Wyk JJ, Smith EP. Insulin-like growth factors and skeletal growth: possibilities for therapeutic interventions. J Clin Endocrinol Metab. 1999;84(12):4349–54.

154. Wallman J, Gottlieb MD, Rajaram V, Fugate-Wentzek LA. Local retinal regions control local eye growth and myopia. Science. 1987;237(4810):73–7.

155. Norton TT, Essinger JA, McBrien NA. Lid-suture myopia in tree shrews with retinal ganglion cell blockade. Vis Neurosci. 1994;11(1):143–53.

156. Troilo D, Wallman J. The regulation of eye growth and refractive state: an experimental study of emmetropization. Vis Res. 1991;31(7–8):1237–50.

157. Saint-Geniez M, Maldonado AE, D'Amore PA. VEGF expression and receptor activation in the choroid during development and in the adult. Invest Ophthalmol Vis Sci. 2006;47(7):3135–42.

158. Frank RN, Amin RH, Eliott D, Puklin JE, Abrams GW. Basic fibroblast growth factor and vascular endothelial growth factor are present in epiretinal and choroidal neovascular membranes. Am J Ophthalmol. 1996;122(3):393–403.

159. Ogata N, Matsushima M, Takada Y, Tobe T, Takahashi K, Yi X, Yamamoto C, Yamada H, Uyama M. Expression of basic fibroblast growth factor mRNA in developing choroidal neovascularization. Curr Eye Res. 1996;15(10):1008–18.

160. Grierson I, Heathcote L, Hiscott P, Hogg P, Briggs M, Hagan S. Hepatocyte growth factor/scatter factor in the eye. Prog Retin Eye Res. 2000;19(6):779–802.

161. Steen B, Sejersen S, Berglin L, Seregard S, Kvanta A. Matrix metalloproteinases and metalloproteinase inhibitors in choroidal neovascular membranes. Invest Ophthalmol Vis Sci. 1998;39(11):2194–200.

162. Rada JA, Huang Y, Rada KG. Identification of choroidal ovotransferrin as a potential ocular growth regulator. Curr Eye Res. 2001;22(2):121–32.

163. Rada JA, Palmer L. Choroidal regulation of scleral glycosaminoglycan synthesis during recovery from induced myopia. Invest Ophthalmol Vis Sci. 2007;48(7):2957–66.

164. Mertz JR, Wallman J. Choroidal retinoic acid synthesis: a possible mediator between refractive error and compensatory eye growth. Exp Eye Res. 2000;70(4):519–27.

165. Summers Rada JA, Hollaway LY, Li N, Napoli J. Identification of RALDH2 as a visually regulated retinoic acid synthesizing enzyme in the chick choroid. Invest Ophthalmol Vis Sci. 2012;53(3):1649–62.

166. McFadden SA, Howlett MH, Mertz JR. Retinoic acid signals the direction of ocular elongation in the guinea pig eye. Vis Res. 2004;44(7):643–53.

167. Troilo D, Nickla DL, Mertz JR, Summers Rada JA. Change in the synthesis rates of ocular retinoic acid and scleral glycosaminoglycan during experimentally altered eye growth in marmosets. Invest Ophthalmol Vis Sci. 2006;47(5):1768–77.

168. Napoli JL. Physiological insights into all-trans-retinoic acid biosynthesis. Biochim Biophys Acta. 2011;1821:152–67.

169. Fischer AJ, Wallman J, Mertz JR, Stell WK. Localization of retinoid binding proteins, retinoid receptors, and retinaldehyde dehydrogenase in the chick eye. J Neurocytol. 1999;28(7):597–609.

170. Bitzer M, Feldkaemper M, Schaeffel F. Visually induced changes in components of the retinoic acid system in fundal layers of the chick. Exp Eye Res. 2000;70(1):97–106.

171. Simon P, Feldkaemper M, Bitzer M, Ohngemach S, Schaeffel F. Early transcriptional changes of retinal and choroidal TGFbeta-2, RALDH-2, and ZENK following imposed positive and negative defocus in chickens. Mol Vis. 2004;10:588–97.

172. Harper AR, Wang X, Moiseyev G, Ma JX, Summers JA. Postnatal chick choroids exhibit increased retinaldehyde dehydrogenase activity during recovery from form deprivation induced myopia. Invest Ophthalmol Vis Sci. 2016;57(11):4886–97.

173. Harper AR, Wiechmann AF, Moiseyev G, Ma JX, Summers JA. Identification of active retinaldehyde dehydrogenase isoforms in the postnatal human eye. PLoS One. 2015;10(3):e0122008.

174. Schroedl F, Kaser-Eichberger A, Trost A, Runge C, Bruckner D, Bogner B, Strohmaier C, Reitsamer HA, Summers JA. Morphological classification of RALDH2-positive cells in the human choroid. Invest Ophthalmol Vis Sci. 2018;59:308.

175. Watson PG, Young RD. Scleral structure, organisation and disease. A review. Exp Eye Res. 2004;78:609–23.

Part II

Ocular Changes in the Development of Pathologic Myopia

Update on the Pathology of Pathological Myopia

8

Alia Rashid and Hans E. Grossniklaus

8.1 Introduction

Pathological myopia is the leading cause of blindness in many developed countries, especially in Asia and the Middle East [1–3]. Pathological myopia has been defined in several different ways but usually combines a high refractive error with degenerative changes. Duke-Elder defined it as a myopia occurring with (predominantly posterior lobe) degenerative changes [4]. In Japan, where pathological myopia affects between 6% and 18% of the myopic population, a high refractive error of > -8 diopters (D) is used as the diagnostic criteria for pathological myopia [5]. High myopia is usually associated with enlargement or elongation of the globe. The mechanical stretching forces associated with this enlargement can lead to several different types of fundus changes which can result in variable amount of visual deterioration.

There have been a number of research studies that have documented the most common histopathological findings in myopic eyes. Most recently, a review of 308 eyes comprehensively delineated the histopathological findings in pathological myopia [6]. These include the tigroid fundus, lacquer cracks, geographic atrophy of RPE and choroid, posterior staphyloma, choroidal neovascularization also known as Fuchs spot, myopic configuration of the optic nerve head including peripapillary changes, macular holes and retinal holes, or detachments, and vitreous, cobblestone, and lattice degeneration (see Table 8.1).

Studies have shown that both genetic and environmental factors both cause and affect the development of pathological myopia [7–10]. Recent studies investigating the genomics of this condition have successfully identified novel loci which may be responsible for the development of this pathological process. With the under-acknowledged but significant impact of pathological myopia in patients, the importance of genomic profiling and early recognition of pathological

Table 8.1 Histopathologic findings in 308 myopic eyes

Finding	Percent of total
Myopic configuration of optic nerve head	37.7
Staphyloma	35.4
Vitreous degeneration (liquefaction, detachment)	35.1
Cobblestone degeneration	14.3
Myopic degeneration of retina	11.4
Retinal detachment	11.4
Retinal pits, holes, or tears	8.1
Subretinal neovascularization	5.2
Lattice degeneration	4.9
Fuchs spot	3.2
Lacquer cracks	0.6

changes in the myopic eye can potentially aid earlier intervention or appropriate alternative therapies to improve the quality of life of these patients. In recent years, various interventional techniques have been tried to control progression myopia in children, including the use of antimuscarinic or cycloplegic drops, bifocal lenses, RGPCLs, and intraocular pressure-lowering drugs. According to a recent Cochrane review, the most promising results were shown in trials using antimuscarinic topical medication. Bifocal lenses and lenses to reshape the corneal surface were deemed to also be promising but in need of further elucidation with clinical trials [11]. Understanding the histopathology of pathological myopia is an important step in being able to focus the future development of appropriate interventions on those tissues that may benefit the most.

8.2 Pathological Findings in Pathological Myopia

8.2.1 Lacquer Cracks

Lacquer cracks are a result of linear breaks forming in the Bruch's membrane. The breaks occur in the posterior pole and clinically appear as a crisscrossed, reticular pattern of subretinal yellowish-white fine irregular lines and are associ-

A. Rashid · H. E. Grossniklaus (✉)
L.F Montogomery Laboratory, Department of Ophthalmology, Emory University School of Medicine, Atlanta, GA, USA
e-mail: arashi6@emory.edu; ophtheg@emory.edu

© Springer Nature Switzerland AG 2021
R. F. Spaide et al. (eds.), *Pathologic Myopia*, https://doi.org/10.1007/978-3-030-74334-5_8

ated with retinal hemorrhage and subretinal neovascularization [12, 13]. Typically, the overlying neuroretina appears normal. The presence of lacquer cracks may have some relation to the stress caused by mechanical forces acting on the ocular tissues from an enlarged eye as typically found in high myopia [6, 14]. Between 1.6% and 4.3% of severely myopic eyes have been shown to have lacquer crack formation pathologically [6, 15]. Curtin et al. noted that axial length showed some correlation with the presence of lacquer cracks, finding that 4.3% of eyes with an axial length greater than 26.5 mm exhibited lacquer cracks and eyes with an axial length of 31.5 mm or more had the highest incidence [16]. Klein et al. found a distinct correlation between the presence and extent of lacquer cracks and worsening visual acuity [15]. Histopathologically, lacquer cracks can be seen as distinct defects in Bruch's membrane, leading to capillary-like vessels extending internally, through the defect to the underlying retinal pigment epithelium. Sometimes these linear tears can be healed by retinal gliosis that fills in the area of the defect. Hyperplasia of the retinal pigment epithelium can also be seen to extend into the choroid through the defects. Clinically this hyperplasia of the RPE can be seen as pigmentary changes in the area of the lacquer cracks. The mechanical forces causing the stretching and hence breakage in the elastic lamina of Bruch's membrane can lead to the formation of choroidal neovascular membranes which may bleed, eventually causing scarring and atrophy of the RPE.

A study by Ohno-Matsui et al. found that subretinal bleeding in the absence of a myopic CNV heralded the development of lacquer cracks [17]. The study prospectively examined 22 highly myopic eyes in 19 patients that had exhibited subretinal bleeding. Ophthalmoscopy and fluorescein funduscopic angiography were used to evaluate the area of the subretinal bleed. 17 of the eyes (77%) developed lacquer cracks in the following 2–6 months (mean 4 months) following the subretinal bleeds. Another study by the same team followed 66 eyes with lacquer cracks for an average of 73 months [18]. Progression of the lacquer cracks was seen in 37 eyes (56.1%), and of these, 37% showed an increase in the number of cracks and evolved into other myopic fundus changes such as patchy atrophy, diffuse atrophy, and Fuchs' spot, in 68%. We know that lacquer cracks are formed when there is a break in Bruch's membrane through the RPE to the choriocapillaris. Laser photocoagulation, used to treat CNV and retinal holes/tears, can also cause fractions in this RPE-Bruch's-choriocapillaris complex. It then stands to reason that laser photocoagulation can lead to the formation of lacquer cracks. Johnson et al. reviewed five eyes treated for myopic CNV with laser photocoagulation and found that the existing lacquer cracks expanded from the laser scar between 10 days and 3 months after treatment [19]. Furthermore, the cracks acted as pathways for recurrence or progression of the myopic CNVs. Ohno-Matsui et al. evaluated 325 highly

myopic eyes and found that of those that were noted to have lacquer cracks, 29.4% went on to develop myopic CNV, showing that lacquer cracks are an important predisposing risk factor for the development of CNV [20].

8.2.2 Geographic Atrophy of RPE and Choroid (Diffuse Versus Patchy)

The degenerative changes that are found in high myopia cause early changes, primarily atrophy of the choriocapillaris and retinal pigment epithelium. The atrophy of the RPE and choriocapillaris leads to a reduction in nutritional support for the retina, and this subsequently also atrophies. The atrophy leads to increased visualization of the choroidal circulation, known as a "tessellated" or "tigroid" fundus appearance.

Chorioretinal degeneration is the most commonly reported clinical finding in pathological myopia [8]. The changes progress from the early findings of a tigroid fundus to lacquer crack and staphyloma formation and then diffuse followed by patchy choroidal atrophy and eventually leading to bare sclera [21, 22]. A study by Ohno-Matsui et al. reviewed 325 eyes with myopic fundus changes over a course of at least 3 years and found that choroidal neovascularization occurred in 3.7% of eyes with diffuse chorioretinal atrophy and in 20% of eyes with patchy atrophy [20].

Kobayashi et al. reviewed the fundus characteristics in children with high myopia and found that only mild chorioretinal atrophy was noted in 16.3% of eyes, and this was located around the optic disc. None of the children exhibited signs of geographic atrophy, suggesting that aging, in addition to mechanical tension, may be an important factor in the development of myopic chorioretinal degeneration [23].

A long-term study (range 5–32 years, mean 12.7 years) of 806 highly myopic eyes in 429 patients found that myopic maculopathy – that is, a tessellated fundus, diffuse or patchy chorioretinal atrophy, CNV, and macular atrophy – was seen to progress in approximately 40% of eyes over time [24]. Additionally, eyes that also had posterior staphyloma were more likely to show progression of maculopathy.

Histopathologically, the study by Grossniklaus et al. found that the RPE did indeed show substantial atrophy, and interestingly they also noted a loss of choroidal melanocytes in the area [6] (see Figs. 8.1, 8.2, 8.3, 8.4, 8.5, 8.6, 8.7, and 8.8). The choriocapillaris has been shown on ultramicroscopy to progressively thin with a graduated blockade of the choriocapillaris [25]. A study to evaluate macular choroidal thickness in eyes with myopic maculopathy found that a thinner macular choroidal thickness was related to more advanced stages of maculopathy and an increased likelihood of the presence of lacquer cracks and a lower BCVA [26]. This finding was confirmed by a recent comparative study of choroidal thickness in highly myopic eyes with emmetropic

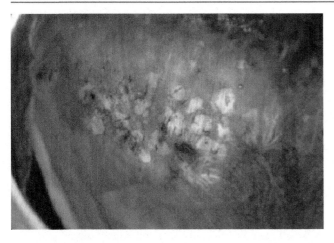

Fig. 8.1 Gross appearance of cobblestone degeneration. There is diffuse and patchy atrophy of the peripheral RPE and outer retina forming cobblestone degeneration

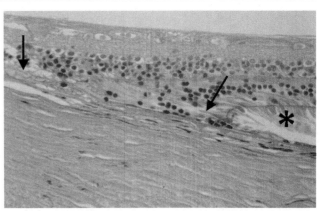

Fig. 8.4 Cobblestone degeneration. This area of cobblestone degeneration is composed of RPE atrophy and overlying atrophy of the outer retinal layers (*between arrows*). Adjacent to the cobblestone degeneration, the photoreceptor outer segments are intact (*asterisk*). *H&E 100×*

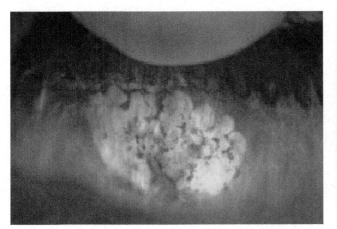

Fig. 8.2 Gross appearance of confluent cobblestone degeneration

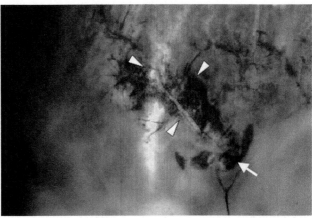

Fig. 8.5 Gross appearance of lattice degeneration. The area of lattice degeneration (*arrowheads*) has an associated retinal hole (*arrow*)

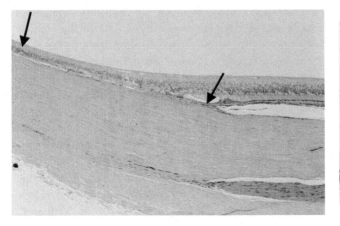

Fig. 8.3 Cobblestone degeneration. Outer retinal atrophy. There is atrophy of the outer retina and retinal pigment epithelium present (*between arrows*). *H&E 25×*

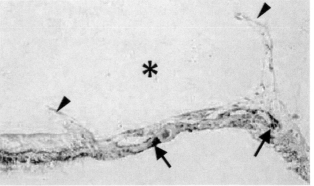

Fig. 8.6 Lattice degeneration. Lattice degeneration in this myopic eye is composed of inner layer atrophy with an overlying pocket of liquid vitreous (*asterisk*) surrounded by tufts of gliotic retina (*arrowheads*). There is RPE hypertrophy and hyperplasia present (*arrows*), and a sclerotic vessel is observed. *H&E 100×*

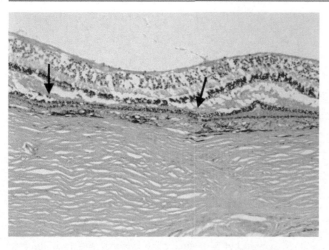

Fig. 8.7 Outer retinal atrophy. The outer retina is atrophic (*between arrows*), and only a thin portion of the outer nuclear layer remains. *H&E 25×*

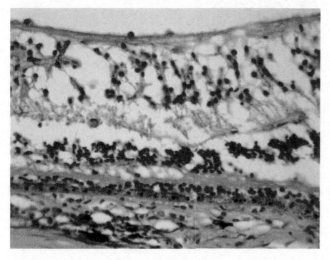

Fig. 8.8 Outer retinal atrophy. The outer retina is atrophic, and only a thin portion of the outer nuclear layer remains. *H&E 100×*

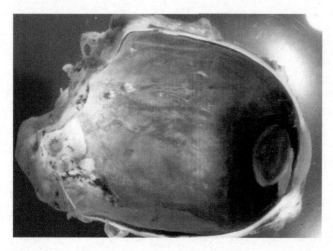

Fig. 8.9 Gross appearance of highly myopic eye with posterior staphyloma. This highly myopic eye exhibits a posterior staphyloma composed of an area of extremely thin sclera with underlying atrophy of the choroid, retinal pigment epithelium, and retina

eyes [27]. Enhanced depth imaging optical coherence tomography (EDI-OCT) was performed on 25 highly myopic eyes and 25 normal eyes. The choroidal thickness in the macula was significantly smaller ($p < 0.0001$) in the highly myopic group as compared to the normal group.

At the edges of the atrophied areas, pigment clumping could be seen, a sign that can also be frequently noted on clinical examination. Animal models of myopia have shown that ultrastructural changes include a reduced density of the choroidal capillaries and irregular, attenuated intercapillary meshes [28].

An early study of 1437 myopic eyes looked at the peripheral retinas and found a statistically significant association between axial length of the eye and white without pressure, pigmentary degeneration, paving stone (or cobblestone) degeneration, and lattice degeneration [29]. These findings have been supported by numerous other studies. Celorio et al. found that 33% of highly myopic eyes had lattice degeneration; however, they found the greatest prevalence (40.9%) in eyes between 26 and 26.9 mm in length and the least (7%) in eyes with axial lengths greater than 32 mm [30]. A study from Japan found that independently of axial length, lattice degeneration was significantly more frequent in eyes that did not have posterior staphylomas, concluding that the type of axial elongation (staphyloma vs. no staphyloma) influenced the formation of lattice degeneration [31].

8.2.3 Posterior Staphyloma

Clinically, staphylomas have been noted in approximately 19% of highly myopic eyes with axial lengths greater 26.5 mm [16] (see Figs. 8.9 and 8.10). In the study by Grossniklaus, the second most common histopathological finding was staphyloma, occurring in 33% of the 369 eyes with pathological myopia [6], indicating that the presence of staphyloma may be underestimated by clinical evaluation. Staphylomas occur most commonly in the posterior pole [32]. In pathological myopia, the sclera has been shown to be abnormal. Histopathologically, the collagen bundles in the sclera are found to be thinner, with fewer striations of collagen, and the lamellar structure of the sclera appears similar to the architecture of the corneal stroma [33] (see Figs. 8.6, 8.7, 8.8, 8.9, 8.10, and 8.11). Ultrastructural investigations have revealed that the scleral collagen in pathological myopia has a more lamellar fiber placement, as well as the appearance of star-shaped collagen fibrils, a decrease in the fibril caliber and number of fibrils, and increased interfibrillary separation [34]. Animal studies have indicated that these changes are due to accelerated collagen turnover and a decrease in the synthesis of collagen [35]. These ultrastructural alterations in the scleral tissue lead to a weaker, less rigid structure that is more susceptible to mechanical stresses and deformation. The histologic evaluation by Grossniklaus

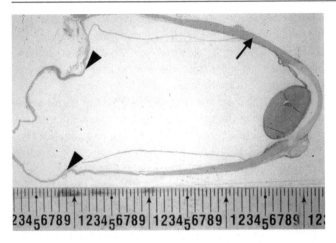

Fig. 8.10 Highly myopic eye with posterior staphyloma. This highly myopic eye is approximately 40 mm in anteroposterior dimension. There is normal sclera anteriorly (*arrow*) and a staphyloma posteriorly where the sclera has thinned and stretched (*between arrowheads*). *H&E 2×*

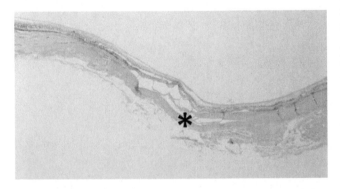

Fig. 8.11 Staphyloma. A staphyloma corresponds to an area of thinned sclera (*asterisk*). *H&E 10×*

found that on gross examination, the mean anteroposterior measurement in pathologically myopic eyes was greater than either the horizontal or vertical measurements (26.5 mm vs. 25.5 mm and 25 mm, respectively), indicating that the eyes were "egg-shaped" with the greatest mechanical forces/deformation occurring in the anteroposterior axis [6]. This finding is in keeping with the fact that the vast majority of staphylomas occur in the posterior pole, where these forces would have the greatest mechanical impact, leading to ectasia of the sclera and formation of a staphyloma.

In 1977, Curtin developed a grading system for posterior staphylomas, determined by the location, size, and severity of the staphyloma [36]. In total, ten types of staphyloma were identified. The primary staphylomas were type I–V, and compound staphylomas were type VI–X. A study by Hsiang et al. using ultrasound B-scans to evaluate posterior staphylomas looked at 209 eyes of 108 patients with pathological myopia [37]. By using ultrasound B-scans, they found that 90% of the eyes had a staphyloma. The study found that the prevalence of staphyloma, as well as the severity, or grading, increased with increasing age. Type II staphy-

lomas were the most common, occurring in 52.7% of eyes, followed by Type I (23.4%) and Type IX (17%). Severe retinal degeneration was noted in 71.9% of the Type IX eyes, in 50% of both Type I and Type III eyes, and in 46.5% of Type II staphyloma eyes. The difference between the Type II and Type IX eyes was statistically significant ($p = 0.01$). Furthermore, when comparing Type II staphyloma eyes to Type IX eyes, the axial length was significantly greater for the latter group, as was the presence of lacquer cracks. These findings, of an increase in the prevalence of staphyloma and chorioretinal atrophy with increasing axial length and increasing age, have been confirmed by other studies [38].

Staphyloma formation in pathological myopia is part of a spectrum of myopic maculopathy, and a variety of features such as retinoschisis, retinal holes and detachments, CNV, and atrophy have been noted to occur in the presence of staphylomas [39–44]. A study by Henaine-Berra et al. has found that the prevalence of macular abnormalities in high myopia, such as foveoschisis, vascular traction, and epiretinal membrane formation, is significantly more frequent in the presence of a posterior staphyloma ($p = 0.0001$) and that 53.65% of eyes with posterior staphyloma were observed to have macular abnormalities [45]. Wu et al. found that foveoschisis and foveal detachment without macular hole were significantly associated with posterior staphyloma ($p = 0.0003$) [46], a finding confirmed by Takano et al. [47]. The question of whether posterior staphyloma influenced the formation of macular holes and retinal detachments (MHRD) in highly myopic eyes was investigated by Oie et al., who found that the type of posterior staphyloma appeared to have some correlation [48]. They found that the percentage of eyes with staphyloma in the group of highly myopic eyes MHRD was significantly higher than in the highly myopic group without MHRD ($p < 0.001$), and furthermore, Type II staphylomas were significantly more prevalent in the MHRD group ($p = 0.01$).

8.2.4 CNV/Fuchs Spot

Macular choroidal neovascularization (CNV), known as Fuchs spot in its later stages, has been reported in between 5% and 10% of cases of pathological myopia [49]. It is the most common cause of vision loss in high myopia [12, 50]. One study found that in persons under the age of 50, myopia accounted for 62% of CNV [51]. The CNV occurring in high myopia is associated with typical pathological findings such as lacquer cracks and patchy atrophy. Drusen and pigment epithelium detachments, which are commonly found with age-related CNV, are rarely found in myopic CNV [52]. Myopic CNV tend to be smaller in dimension and with a smaller extent of leakage when compared to the age-related form of CNV. Subsequently, the areas of atrophy that develop over these CNV locations in myopia will initially be smaller.

Later on, however, there is a well-documented tendency for areas of atrophy and scarring in myopic eyes to increase in size, a phenomenon known as "atrophic creep." This phenomenon is especially well recognized as a sequela of laser treatment in eyes with pathological myopia with several studies showing that >90% of myopic eyes treated with laser of varying wavelengths will suffer from laser scar expansion [53–56]. An explanation for this phenomenon is that of mechanical stretching of the chorioretinal complex, which has been noted to occur in highly myopic eyes. The combination of thinning of the chorioretinal complex, along with the likely concomitant presence of a staphyloma, can often make the task of early detection of a myopic CNV a difficult one [52]. Chorioretinal atrophy itself is very common in the areas around a regressed CNV, with one study quoting the frequency as high as 96% at 5–10 years after onset of the CNV [57].

CNV may occur more frequently in the presence of chorioretinal atrophy and lacquer cracks [24, 58, 59]. A study by Ohno-Matsui et al. found that of those eyes with chorioretinal atrophy, only 3.7% progressed to CNV formation. This increased dramatically with patchy atrophy – with 20% of those eyes developing CNV – and in the eyes with lacquer cracks, 29.4% developed CNV [20].

There are differences between myopic CNV in patients depending on age – younger patients (<55 years) have been shown to develop significantly smaller lesions than older patients (p < 0.05) [60]. In younger patients, myopic CNVs tend to occur close to the fovea, and one study revealed that 83% of myopic CNVs appear to be smaller "classic" lesions [61]. Extrafoveal locations for myopic CNV are less common, with a study by Yoshida et al. finding that about 20% were not located in the foveal region [62]. Older patients tend to form more extensive and exudative myopic CNVs which can subsequently form large disciform scars which can easily be mistaken for those of neovascular age-related macular degeneration [62]. Histopathologically, the differences between the two processes can be determined more easily: in the majority of cases, myopic CNV is located between the neurosensory retina and the RPE, making it a Type 2 CNV, whereas the vast majority of AMD-related CNV are classified as Type 1 CNV, as they are sub-RPE lesions [63]. Myopic CNV is also characterized by several unique features: Bruch's membrane typically does not display diffuse thickening, the RPE and inner collagenous layer of Bruch's membrane tend not to cleave apart resulting in the formation of pigment epithelial detachments, and widespread deposits of extraneous extracellular matrix are not present [64]. Retinal hemorrhages are less common, and neurosensory detachments are typically shallower than those found in AMD-related CNV and are also much shallower in depth. Subretinal and intraretinal fluid accumulation is very limited and usually insignificant [64]. Once the myopic CNV

starts to regress, there may be some hyperpigmentation visible, and eventually this leads to fibrotic tissue scarring and subsequently thinning and atrophy of the chorioretinal complex. In the very end stages, the atrophy may be so severe as to result in exposure of bare sclera.

Light microscopy of a myopic CNV will show a thin fibrovascular membrane overlying RPE. The membrane may show small collagen bundles, fibroblasts, and nonuniformly distributed small blood vessels in a homogeneous matrix. Typically there is no evidence of inflammatory cells or thrombotic vessels [65] (see Figs. 8.12 and 8.13).

An interesting subtype of myopic CNV is the periconus CNV – that is, an extrafoveal CNV located next to a myopic conus. Nagaoka et al. looked at 260 eyes with myopic CNV

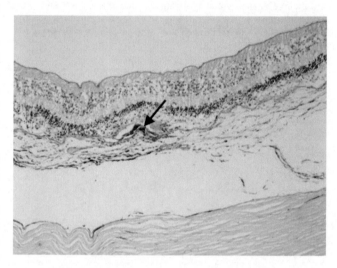

Fig. 8.12 Fuchs spot. The Fuchs spot is composed of a focal area of choroidal neovascularization surrounded by hyperplastic retinal pigment epithelium (*arrow*). *PAS 25×*

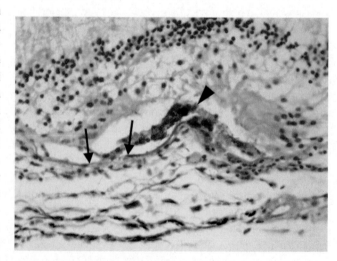

Fig. 8.13 Fuchs spot. There is a break in Bruch's membrane (*between arrows*) and a choroidal neovascular membrane surrounded by retinal pigment epithelium which extends through the break (*arrowhead*). *PAS 100×*

and found only 4.2% exhibited a periconus CNV [66]. They found that this subtype was more likely to occur in eyes that had a large myopic conus, and furthermore, the eyes with a periconus CNV had a significantly larger conus than those eyes that had subfoveal CNV. Axial length and degree of myopia were not associated with the formation of a periconus CNV, suggesting the spatial characteristics of the eye did not have any effect on the formation of CNV in this location. The study also found that just under half of the patients with periconus CNV experienced sudden regression, and the rest resolved after a single treatment to the CNV. Chorioretinal atrophy developed in three eyes (27%).

8.2.5 Retinal and Macular Hole/Schisis/ Detachment

Changes in the vitreoretinal interface at the posterior pole can manifest as a macular hole, which can subsequently lead to retinal detachment in highly myopic eyes. Vector forces from axial elongation or staphyloma formation in highly myopic eyes, increased vitreous liquefaction, and atrophy of the chorioretinal complex which is common in pathological myopia may combine to form the perfect storm of which the unfortunate outcome is the formation of a macular hole.

A study by Gass looking at the mechanism of formation of macular hole in non-myopic eyes found that the posterior vitreous cortex would pull on the connections at the vitreoretinal interface, with the ensuing traction resulting in a hole being torn in the macula as the vitreous was pulled away [67]. It is easy to hypothesize that the space formed by the retraction of the vitreous from the retinal surface would cause a negative pressure space into which the liquefied vitreous could move, coursing through the newly formed macular hole and under the retina and inducing a retinal detachment.

There are several stages of foveal or macular change in this process: epiretinal membrane; macular schisis; partial and full-thickness macular hole, with or without PVD; and posterior macular retinal detachments (see Figs. 8.14, 8.15, 8.16, and 8.17). One study looked at 214 eyes with pathological myopia and staphyloma and noted there to be vitreoretinal abnormalities in 56.8% of those patients [68].

Myopic foveoschisis was assessed using FD-OCT by Sayanagi et al. to evaluate the pathological features in this condition [69]. They found that defects in the inner and outer photoreceptor segments of foveal detachment type were seen in 3 of 6 eyes (50%), and IS/OS (foveoschisis type) was seen in 2 of 11 eyes (18%). Diffuse atrophy with the myopic foveoschisis was seen in 24%, and patchy atrophy was also observed in 24%.

A study by Takano et al. looked at 32 eyes of 19 patients with severe myopia and posterior staphyloma [47]. Using

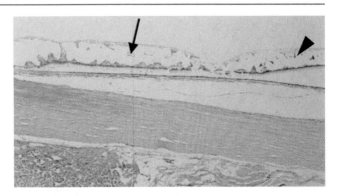

Fig. 8.14 Retinoschisis. An area of retinoschisis (*arrow*) is seen adjacent to an area of typical peripheral cystoid degeneration (*arrowhead*). *H&E 10×*

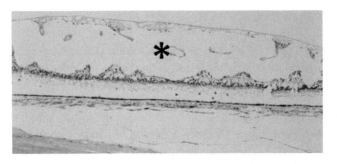

Fig. 8.15 Retinoschisis. Higher magnification shows the area of retinoschisis (*asterisk*) formed where there are interruptions of the bridges of Müller cells. *H&E 25×*

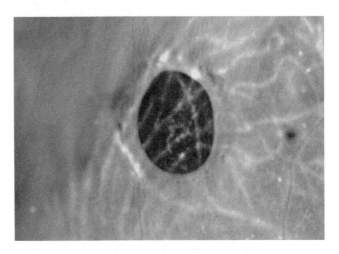

Fig. 8.16 Gross appearance of a full-thickness myopic retinal hole

OCT, they found 11/32 eyes (34%) to have foveal retinoschisis or detachment. Of these 8/32 eyes had foveal retinoschisis and retinal detachment, and 1/32 had only a foveal retinal detachment without schisis formation. 2/32 had only retinoschisis. The remaining 21/32 eyes with neither retinoschisis nor retinal detachment were all found to have macular thinning using OCT measurements of about 100–150 μm at the fovea. The results of this study suggest that a macular hole is

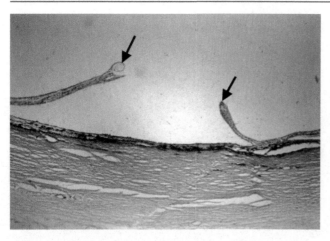

Fig. 8.17 Retinal hole. The full-thickness hole exhibits rounded edges of the surrounding retina (*arrows*). *H&E 100×*

not a prerequisite for retinoschisis or retinal detachment formation in severely myopic eyes that have a posterior staphyloma. It is possible that the tractional forces from the posterior staphyloma may cause a "stretch retinoschisis," leading to foveal detachment instead, followed by macular hole formation as these posteriorly located forces continue to act, pulling the macular retina away from the vitreous cortex.

Similarly, studies of myopic traction maculopathy using OCT have found that macular traction seems to be associated with a schisis, suggesting that the etiology of macular schisis may be a result of pre- or extraretinal traction due to the stretching forces experienced by an enlarged highly myopic eye [70, 71]. Following on from this finding, another study reviewed the prevalence of macular holes in highly myopic eyes and found that the macular holes were present in 6.26% of the eyes [72]. The most frequent vitreoretinal abnormalities associated with the macular holes was a schisis, found in 75% of that subgroup. 20.8% of the eyes with macular hole showed progression over a mean follow-up time of 30.2 months, in the form of enlargement of the hole, or a posterior retinal detachment.

In the study by Grossniklaus et al., the prevalence of retinal pits, holes, or tears seen on histologic section in the 369 eyes evaluated was 8.4% [6]. Previous studies have shown a link between myopic eyes and an increased risk for retinal hole formation [73, 74] and a significant correlation between retinal detachment and high myopia [75]. Retinal detachments were seen in 12.2% of eyes in the Grossniklaus study; however, the authors also considered the fact that a number of eyes in the study had at some point undergone a retinal detachment repair procedure, which increased the prevalence of retinal detachment occurrence in the study population of highly myopic eyes to 20%. One study found several factors that were associated with myopia and the formation of retinal detachments, including lattice degeneration,

asymptomatic retinal breaks, increased frequency of posterior vitreous detachment, and vitreous liquefaction [76].

A large Scottish study of 1202 cases of retinal detachment found that 18.7% of the eyes exhibited lattice degeneration [77]. Of these, retinal hole-related RD was significantly more common (35.7%) than horseshoe-tear RD (19.3%) and occurred mostly in more myopic patients. Furthermore, >85% of the RD were associated with PVD and related tractional abnormalities. These results are similar to another British study which found that retinal hole-related RD were more common in younger patients (median age 28.9 years) with a high degree of myopia (−5.5 D, range −1 to −18 D), and about 50% of the cases exhibited lattice degeneration [78].

8.2.6 Myopic Configuration of the Optic Nerve Head, Including Peripapillary Changes

In the American histopathological study of highly myopic eyes by Grossniklaus, the most common finding was of myopic configuration of the optic nerve head, found in 40% of the eyes [6]. A clinical study of pathological myopia fundus changes from Singapore found that peripapillary atrophy was the most common finding by far, in 81.2% of eyes, followed by disc tilt, found in 57.4% of eyes, and furthermore was found to be more common in teenaged high-myopes than in adults and those of Chinese descent [38]. Clinically, this myopic configuration appears as a tilted disc with the retina, RPE, and choroid extending over the disc nasally and the retina falling short of the optic disc on the temporal side. This combination gives rise to the appearance of a temporal crescent at the optic disc, although it can occasionally be seen nasally, or inferiorly, or in about 10% of cases surrounding the disc completely [22, 79]. These findings can all be seen clearly on histopathological examination, and in addition, the peripapillary sclera is often found to be stretched with a widening of the vaginal space between the subdural and subarachnoid spaces (see Figs. 8.18, 8.19, 8.20, 8.21, and 8.22). In addition, they found that when the optic nerve head was involved in the area of a staphyloma, it was typically enlarged.

A study by Jonas et al. compared the optic discs of highly myopic eyes to those of normal eyes [79]. They found that highly myopic eyes had significantly ($p < 0.000001$) larger and more oval-shaped optic discs than normal eyes and suggested that highly myopic optic discs could be regarded as secondary acquired macrodiscs, whereby the size of the disc could be correlated with refractive error and age.

A similar study by Fulk et al. attempted to correlate optic disc crescents with axial length and refractive error [80]. The study found that crescent size was significantly associated

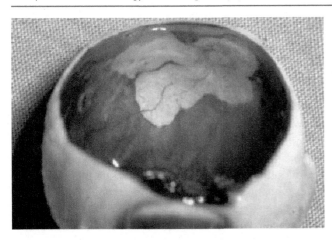

Fig. 8.18 Gross appearance of myopic degeneration of the optic nerve head. There is a myopic conus present surrounding the optic nerve. This is manifested by peripapillary atrophy and thinning of the sclera

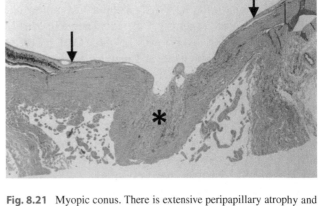

Fig. 8.21 Myopic conus. There is extensive peripapillary atrophy and thinning (*arrows*) which corresponds to a myopic conus. The bare sclera is seen surrounding an atrophic optic nerve (*asterisk*). *H&E 10×*

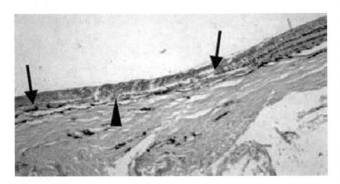

Fig. 8.19 Myopic degeneration. The peripapillary myopic conus corresponds to where the retina is reduced to a thin gliotic band (*between arrows*), and there is underlying atrophy of the retinal pigment epithelium and choroid (*arrowhead*). *H&E 100×*

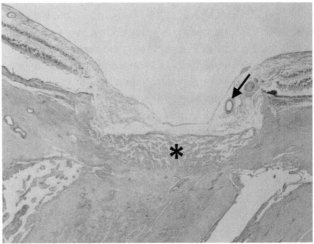

Fig. 8.22 Optic nerve degeneration. There is optic nerve atrophy down to the lamina cribrosa (*asterisk*) and only a vestigial blood vessel remains (*arrow*) in the atrophic tissue. *PAS 5×*

with both parameters ($p = 0.02$). For crescents ≥ 0.2 mm in width, each millimeter increase in axial length correlated to an average 1.26 D increase in myopic shift, but for those with <0.2 mm of crescent, each millimeter increase in axial length only correlated to about 0.66 D of myopic shift. The results also suggested that male gender and refractive error were directly associated with a large optic nerve crescent.

Nakazawa et al. did a long-term study to assess changes in optic nerve crescents in myopic eyes [81] and found that the degree of disc deviation correlated significantly to myopic progression ($p < 0.0001$). The optic discs observed were noted to deviate nasally in most cases as the myopia progressed, with subsequent formation of a peripapillary crescent on the temporal side of the disc.

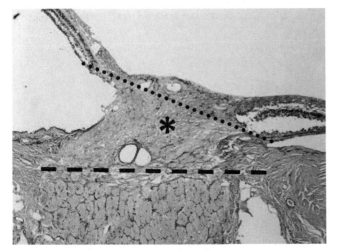

Fig. 8.20 Oblique optic nerve head. The optic nerve head (*asterisk*) enters the eye at an oblique angle (*dotted line*) compared to the lamina cribrosa (*dashed line*). *H&E 10×*

The lamina cribrosa is known to be affected by myopic degeneration [82, 83]. Both high myopia and glaucomatous change are independently significantly correlated with thinning of the lamina cribrosa [82]. In addition, numerous studies have shown that the peripapillary retinal nerve fiber layer is changed in highly myopic eyes [84–86]. OCT has been used to image the optic nerve and peripapillary regions of highly myopic eyes to reveal that the RNFL is typically thickened temporally and thinned nasally in eyes with tilted nerves [86]. Additionally, a thicker mean RNFL significantly correlated with both a lower degree of myopia and greater optic nerve disc and rim areas [85]. Superior and inferior RNFL thickness was not found to be significantly different between myopic and emmetropic eyes [84].

A histologic review of the peripapillary area in highly myopic eyes by Jonas et al. revealed that the distance between the border of the optic nerve and the dura mater, also known as the scleral flange, showed a significant increase with increasing axial length and decrease in length relative to the thickness of the flange area [87]. Furthermore, they discovered that 42% of the highly myopic eyes had a space >0.5 mm between the border of the optic nerve and the start of Bruch's membrane, where the flange was both elongated and thinned and a retrobulbar cerebrospinal fluid space was found to extend into the retroparapapillary region. Notably, the parapapillary region in these eyes only contained the RNFL or its remnants, with no detectable Bruch's membrane or choroid.

The peripapillary region in highly myopic eyes also exhibits other changes such as cavitations or pits. Wei et al. used OCT to evaluate these peripapillary intrachoroidal cavitations which appear as elevated, patchy, yellowish lesions on fundoscopic examination [88]. OCT revealed these lesions to be intrachoroidal spaces located below the RPE. About half of the cases showed evidence of communicating channels leading from the vitreous to the intrachoroidal cavitation, and one quarter also revealed intrachoroidal splitting. Wei et al. hypothesized that these peripapillary lesions could represent either a cavitation or choroidal schisis, with the possibility that they could both be part of a spectrum of the same pathological process.

Another finding in the optic nerve and peripapillary region of highly myopic eyes is that of pitlike structures. One study found that pits were found at the optic nerve border or peripapillary area in 16.2% of highly myopic eyes and that these eyes also were more highly myopic and had significantly larger optic discs and longer axial lengths than highly myopic eyes that did not have any pits [89]. In about a third of cases, the pits were located at the optic disc, where they were present at either the superior or inferior border, and in two-thirds, the pits were located in the peripapillary conus. The conus pits were associated with Type IX staphyloma, and the pitting was evident in between the optic nerve border and the scleral ridge and appeared to have developed from a staphyloma-induced schisis.

8.2.7 Vitreous Degeneration

It is known that vitreous syneresis occurs earlier in myopia and, additionally, is more extensive and increases as the myopia worsens [90]. Both vitreous liquefaction and posterior vitreous detachment are common clinical findings with pathological myopia as the increased intraocular volume of an enlarged myopic eye contributes to the development of vitreous degeneration [91]. In the study by Grossniklaus, central vitreous liquefaction was found on histopathological examination in all the myopic eyes examined and posterior vitreous detachment in 33% of the eyes [6]. In most cases, only the cortical vitreous remained intact (see Fig. 8.23). In several cases, they also noted that the posterior vitreous traction had caused retinal holes, cystic degeneration, and retinoschisis. Although increased age is known to be a risk factor for the formation of posterior vitreous detachment, one study compared 224 eyes with high myopia (−6 D or greater) with emmetropic eyes and found that the prevalence of PVD was higher in the myopic group at every age group [92].

Animal models have found that faulty proteins encoding for the inner limiting membrane (ILM) and vitreous body lead to a 50% increase in eye size within 4 days, a process which was only slowed by reconstituting the ILM [93]. The results indicate that congenital high myopia can be affected by the integrity of the vitreoretinal border. A study by Chuo et al. found a significant association between myopic refraction and the formation of a posterior vitreous detachment (OR = 4.32, $p < 0.0005$) [94].

A study by Stirpe et al. looked at 496 highly myopic eyes that underwent surgical treatment for retinal detachments [95]. They noticed five characteristic appearances for the vitreous and retina: (1) uniform PVD (21.8%), (2) PVD spreading to upper quadrants (46.5%), (3) extensive liquefaction

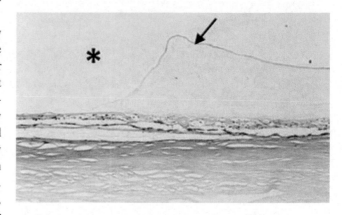

Fig. 8.23 Posterior vitreous detachment. The posterior vitreous is liquefied (*asterisk*), and the vitreous has been dragged forward (*arrow*). *PAS 100×*

and condensations of the vitreous base (10.2%), (4) posterior vitreous lacuna (17.5%), and (5) very limited PVD (3.8%). The group with posterior vitreous lacuna was found to have a higher degree of myopia and more pronounced staphylomas.

8.3 Conclusion

The histopathology of pathological myopia plays an important role in understanding the mechanisms by which this condition can affect vision. There have been several excellent and extensive histopathological studies of highly myopic eyes, but in recent years, the use of other imaging modalities such as OCT, fluorescein angiograms, and ICG has become more commonplace in trying to elucidate the nature of the pathological processes. It is important to be able to use these imaging studies in combination with the histopathological descriptions in order to be able to better understand the disease processes and spectrum.

References

1. Foster PJ. Myopia in Asia. Br J Ophthalmol. 2004;88(4):443–4. PubMed PMID: 15031147. Pubmed Central PMCID: 1772076.
2. Ghafour IM, Allan D, Foulds WS. Common causes of blindness and visual handicap in the west of Scotland. Br J Ophthalmol. 1983;67(4):209–13. PubMed PMID: 6830738. Pubmed Central PMCID: 1040020.
3. Sperduto RD, Seigel D, Roberts J, Rowland M. Prevalence of myopia in the United States. Arch Ophthalmol. 1983;101(3):405–7. PubMed PMID: 6830491.
4. Duke Elder S. Pathological refractive errors. In: Ophthalmic optics and refraction, system of ophthalmology, vol. V. St. Louis: Mosby; 1970. p. 297–373.
5. Tokoro T. On the definition of pathologic myopia in group studies. Acta Ophthalmol Suppl. 1988;185:107–8. PubMed PMID: 2853512.
6. Grossniklaus HE, Green WR. Pathologic findings in pathologic myopia. Retina. 1992;12(2):127–33. PubMed PMID: 1439243. Epub 1992/01/01.
7. Curtin BJ. The etiology of myopia. In: The myopias: basic science and clinical management. Philadelphia: Harper and Row; 1985. p. 61–113.
8. Curtin BJ. Physiologic vs pathologic myopia: genetics vs environment. Ophthalmology. 1979;86(5):681–91. PubMed PMID: 397448.
9. Zejmo M, Forminska-Kapuscik M, Pieczara E, Filipek E, Mrukwa-Kominek E, Samochowiec-Donocik E, et al. Etiopathogenesis and management of high myopia. Part II. Med Sci Monit. 2009;15(11):RA252–5. PubMed PMID: 19865068.
10. Zejmo M, Forminska-Kapuscik M, Pieczara E, Filipek E, Mrukwa-Kominek E, Samochowiec-Donocik E, et al. Etiopathogenesis and management of high-degree myopia. Part I. Med Sci Monit. 2009;15(9):RA199–202. PubMed PMID: 19721411.
11. Walline JJ, Lindsley K, Vedula SS, Cotter SA, Mutti DO, Twelker JD. Interventions to slow progression of myopia in children. Cochrane Database Syst Rev. 2011;(12):CD004916. PubMed PMID: 22161388.
12. Avila MP, Weiter JJ, Jalkh AE, Trempe CL, Pruett RC, Schepens CL. Natural history of choroidal neovascularization in degenerative myopia. Ophthalmology. 1984;91(12):1573–81. PubMed PMID: 6084222.
13. Klein RM, Green S. The development of lacquer cracks in pathologic myopia. Am J Ophthalmol. 1988;106(3):282–5. PubMed PMID: 3421288.
14. Pruett RC, Weiter JJ, Goldstein RB. Myopic cracks, angioid streaks, and traumatic tears in Bruch's membrane. Am J Ophthalmol. 1987;103(4):537–43. PubMed PMID: 3565514.
15. Klein RM, Curtin BJ. Lacquer crack lesions in pathologic myopia. Am J Ophthalmol. 1975;79(3):386–92. PubMed PMID: 1121996.
16. Curtin BJ, Karlin DB. Axial length measurements and fundus changes of the myopic eye. Am J Ophthalmol. 1971;71(1 Pt 1):42–53. PubMed PMID: 5099937.
17. Ohno-Matsui K, Ito M, Tokoro T. Subretinal bleeding without choroidal neovascularization in pathologic myopia. A sign of new lacquer crack formation. Retina. 1996;16(3):196–202. PubMed PMID: 8789857. Epub 1996/01/01.
18. Ohno-Matsui K, Tokoro T. The progression of lacquer cracks in pathologic myopia. Retina. 1996;16(1):29–37. PubMed PMID: 8927806. Epub 1996/01/01.
19. Johnson DA, Yannuzzi LA, Shakin JL, Lightman DA. Lacquer cracks following laser treatment of choroidal neovascularization in pathologic myopia. Retina. 1998;18(2):118–24. PubMed PMID: 9564691. Epub 1998/06/27.
20. Ohno-Matsui K, Yoshida T, Futagami S, Yasuzumi K, Shimada N, Kojima A, et al. Patchy atrophy and lacquer cracks predispose to the development of choroidal neovascularisation in pathological myopia. Br J Ophthalmol. 2003;87(5):570–3. PubMed PMID: 12714395. Pubmed Central PMCID: 1771643. Epub 2003/04/26.
21. Noble KG, Carr RE. Pathologic myopia. Ophthalmology. 1982;89(9):1099–100. PubMed PMID: 7177575.
22. Rabb MF, Garoon I, LaFranco FP. Myopic macular degeneration. Int Ophthalmol Clin. 1981;21(3):51–69. PubMed PMID: 6169677.
23. Kobayashi K, Ohno-Matsui K, Kojima A, Shimada N, Yasuzumi K, Yoshida T, et al. Fundus characteristics of high myopia in children. Jpn J Ophthalmol. 2005;49(4):306–11. PubMed PMID: 16075331.
24. Hayashi K, Ohno-Matsui K, Shimada N, Moriyama M, Kojima A, Hayashi W, et al. Long-term pattern of progression of myopic maculopathy: a natural history study. Ophthalmology. 2010;117(8):1595–611, 611.e1–4. PubMed PMID: 20207005.
25. Okabe S, Matsuo N, Okamoto S, Kataoka H. Electron microscopic studies on retinochoroidal atrophy in the human eye. Acta Med Okayama. 1982;36(1):11–21. PubMed PMID: 7064730.
26. Wang NK, Lai CC, Chu HY, Chen YP, Chen KJ, Wu WC, et al. Classification of early dry-type myopic maculopathy with macular choroidal thickness. Am J Ophthalmol. 2012;153(4):669–77, 77.e1–2. PubMed PMID: 22071232.
27. Ohsugi H, Ikuno Y, Oshima K, Tabuchi H. 3-D choroidal thickness maps from EDI-OCT in highly myopic eyes. Optom Vis Sci. 2013;90:599–606. PubMed PMID: 23604298.
28. Hirata A, Negi A. Morphological changes of choriocapillaris in experimentally induced chick myopia. Graefes Arch Clin Exp Ophthalmol. 1998;236(2):132–7. PubMed PMID: 9498124.
29. Karlin DB, Curtin BJ. Peripheral chorioretinal lesions and axial length of the myopic eye. Am J Ophthalmol. 1976;81(5):625–35. PubMed PMID: 1275043.
30. Celorio JM, Pruett RC. Prevalence of lattice degeneration and its relation to axial length in severe myopia. Am J Ophthalmol. 1991;111(1):20–3. PubMed PMID: 1985485.
31. Yura T. The relationship between the types of axial elongation and the prevalence of lattice degeneration of the retina. Acta Ophthalmol Scand. 1998;76(1):90–5. PubMed PMID: 9541442.
32. Curtin BJ. Posterior staphyloma development in pathologic myopia. Ann Ophthalmol. 1982;14(7):655–8. PubMed PMID: 6982020.

33. Curtin BJ, Teng CC. Scleral changes in pathological myopia. Trans Am Acad Ophthalmol Otolaryngol. 1958;62(6):777–88; discussion 88–90. PubMed PMID: 13625324.

34. Curtin BJ, Iwamoto T, Renaldo DP. Normal and staphylomatous sclera of high myopia. An electron microscopic study. Arch Ophthalmol. 1979;97(5):912–5. PubMed PMID: 444126.

35. Gentle A, Liu Y, Martin JE, Conti GL, McBrien NA. Collagen gene expression and the altered accumulation of scleral collagen during the development of high myopia. J Biol Chem. 2003;278(19):16587–94. PubMed PMID: 12606541.

36. Curtin BJ. The posterior staphyloma of pathologic myopia. Trans Am Ophthalmol Soc. 1977;75:67–86. PubMed PMID: 613534. Pubmed Central PMCID: 1311542.

37. Hsiang HW, Ohno-Matsui K, Shimada N, Hayashi K, Moriyama M, Yoshida T, et al. Clinical characteristics of posterior staphyloma in eyes with pathologic myopia. Am J Ophthalmol. 2008;146(1):102–10. PubMed PMID: 18455142.

38. Chang L, Pan CW, Ohno-Matsui K, Lin X, Cheung GC, Gazzard G, et al. Myopia-related fundus changes in Singapore adults with high myopia. Am J Ophthalmol. 2013;155:991–9.e1. PubMed PMID: 23499368.

39. Moriyama M, Ohno-Matsui K, Futagami S, Yoshida T, Hayashi K, Shimada N, et al. Morphology and long-term changes of choroidal vascular structure in highly myopic eyes with and without posterior staphyloma. Ophthalmology. 2007;114(9):1755–62. PubMed PMID: 17368542.

40. Quaranta M, Brindeau C, Coscas G, Soubrane G. Multiple choroidal neovascularizations at the border of a myopic posterior macular staphyloma. Graefes Arch Clin Exp Ophthalmol. 2000;238(1):101–3. PubMed PMID: 10664062.

41. Mehta P, Dinakaran S, Squirrell D, Talbot J. Retinal pigment epithelial changes and choroidal neovascularisation at the edge of posterior staphylomas; a case series and review of the literature. Eye. 2006;20(2):150–3. PubMed PMID: 15776012.

42. Ohno-Matsui K, Akiba M, Moriyama M, Ishibashi T, Hirakata A, Tokoro T. Intrachoroidal cavitation in macular area of eyes with pathologic myopia. Am J Ophthalmol. 2012;154(2):382–93. PubMed PMID: 22541655.

43. Leys AM, Cohen SY. Subretinal leakage in myopic eyes with a posterior staphyloma or tilted disk syndrome. Retina. 2002;22(5):659–65. PubMed PMID: 12441740.

44. Gaucher D, Erginay A, Lecleire-Collet A, Haouchine B, Puech M, Cohen SY, et al. Dome-shaped macula in eyes with myopic posterior staphyloma. Am J Ophthalmol. 2008;145(5):909–14. PubMed PMID: 18342827.

45. Henaine-Berra A, Zand-Hadas IM, Fromow-Guerra J, Garcia-Aguirre G. Prevalence of macular anatomic abnormalities in high myopia. Ophthalmic Surg Lasers Imaging Retina. 2013;44(2):140–4. PubMed PMID: 23438042.

46. Wu PC, Chen YJ, Chen YH, Chen CH, Shin SJ, Tsai CL, et al. Factors associated with foveoschisis and foveal detachment without macular hole in high myopia. Eye. 2009;23(2):356–61. PubMed PMID: 18064059.

47. Takano M, Kishi S. Foveal retinoschisis and retinal detachment in severely myopic eyes with posterior staphyloma. Am J Ophthalmol. 1999;128(4):472–6. PubMed PMID: 10577588.

48. Oie Y, Ikuno Y, Fujikado T, Tano Y. Relation of posterior staphyloma in highly myopic eyes with macular hole and retinal detachment. Jpn J Ophthalmol. 2005;49(6):530–2. PubMed PMID: 16365803.

49. Tano Y. Pathologic myopia: where are we now? Am J Ophthalmol. 2002;134(5):645–60. PubMed PMID: 12429239.

50. Neelam K, Cheung CM, Ohno-Matsui K, Lai TY, Wong TY. Choroidal neovascularization in pathological myopia. Prog Retin Eye Res. 2012;31(5):495–525. PubMed PMID: 22569156.

51. Cohen SY, Laroche A, Leguen Y, Soubrane G, Coscas GJ. Etiology of choroidal neovascularization in young patients. Ophthalmology. 1996;103(8):1241–4. PubMed PMID: 8764794.

52. Inhoffen W, Ziemssen F. Morphological features of myopic choroidal neovascularization: differences to neovascular age-related macular degeneration. Ophthalmologe. 2012;109(8):749–57. PubMed PMID: 22911352. Morphologische Charakteristika der myopen choroidalen Neovaskularisation: Unterschiede zur neovaskularen altersabhangigen Makuladegeneration.

53. Jalkh AE, Weiter JJ, Trempe CL, Pruett RC, Schepens CL. Choroidal neovascularization in degenerative myopia: role of laser photocoagulation. Ophthalmic Surg. 1987;18(10):721–5. PubMed PMID: 2448722.

54. Brancato R, Pece A, Avanza P, Radrizzani E. Photocoagulation scar expansion after laser therapy for choroidal neovascularization in degenerative myopia. Retina. 1990;10(4):239–43. PubMed PMID: 1708513.

55. Pece A, Brancato R, Avanza P, Camesasca F, Galli L. Laser photocoagulation of choroidal neovascularization in pathologic myopia: long-term results. Int Ophthalmol. 1994;18(6):339–44. PubMed PMID: 7543889.

56. Morgan CM, Schatz H. Atrophic creep of the retinal pigment epithelium after focal macular photocoagulation. Ophthalmology. 1989;96(1):96–103. PubMed PMID: 2919053.

57. Yoshida T, Ohno-Matsui K, Yasuzumi K, Kojima A, Shimada N, Futagami S, et al. Myopic choroidal neovascularization: a 10-year follow-up. Ophthalmology. 2003;110(7):1297–305. PubMed PMID: 12867382.

58. Kim YM, Yoon JU, Koh HJ. The analysis of lacquer crack in the assessment of myopic choroidal neovascularization. Eye. 2011;25(7):937–46. PubMed PMID: 21527958. Pubmed Central PMCID: 3178161.

59. Ikuno Y, Sayanagi K, Soga K, Sawa M, Gomi F, Tsujikawa M, et al. Lacquer crack formation and choroidal neovascularization in pathologic myopia. Retina. 2008;28(8):1124–31. PubMed PMID: 18779719.

60. Leveziel N, Caillaux V, Bastuji-Garin S, Zmuda M, Souied EH. Angiographic and optical coherence tomography characteristics of recent myopic choroidal neovascularization. Am J Ophthalmol. 2013;155(5):913–9 e1. PubMed PMID: 23352343.

61. Verteporfin in Photodynamic Therapy Study Group. Photodynamic therapy of subfoveal choroidal neovascularization in pathologic myopia with verteporfin. 1-year results of a randomized clinical trial – VIP report no. 1. Ophthalmology. 2001;108(5):841–52. PubMed PMID: 11320011.

62. Yoshida T, Ohno-Matsui K, Ohtake Y, Takashima T, Futagami S, Baba T, et al. Long-term visual prognosis of choroidal neovascularization in high myopia: a comparison between age groups. Ophthalmology. 2002;109(4):712–9. PubMed PMID: 11927428.

63. Grossniklaus HE, Gass JD. Clinicopathologic correlations of surgically excised type 1 and type 2 submacular choroidal neovascular membranes. Am J Ophthalmol. 1998;126(1):59–69. PubMed PMID: 9683150.

64. Baba T, Ohno-Matsui K, Yoshida T, Yasuzumi K, Futagami S, Tokoro T, et al. Optical coherence tomography of choroidal neovascularization in high myopia. Acta Ophthalmol Scand. 2002;80(1):82–7. PubMed PMID: 11906310.

65. Scupola A, Ventura L, Tiberti AC, D'Andrea D, Balestrazzi E. Histological findings of a surgically excised myopic choroidal neovascular membrane after photodynamic therapy. A case report. Graefes Arch Clin Exp Ophthalmol. 2004;242(7):605–10. PubMed PMID: 14986008.

66. Nagaoka N, Shimada N, Hayashi W, Hayashi K, Moriyama M, Yoshida T, et al. Characteristics of periconus choroidal neovascularization in pathologic myopia. Am J Ophthalmol. 2011;152(3):420–7 e1. PubMed PMID: 21696698.

67. Gass JD. Idiopathic senile macular hole: its early stages and pathogenesis. 1988. Retina. 2003;23(6 Suppl):629–39.

68. Ripandelli G, Rossi T, Scarinci F, Scassa C, Parisi V, Stirpe M. Macular vitreoretinal interface abnormalities in highly myopic eyes with posterior staphyloma: 5-year follow-up. Retina. 2012;32(8):1531–8. PubMed PMID: 22614742.

69. Sayanagi K, Ikuno Y, Soga K, Tano Y. Photoreceptor inner and outer segment defects in myopic foveoschisis. Am J Ophthalmol. 2008;145(5):902–8. PubMed PMID: 18342829.

70. Robichaud JL, Besada E, Basler L, Frauens BJ. Spectral domain optical coherence tomography of myopic traction maculopathy. Optometry. 2011;82(10):607–13. PubMed PMID: 21840263.

71. Konidaris V, Androudi S, Brazitikos P. Myopic traction maculopathy: study with spectral domain optical coherence tomography and review of the literature. Hippokratia. 2009;13(2):110–3. PubMed PMID: 19561782. Pubmed Central PMCID: 2683149.

72. Coppe AM, Ripandelli G, Parisi V, Varano M, Stirpe M. Prevalence of asymptomatic macular holes in highly myopic eyes. Ophthalmology. 2005;112(12):2103–9. PubMed PMID: 16225922.

73. Ripandelli G, Coppe AM, Parisi V, Stirpe M. Fellow eye findings of highly myopic subjects operated for retinal detachment associated with a macular hole. Ophthalmology. 2008;115(9):1489–93. PubMed PMID: 18439680.

74. Tsujikawa A, Kikuchi M, Ishida K, Nonaka A, Yamashiro K, Kurimoto Y. Fellow eye of patients with retinal detachment associated with macular hole and bilateral high myopia. Clin Exp Ophthalmol. 2006;34(5):430–3. PubMed PMID: 16872338.

75. Tornquist R, Stenkula S, Tornquist P. Retinal detachment. A study of a population-based patient material in Sweden 1971–1981. I. Epidemiology. Acta Ophthalmol (Copenh). 1987;65(2):213–22.

76. Michels RG, Wilkinson CP, Rice TA. Retinal detachment. St. Louis: Mosby; 1990. p. 76–84.

77. Mitry D, Singh J, Yorston D, Siddiqui MA, Wright A, Fleck BW, et al. The predisposing pathology and clinical characteristics in the Scottish retinal detachment study. Ophthalmology. 2011;118(7):1429–34. PubMed PMID: 21561662.

78. Williams KM, Dogramaci M, Williamson TH. Retrospective study of rhegmatogenous retinal detachments secondary to round retinal holes. Eur J Ophthalmol. 2012;22(4):635–40. PubMed PMID: 22081671.

79. Jonas JB, Gusek GC, Naumann GO. Optic disk morphometry in high myopia. Graefes Arch Clin Exp Ophthalmol. 1988;226(6):587–90. PubMed PMID: 3209086.

80. Fulk GW, Goss DA, Christensen MT, Cline KB, Herrin-Lawson GA. Optic nerve crescents and refractive error. Optom Vis Sci. 1992;69(3):208–13. PubMed PMID: 1565418.

81. Nakazawa M, Kurotaki J, Ruike H. Long term findings in peripapillary crescent formation in eyes with mild or moderate myopia. Acta Ophthalmol. 2008;86(6):626–9. PubMed PMID: 18577184.

82. Jonas JB, Berenshtein E, Holbach L. Lamina cribrosa thickness and spatial relationships between intraocular space and cerebrospinal fluid space in highly myopic eyes. Invest Ophthalmol Vis Sci. 2004;45(8):2660–5. PubMed PMID: 15277489.

83. Kubena K, Rehak S. Collagen architecture of the lamina cribrosa of the human eye in glaucoma and severe myopia. Cesk Oftalmol. 1984;40(2–3):73–8. PubMed PMID: 6488366. Kolagenni architektura lamina cribrosa lidskeho oka pri glaukomu a tezke myopii.

84. Hsu SY, Chang MS, Ko ML, Harnod T. Retinal nerve fibre layer thickness and optic nerve head size measured in high myopes by optical coherence tomography. Clin Exp Optom. 2013;96:373–8. PubMed PMID: 23561012.

85. Hwang YH, Kim YY. Correlation between optic nerve head parameters and retinal nerve fibre layer thickness measured by spectral-domain optical coherence tomography in myopic eyes. Clin Exp Ophthalmol. 2012;40(7):713–20. PubMed PMID: 22429807.

86. Hwang YH, Yoo C, Kim YY. Characteristics of peripapillary retinal nerve fiber layer thickness in eyes with myopic optic disc tilt and rotation. J Glaucoma. 2012;21(6):394–400. PubMed PMID: 21946540.

87. Jonas JB, Jonas SB, Jonas RA, Holbach L, Panda-Jonas S. Histology of the parapapillary region in high myopia. Am J Ophthalmol. 2011;152(6):1021–9. PubMed PMID: 21821229.

88. Wei YH, Yang CM, Chen MS, Shih YF, Ho TC. Peripapillary intrachoroidal cavitation in high myopia: reappraisal. Eye. 2009;23(1):141–4. PubMed PMID: 17721499.

89. Ohno-Matsui K, Akiba M, Moriyama M, Shimada N, Ishibashi T, Tokoro T, et al. Acquired optic nerve and peripapillary pits in pathologic myopia. Ophthalmology. 2012;119(8):1685–92. PubMed PMID: 22494632.

90. Soubrane G, Coscas G, Kuhn D. Myopia. In: Retina-vitreous-macula [internet]. Philadelphia: WB Saunders Co; 1999. p. 189–205.

91. Curtin BJ. Pathology. In: The myopias: basic science and clinical management [internet]. Philadelphia: Harper and Row; 1985. p. 247–67.

92. Akiba J. Prevalence of posterior vitreous detachment in high myopia. Ophthalmology. 1993;100(9):1384–8. PubMed PMID: 8371928.

93. Halfter W, Winzen U, Bishop PN, Eller A. Regulation of eye size by the retinal basement membrane and vitreous body. Invest Ophthalmol Vis Sci. 2006;47(8):3586–94. PubMed PMID: 16877433. Epub 2006/08/01.

94. Chuo JY, Lee TY, Hollands H, Morris AH, Reyes RC, Rossiter JD, et al. Risk factors for posterior vitreous detachment: a case–control study. Am J Ophthalmol. 2006;142(6):931–7. PubMed PMID: 17157578. Epub 2006/12/13.

95. Stirpe M, Heimann K. Vitreous changes and retinal detachment in highly myopic eyes. Eur J Ophthalmol. 1996;6(1):50–8. PubMed PMID: 8744851. Epub 1996/01/01.

The Sclera and Induced Abnormalities in Myopia

Richard F. Spaide

The main constructural element of the eye is the sclera, a tough, translucent fibrous coat that provides a set shape and volume of the eye and functions as a protective casing to its fragile internal contents. The sclera is a composite of an interwoven network of collagen fibers (mostly Type I) embedded in a hypocellular ground substance matrix. The sclera has some similarities to a pneumatic tire. The collagen fibers are analogous to the plies in a tire; they are relatively less distensible fibers embedded in a matrix that is more distensible. A pneumatic tire is inflated by air, while the sclera is inflated by the intraocular pressure. The mechanical engineering advantages of this arrangement include strength, sufficient rigidity without brittleness, and little need for intrinsic blood supply or cellular turnover. Because the eye has structural rigidity, the length and shape of the eye are not altered with eye movement or diurnal changes in intraocular pressure. On the other hand, the eye is easily deformable without suffering internal or external damage during ordinary use in life. Blood vessels and nerves of various sizes penetrate the sclera, and design features of the scleral openings help mitigate against loss of the intraocular contents. The muscles of the iris and ciliary body attach to the sclera as do the extraocular muscles used for movement of the globe. The sclera, which accounts for more than 90% of the surface area of the eye [1], merges anteriorly with the optically clear specialization, the cornea.

Many changes occur in the sclera of high myopes, and these changes and the abnormalities they may induce are the focus of this chapter. In most high myopes, the eye undergoes normal development in utero and early childhood to be followed later by progressive scleral thinning and ocular expansion. With knowledge of the base anatomy and the induced alterations caused by the expansion, the subsequent abnormalities associated with myopia are eas-ier to understand. As such, this chapter starts with a review of the embryology and development of the sclera, its anatomy, and mechanical properties. Features of what happens in myopization will then be presented, followed by how these forces cause specific clinically recognizable alterations in the sclera and associated structures. One specific and important induced alteration, the staphyloma, is sufficiently complex as to require treatment in two accompanying chapters.

9.1 Embryology and Development of the Sclera

The evagination of the optic vesicle starts in the fourth week and invaginates to form the optic cup in the fifth week. A thickening of the overlying ectoderm called the lens placode develops around this time and will eventually invaginate to form the primordial lens. The sclera is derived from the neural crest, and to a much lesser extent the mesoderm, starting in the sixth week as waves of invading cells form a condensation on the optic cup (Fig. 9.1). It appears that the pigment epithelium and the uvea are required to induce formation of the posterior sclera. Incomplete closure of the fetal fissure causes colobomas to occur, and these colobomas influence development of the nascent sclera. The sclera develops anterior to posterior, but also in an inner to outer scleral vector as well [2]. Over the next months, the thickness of the collagen fibers increases so that by week 24, the fibers are three times thicker than they were at week 6 [2]. In a normal eye, the anterior sclera reaches adult size by age 2, while the posterior sclera does so by age 13. The axial length of a term infant is about 17 mm and is destined to reach 23 mm by age 13 years [3]. Considered as a simple sphere, the eye expands 2.5 times in volume over this time. The remarkable aspect of ocular growth is that the eye can remain emmetropic even though the individual components of the eye are growing at their own individual rate.

R. F. Spaide (✉)
Vitreous, Retina, Macula Consultants of New York,
New York, NY, USA

© Springer Nature Switzerland AG 2021
R. F. Spaide et al. (eds.), *Pathologic Myopia*, https://doi.org/10.1007/978-3-030-74334-5_9

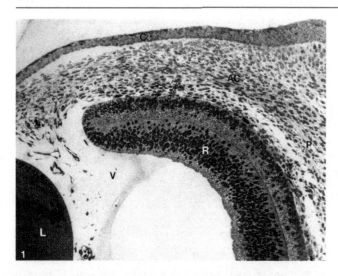

Fig. 9.1 At week 6.4, there is a condensation of mesenchyme (AC) around the optic cup. The cell density in the mesenchyme is somewhat lower posteriorly (P) in this section. The retina (R) is undergoing differentiation and is in contact with the vitreous (V). The lens (L) is visible at the bottom left. (Derived from Ref. [2])

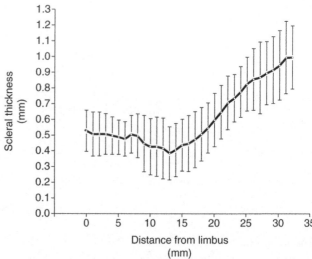

Fig. 9.2 Graphical representation of the scleral thickness in normal eyes extending from the surgical limbus (left) toward the optic nerve (right). (Derived from Ref. [1])

9.2   Gross Scleral Anatomy of an Emmetropic Eye

In an emmetropic eye, the sclera shell has a diameter of approximately 24 mm and a surface area of approximately 17 square centimeters [1]. The sclera has no lymphatics or cellular boundary. The thickness of the sclera in a nonmyopic eye varies considerably with location; the thickest is around the optic nerve where it can be slightly more than 1 mm, while immediately under the rectus muscle insertions, it can be as little as 0.3 mm thick. In the submacular region, the sclera has a thickness of about 0.9 mm in normal eyes (Fig. 9.2). On the outer surface of the scleral stroma is the episclera, a loose connective tissue. Anteriorly the episclera contains a plexus of capillaries, but no lymphatics. The sclera is enveloped by Tenon's capsule, a double layer of fibrous tissue with a smooth inner border separated from the eye by a potential space occasionally traversed by diaphanous strands of the episclera [4]. Tenon's capsule merges with the dura mater of the optic nerve posteriorly and the muscle capsules. The inner surface of the sclera is composed of a thin layer containing melanocytes, giving it a brown color and its name, lamina fusca.

The anterior portion of the sclera terminates at the posterior boundary of the cornea at what is called the anterior scleral foramen. The limbus forms the transitional zone between the sclera and the cornea. The largest opening in the sclera posteriorly is the scleral canal, which exists to allow exit of the optic nerve. The retinal nerve fiber layer changes direction by bending around the inner opening of the optic canal, formed by Bruch's membrane and the scleral ring to

head posteriorly out of the eye. The inner opening of the optic canal is approximately 1.8 mm in diameter. Somewhat anterior to the midpoint of the optic canal, there is a sieve-like network of fibers, called the lamina cribrosa, which crisscross the breadth of the canal. The openings, or pores, are bordered by these fibers within each plate of the lamina. The pores in an emmetropic nonglaucomatous eye are round or oval, and the pores are nearly aligned in a vertical sense from one plate to another, except toward the periphery of the lamina cribrosa. The resultant openings allow the nerve fibers to exit the eye. A central opening in the lamina is larger than the surrounding to allow passage of the central retinal artery and vein. The pores in the lamina are largest superiorly and inferiorly, where the predominate number of nerve fibers are seen to enter the optic canal [5]. Providing additional structural and metabolic support in this region are the closely associated glial cells [6, 7]. Surrounding the optic nerve as it transits the lamina is the border tissue of Elschnig. The diameter of the canal increases posteriorly to accommodate the larger diameter of the retrolaminar optic nerve, which contrary to the prelaminar portion of the optic nerve is myelinated. The posterior optic nerve canal is approximately 3.5 mm wide. The optic nerve has a dura mater covering. The outer two-thirds of the scleral collagen merge with the fibers of the dura mater.

Arteries, vein, and nerves course through smaller openings in the sclera. These openings, or emissaries, are often placed at an angle to the thickness of the sclera, apparently to reduce the likelihood of loss of intraocular contents with increased pressure in the eye. The 15–20 short posterior artery emissaries aggregate around the optic nerve and macular regions. Using optical coherence tomography (OCT) with deeper imaging capabilities, it is common to see branching of some of the posterior vessels in the sclera. Therefore, there are at least as many internal openings of the emissary as there are external openings in the sclera. Most of the emissaries in the posterior pole are for the short posterior ciliary arteries to bring blood flow into the choroid. Branches from short posterior ciliary arteries, with possible contributions from the choroidal circulation, form a ring, often incomplete, around the prelaminar portion of the optic nerve known as the circle of Zinn-Haller. This circle is located a mean of 403 microns from the outer portion of the optic nerve in normal eyes. The mean vascular diameter was 123 microns but ranges from 20 to 230 microns in diameter [7]. There is variation to the depth that the circle of Zinn-Haller is located but may be as much as 345 microns below the inner scleral surface [8]. This structure is visible with angiography [9, 10]. The long posterior ciliary arteries enter the sclera nasal and temporal to the optic nerve and do not fully penetrate the inner portion of the sclera until the equator. The main venous drainage of the choroid occurs through the vortex veins, the ampullae of which are found at the equator of the eye. The vortex veins travel obliquely through the sclera to exit the eye posterior to the equator. Associated with the insertions of the rectus muscles are the anterior ciliary arteries, which bring blood flow to the ciliary body. Superficial branches of these arteries contribute to the episcleral circulation. There is also a copious supply of nerves as evidenced by the pain associated with trauma or inflammation of the sclera.

9.3 Fine Anatomy of the Sclera

The sclera is composed of collagen fibers of varying sizes, but the inner fibers are smaller, about 62 nanometers, than the outer fibers, which are about 125 nanometers [11] (Fig. 9.3). The fibrils are composed of Type I collagen and consequently have high proportions of proline, hydroxyproline, and hydroxylysine. The presence of hydroxylysine provides for the possibility of molecular cross-linking, which increases the tensile strength and mechanical stability of the sclera. These structural modifications can come at the expense of increased rigidity. The collagen fibers are embedded in the interfibrillary matrix composed of proteoglycans. Proteoglycans have a protein core that is attached to varying numbers of glycosaminoglycans, which are long molecules composed of sugar subunits. Proteoglycans are classified by the nature of the core protein and by the number and types of attached glycosaminoglycans. The two main glycosaminoglycans in the sclera are chondroitin sulfate and dermatan sulfate, which alone or in combination contribute to the formation of the major proteoglycans, biglycan, aggrecan, and decorin [13]. The remarkable attribute of proteoglycans,

conferred by their glycosaminoglycan constituents, is the ability to bind to large amounts of water. This allows proteoglycan fraction to occupy large volumes with little dry weight. The proteoglycan gel resists compression and maintains the composite structure of the sclera with the embedded collagen fibers. The predominant glycosaminoglycan appears to vary somewhat with topographical location in the sclera [14]. Estimates of the proportions of the constituent parts of the sclera vary, but as a rough guide, the sclera is composed of roughly 68% water, 24% collagen, 1.5% elastin, 1.5% proteoglycans, and the remainder fibroblasts, nerve tissue, blood vessels, and salts. The inner surface of the sclera, the lamina fusca, has a large number of elastin fibers [15]. Elastin has a high proportion of hydrophobic amino acids and contains a low proportion of hydroxyproline and hydroxylysine. It does have desmosine, which is a derivative of lysine and is used to make cross-links between elastin fibers. Also contained within the sclera are matrix metalloproteinases, which are enzymes that are capable of degrading proteoglycans and collagen. These enzymes are stored in an inactive form and can be activated during inflammation and growth.

The cores of the lamina cribrosa fibers are composed of elastin surrounded by collagen fibers. Encircling the optic nerve in the region of the lamina are layers of concentrically arranged collagen fibers and elastin fibers [16]. At the outer surface of the elastin fibers, ring merges into the sclera. Elastin fibers of the lamina merge into the inner portion of the surrounding elastin fibers. Glial cell processes extend from the lamina cribrosa into the concentric elastin fibers and also appear to help anchor the lamina. The arrangement of elastic fibers would seem to serve as a buffer against trauma from rapid changes in intraocular pressure.

A number of molecular changes happen in the sclera with age. The cross-linking between adjacent collagen fibers increases and so does glycosylation and accumulation of advanced glycation end products [17]. There is a decrease in the amount of Type I collagen present, the diameters of the collagen fibers increase, and there is a greater variability in the sizes of the fibers with age [18] (Fig. 9.3). The amount of decorin and biglycan decreases with age, as does sclera hydration [19, 20]. There is a decrease in the amount of elastin with age. These contribute to the altered biomechanical characteristics of the sclera with age, particularly an increase in stiffness [20–23]. The amount of collagen in the lamina cribrosa increases, as does the cross-linked proportion [24].

As compared with the transparent cornea, the white relatively opaque nature of the sclera is related to the more randomly oriented and larger diameter collagen fibers and the greater amount of water bound. A common occurrence in retinal detachment surgery is a localized drying of the

a   Development of fibril diameter gradient

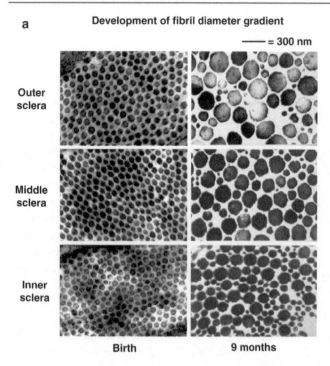

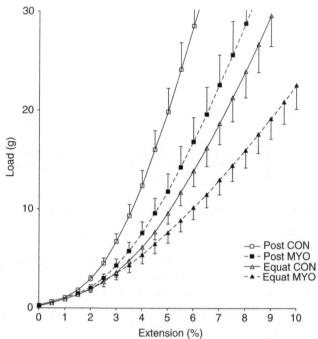

Fig. 9.4 The elastic properties of the sclera. The amount of expansion (strain) for increasing amounts of load (stress) is shown graphically for the control normal strips (CON) and the myopic eyes (MYO) for both the posterior pole (Post) and the equatorial region (Equat). (Derived from Ref. [12])

b

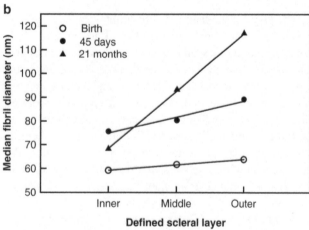

Fig. 9.3 (a) The cross-sectional thickness of collagen fibers in the outer, middle, and inner sclera at birth and at 9 months. (b) The median cross-sectional diameter is shown graphically at birth, 45 days, and 21 months for the tree shrew. (Derived from Ref. [12])

sclera allowing some visualization of the underlying choroid. With rehydration, the sclera becomes whiter and less translucent.

9.4   Mechanical Properties of the Sclera

The sclera is a viscoelastic substance. Over smaller ranges of tensile pulling, or stress, a sample of sclera will lengthen or show strain [25] (Fig. 9.4). Release of the stress after a short period of time leads to a recoil in the length of the sample. The same load applied over a longer period of time will

result in more tissue extension than just the elastic stretching. The difference over time is called creep rate of a viscoelastic tissue (Fig. 9.5). A commonly seen practical example of the viscoelastic properties of sclera is shown by how the height of a scleral buckle will seem to increase over days following surgery. The initial buckling effect is from the elastic strain, while the increase in size of the buckling effect in the subsequent days is due to a slower creep of the viscoelastic sclera.

The relationship between stress and strain provides a measure of the stiffness of a material. The sclera shows increasing stiffness with age. In babies, the sclera is highly distensible. The newborn's eye can expand and adopt a bovine appearance from congenital glaucoma (buphthalmos – which means "ox eye"). Over life, the sclera loses some of its dispensability, and interestingly the change in stiffness is highly dependent on location in the eye. In a study by Geragthy et al., the change in stiffness with age of the anterior sclera was much more pronounced than the posterior sclera, and the change was statistically significant only for the anterior sclera [21]. Pressure loading of the eye causes a variable amount of stiffness increase in eyes. The collagen fibers in the sclera show interweaving, which has the effect of increasing stiffness of the fibers for any given collagen volume fraction [26].

The biomechanical behavior of the posterior sclera to increased pressure shows variation from one person to the

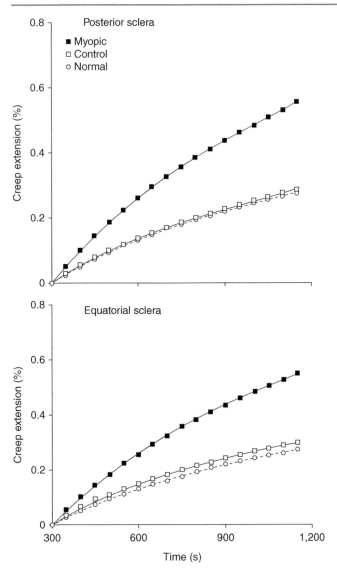

Fig. 9.5 The viscoelastic properties of sclera. With a constant applied load, the sclera will show increasing amounts of strain over time. This slow extension is called creep. Note the increased amount of creep for myopic samples as compared with normal or contralateral control eyes. The top graph is the posterior pole and the bottom for sclera strips obtained from the equator. (Derived from Ref. [12])

next but is nonlinear and anisotropic [27]. Experiments on isolated eyeballs may overstate some induced biomechanical properties of the eye because under ordinary circumstances, the eye is suspended in extraocular tissue, which has a pressure of its own. The extraorbital pressure is estimated as being about 20% of the intraocular pressure. That means the pressure gradient across the sclera is lower than the intraocular pressure posteriorly within the orbit, but not anteriorly along the external surface of the eye.

The main source of resistance of passage of both water and larger molecules through the cornea is the corneal epithelium [28]. The corneal endothelium is also a source of resistance albeit quite a bit lower than the corneal epithe-

lium. The sclera has neither an epithelium nor endothelium and consequently is quite permeable to the flow of water and larger molecules through its substance [29, 30]. Contained within the eye is the choroid, which is a densely packed permeable layer of blood vessels without a lymphatic system. Consequently, protein, fluid, and other intravascular elements that have leaked into the extravascular space in the choroid not removed by reabsorption by the choroidal vessels are removed by diffusion posteriorly through the sclera into Tenon's space.

The scleral stroma receives oxygen and nutrition externally from the episclera and Tenon's capsule externally. An interesting possibility is the stroma receives oxygen from the choroid internally. The passive diffusion of proteins and the like from the choroidal circulation may serve as a source of metabolic building blocks for the few stromal fibroblasts present. The amount of fluid requiring drainage is probably related to the thickness of the choroid and the permeability of the vessels in the choroid. The resistivity to flow out through the sclera is likely to depend on thickness and exact composition of the sclera itself. In eyes with uveal effusion syndrome, the choroid is thick, as is the sclera [31]. The collagen fibril diameters are larger and more variable [32], and there appears to be decreased diffusion of larger molecular weight substances such as albumin through the sclera in eyes with uveal effusion [33]. When areas of sclera are excised from the sclera such that the remaining thickness is a fraction of the original thickness, fluid can be seen to seep through the window created.

9.5 Emmetropization and Myopization

The axial length of the eye increases by about 35% from infancy to adulthood [3, 34], and the individual components of the eye that have an effect on refractive error change at slightly different rates [35–38]. Each of these components eventually adopts a Gaussian distribution. Even though the pooled variance would be expected to be a Gaussian distribution as a function of all of the individual variances, the measured refractive errors actually shows a peaked, or leptokurtic, distribution with far too many eyes having emmetropia or slight hyperopia. Although the individual components vary, they all work together in concert to achieve an eye that has little refractive error in most cases. The obvious exception is that the curve shows a skew toward myopic refractive errors. Although emmetropization is amazing, it is a logical consequence of evolutionary pressures: if vision is an advantageous thing, then good vision is even more so.

The process of emmetropization appears to be an active process that is largely mediated by changes in the choroid and sclera [39] (Fig. 9.6). Occlusion, form deprivation, and imposition of refractive lenses all cause alterations in the

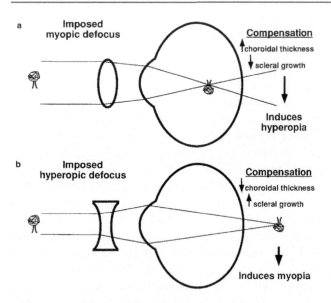

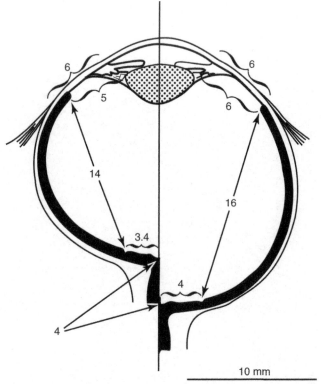

Fig. 9.6 The compensatory changes induced by forced wearing of spectacle refraction as evidence of active emmetropization. (**a**) Forced wearing of a plus lens brings the image plane in front of the retina. In compensation, the eye shows increased choroidal thickness. In birds, this can be dramatic and can account for one-half of the early compensatory response. Eventually there is a decrease in scleral growth rate. (**b**) A negative lens shifts the focal plane behind the retina, and the eye shows decreased choroidal thickness and scleral remodeling to include increased growth of the posterior sclera. In each case, the eye changes in character to move the level of the retina toward the focal plane of the combined lens and dioptric mechanism of the eye. In addition, removal of the spectacle lens leads to the exact opposite of the induced effects to occur. For example, removing the plus lens will cause the choroid to become thinner and the eye to expand toward its normal size [39]

Fig. 9.7 Eyelid fusion in monkeys causes an expansion of the posterior sclera (right side as compared with the normal left), but virtually no change in the anterior segment. (From Ref. [53])

refractive capabilities of animal eyes after birth. Form deprivation and lens-induced refractive change has been demonstrated in animals ranging from fish, chick, kestrel, squirrel, mouse, guinea pig, cat, tree shrew, to monkey and appears to be true in humans as well [40–57]. The first changes include alterations in the thickness of the choroid [55, 58–60]. In eyes becoming more myopic, the choroid becomes thinner as compared to those eyes becoming hyperopic. Removal of the stimulus stops the induced alteration in refractive error. The choroid thickness change normalizes, and the direction of the choroidal thickness change is always in the correct direction [58–61].

Longer-term application of either form deprivation or lens-induced errors is followed by axial length changes of the eye, shortening in the case of hyperopia and lengthening in the case of myopia (Fig. 9.7). These changes are also reversible in that removal of the stimulus causes an acceleration or retardation in the growth of the eye to the extent it approaches emmetropia over time. Optic nerve sectioning or destruction of the ciliary nerve does not prevent the development of experimental myopia [41, 44, 62]. Form deprivation of a hemifield produces expansion of the eye conjugate with that hemifield [56, 63, 64]. These findings all support a

hypothesis that remodeling of the eye occurs due to local effects within the eye starting with signaling that originates in the retina that eventually affects the choroid and sclera.

The modulation of ocular components such as the choroid and sclera are bidirectional and precise [65]. Exposure of the retina to different signs of optical defocus in the same eye induced compensatory regional changes [64, 66]. The direction of emmetropization to either positive or negative optical defocus appears to occur by different pathways. In marmosets, the retinal response to negative defocus appears to involve at least 12 different pathways, while positive defocus involves at least 14 (as reviewed in Ref. [67]). This messaging is conducted through multiple layers, not only the retina but the retinal pigment epithelium choroid and finally the sclera. Negative defocus leads to thinning of the choroid and sclera, increased elasticity of the sclera, and expansion of the eye. Positive defocus leads to the opposite effects.

Experimental myopia induces several changes in the composition of the sclera. There is a general loss of collagen and proteoglycans. With the start of experimental myopia, there is a reduction in ongoing Type I collagen synthesis, and existing collagen and proteoglycans are degraded by matrix metalloproteinases [68–70]. After a significant amount of myopia has developed, the collagen fibril diameter decreases, particularly in the outer portions of the sclera [68]. The decreased and altered collagen appears to be responsible for changes in the biomechanical characteristics of the sclera [12, 71]. Myopic sclera shows more elasticity and greater viscoelastic creep over time (Figs. 9.3 and 9.4). This could suggest passive expansion of the eye occurs as the result of intraocular pressure. However, administration of timolol decreased intraocular pressure but did not affect the development of myopia in a chick model [72]. This implies there may be a control mechanism that drives the amount of axial lengthening and thereby the amount of myopia.

9.6 Human Myopia

Myopia seen from an epidemiological standpoint is an increasing problem related to modern society. Sweeping changes in the pattern of refractive error have been seen in populations changing from agrarian to urban-based living [73–77]. Urban children spend more time indoors occupied with near activities and less time outdoors [78–81]. Eskimo populations showed shift of refractive error from hyperopic to myopic in the early and mid-twentieth century coincident with the introduction of schooling [82, 83]. Although there is a modest inheritable effect for myopia [84], the strongest predictors of developing myopia appear to be near work and decreased times spent outdoors when young [79, 81]. The time outdoors exposes the eye to a reduced dioptric range and also to increased amounts of shorter wavelength light as compared with indoor lighting. The effect of time outdoors may be mediated, in part, by dopamine [85], and is modest: increased outdoor exposure is associated with reduction of myopia progression by about 0.2 diopters per year [86–89].

The development of high myopia seems to be driven by processes related to emmetropization with the less desirable effect of producing a radically incorrect refractive error – for distance acuity that is. On the other hand, close work as a risk factor would seem to be an adaptive mechanism. The receptive part of the eye is being shifted to the most common focal plane of the eye. Because close work has been associated with accommodation, the idea of preventing accommodation as a way of decreasing the progression of myopia has been considered for more than a century. In 1876, Loring discussed possible mechanisms by which myopia could develop and the potential pharmacotherapeutic effects of atropine in a very interesting review [90]. In 1891, Taylor recommended atropine, blue glasses, and leaches as a treatment of progressive myopia [91]. In 1979, Bedrossian reported eyes treated with atropine were less likely to show progression of myopia as compared with untreated eyes [92]. McBrien and coworkers demonstrated atropine could blunt the development of form deprivation myopia in a mechanism that was independent of accommodation [93]. There is a dose response between atropine concentration and the retardation of myopia. Following cessation of topical atropine,

there is a rebound effect in which the eye becomes more myopic. The rebound effect shows a relationship as well; the eyes receiving 1% atropine had much more of a rebound effect than those receiving 0.01% atropine [94]. The net effect of the drug plus rebound appears to be greater with 0.01% atropine than 0.1 or 1% [94]. Lower doses of atropine are also associated with minimal pupillary dilation and less loss of accommodation as compared with higher doses. The ideal drug does is not without controversy, as some authorities recommend a higher dose [95].

In the process of myopization in humans, there is expansion of the posterior sclera and expansion of the vitreous cavity. Associated with the increasing myopia is thinning of the choroid [96–98], but as was seen in animal models, thinning of the choroid precedes scleral enlargement. There does seem to be control mechanisms involving the sclera that are mediated by or at least are influenced by the choroid. This raises the question: do abnormalities of the choroid contribute to the progression of myopia? This is an important question, given the potential for undesirable feedback loops to occur in progressive myopia. Indeed, myopia is a common association with many diseases that affect the choroid or retina and then secondarily the choroid such as choroideremia, gyrate atrophy, retinitis pigmentosa, congenital stationary night blindness, Kearns-Sayre syndrome, progressive bifocal chorioretinal atrophy, achromatopsia, and fundus flavimaculatus [99–106]. With increasing myopia, the choroid ordinarily becomes quite thin and can disappear in patches altogether. Eventually, the patches become larger and confluent, resulting in broad white areas of absent choroid, with a loss of the overlying retinal pigment epithelium and outer retina as well. These same eyes are often the ones with the most exaggerated findings in the sclera [107]. Whether or not relevant signaling originating from the choroid is correct when the choroid is in the last throes of existence is not known.

The expansion and stretching of the posterior pole induced in myopia affects every aspect of the sclera. The wall thickness decreases, the curvatures change, the emissary openings widen, and the scleral canal can enlarge and become tilted and distorted. Local exacerbation of ocular expansion is manifested as regional outpouchings, staphylomas. In the following sections, the clinical manifestations of these changes will be shown.

9.7 Ocular Shape

Along with location, rotation, and size, shape is one of the elemental features of an object. Shape can be difficult to describe, but the eye has a general ellipsoidal shape and therefore is potentially easier to model. The most exacting representation would be in the form of a mathematical statement, but mathematical equations are difficult to incorporate into everyday speech. Verbal simplifications of shape commonly have been substituted, sometimes to the extent of ineffective oversimplification. In most publications, the three-dimensional characteristics of the shape were reduced to cardinal planes for description and analysis. The analysis of these planes varied in sophistication from measuring linear distances and angles to fitting curves to the shapes. One common method of describing spheroids is to use the terms oblate and prolate. Oblate spheroids are obtained by rotating an ellipsoid along its minor axis. The resultant eye shape would be flatter in the posterior pole and would steepen toward the equator. The flatter side of an egg has an oblate shape. A prolate shape is obtained by rotating an ellipse along its major axis and thus is lengthened in the direction of its polar diameter. The pointy side of an egg has a prolate shape. There are two main approaches to estimate the shape of the eye. One method, which initially may seem to be the more precise and useful of the two, is to image the eye with a tomographic means such as with computed axial tomography or magnetic resonance imaging. The second way is to measure the refractive error and to make assumptions about the eye from these measurements. Widefield refractive error

measurements may supply information that is more useful in regard to physiological processes that influence the development of myopia. The size estimates in these papers are of secondary importance since the refractive error across the expanse of the retina has been shown to have extremely important consequences as will be described below (Fig. 9.8).

Cheng and associates [108] obtained multislice magnetic resonance images and measured the diameters in the sagittal, coronal, and transverse planes. The eye shape for hyperopic and emmetropic eyes was similar, and both had a coronal diameter greater than the transverse or sagittal diameters. Myopes had the same basic eye shape but appeared to be larger in every radius. Atchison and coworkers [109] fitted symmetrical ellipsoids to the transverse and sagittal images of emmetropic, and myopic eyes derived from magnetic resonance imaging. They found considerable variation in shape, but most emmetropes had an oblate shape, that is, one that was flatter in the posterior pole. Myopes showed an increase in all dimensions with a loss of oblateness. Only a few of the myopic eyes demonstrated a frank prolate shape, however.

Lim and colleagues [110] looked at a subset of Singaporean Chinese boys enrolled in a population-based study in Singapore. Eye shape was assessed from three-

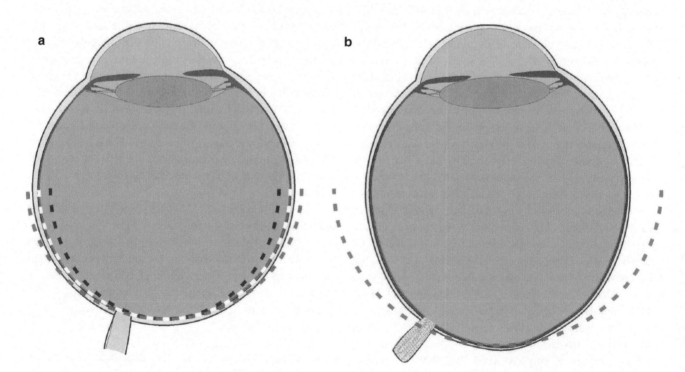

Fig. 9.8 (**a**) Shows the cross-section of an emmetropic eye with its typical mild oblate shape. Three different image planes are shown by the dashed lines, all of which intersect the fovea posteriorly. The white dashed line falls on the peripheral retina as well. The blue dashed line demonstrates an image plane in which the periphery is relatively myopic as compared to the posterior pole. This is a common occurrence in emmetropes, particularly if there is accommodation. The red dashed line shows the image plane that falls behind the retinal surface in the

periphery. In this case, the periphery is relatively hyperopic as compared with the posterior pole. (**b**) In highly myopic eyes, the eye shape is more prolate. This causes an exaggerated amount of peripheral hyperopia, which is common in high myopes. The significance of this occurrence is in emmetropization, which seems to strike a balance minimizing the refractive error across the whole eye, even though we consider foveal vision to be the most important. The peripheral hyperopia may create a drive toward increasing myopization of the posterior pole

dimensional models, and the diameters along the cardinal axes were recorded. Myopic eyes were larger and had greater surface area, as would be expected. The eyes were larger along the longitudinal axial length and transverse diameter, but apparently not the vertical diameter in the coronal plane. The myopic eyes had a prolate profile in the axial plane. Thus, even in younger individuals, the eyes appeared to have differing size and shape. Ohno-Matsui and associates [107] evaluated myopic eyes and divided the posterior curvature of the eye into four types. The first three types all appear to be variations on a prolate shape with the apex of the curve located at the optic nerve, the central macula, or just temporal to the center of the macula, but the presence or absence of staphylomas as an influencing characteristic was not stated. The fourth shape was termed irregular, because the curvature was not uniform. Eyes with irregular curvature were significantly older, had longer axial lengths, and were more likely to have myopic fundus lesions. It is not clear if the myopic fundus lesions were primarily associated with the irregular shape or the increased axial length and age.

Tomographic means show the general shape of the eye, but to be able to determine regional refractive effects the shape abnormalities could have would require knowledge of the corneal shape and the refractive powers of the crystalline lens in different meridia, which cannot be determined with sufficient accuracy from the tomographic images. Ordinary refractive evaluation and correction of the eye seeks to correct defocus and astigmatism of the image on the macula. That is, only the central acuity is optimized. An ideal lens in a camera system would form an image of a flat plane as a flat plane. With actual simple lenses, the image formed is a curved image plane. The field curvature makes it difficult for a rigid flat sensor such as a digital sensor to produce a uniformly sharp image across this field. The eye has a curvature inherent in its anatomy, so field curvature potentially is a desirable characteristic. The important consideration, of course, is if the field curvature of the dioptric mechanism of the eye matches the anatomic curvature of the eye (Fig. 9.9). In many emmetropic eyes, the periphery is relatively myopic, and this relative myopia increases with accommodation [111]. In high myopia, there is an axial lengthening of the eye so that there is an increasing difference between the distance from the nodal point of the eye and the posterior pole as compared with the equatorial regions. This means the periphery is typically relatively hyperopic as compared with the posterior pole in high myopes, with the amount of relative hyperopia increases with the increase in myopia because the eye does not expand symmetrically in axial myopia. As eyes become more prolate, the differences in refraction become more evident [112–117]. Relative hyperopia of the

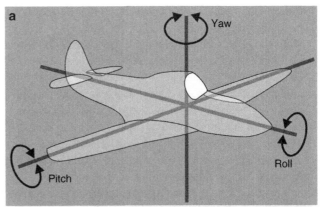

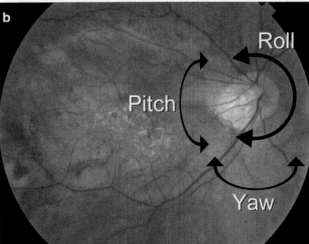

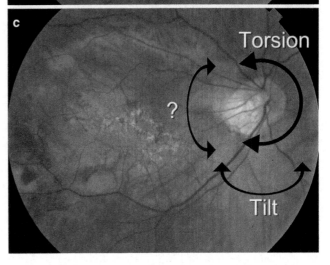

Fig. 9.9 Terminology used to describe axes of rotation. (**a**) With an airplane, the movement around the three axes of rotation are termed yaw, roll, and pitch. (**b**) Overlaying this to optic nerve highlights the three axes of rotation. (**c**) The terminology employed in ophthalmology uses the term tilt to signify yaw, although the term also has been used to refer to what is better termed torsion, which corresponds to roll. There is no term used at present that is analogous to pitch. The imprecision induced by the lack of terminology means many authors use the term tilt to signify a variety of different things

periphery has been documented in many large studies [112–120].

Animal models of myopia show that both defocus and form deprivation lead to myopia, even if the fovea is ablated [120–124]. After foveal ablation, monkeys reared with occluders that caused form deprivation only in the periphery developed myopia to the same degree as animals not undergoing foveal ablation that still had peripheral occlusion [121]. Animals undergoing foveal ablation that were not hindered in emmetropization [122] and generalized form deprivation still caused myopia. The peripheral refractive errors were not different in eyes having foveal ablation as compared with those who did not [123]. These findings establish the importance of the periphery in the development of form deprivation myopia. Chicks reared with concentric two zone lenses were evaluated for amount of emmetropization in the face of varying imposed refractions [125]. The posterior portion of the eye appeared to contribute to the overall refraction of the eye in proportion to its surface area. The eye has local mechanisms that influence eye growth, but there appears to be some larger acting mechanisms that extend beyond these local regions to affect growth of the posterior portion of the eye. In terms of surface area, the periphery is the most important, but in everyday life, refraction of the eye is optimized for the fovea. This same optical correction may then place the periphery at increased amount of hyperopic defocus. The drive toward emmetropization appears to involve the whole eye, weighing the periphery and posterior pole on a surface area basis. Therefore, while the eye may be grossly large, and the macula has a myopic refractive error, the periphery is still hyperopic because of the shape of the eye and field curvature (Fig. 9.8). This may compound the propensity to develop increasing amounts of myopia.

Because of the significance of the periphery in the development of axial myopia, some studies have tested the hypothesis that peripheral hyperopia may precede or at least be predictive of the development of axial myopia. The effect, if present, seems relatively small. Relative peripheral hyperopia was seen to precede the development of axial myopia in a prospective study over 8 years involving 605 children [115]. A study of 105 children over a period of 1.26 years did not find evidence of the same, although the statistical power of this study was limited [126]. A larger study done by Mutti of 774 myopic children followed from grades 1–8 found a modest predictive effect for myopia by peripheral hyperopia [120]. The risk appeared to vary by ethnic group. A limitation of this line of reasoning is the image quality in the periphery is a function of a number of features such as defocus, oblique astigmatism, spherical aberration, coma, and chromatic aberration [127–130]. It appears likely that peripheral image degradation contributes to the formation of myopia, but simple defocus is only one of many potential contributors to decreased image quality. Indeed, the peripheral retina appears to weigh the amounts of image blur caused by radial versus tangential astigmatism as one means of providing a feedback signal [114, 131].

The shape of the eye, as manifested by scleral expansion, is at the heart of myopia. The experiments in animals are relatively recent in human scientific endeavors and are likely to hold the keys to unlocking many of the mysteries of myopia. Animal experiments may have limited utility as they apply to humans. If the fovea contributes to the signal modulating eye expansion in relation to its surface area, the periphery would be more important just because of area reasons alone. A second important point is humans, who depend extensively on fovea vision for reading and other close tasks, may differ from monkeys in the relative proportion that the periphery accounts for in the development of myopia. Of interest though is that the list of chorioretinal conditions associated with myopia previously mentioned in this chapter was predominated by diseases that primarily affect the peripheral vision first. Thus, evaluation of the peripheral visual function appears to be an important area for future myopia research.

9.8 Shape Alterations Across Smaller Units of Scale

After evaluating the general shape of the eye, the next lower unit of scale would be to evaluate regional variations. Large regional variations in eye shape usually are manifested as outpouchings of the eye. These outpouchings are known as staphylomas. The principle area affected by staphylomas is the same as that affected by general expansion of the eye, namely, the posterior portion of the eye. Ocular abnormalities associated with staphylomas include subretinal fluid [132, 133], choroidal neovascularization [134], polypoidal choroidal vasculopathy [135], retinal detachment [136], myopic macular schisis [137, 138], peripapillary intrachoroidal cavitation [139], macula intrachoroidal cavitation [140], choroidal folds [141], and tilted optic nerve appearance. For the most part, these topics are discussed in the chapter devoted to staphylomas. Tilting of the optic nerve will be covered in part here, but for the most part in the Chap. 25, Myopic Optic Neuropathy.

The nonuniform mechanical expansion of the eye shifts the plane of the optic nerve from pointing toward the geometric center of the vitreous cavity to point toward the nearest foci of the ellipse describing the shape of the posterior pole. Since the shape of the posterior portion of the eye in high myopia is prolate, the nerve shifts such that a normal to its surface points more posteriorly. This causes the anterior edge to be forward of the posterior edge along a transverse plane than what would be seen in an emmetrope. This shifting of orientation is compounded by the frequent development of distension of the globe with coexistent atrophy of the choroid and retinal pigment epithelium by a roughly triangular shaped area inferotemporal to the optic disc known as the conus.

The effects related to ocular expansion of the posterior segment may produce recognizable alterations on even smaller units of scale.

9.9 Ectasia of the Sclera and Intrascleral Cavitations Related to Emissary Openings

With expansion of the eye, the sclera becomes thinner. Emissary vessels ordinarily penetrate the eye, often at oblique angles and course through the sclera toward the choroid. With scleral thinning, these passageways become much shorter. The internal openings of the emissary openings seem to become stretched and enlarged (Figs. 9.10, 9.11, and 9.12). Concurrently the structures supplied by arterioles, such as the choroid, are thin and in some areas are obliterated. As a consequence, the vessels that used to supply these structures also become attenuated. These emissary openings are evident as funnel-shaped depressions associated with threadlike vessels emanating from the deeper sclera. Because the course of the emissary passageway often is at a shallow angle to the sclera, the opening of the emissary itself can be tilted. These openings typically are noticed in the context of profound atrophy of the choroid, retinal pigment epithelium, and overlying retina. In some cases, there can be a full-thickness defect of the overlying retina. Successive OCT scans across the opening reveals retinal tissue and then also inner lamellae of sclera over the passageway as the region of interest approaches the inner edge of the funnel. The draping of retinal tissue creates a closed space in which three sides

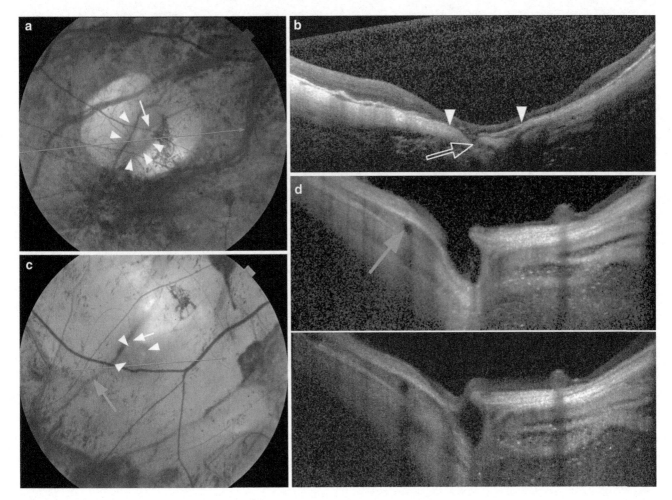

Fig. 9.10 Expansion of scleral emissary passageways and openings. (**a**) This patient had an oval depression (arrowheads) that allowed the passage of a blood vessel (arrow). (**b**) The corresponding OCT scan shows the depression between the arrowheads but also shows the expansion of the emissary passageway (open arrow) such that there was a full-thickness defect in the sclera visible. Note how thin the sclera is temporal to the opening. (**c**) This eye had a circular depression as outlined by the arrowheads. There was a barely visible vessel coming from the emmisary opening (white arrow). Note the absence of the choroid and the visibility of a deeper vessel (cyan arrow). (**d**) Upper OCT taken at the cyan arrow in (**c**) shows the deep depression, scleral ectasia present, and the intrascleral vessel (cyan arrow). The lower OCT was taken slightly inferior to the upper OCT and shows retina draping across the scleral opening

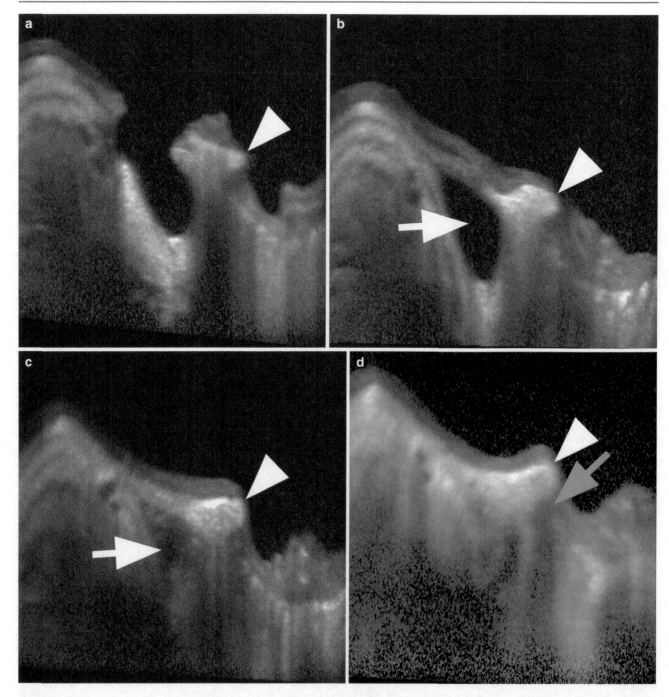

Fig. 9.11 Successive scans spaced 300 microns apart near the optic nerve in a highly myopic eye. (**a**) In this picture and all the remaining ones, the scleral ring at the border of the optic nerve is shown by the arrowhead. On either side is a pitlike depression. To the left is a depression related to an emissary opening, and to the right is an acquired pit in the nerve. (**b**) A scan taken 300 microns inferior to (**a**) shows a band of retinal tissue over the emissary passageway (arrow). (**c**). Inferior to (**b**), there appears to be scleral tissue over the passageway creating an intrascleral cavity. (**d**) Inferior to (**c**), the emissary is exposed to the outer portion of the sclera. Note the tear in the lamina cribrosa (cyan arrow)

are the cavity in the sclera and the roof is the retina. The addition of scleral fibers creates a true intrascleral cavitation. These exaggerated openings are found in regions where there are numerous emissaries, profound atrophy, and marked ocular expansion and thus are most commonly found near the nerve [142]. However, they can be found well away from the nerve as illustrated in Fig. 9.10.

9.10 Irregularities of the Thinned Sclera

With ocular expansion, the sclera becomes increasingly thinned, probably as the combined result of stretching and remodeling. The effects of this thinning do not appear to be uniform, and the resultant sclera, as visualized using

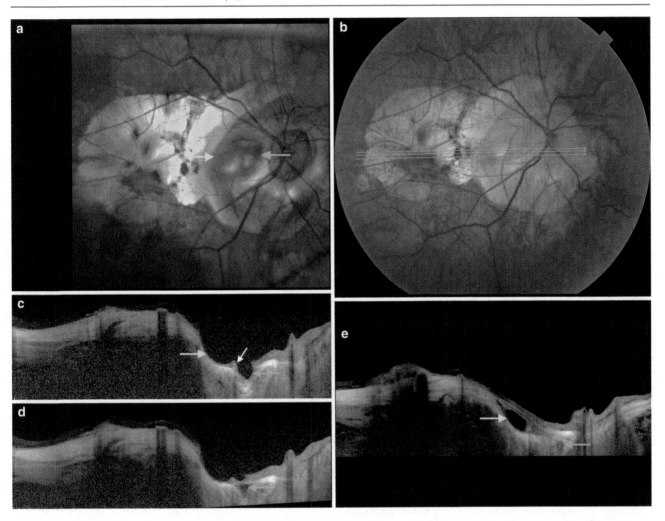

Fig. 9.12 (**a**) This eye shows a complex depression temporal to the nerve with two main components (yellow and cyan arrows) in the scanning laser ophthalmoscopic image. (**b**) The corresponding color fundus photograph is shown along with the scan lines shown as green arrows. (**c**) This scan corresponds to the upper scan line in (**b**) and shows two pitlike depressions; the temporal one is broader (yellow arrow) separated from the smaller, deeper pit (cyan arrow) by a ridge (white arrow). (**d**) The middle scan line in (**b**) shows tissue had covered the nasal pit (cyan arrow) while the temporal depression remains. (**e**) Immediately inferior to (**d**) intact retina is draped over the temporal depression (yellow arrow). Note the continuation of the cavity seen in (**d**) as an intrascleral cavity in (**e**) as demonstrated by the cyan arrow. The large cavity in (**e**) could conceivably be mistaken for an intrachoroidal cavitation, but there is no choroid present in the region around the cavity in (**e**), and the mechanism of formation is different as well

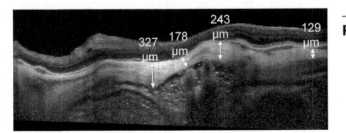

Fig. 9.13 In high myopia, the posterior sclera is thinned through a process of stretching and remodeling. The remaining sclera shows a large variation in thickness

OCT techniques that enable deeper visualization, shows remarkable variation in thickness in many high myopes (Fig. 9.13).

References

1. Olsen TW, Aaberg SY, Geroski DH, Edelhauser HF. Human sclera: thickness and surface area. Am J Ophthalmol. 1998;125(2):237–41.
2. Sellheyer K, Spitznas M. Development of the human sclera: a morphological study. Graefes Arch Clin Exp Ophthalmol. 1988;226:89–100.
3. Fledelius HC, Christensen AC. Reappraisal of the human ocular growth curve in fetal life, infancy, and early childhood. Br J Ophthalmol. 1996;80:918–21.
4. Kakizaki H, Takahashi Y, Nakano T, Asamoto K, Ikeda H, Ichinose A, Iwaki M, Selva D, Leibovitch I. Anatomy of tenons capsule. Clin Exp Ophthalmol. 2012;40(6):611–6.
5. Quigley HA, Addicks EM. Regional differences in the structure of the lamina cribrosa and their relation to glaucomatous optic nerve damage. Arch Ophthalmol. 1981;99(1):137–43.

6. Anderson DR. Ultrastructure of human and monkey lamina cribrosa and optic nerve head. Arch Ophthalmol. 1969;82(6):800–14.

7. Ko MK, Kim DS, Ahn YK. Morphological variations of the peripapillary circle of Zinn-Haller by flat section. Br J Ophthalmol. 1999;83(7):862–6.

8. Gauntt CD. Peripapillary circle of Zinn-Haller. Br J Ophthalmol. 1998;82(7):849.

9. Ko MK, Kim DS, Ahn YK. Peripapillary circle of Zinn-Haller revealed by fundus fluorescein angiography. Br J Ophthalmol. 1997;81(8):663–7.

10. Ohno-Matsui K, Futagami S, Yamashita S, Tokoro T. Zinn-Haller arterial ring observed by ICG angiography in high myopia. Br J Ophthalmol. 1998;82(12):1357–62.

11. Spitznas M. The fine structure of human scleral collagen. Am J Ophthalmol. 1971;71(1 Pt 1):68.

12. McBrien NA, Jobling AI, Gentle A. Biomechanics of the sclera in myopia: extracellular and cellular factors. Optom Vis Sci. 2009;86(1):E23–30.

13. Rada JA, Achen VR, Perry CA, Fox PW. Proteoglycans in the human sclera. Evidence for the presence of aggrecan. Invest Ophthalmol Vis Sci. 1997;38(9):1740–51.

14. Trier K, Olsen EB, Ammitzbøll T. Regional glycosaminoglycans composition of the human sclera. Acta Ophthalmol. 1990;68(3):304–6.

15. Anatomical, physiological, and comparative aspects. In: Watson PG, Hazleman BL, McCluskey P, Pavesio CE, editors. The sclera and systemic disorders. 3rd ed. London: JP Medical Publishers; 2012. p. 11–45.

16. Hernandez MR, Luo XX, Igoe F, Neufeld AH. Extracellular matrix of the human lamina cribrosa. Am J Ophthalmol. 1987;104(6):567–76.

17. Beattie JR, Pawlak AM, McGarvey JJ, Stitt AW. Sclera as a surrogate marker for determining AGE-modifications in Bruch's membrane using a Raman spectroscopy-based index of aging. Invest Ophthalmol Vis Sci. 2011;52(3):1593–8.

18. Watson PG, Young RD. Scleral structure, organisation and disease. A review. Exp Eye Res. 2004;78(3):609–23.

19. Rada JA, Achen VR, Penugonda S, Schmidt RW, Mount BA. Proteoglycan composition in the human sclera during growth and aging. Invest Ophthalmol Vis Sci. 2000;41(7):1639–48.

20. Brown CT, Vural M, Johnson M, Trinkaus-Randall V. Age-related changes of scleral hydration and sulfated glycosaminoglycans. Mech Ageing Dev. 1994;77(2):97–107.

21. Geraghty B, Jones SW, Rama P, Akhtar R, Elsheikh A. Age-related variations in the biomechanical properties of human sclera. J Mech Behav Biomed Mater. 2012;16:181–91.

22. Girard MJ, Suh JK, Bottlang M, Burgoyne CF, Downs JC. Scleral biomechanics in the aging monkey eye. Invest Ophthalmol Vis Sci. 2009;50(11):5226–37.

23. Elsheikh A, Geraghty B, Alhasso D, Knappett J, Campanelli M, Rama P. Regional variation in the biomechanical properties of the human sclera. Exp Eye Res. 2010;90(5):624–33.

24. Albon J, Karwatowski WS, Avery N, Easty DL, Duance VC. Changes in the collagenous matrix of the aging human lamina cribrosa. Br J Ophthalmol. 1995;79(4):368–75.

25. Curtin BJ. Physiopathologic aspects of scleral stress-strain. Trans Am Ophthalmol Soc. 1969;67:417–61.

26. Wang B, Hua Y, Brazile BL, Yang B, Sigal IA. Collagen fiber interweaving is central to sclera stiffness. Acta Biomater. 2020;113:429–37.

27. Girard MJ, Suh JK, Bottlang M, Burgoyne CF, Downs JC. Biomechanical changes in the sclera of monkey eyes exposed to chronic IOP elevations. Invest Ophthalmol Vis Sci. 2011;52(8):5656–69.

28. Prausnitz MR, Noonan JS. Permeability of cornea, sclera, and conjunctiva: a literature analysis for drug delivery to the eye. J Pharm Sci. 1998;87:1479–88.

29. Ambati J, Canakis CS, Miller JW, Gragoudas ES, Edwards A, Weissgold DJ, Kim I, Delori FC, Adamis AP. Diffusion of high molecular weight compounds through sclera. Invest Ophthalmol Vis Sci. 2000;41(5):1181–5.

30. Anderson OA, Jackson TL, Singh JK, Hussain AA, Marshall J. Human transscleral albumin permeability and the effect of topographical location and donor age. Invest Ophthalmol Vis Sci. 2008;49(9):4041–5.

31. Harada T, Machida S, Fujiwara T, Nishida Y, Kurosaka D. Choroidal findings in idiopathic uveal effusion syndrome. Clin Ophthalmol. 2011;5:1599–601.

32. Stewart DH 3rd, Streeten BW, Brockhurst RJ, Anderson DR, Hirose T, Gass DM. Abnormal scleral collagen in nanophthalmos. An ultrastructural study. Arch Ophthalmol. 1991;109(7):1017–25.

33. Jackson TL, Hussain A, Salisbury J, Sherwood R, Sullivan PM, Marshall J. Transscleral albumin diffusion and suprachoroidal albumin concentration in uveal effusion syndrome. Retina. 2012;32(1):177–82.

34. Mayer DL, Hansen RM, Moore BD, Kim S, Fulton AB. Cycloplegic refractions in healthy children aged 1 through 48 months. Arch Ophthalmol. 2001;119:1625–8.

35. Jones LA, Mitchell GL, Mutti DO, Hayes JR, Moeschberger ML, Zadnik K. Comparison of ocular component growth curves among refractive error groups in children. Invest Ophthalmol Vis Sci. 2005;46:2317–27.

36. Stenstrom S. Investigation of the variation and the correlation of the optical elements of human eyes. Am J Optom Arch Am Acad Optom. 1948;25:496–504.

37. Sorsby A, Leary GA, Fraser GR. Family studies on ocular refraction and its components. J Med Genet. 1966;3:269–73.

38. Zadnik K, Manny RE, Yu JA, Mitchell GL, Cotter SA, Quiralte JC, Shipp M, Friedman NE, Kleinstein RN, Walker TW, Jones LA, Moeschberger ML, Mutti DO. Ocular component data in schoolchildren as a function of age and gender. Optom Vis Sci. 2003;80:226–36.

39. Wildsoet CF. Active emmetropization--evidence for its existence and ramifications for clinical practice. Ophthalmic Physiol Opt. 1997;17(4):279–90; Shen W, Vijayan M, Sivak JG. Inducing form-deprivation myopia in fish. Invest Ophthalmol Vis Sci. 2005;46(5):1797–803.

40. Shen W, Sivak JG. Eyes of a lower vertebrate are susceptible to the visual environment. Invest Ophthalmol Vis Sci. 2007;48:4829–37.

41. Wildsoet CF, Schmid KL. Optical correction of form deprivation myopia inhibits refractive recovery in chick eyes with intact or sectioned optic nerves. Vis Res. 2000;40(23):3273–82.

42. Wallman J, Adams JI. Developmental aspects of experimental myopia in chicks: susceptibility, recovery and relation to emmetropization. Vis Res. 1987;27:1139–63.

43. Troilo D, Gottlieb MD, Wallman J. Visual deprivation causes myopia in chicks with optic nerve section. Curr Eye Res. 1987;6:993–9.

44. McBrien NA, Moghaddam HO, New R, Williams LR. Experimental myopia in a diurnal mammal (Sciurus carolinensis) with no accommodative ability. J Physiol. 1993;469:427–41.

45. Andison ME, Sivak JG, Bird DM. The refractive development of the eye of the American kestrel (Falco sparverius): a new avian model. J Comp Physiol A. 1992;170:565–74.

46. Tejedor J, de la Villa P. Refractive changes induced by form deprivation in the mouse eye. Invest Ophthalmol Vis Sci. 2003;44:32–6.

47. Howlett MH, McFadden SA. Form-deprivation myopia in the guinea pig (Cavia porcellus). Vis Res. 2006;46:267–83.

48. Kirby AW, Sutton L, Weiss H. Elongation of cat eyes following neonatal lid suture. Invest Ophthalmol Vis Sci. 1982;22:274–7.

49. Sherman SM, Norton TT, Casagrande VA. Myopia in the lid-sutured tree shrew (Tupaia glis). Brain Res. 1977;124:154–7.

50. Norton TT, Essinger JA, McBrien NA. Lid-suture myopia in tree shrews with retinal ganglion cell blockade. Vis Neurosci. 1994;11(1):143–53.

51. Siegwart JT Jr, Norton TT. The susceptible period for deprivation-induced myopia in tree shrew. Vis Res. 1998;38:3505–15.

52. McBrien NA, Lawlor P, Gentle A. Scleral remodeling during the development of and recovery from axial myopia in the tree shrew. Invest Ophthalmol Vis Sci. 2000;41:3713–9.

53. Wiesel TN, Raviola E. Myopia and eye enlargement after neonatal lid fusion in monkeys. Nature. 1977;266:66–8.

54. Smith EL III, Hung LF, Harwerth RS. Effects of optically induced blur on the refractive status of young monkeys. Vis Res. 1994;34:293–301.

55. Hung LF, Wallman J, Smith EL 3rd. Vision-dependent changes in the choroidal thickness of macaque monkeys. Invest Ophthalmol Vis Sci. 2000;41:1259–69.

56. Smith EL III, Hung LF, Huang J, Blasdel TL, Humbird TL, Bockhorst KH. Effects of optical defocus on refractive development in monkeys: evidence for local, regionally selective mechanisms. Invest Ophthalmol Vis Sci. 2010;51:3864–73.

57. von Noorden GK, Lewis RA. Ocular axial length in unilateral congenital cataracts and blepharoptosis. Invest Ophthalmol Vis Sci. 1987;28(4):750–2.

58. Wallman J, Wildsoet C, Xu A, et al. Moving the retina: choroidal modulation of refractive state. Vis Res. 1995;35:37–50.

59. Nickla DL, Wildsoet C, Wallman J. Compensation for spectacle lenses involves changes in proteoglycan synthesis in both the sclera and choroid. Curr Eye Res. 1997;16(4):320–6.

60. Troilo D, Nickla DL, Wildsoet CF. Choroidal thickness changes during altered eye growth and refractive state in a primate. Invest Ophthalmol Vis Sci. 2000;41:1249–58.

61. Zhu X, Park TW, Winawer J, Wallman J. In a matter of minutes, the eye can know which way to grow. Invest Ophthalmol Vis Sci. 2005;46(7):2238–41.

62. Schmid KL, Wildsoet CF. Effects on the compensatory responses to positive and negative lenses of intermittent lens wear and ciliary nerve section in chicks. Vis Res. 1996;36(7):1023–36.

63. Smith EL 3rd, Huang J, Hung LF, Blasdel TL, Humbird TL, Bockhorst KH. Hemiretinal form deprivation: evidence for local control of eye growth and refractive development in infant monkeys. Invest Ophthalmol Vis Sci. 2009;50(11):5057–69.

64. Diether S, Schaeffel F. Local changes in eye growth induced by imposed local refractive error despite active accommodation. Vis Res. 1997;37(6):659–68.

65. Wildsoet C, Wallman J. Choroidal and scleral mechanisms of compensation for spectacle lenses in chicks. Vis Res. 1995;35(9):1175–94.

66. Smith EL 3rd, Hung LF, Huang J, et al. Effects of local myopic defocus on refractive development in monkeys. Optom Vis Sci. 2013;90(11):1176–86.

67. Tkatchenko TV, Tkatchenko AV. Pharmacogenomic approach to antimyopia drug development: pathways lead the way. Trends Pharmacol Sci. 2019;40(11):833–52.

68. Gentle A, Liu Y, Martin JE, et al. Collagen gene expression and the altered accumulation of scleral collagen during the development of high myopia. J Biol Chem. 2003;278(19):16587–94.

69. Rada JA, Brenza HL. Increased latent gelatinase activity in the sclera of visually deprived chicks. Invest Ophthalmol Vis Sci. 1995;36(8):1555–65.

70. Guggenheim JA, McBrien NA. Form-deprivation myopia induces activation of scleral matrix metalloproteinase-2 in tree shrew. Invest Ophthalmol Vis Sci. 1996;37(7):1380–95.

71. Rada JA, Shelton S, Norton TT. The sclera and myopia. Exp Eye Res. 2006;82(2):185–20.

72. Schmid KL, Abbott M, Humphries M, Pyne K, Wildsoet CF. Timolol lowers intraocular pressure but does not inhibit the development of experimental myopia in chick. Exp Eye Res. 2000;70(5):659–66.

73. Lin LL, Shih YF, Hsiao CK, Chen CJ, Lee LA, Hung PT. Epidemiologic study of the prevalence and severity of myopia among schoolchildren in Taiwan in 2000. J Formos Med Assoc. 2001;100(10):684–91.

74. Saw SM. A synopsis of the prevalence rates and environmental risk factors for myopia. Clin Exp Optom. 2003;86(5):289–94.

75. Lin LL, Shih YF, Hsiao CK, Chen CJ. Prevalence of myopia in Taiwanese schoolchildren: 1983 to 2000. Ann Acad Med Singap. 2004;33(1):27–33.

76. He M, Zheng Y, Xiang F. Prevalence of myopia in urban and rural children in mainland China. Optom Vis Sci. 2009;86(1):40–4.

77. Shih YF, Chiang TH, Hsiao CK, Chen CJ, Hung PT, Lin LL. Comparing myopic progression of urban and rural Taiwanese schoolchildren. Jpn J Ophthalmol. 2010;54(5):446–51.

78. Saw SM, Hong RZ, Zhang MZ, Fu ZF, Ye M, Tan D, Chew SJ. Near-work activity and myopia in rural and urban schoolchildren in China. J Pediatr Ophthalmol Strabismus. 2001;38(3):149–55.

79. Ip JM, Rose KA, Morgan IG, Burlutsky G, Mitchell P. Myopia and the urban environment: findings in a sample of 12-year-old Australian school children. Invest Ophthalmol Vis Sci. 2008;49(9):3858–63.

80. Guo Y, Liu LJ, Xu L, Lv YY, Tang P, Feng Y, Meng M, Jonas JB. Outdoor activity and myopia among primary students in rural and urban regions of Beijing. Ophthalmology. 2012. pii: S0161-6420(12)00750-6. https://doi.org/10.1016/j.ophtha.2012.07.086. [Epub ahead of print].

81. Guggenheim JA, Northstone K, McMahon G, Ness AR, Deere K, Mattocks C, Pourcain BS, Williams C. Time outdoors and physical activity as predictors of incident myopia in childhood: a prospective cohort study. Invest Ophthalmol Vis Sci. 2012;53(6):2856–65.

82. Young FA, Leary GA, Baldwin WR, West DC, Box RA, Goo FJ, Harris E, Johnson C. Refractive errors, reading performance, and school achievement among Eskimo children. Am J Optom Arch Am Acad Optom. 1970;47(5):384–90.

83. Young FA, Leary GA, Baldwin WR, West DC, Box RA, Harris E, Johnson C. The transmission of refractive errors within Eskimo families. Am J Optom Arch Am Acad Optom. 1969;46(9):676–85.

84. Tsai MY, Lin LL, Lee V, Chen CJ, Shih YF. Estimation of heritability in myopic twin studies. Jpn J Ophthalmol. 2009;53(6):615–22.

85. French AN, Ashby RS, Morgan IG, Rose KA. Time outdoors and the prevention of myopia. Exp Eye Res. 2013;114:58–68.

86. Chakraborty R, Ostrin LA, Nickla DL, Iuvone PM, Pardue MT, Stone RA. Circadian rhythms, refractive development, and myopia. Ophthalmic Physiol Opt. 2018;38(3):217–45.

87. Read SA, Collins MJ, Vincent SJ. Light exposure and eye growth in childhood. Invest Ophthalmol Vis Sci. 2015;56(11):6779–87.

88. Wu PC, Tsai CL, Wu HL, Yang YH, Kuo HK. Outdoor activity during class recess reduces myopia onset and progression in school children. Ophthalmology. 2013;120(5):1080–5.

89. He M, Xiang F, Zeng Y, et al. Effect of time spent outdoors at school on the development of myopia among children in China: a randomized clinical trial. JAMA. 2015;314(11):1142–8.

90. Loring EG. Are progressive myopia and conus (posterior staphyloma) due to hereditary predisposition or can they be induced by defect of refraction acting through the influence of the ciliary muscle? In: Shahurst Jr J, editor. Tansactions of the Internation Medical Congress of Philadelphia. Philadelphia: Collins, Printer 1877; 1876. p. 923–41.

91. Taylor CB. Lectures on diseases of the eye. London: Kegan Paul, Trench and Co; 1891. p. 110.

92. Bedrossian RH. The effect of atropine on myopia. Ophthalmology. 1979;86(5):713–9.

93. McBrien NA, Moghaddam HO, Reeder AP. Atropine reduces experimental myopia and eye enlargement via a nonaccommodative mechanism. Invest Ophthalmol Vis Sci. 1993;34(1):205–15.

94. Chia A, Lu QS, Tan D. Five-year clinical trial on atropine for the treatment of myopia 2: myopia control with atropine 0.01% eyedrops. Ophthalmology. 2016;123(2):391–9.

95. Khanal S, Phillips JR. Which low-dose atropine for myopia control? Clin Exp Optom. 2020;103(2):230–2.

96. Fujiwara T, Imamura Y, Margolis R, Slakter JS, Spaide RF. Enhanced depth imaging optical coherence tomography of the choroid in highly myopic eyes. Am J Ophthalmol. 2009;148:445–50.

97. Ikuno Y, Tano Y. Retinal and choroidal biometry in highly myopic eyes with spectral-domain optical coherence tomography. Invest Ophthalmol Vis Sci. 2009;50(8):3876–80.

98. Nishida Y, Fujiwara T, Imamura Y, Lima LH, Kurosaka D, Spaide RF. Choroidal thickness and visual acuity in highly myopic eyes. Retina. 2012;32:1229–36.

99. Burke MJ, Choromokos EA, Bibler L, Sanitato JJ. Choroideremia in a genotypically normal female. A case report. Ophthalmic Paediatr Genet. 1985;6(3):163–8.

100. Hayasaka S, Shiono T, Mizuno K, Sasayama C, Akiya S, Tanaka Y, Hayakawa M, Miyake Y, Ohba N. Gyrate atrophy of the choroid and retina: 15 Japanese patients. Br J Ophthalmol. 1986;70(8):612–4.

101. Sieving PA, Fishman GA. Refractive errors of retinitis pigmentosa patients. Br J Ophthalmol. 1978;62(3):163–7.

102. Pruett RC. Retinitis pigmentosa: clinical observations and correlations. Trans Am Ophthalmol Soc. 1983;81:693–735.

103. Nemet P, Godel V, Lazar M. Kearns-Sayre syndrome. Birth Defects Orig Artic Ser. 1982;18(6):263–8.

104. Godley BF, Tiffin PA, Evans K, Kelsell RE, Hunt DM, Bird AC. Clinical features of progressive bifocal chorioretinal atrophy: a retinal dystrophy linked to chromosome 6q. Ophthalmology. 1996;103(6):893–8.

105. Haegerstrom-Portnoy G, Schneck ME, Verdon WA, Hewlett SE. Clinical vision characteristics of the congenital achromatopsias. I. Visual acuity, refractive error, and binocular status. Optom Vis Sci. 1996;73(7):446–56.

106. Doka DS, Fishman GA, Anderson RJ. Refractive errors in patients with fundus flavimaculatus. Br J Ophthalmol. 1982;66(4):227–9.

107. Ohno-Matsui K, Akiba M, Modegi T, Tomita M, Ishibashi T, Tokoro T, Moriyama M. Association between shape of sclera and myopic retinochoroidal lesions in patients with pathologic myopia. Invest Ophthalmol Vis Sci. 2012;53(10):6046–61.

108. Cheng HM, Singh OS, Kwong KK, Xiong J, Woods BT, Brady TJ. Shape of the myopic eye as seen with high-resolution magnetic resonance imaging. Optom Vis Sci. 1992;69(9):698–701.

109. Atchison DA, Pritchard N, Schmid KL, Scott DH, Jones CE, Pope JM. Shape of the retinal surface in emmetropia and myopia. Invest Ophthalmol Vis Sci. 2005;46(8):2698–707.

110. Lim LS, Yang X, Gazzard G, Lin X, Sng C, Saw SM, Qiu A. Variations in eye volume, surface area, and shape with refractive error in young children by magnetic resonance imaging analysis. Invest Ophthalmol Vis Sci. 2011;52(12):8878–83.

111. Lundström L, Mira-Agudelo A, Artal P. Peripheral optical errors and their change with accommodation differ between emmetropic and myopic eyes. J Vis. 2009;917:1–11.

112. Schmid GF. Variability of retinal steepness at the posterior pole in children 7-15 years of age. Curr Eye Res. 2003;27(1):61–8.

113. Atchison DA, Jones CE, Schmid KL, Pritchard N, Pope JM, Strugnell WE, Riley RA. Eye shape in emmetropia and myopia. Invest Ophthalmol Vis Sci. 2004;45(10):3380–6.

114. Faria-Ribeiro M, Queirós A, Lopes-Ferreira D, Jorge J, González-Méijome JM. Peripheral refraction and retinal contour in stable and progressive myopia. Optom Vis Sci. 2013;90:9–15.

115. Mutti DO, Sholtz RI, Friedman NE, Zadnik K. Peripheral refraction and ocular shape in children. Invest Ophthalmol Vis Sci. 2000;41(5):1022–30.

116. Mutti DO, Hayes JR, Mitchell GL, Jones LA, Moeschberger ML, Cotter SA, Kleinstein RN, Manny RE, Twelker JD, Zadnik K, CLEERE Study Group. Refractive error, axial length, and relative peripheral refractive error before and after the onset of myopia. Invest Ophthalmol Vis Sci. 2007;48(6):2510–9.

117. Logan NS, Gilmartin B, Wildsoet CF, Dunne MCM. Posterior retinal contour in adult human anisomyopia. Invest Ophthalmol Vis Sci. 2004;45:2152–62.

118. Seidemann A, Schaeffel F, Guirao A, Lopez-Gil N, Artal P. Peripheral refractive errors in myopic, emmetropic and hyperopic young subjects. J Opt Soc Am A Opt Image Sci. 2002;19:2363–73.

119. Sng CC, Lin XY, Gazzard G, Chang B, Dirani M, Chia A, Selvaraj P, Ian K, Drobe B, Wong TY, Saw SM. Peripheral refraction and refractive error in Singapore Chinese children. Invest Ophthalmol Vis Sci. 2011;52(2):1181–90.

120. Mutti DO, Sinnott LT, Mitchell GL, Jones-Jordan LA, Moeschberger ML, Cotter SA, Kleinstein RN, Manny RE, Twelker JD, Zadnik K, CLEERE Study Group. Relative peripheral refractive error and the risk of onset and progression of myopia in children. Invest Ophthalmol Vis Sci. 2011;52(1):199–205.

121. Smith EL III, Kee CS, Ramamirtham R, Qiao-Grider Y, Hung LF. Peripheral vision can influence eye growth and refractive development in infant monkeys. Invest Ophthalmol Vis Sci. 2005;46:3965–72.

122. Smith EL 3rd, Ramamirtham R, Qiao-Grider Y, Hung LF, Huang J, Kee CS, Coats D, Paysse E. Effects of foveal ablation on emmetropization and form-deprivation myopia. Invest Ophthalmol Vis Sci. 2007;48(9):3914–22.

123. Huang J, Hung LF, Smith EL 3rd. Effects of foveal ablation on the pattern of peripheral refractive errors in normal and form-deprived infant rhesus monkeys (Macaca mulatta). Invest Ophthalmol Vis Sci. 2011;52(9):6428–34.

124. Smith EL 3rd, Hung LF, Huang J. Relative peripheral hyperopic defocus alters central refractive development in infant monkeys. Vis Res. 2009;49(19):2386–92.

125. Tse DY, To CH. Graded competing regional myopic and hyperopic defocus produce summated emmetropization set points in chick. Invest Ophthalmol Vis Sci. 2011;52(11):8056–62.

126. Sng CC, Lin XY, Gazzard G, Chang B, Dirani M, Lim L, Selvaraj P, Ian K, Drobe B, Wong TY, Saw SM. Change in peripheral refraction over time in Singapore Chinese children. Invest Ophthalmol Vis Sci. 2011;52(11):7880–7.

127. Ferree CE, Rand G. Interpretation of refractive conditions in the peripheral field of vision. Arch Ophthalmol. 1933;9:925–37.

128. Williams DR, Artal P, Navarro R, McMahon MJ, Brainard DH. Off-axis optical quality and retinal sampling in the human eye. Vis Res. 1996;36:1103–14.

129. Guirao A, Artal P. Off-axis monochromatic aberrations estimated from double pass measurements in the human eye. Vis Res. 1999;39:4141–4.

130. Gustafsson J, Terenius E, Buchheister J, Unsbo P. Peripheral astigmatism in emmetropic eyes. Ophthalmic Physiol Opt. 2001;21:393–400.

131. Rosén R, Lundström L, Unsbo P. Sign-dependent sensitivity to peripheral defocus for myopes due to aberrations. Invest Ophthalmol Vis Sci. 2012;53(11):7176–82.

132. Cohen SY, Quentel G, Guiberteau B, Delahaye-Mazza C, Gaudric A. Macular serous retinal detachment caused by subretinal leakage in tilted disc syndrome. Ophthalmology. 1998;105:1831–4.

133. Nakanishi H, Tsujikawa A, Gotoh N, et al. Macular complications on the border of an inferior staphyloma associated with tilted disc syndrome. Retina. 2008;28(10):1493–501.

134. Quaranta M, Brindeau C, Coscas G, Soubrane G. Multiple choroidal neovascularizations at the border of a myopic poste-

rior macular staphyloma. Graefes Arch Clin Exp Ophthalmol. 2000;238:101–3.

135. Becquet F, Ducournau D, Ducournau Y, Goffart Y, Spencer WH. Juxtapapillary subretinal pigment epithelial polypoid pseudocysts associated with unilateral tilted optic disc: case report with clinicopathologic correlation. Ophthalmology. 2001;108(9):1657–62.

136. Baba T, Ohno-Matsui K, Futagami S, Yoshida T, Yasuzumi K, Kojima A, Tokoro T, Mochizuki M. Prevalence and characteristics of foveal retinal detachment without macular hole in high myopia. Am J Ophthalmol. 2003;135(3):338–42.

137. Dałkowska A, Smogulecka E, Dziegielewska J. Retinoschisis in myopic eye. Klin Ocz. 1979;81(1):17–9.

138. Takano M, Kishi S. Foveal retinoschisis and retinal detachment in severely myopic eyes with posterior staphyloma. Am J Ophthalmol. 1999;128(4):472–6.

139. Spaide RF, Akiba M, Ohno-Matsui K. Evaluation of peripapillary intrachoroidal cavitation with swept source and enhanced depth imaging optical coherence tomography. Retina. 2012;32(6):1037–44.

140. Ohno-Matsui K, Akiba M, Moriyama M, Ishibashi T, Hirakata A, Tokoro T. Intrachoroidal cavitation in macular area of eyes with pathologic myopia. Am J Ophthalmol. 2012;154(2):382–93.

141. Cohen SY, Quentel G. Chorioretinal folds as a consequence of inferior staphyloma associated with tilted disc syndrome. Graefes Arch Clin Exp Ophthalmol. 2006;244:1536–8.

142. Ohno-Matsui K, Akiba M, Moriyama M, Shimada N, Ishibashi T, Tokoro T, Spaide RF. Acquired optic nerve and peripapillary pits in pathologic myopia. Ophthalmology. 2012;119(8):1685–92.

The Choroid

Richard F. Spaide

The choroid is situated between the sclera and Bruch's membrane, and most of its substance is occupied by blood vessels; more than 70% of all of the blood flow to the eye goes to the choroid [1]. The photoreceptors have the highest rate of oxygen use per unit weight of tissue in the body [2], and nearly all of that is accounted for by the mitochondria of the inner segments. The retinal circulation, which is about 5% of the blood flow to the eye, supplies the inner retina, but the choroid supplies the oxygen used by the outer retina, including the inner segments. The choroid is the only source for the avascular fovea. The choroid has additional functions including acting as a heat sink [3] and absorbing stray light, participating in immune response, and host defense [4] and is an integral part in the process of emmetropization [5]. Although the ocular manifestations of high myopia have become apparent over the past centuries, appreciation of the abnormalities within the choroid has occurred only recently. High myopia is associated with profound changes in the choroid that are important in the pathogenesis of many important visually significant abnormalities. Advances in imaging have greatly increased our ability to visualize the choroid, providing an opportunity to better understand the choroid in health and disease.

10.1 The Embryology and Anatomy of the Choroid

10.1.1 Embryology

Each optic vesicle forms as outpouching of the forebrain. This vesicle invaginates to form a double-walled optic cup. The inner layer of the cup is destined to form the retina and the outer layer the retinal pigment epithelium (RPE). The inferior portion of the cup initially has a gap that forms the choroidal fissure, which allows access for the hyaloid artery to enter the eye. Eventually the gap closes. The uvea develops from the mesoderm and migrating neuroectoderm that surround the optic cup. Mesodermal cells start to differentiate into vessels around the same time that the RPE appears. The choriocapillaris starts to form at about the fifth to sixth week. The basal lamina of the RPE and of the choriocapillaris define the boundaries of the developing Bruch's membrane by week 6 [6]. The choriocapillaris becomes organized with luminal networks well before the rest of the choroidal vasculature develops. The posterior ciliary arteries enter the choroid during the eighth week of gestation, but it takes until week 22 before arteries and the veins become mature. Melanocytes precursors migrate into the uveal primordia from the neural crest at the end of the first month but start differentiating at the seventh month. The pigmentation of the choroid begins at the optic nerve and extends anteriorly to the ora serrata. This process is complete by about 9 months [7]. The sclera is derived from mesenchymal condensation starting anteriorly and completing posteriorly by week 12.

10.1.2 Choroidal Anatomy

The choroid is an unusual structure primarily composed of blood vessels but also has connective tissue, melanocytes, and intrinsic choroidal neurons. Birds have fluid-filled lacunae identified as true functional lymphatic system in their choroid [8]. Although humans don't have a lymphatic system in the eye, Schroedl and associates found human choroids have macrophage-like cells that stain positively for a lymphatic endothelium-specific marker, lymphatic vessel endothelial hyaluronic acid receptor [9]. Humans also have cells with nonvascular smooth muscle-like elements in the choroid [10, 11]. These cells are located around the entry of posterior ciliary vessels and nerves, along the vessels in the posterior segment, and under the foveal region. It has been proposed that the arrangement suggests the cells, which have actin contractile elements, may help stabilize the position of

R. F. Spaide (✉)
Vitreous, Retina, Macula Consultants of New York,
New York, NY, USA

R. F. Spaide et al. (eds.), *Pathologic Myopia*, https://doi.org/10.1007/978-3-030-74334-5_10

the fovea during accommodation [12]. The human choroid has intrinsic choroidal neurons, the functions of which are not known with certainty [13]. The choroid is attached to the sclera by strands of connective tissue which are easily separated anteriorly creating a potential space between them, the suprachoroidal space.

The blood from the short PCAs enters the eye and travels through successively smaller branches of arterioles within the choroid. The choroid is traditionally thought to be arranged in layers of vessels from the outer to inner part of the choroid labeled as Haller's layer, Sattler's layer, and the choriocapillaris. Haller's layer contains larger choroidal veins, while Sattler's layer has medium-sized vessels that branch inward to supply the choriocapillaris. There is no distinct border between Haller's and Sattler's layers or even an established definition of what is meant by large or medium. The pressure of the blood is reduced from about 75% of the systemic blood pressure at the short PCAs to that in the choriocapillaris, which has been measured in rabbits to be a few mm Hg greater than the intraocular pressure [14]. Increases in the intraocular pressure cause a proportional increase in the blood pressure in the choriocapillaris [14]. There does not appear to be effective autoregulation in the choroid, although myogenic mechanisms may be present. There is a sophisticated neural innervation that provides partial control. Like the brain, the eye has a high pulsatile blood flow rate and is encased in a noncompliant casing. As part of modulating pulsatile pressure in the cranium, the brain uses venous storage and a Starling resistor effect, to modulate venous outflow. An analogous function in the eye could be provided by the choroid, which contains fascicles of large veins that converge in vortices to drain out of the eye. This vortex area appears to be where the Starling resistor effect is possible.

The choriocapillaris is a planar plexus of small vessels with a lumen slightly larger than a typical capillary. The network of vessels in the choriocapillaris is tightly packed in the posterior portion of the eye, but the structure becomes looser in the periphery. The efferent and afferent vessels set up pressure gradients within the choriocapillaris to create a lobular flow. The flow characteristics are thought to be more dependent on complex gradients rather than anatomic patterns strictly dictated by choriocapillaris anatomy [15].

The vitality of the choriocapillaris is maintained in part by constitutive secretion of vascular endothelial growth factor (VEGF) by the RPE [16]. The choriocapillaris is highly polarized [17] with the internal surface having localized multiple localized areas of thinning of the capillary wall known as fenestrations. These thinner areas appear to facilitate the passage of material out of the capillaries and direct the flow toward the RPE. The number of fenestrations is more prominent in the submacular area as compared with the mid- or far periphery [18]. Similarly sized vessels in the retina do not have fenestrations. Soluble VEGF isoforms are required for fenestrations to occur in the choriocapillaris

[14], and these fenestrations disappear with VEGF withdrawal [19]. In experimental myopia, the choriocapillaris becomes less dense (Fig. 10.1), with decreased capillary lumens and a loss of fenestrations [20]. Also in myopes, as will be seen, the choroid is thinner than in emmetropes, and the vascular diameter of larger choroidal blood vessels is less as well.

Blood from the choriocapillaris collects into venules that lead into larger venules that course in the outer choroid toward the ampulla of the vortex veins. The typical vortex vein passes obliquely through the sclera for a distance of about 4.5 mm as it exits the eye. Some drainage of the anterior choroid occurs through the anterior ciliary veins into the ciliary body. There are often four vortex veins per eye, with the ampulla of the vortex veins lying at the equator of the eye. The number can range from three to eight [21]; in high myopes, there is often more than four, and there may be posterior vortex veins known as ciliovaginal veins, which drain near or through the optic nerve foramen (Fig. 10.2). The number and configuration of vortex veins is different in myopia; since myopia develops over time, the implication is what appears to be additional vortex veins in myopia are acquired. The superior vortex veins drain into the superior and the inferior vortex veins into the inferior ophthalmic veins, although anastomoses occur between these two main drainage pathways in the orbit [14].

10.2 Blood Flow Within the Choroid

Hayreh discovered many of the fascinating features of the choroidal blood flow from his observations of humans and monkeys [22, 23]. Although there are limited anastomotic connections, the arterial supply in the choroid is segmental as is the venous drainage; however, these segmental distributions do not correspond with each other. The choroid has high blood flow to deliver oxygen and metabolites to the retina and act as a heat sink. Blood is delivered to the choroid via the ophthalmic artery that branches to form (typically) two posterior ciliary arteries [23], which in turn branch to form many short posterior ciliary arteries and two long posterior ciliary arteries. There are no direct anastomoses between the PCAs or in arterial supply within the choroid. There is potential for local flow alterations to occur in the choriocapillaris based on pressure fluctuations. Once the blood leaves the choriocapillaris, it enters another segmented system, the venous outflow from the eye. The segmentation of the venous system is different from that of the arterial system, and the choroid is one of the few places in the body where this is true.

In the early phase of fluorescein angiography, it is common to see areas of the choroid that do not appear to fill with dye as quickly as adjacent regions. The designation of a watershed filling defect is made if the region of choroidal

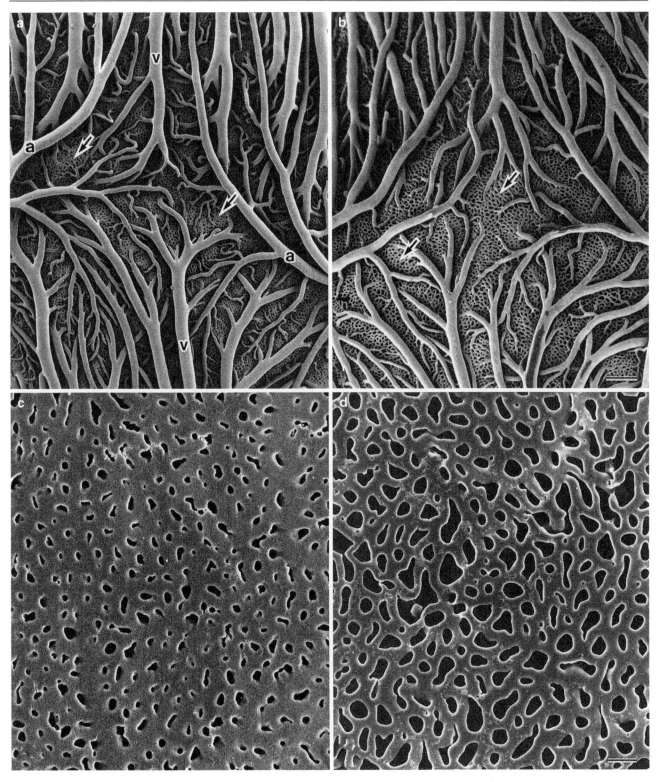

Fig. 10.1 Scanning electron micrographs of corrosion casts of the choroidal vasculature in control and myopic chick eyes at the fourth week. (**a, b**) The control eye (left) has a greater vascular density of larger vessels serving the choriocapillaris (arrows) than the myopic eye. The arterioles are designated by (a) and the venules (b). (**c**) The choriocapillaris seen en face in a control eye has the expected high vascular density. (**d**) In a representative myopic eye, the individual vessels of the choriocapillaris have a lower packing density, and the vessels are smaller and more tubelike. (Derived from reference [20])

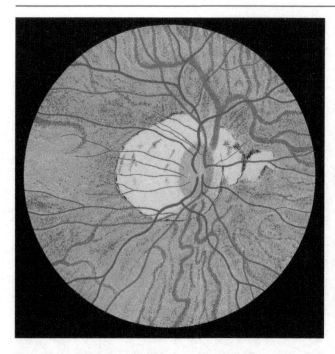

Fig. 10.2 Otto Haab, a prominent Swiss ophthalmologist, described posterior venous drainage in high myopes and called the vessels posterior vortex veins, a name still used today. In this color drawing, taken from the third edition of Haab's atlas, a prominent vein is seen to exit the choroid superonasal to the nerve. Two smaller vessels are seen at the inferior border of the nerve. The drawing is an accurate reflection of the posterior venous drainage in high myopes. Unlike the typical vortex veins in the periphery, the posterior vortex veins do not have an ampulla or a spray of contributing vessels

filling is delayed past the laminar flow stage of the retinal veins [24]. A common appearance of a watershed zone is a stripe, one to several millimeters wide, running vertically at the temporal border of the optic disc in which the choroid is not as hyperfluorescent as surrounding areas [22]. This watershed zone is thought to be the boundary between areas of the choroid supplied by the medial and lateral PCAs. Eyes with more than two PCAs have more watershed zones, with a vertical stripe involving the optic nerve region and a number of radiating lines extending from the nerve seen dependent on the actual number of PCAs. Venous watershed zones exist for the venous circulation and form a cruciate pattern centered slightly temporal to the optic nerve [22]. In times of decreased perfusion, watershed zones may represent the regions with the poorest flow since they are at the shared boundaries of non-overlapping systems.

10.3 The Regulation of Choroidal Blood Flow

The retina has autoregulation of blood flow, but no autonomic nervous systems control within the eye. The retinal vessels are embedded in the retinal tissue and can respond to metabolic demands and neurovascular coupling. The choroid is separated by several layers from the tissue it supplies, potentially limiting metabolic feedback mechanisms. The choroid has no autoregulation in the usual sense but is supplied by sympathetic, parasympathetic, and sensory nerve fibers [25]. These fibers are associated with the arteries and vein, but not the choriocapillaris. There are a variety of mediators that can be potentially released: the sympathetic nerve terminals release norepinephrine and neuropeptide Y [26, 27], the parasympathetic acetylcholine and also vasoactive intestinal polypeptide and neuronal nitric oxide synthase, and the sensory fibers substance P and calcitonin gene-related peptide [25]. Sympathetic stimulation causes a decrease in choroidal flow, which is potentially helpful in preventing overload in the choroid in "fight or flight" situations. Systemic increases in blood pressure would be countered by constriction of the choroidal arterioles. Stimulation of sympathetic innervation increases vascular resistance and decreases blood flow in the choroid. This is due to the release of norepinephrine and, possibly, neuropeptide Y release [28]. Parasympathetic stimulation causes choroidal vascular dilation [29]. The parasympathetic system is more dominant in "rest and digest" times and counterbalances the effects of sympathetic activation. The vascular tone in the choroid is modulated by acetylcholine, vasoactive intestinal polypeptide, and NO release from the parasympathetic nerve terminals.

The venous outflow from the choroid has an unusual anatomic arrangement. Blood form groups of choriocapillaris lobules are collected by draining venules, which consolidate to form larger veins. These larger veins do not continue to join other veins to form larger draining veins. Instead they course in a parallel fashion with minimal if any anastomosis with similarly sized veins until they converge on the ampulla of the vortex veins. Whereas blood vessel systems in the body form self-similar networks to form fractal-like arrangements, the choroidal veins do not follow allometric scaling laws. It has been proposed that this system can store venous blood to mitigate pulse pressure spikes during arterial inflow of blood during systole. A similar process occurs in the cranium, with the cerebral veins controlling blood flow into the superior sagittal sinus to help reduce pulse-related increases in intracranial pressure. The pressure in the vortex veins after they leave the eye is approximately 3 mm Hg, even though venous pressure in the choroid can be much higher than that. It has been proposed the venous outflow is controlled by a Starling resistor and is integrally related to intraocular pressure [14].

Perfusion in normal tissues in the body usually keeps the oxygen partial pressure at a relatively low level. The choroid is different – the oxygen partial pressure is very high, which from a teleologic standpoint is desirable so that the outer retina may receive as much oxygen as possible. The RPE secretes vascular endothelial growth factor (VEGF) to help maintain the choriocapillaris. CD-36 is a scavenger receptor expressed in the basal RPE. Houssier and associates showed that CD-36-deficient mice fail to induce COX-2 and subsequent VEGF synthesis at the level of the RPE and develop progressive degeneration of the choriocapillaris [30]. Therefore, CD-36 binding by the RPE, such as what happens in the normal process of phagocytosis of the photoreceptor outer segments, seems to be one of the factors maintaining the vessels of the inner choroid.

10.4 Other Choroidal Functions

There have been other reasons proposed for the large blood flow in the choroid. The amount of light energy delivered to the retina by incoming light is insufficient to cause a significant elevation in temperature and thus is an unlikely explanation [31]. It is possible that the high metabolism in the outer retina may produce enough heat to require mechanisms to reduce the local temperature. The high blood flow may help conduct heat away from the outer retina/RPE complex. The choroid contains melanocytes which improve optical function by absorbing scattered light and may also indirectly protect against oxidative stress. These melanocytes exist in an environment of high O_2 partial pressure, which, along with the light exposure, may be a risk factor for malignant transformation to melanoma. Melanocytes in human RPE are particularly rich in zinc and may serve as a reservoir for this metal ion [32–34].

10.5 Imaging the Choroid

Because of its localization between the overlying pigmented RPE and the underlying opaque and rigid fibrous sclera, the choroid is difficult to visualize with conventional imaging. Methods employing light reflection or fluorescence generation are impeded by the pigment in the RPE and choroid. Conventional OCT is affected by the effects of melanin and also the scattering properties of the blood and blood vessels. The choroid is a deeper structure and the depth, which affects the detection sensitivity.

10.5.1 Angiography

Fluorescein is stimulated by blue light with a wavelength between 465 and 490 nm and emits at a green light with the peak of the emission spectral curve ranging between 520 and 530 nm and a curve extending to approximately 600 nm. Both the excitation and emission spectra from fluorescein are blocked in part by melanin pigment, which acts to decrease visualization of the choroid. Fluorescein extravasates rapidly from the choriocapillaris and fluoresces in the extravascular space, and this also prevents delineation of the choroidal anatomy. The analysis of the choroid using fluorescein angiography is also limited by light absorption and scattering by the pigment in the RPE and choroid and by the blood in the choroid. Gross filling of the choroid can be seen, as can the converse, choroidal filling defects. Diseases causing arteritis, such as giant cell arteritis or Wegener's granulomatosis can cause regions of decreased perfusion of the choroid, but actual vessels are not visualized. Therefore, estimations of vascular density of the choroid are not easily done with fluorescein angiography. On the other hand, fluorescein angiography is good for visualizing retinal vascular abnormalities and many forms of choroidal neovascularization (CNV), particularly Type 2 CNV.

Indocyanine green (ICG) absorption peak is between 790 and 805 nm, and it fluoresces in a somewhat longer wavelength range, depending on the protein content and pH of the local environment. The longer wavelengths used have the attribute of penetrating the pigmentation of the eye better than the wavelengths used with fluorescein angiography. The retinal pigment epithelium and the choroid absorbs up to 75% of blue-green light used for fluorescein angiography but only up to 38% of the near infrared light used for ICG angiography [35]. ICG is 98% protein bound, with 80% binding to larger proteins such as globulins and alpha-1-lipoproteins [36, 37]. The amount of fluorescence derived from ICG during typical angiographic examination is much less than that obtained from fluorescein, and the resultant light is in the near infrared wavelengths. Because of the poor sensitivity to near infrared light by photographic film, the first practical imaging of ICG fluorescence in the clinic awaited commercial availability of digital charged couple devices (CCDs). Optical resolution is related to wavelength, and so, the resolution of ICG angiography is lower than fluorescein angiography.

ICG is highly protein bound, so there is less opportunity for the dye to leak from the normal choroidal vessels. During the earlier phases of ICG angiography, the choroidal vessels are visible. The vertical summation of the choroid is seen, making it difficult to delineate individual layers of vessels. Over the course of the angiogram, some staining of the extravascular tissue particularly Bruch's membrane occurs, obscuring visualization of deeper structures. This means flow can be estimated by looking at the early frames of the ICG angiogram, but later phases cannot be used for the same purpose.

Early after the availability of ICG angiography, many diseases were investigated, and new information that was not obtainable by fluorescein angiography was generated. Much of this information was interesting from a research standpoint but did not have practical clinical utility. For real-world use, ICG is most helpful in diagnosing and evaluating polypoidal choroidal vasculopathy and central serous chorioretinopathy. Secondary uses include evaluation of choroidal inflammatory diseases, angioid streaks, and choroidal tumors and in providing rough estimates of choroidal blood flow. The advent of widespread use of autofluorescence imaging and optical coherence tomography (OCT) methods to evaluate the choroid has largely supplanted ICG angiography for these secondary uses.

10.5.2 Ultrasonography

Contact B-scan ultrasonography typically uses a 10–12 megahertz probe placed on the eyelid. The probe used contains a piezoelectric crystal that is stimulated to vibrate by a short duration of an electrical driving current. Reflected sound waves cause the crystal to vibrate, which through the piezoelectric effect causes an electrical current. Sound decreases in intensity with increasing distance because of divergence of the sound beam and attenuation of the sound by the intervening tissue. Thus, reflected sound waves vary in strength with the depth of the reflecting structure in the eye. To compensate for the decrease in signal strength with time of flight, the gain of the amplifier is increased over the detection interval. Depth information is derived directly from time of flight information and the speed of sound through the medium involved. The direction of the crystal then is rotated slightly by a motor within the probe to successively build a two-dimensional image, a B-scan.

Although each A-scan is shown as a needle thin line within the B-scan image, the actual situation is far different. The piezoelectric crystal has some focusing ability, but in reality the sound beam produced by a piezoelectric crystal in a conventional B-scan probe has a main lobe and several side lobes [38]. Even the main lobe can be 1 mm in diameter at the surface of the retina. The side lobes add to the ambiguity of the reflection as does scattering within the eye. Given the eye is a curved structure, the wide probing beam produces a returning echo from any given region in the posterior portion of the eye that is smeared over an interval of time. The wavelengths used in ultrasonography dictate a theoretical axial resolution of about 150 microns, but the actual resolution in clinical use is much lower. For example, a typical B-scan of the optic nerve will not show the cup unless there is a high cup-to-disc ratio because of the broad diameter of the curved target that is imaged. Another significant problem with ultrasonography is that the exact location of the image obtained is not known. The general region can be estimated by evaluating relationships with neighboring structures and by trying to imagine where the probe is aimed.

In non-pathologic conditions, the reflectivity of the choroid is difficult to distinguish from the overlying retina and the underlying sclera. In high myopes, the thickness of the choroid can easily be less than the resolution of contact B-scan ultrasonography making any meaningful imaging of the choroid in populations of high myopes impossible. Contact B-scan ultrasonography is useful to examine the general contour of the eyewall and the visualize staphylomata.

10.5.3 Optical Coherence Tomography

10.5.3.1 Interferometry

In dry air, the speed of sound is 343.2 meters per second. The sound velocity in an average phakic eye is 1555 meters per second [39]. This means that the time it takes sound to travel the length of a phakic eye with an axial length of 24 mm is approximately 15.4 microseconds, which is easy to measure. Because light travels very rapidly (3×10^8 m/sec), it is not possible to measure the time-of-flight delay on a micron-scale level of resolution using an external system of time measurement. The time it takes light to travel a micron is the same or less than it would take an electron to travel the same distance in an electronic circuit. Measurement of multiple reflections with a detector and the subsequent required electronic circuitry requires conduction paths for electrons that are much longer than the variations in path length of the light rays. However, light rays have a repeating characteristic inherent in their own wave properties. A clever way to time how long light takes to travel a given distance is to use the wave-like character of the light itself as its own internal clock. Phase differences in waveforms can be detected and reveal very small changes in time of flight. That is what a Michelson interferometer does; the wavelength of the light is used as its own timing standard. The micron-scale resolution is achieved by comparing the time of flight of the sample reflection with the known delay of a reference reflection by using interference to find phase differences in the light waves.

Coherency of light is a measure of how correlated one wave of light is with another. Temporal coherency is a measure of how correlated one wave of light is with another generated at a different time. Coherence length is the distance light would travel during the coherence time. Light produced by a conventional laser has a long coherence time because one wave of light is similar to other waves of light produced at times before or after. It is possible to produce light with a short coherence length. In this situation, the waveform of light produced is the same for all of the light rays produced at any one instance, but this waveform is different from other waveforms produced at other times. This approach essentially puts a time stamp on the waveform. Low coherence light split into a reference arm can only interfere with light from the sample arm if the path lengths are the same or are nearly the same.

In time domain OCT, each point in the tissue is sampled one at a time. The probing beam illuminates the tissue, but information is obtained from a small portion of the tissue at any given instant. This means time domain OCT is less efficient at extracting information from tissue at any given total light exposure. The total amount of light that can be delivered to tissue is limited by safety standards. Spectral domain (SD) OCT takes the light from the interferometer and passes it through a grating to separate out the component wavelengths. Using a Fourier transform, it is possible to determine where, and how strongly, different reflections in the sample arm originated from simultaneously. In effect, all layers produce signal during each A-scan. Because of this feature, SD-OCT devices are much more efficient at extracting information from tissue at any given light exposure. This increase in efficiency is often translated to increased scanning speeds such that SD-OCT instruments typically scan the eye with speeds up to 100 times faster than time-domain OCT instruments. There are some problems inherent in SD technology. The deeper tissues produce higher-frequency signals, but the way the grating and detector sample this frequency is not linear. The higher frequencies are bunched together to a greater extent than lower frequencies. In addition, the sensitivity of the detection decreases with increasing frequency. This causes SD-OCT to have decreasing sensitivity and resolution with increasing depth.

A consequence of the decreasing sensitivity is that the choroid cannot be imaged in many emmetropes with convention SD-OCT. Eyes with high myopia have thinner choroids and a relative depigmentation, making it possible to visualize the full thickness of the choroid in many eyes with conventional SD-OCT. Because a Fourier transform is used, two conjugate images are developed from the interferometric signal. In practical use, only one of these two images are shown, typically with the retina facing toward the top of the screen. If the peak sensitivity is placed posteriorly typically at the inner sclera, deeper structures such as the choroid can be seen. This method of imaging the choroid is called enhanced depth imaging (EDI) OCT. [40] It is now simply performed with SD-OCT instruments, often by just selecting EDI in the software of the instrument. To improve the signal-to-noise ratio and therefore image appearance, many B-scans can be averaged together, typically using 50 to 100 images. Segmentation of OCT images allows visualization and measurement of various layers in the eye. In high myopes, the choroid can be extremely thin, making it difficult to segment volume scans without attendant segmentation errors.

Swept-source OCT (SS OCT) uses a frequency-swept light source and detectors, which measure the interference output as a function of time [41, 42]. The sensitivity of SS-OCT varies with depth as well, but the roll-off in sensitivity is not as great as seen with SD-OCT. Current implementations of SS-OCT have light sources that use a longer center wavelength, which has improved ability to penetrate through tissue. Therefore, both the vitreous and choroid can be imaged simultaneously; there is no need to pick one or the other. There are trade-offs with swept source OCT that have to be considered. Although longer wavelengths of light may penetrate tissue to a greater degree, the problem is water absorbs longer wavelengths of light. This restricts the range, or bandwidth of wavelengths that can be used in the eye, since the vitreous is mostly water. Increasing the center wavelength has the effect of decreasing the resolution for any given bandwidth. Water absorption of longer wavelengths is an important impediment to expanding the bandwidth of current 1 micron swept light sources, which limits the ability to overcome the decrease in resolution by increasing the bandwidth. Newer light sources operating at shorter wavelengths are being developed, and these light sources may avoid the problem of water absorption. For example, a SS-OCT using a large bandwidth light source with a center wavelength of 850 nm could provide very high-speed, high-resolution imaging with potentially less fall-off in sensitivity with depth as compared with SD-OCT implementations.

No matter what the imaging modality, high myopia represents special challenges for OCT. The extreme axial length of highly myopic eyes can represent difficulties in obtaining a usable image. The posterior portion of the highly myopic eye often has staphylomata, and curvatures of the eyewall appear exaggerated in OCT renderings. The depth in which images are obtained in most commercial OCT instruments is approximately 2–3 mm. Wide-angle scans image enough of the extent of a highly myopic eye that the vertical range of tissue can exceed the available depth range. Imaging of the areas outside of this 2 mm are seen as upside down conjugates. This produces artifactual image folding or mirroring. Imaging high myopes presents interesting opportunities, however. The choroid is thin and doesn't have much pigment, so with EDI-OCT or SS-OCT it is possible to visualize the full thickness of the sclera and even to see into the subarachnoid space around the optic nerve (Fig. 10.3) [43].

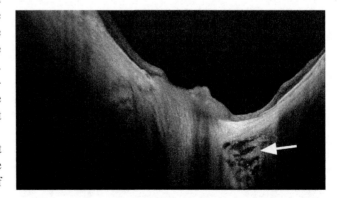

Fig. 10.3 Swept source OCT is able to provide visualization of the subarachnoid space if there is peripapillary atrophy, which there usually is, particularly in the region of the conus. Note the beams of tissue visible (arrow)

10.6 Measurements and Reproducibility of Choroidal Thickness

There is a very good intersystem [44, 45], inter-observer, and inter-visit reproducibility [45] of manual choroidal thickness measurements. The inter-observer repeatability is good using EDI-OCT [45, 46], Cirrus HD OCT [44, 47], Optovue RTVue [45], and SS OCT. [45, 48] The intersystem reproducibility of choroidal thickness measurements has been assessed between EDI-OCT and SS OCT [45] and also between three different SD-OCT devices: Cirrus HD-OCT, Spectralis using EDI module, and RTVue [44]. Tan and associates found the intraclass correlation coefficient for inter-observer reproducibility of 0.994 but also the value of the mean difference between choroidal thickness measurements between graders that was 2.0 μm for 24 normal eyes of 12 healthy subjects [46]. These levels of agreement are smaller than the diurnal variation in choroidal thickness in humans [46]. Automated segmentation methods are generally faster but substitute idiosyncrasies and biases of the coded algorithm for idiosyncrasies and biases of a human observer.

10.7 Normal Subfoveal Choroidal Thickness

Margolis and Spaide investigated 54 normal, non-myopic eyes with a mean age of 50.4 years using the EDI-OCT and reported a mean subfoveal choroidal thickness of 287 microns (Fig. 10.4) [49]. Normal was defined as patients without any significant retinal or choroidal pathologic features, uncontrolled diabetes or hypertension, and a refractive error less than 6 diopters of spherical equivalent. The choroidal-scleral interface has been identified in 100% of subjects in this study [49]. The authors showed that increasing age was correlated significantly with decreasing choroidal thickness at all points measured. The subfoveal choroidal thickness was found to decrease by 15.6 microns for each decade of age [49]. Ikuno and associates investigated 86 non-myopic eyes of healthy Japanese patients with SS-OCT with a mean age of 39.4 years and found a subfoveal choroidal thickness of 354 microns.

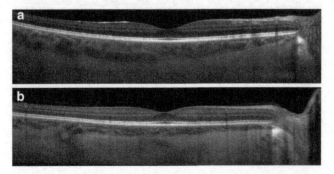

Fig. 10.4 Choroidal thickness in (**a**) a 31-year-old emmetrope and (**b**) a 29-year-old −6 myope. Note the subfoveal choroidal thickness is decreased in the myope as compared with the emmetrope despite their relatively young ages

Ikuno and associates found that the choroidal thickness decreased by 14 microns for each decade of age [50]. The mean subfoveal choroidal thickness has been found to vary among studies from 203.6 microns in 31 eyes with a mean age of 64.6 years [48] to 448.5 microns in 22 eyes with a mean age of 35.7 years [51]. The refractive error and age has to be taken into account, as does diurnal variation, making comparison of general mean values impossible for many studies. These comparisons are further hindered by some studies reporting choroidal thickness in patient groups using techniques that could not visualize the choroidal scleral junction in all eyes. The percentage of identification of the scleral choroidal interface was 74% of 34 eyes in one series using SD-OCT [47], for example. Some studies excluded patients with ocular disorders [47–49], some excluded patients with ocular and systemic disorders [50, 52], and some mentioned they excluded patients with systemic disorders that might affect choroidal thickness [48, 49]. Even though these studies propose to evaluate normal eyes, some of them included highly myopic eyes with a spherical equivalent error greater than −6 diopters [48, 52, 53].

There are several possible reasons for the decrease in subfoveal choroidal thickness with age, such as loss of choriocapillaris, a decrease in the diameter of the choriocapillary vessels, decrease in luminal diameter of blood vessels, and, in some cases, a diminution of the middle layer of the choroid[52] [54, 55]. Histologic evaluation of eye bank and autopsy eyes found a yearly decrease in choroidal thickness of 1.1 microns per year, which was less than the amount measured in vivo [49]. The differences may be related to measurement technique as the histologic specimens were measured in autopsy eyes, which by default had no blood pressure and the choroid is an inflated structure [54–56].

The choroidal thickness has also been found to fluctuate with defocus in humans [46, 57]. Maintenance of emmetropia is now known to depend on active mechanisms that sense image blur and then take steps to improve the image to include moving retina to reduce the blur and permanently altering ocular dimensions. Among the first changes are an active increase or decrease in choroidal thickness that moves the retina, as shown in laboratory investigations in chickens [58, 59] and primates [60, 61]. Read and associates demonstrated that similar changes in choroidal thickness occur in humans in response to short-term unilateral image blur [57]. The choroid was found to thicken with the myopic defocus condition and to become thinner with the hyperopic defocus [62]. Humans have a diurnal variation in choroidal thickness [46, 63] that is related in magnitude to the baseline thickness of the choroid and systolic blood pressure [46].

10.8 Topography of Choroidal Thickness

In emmetropic eyes, the choroid thickness varies topographically within the posterior pole: the choroid was thickest under the fovea with a mean value, and the choroidal thickness decreased rapidly in the nasal direction. The choroidal thickness appears to be thinner in the inferior macula as compared with the superior macula [47, 48, 50, 52]. The inferior peripapillary choroid is thinner than all other quadrants around the nerve [64] [65]. The reason for this finding is not known, but the optic fissure is located in the inferior aspect of the optic cup and is the last part to close during embryology of the eye. Another factor may be this area is in the typical watershed zone in the choroidal circulation. In their study, Ho and associates found that the choroidal thickness increases radially from the optic nerve in all directions in normal emmetropic patients and eventually approaches a plateau [64].

10.9 Imaging the Internal Structure of the Choroid

The basement membrane of the choriocapillaris is attached to the outer layer of the trilayer Bruch's membrane. The intercapillary pillars separate the vessels of the choriocapillaris. The outer band of reflectivity from the outer retina is ascribed to the RPE, but it is likely that Bruch's membrane, and therefore the choriocapillaris is incorporated in the summation of reflection attributed to the RPE obtained with commercially available OCTs. Fong and associates have hypothesized that hyperreflective foci visualized beneath the Bruch membrane line represent cross sections of feeding and draining arterioles and venules [66]. Larger choroidal vessels have hyporeflective cores with surrounding hyperreflective walls. The luminal diameter of the images probably is proportional, but not necessarily exactly equal to the lumen diameter of the corresponding vessel. It is possible that some portion of the outer blood column could be imaged as being part of the wall.

10.10 Optical Coherence Tomography Angiography

In successive OCT images of the eye, provided the patient does not move, there is little change from one image to the next, except for blood flow. By obtaining several B-scans over a short time interval and computing the change over time, a flow signal can be detected [67]. Using many B-scans produces a 3-D block of flow information. In practical use, slabs of this block are condensed to produce en face representations of flow. The slabs selected typically are based on the anatomy of the retina or choroid. OCT angiography images of the choriocapillaris are noisy and in the past were analyzed based on areas of where flow signal was not detected. These are called flow deficits or signal deficits. Frame averaging of the choriocapillaris scans produces images of the choriocapillaris that can be binarized and then skeletonized. The capillary segments in the mesh can be quantitatively evaluated. Analyzing the choriocapillaris is done using slabs that are 10–20 μm thick. As the total choroidal thickness of high myopes, particularly older subjects, may not be that much thicker, the choriocapillaris images also contain flow information from other layers in the choroid.

10.11 The Choroid in High Myopia

The thickness of the choroid has been found to vary inversely with the age of the subject and the amount of myopic refractive error (Tables 10.1 and 10.2). The choroidal thickness varies inversely with the axial length, with the regression models being nearly equivalent to those using refractive error. This is probably because high myopes seen in a retina

Table 10.1 Determinants of Choroidal Thickness

Parameter estimates							
			95% Wald confidence interval		Hypothesis test		
Parameter	B	Std. error	Lower	Upper	Wald Chi-Square	df	Sig.
(Intercept)	310.693	27.3223	257.142	364.244	129.309	1	<0.001
Age	−1.550	0.4064	−2.347	−0.754	14.553	1	<0.001
Refraction	8.133	1.8408	4.525	11.741	19.520	1	<0.001

Dependent variable = subfoveal choroidal thickness
Predictors of subfoveal choroidal thickness of a group of 145 highly myopic eyes with no macular pathology. Each year of age is associated with a decrease of 1.55 μm of choroidal thickness, while each diopter of myopic refractive error is associated with a decrease of 8.13 μm. From reference [77]

Table 10.2 Visual Acuity and Choroidal Thickness

Parameter estimates							
			95% Wald confidence interval		Hypothesis test		
Parameter	B	Std. error	Lower	Upper	Wald Chi-Square	df	Sig.
(Intercept)	0.287	0.0630	0.163	0.410	20.689	1	<0.001
Subfoveal choroidal thickness	−0.0011	0.0003	−0.002	0.000	13.397	1	<0.001

Dependent variable: logarithm of minimal angle of resolution (logMAR)
Predictors of log MAR visual acuity in a group of 145 highly myopic eyes. Only the subfoveal choroidal thickness proved predictive. From reference [77]

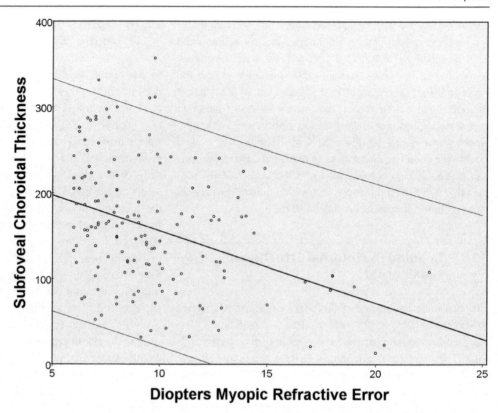

Fig. 10.5 Subfoveal choroidal thickness versus myopic refractive error in a group of 145 highly myopic eyes with no macular pathology. The trendline demonstrates the decrease in thickness with increasing refractive error, and the thinner bordering lines show the 95% confidence interval of the trend line

clinic are almost always axial myopes; as such, this observation might not apply universally to the general pool of high myopes. In the process of becoming highly myopic, the eye appears to expand, but does not make additional tissue. For example, the collagen weight of the sclera does not increase with the development of experimental myopia; it actually decreases. The choroid may well be stretched to a certain degree by the development of myopia without the creation of additional vasculature. This determination has not been made yet and would be best modeled over the expanse of the eye and not just the limited area currently imaged with commercial OCT instruments. The decrease in thickness of the choroid in high myopes has, appropriately enough, been called myopic choroidal thinning (Fig. 10.5) [68]. The expansion of the eye seems to cause a decrease in the packing density of the photoreceptors [69], with retention of the same visual acuity because the extension of the axial length also causes a proportional enlargement of the projected image. Although the choroid is thinner, the oxygen requirements per unit area of outer retina may be decreased because of the reduced packing density (Fig. 10.6). However, the reduction in thickness of the choroid with age continues in non-myopes and myopes alike. Curiously the diminution in choroidal thickness with age is approximately the same in absolute amounts in high myopes as in eyes that do not have high myopia (Fig. 10.7) [68]. High myopes start out with attenuated thicknesses and progress to remarkably thin or even absent areas of choroid. At some threshold, the choroid would have some difficulty in supplying enough oxygen and other metabolites. From that point, the term myopic choroidal atrophy is appropriate [68]. In elderly people without high myopia, the choroid may show reduced thickness in a process known as age-related choroidal atrophy (ARCA) [70]. These patients have normal axial lengths but show tessellation of the fundus, much the same as older high myopes, and beta-zone peripapillary atrophy. Eyes with decreased choroidal thickness as part of ARCA are more likely to have pseudodrusen, while highly myopic eyes almost never have pseudodrusen [71]. ARCA has been defined as a choroidal thickness of less than 125 microns based on population studies, while myopic choroidal atrophy has not had a thickness definition published.

Animal models of myopia were found to have decreased choriocapillaris density and diameter [20]. Angiographic studies of the choroid with ICG have also found that the choroidal vasculature was altered in highly myopic eyes [72, 73]. A color Doppler ultrasonographic study found that the choroidal circulation was decreased in highly myopic eyes [74]. The choroid of highly myopic patients is significantly thinner than the choroid of normal eyes [68, 75]. As the choroid supplies oxygen and nutrition to the retinal pigment epithelial cells and the outer retina, compromised choroidal circulation may account, in part, for the retinal dysfunction and vision loss that is seen in high myopia.

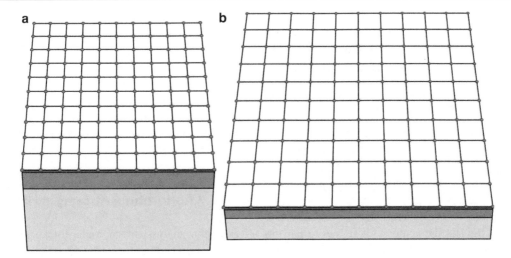

Fig. 10.6 Hypothetical explanation for choroidal thinning and supply of oxygen and metabolites to the retina. (**a**) In an emmetropic eye, the photoreceptors (blue dots) have a certain packing density. These are arranged on the retinal pigment epithelium (brown layer), which in turn is on the choroid (orange-red layer). The sclera is depicted by the gray structure. In a high myope, (**b**) the posterior pole is stretched resulting in a lower packing density of the photoreceptors. The choroid is thinner than an emmetrope. However, the ratio of the choroid's ability to supply oxygen and metabolites as compared with the packing density of the photoreceptors may not be adversely affected in high myopes, as evidenced by their good visual function, at least when young. With increasing age, the choroid thins, and later in life there is potential for decreased visual function as a consequence of choroidal atrophy

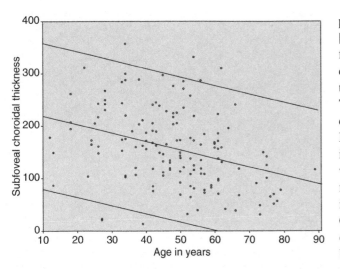

Fig. 10.7 Subfoveal choroidal thickness versus age in a group of 145 highly myopic eyes with no macular pathology. The trendline demonstrates the decrease in thickness with age, and the thinner bordering lines show the 95% confidence interval. The Y-axis shows the thickness of the choroid in microns

10.12 Biometric Choroidal Changes and Their Clinical Significance

A group of 18 patients (31 eyes), with a mean age of 51.7 years and a mean refractive error of −15.5 D, was evaluated with regular SD-OCT. The mean subfoveal choroidal thickness was only 100.5 μm and was even thinner in older patients and those with greater posterior staphyloma height [76]. The authors defined staphyloma height as the sum of four vertical measurements on SD-OCT foveal scans: the distance from the RPE line beneath the fovea to the nasal, temporal, superior, and inferior edges of the OCT image. This method does not mention how the presence, shape, and exact location of the posterior staphyloma were determined. By definition, a staphyloma is an outpouching of the eye and is a region where there is an exaggerated curvature of the wall of the eye. Any eye, whether it is myopic or not, is not a flat structure, and as such, it should have some "height" as it is defined by this SD-OCT method of measurement. Conventional SD-OCT allows a relatively good visualization of the choroidal-scleral interface in highly myopic eyes because of the dramatic choroidal thinning [75]. Ikuno and associates reported the scleral interface was undetectable in eyes with a choroidal thickness greater than 300 μm with regular SD-OCT. [75] Visualization would be expected to be dependent on the amount of pigmentation of the RPE and choroid. Another group of 31 patients (55 eyes) with a mean age of 59.7 years and a mean refractive error of −11.9 D was evaluated with EDI-OCT. The mean subfoveal choroidal thickness was 93.2 μm and was negatively correlated with age ($P = 0.006$) and refractive error ($P < 0.001$) [68]. Eyes with a history of choroidal neovascularization also had a thinner choroid ($P = 0.013$), but the patients in this study were treated with photodynamic therapy, which may have damaged the choroid [68]. In this EDI-OCT study, subfoveal choroidal thickness was found to decrease by 12.7 μm for each decade of life and by 8.7 µm for each diopter of myopia. Nishida and associates evaluated 145 highly myopic eyes and found the choroidal thickness decreased by 15.5 µm per decade of age and 8.13 µm for each diopter of myopia [77].

Given the knowledge that choroidal thickness decreases with both age and myopia, a study was done to look at factors related to visual acuity in highly myopic eyes with no other evident pathology. Two groups of patients, one from New York and the other Japan, were evaluated separately and as a pooled group [77]. Various features were measured in OCT scans by two masked readers. The only predictor of visual acuity, in each of the patient populations and in the pooled data, was the subfoveal choroidal thickness. The thinner the choroid, the less the acuity, although even patients with pronounced thinning of the choroid had what would seem like modest reductions in acuity. Of interest are measures of utility of vision, which show disproportionate loss with even mild changes in acuity. For example, the utility loss of an eye going from 20/20 to 20/40 is about the same as an eye going from 20/40 to 20/200. A study of 60 eyes of highly myopic patients without evidence of maculopathy found a negative correlation between visual acuity and macular choroidal thickness, subfoveal choroidal thickness, and photoreceptor/RPE aggregate thickness [78]. A study of 37 highly myopic eyes as compared with 86 normal eyes found an inverse correlation between choroidal thickness and visual acuity [79]. A case control study found axial length to be negatively correlated with visual acuity after adjusting for age. Addition of choroidal thickness did not cause a statistically significant change. In a study of 105 extremely high myopic subjects, choroidal thickness is inversely correlated with visual acuity, but following correction for spherical equivalent, among other things, the correlation was no longer significant [80]. Note the biggest predictors for choroidal thickness are age and refractive error (or axial length). That means if these variables are included in a regression equation, adding choroidal thickness on top of that as a variable would then only evaluate the shared variance in the variable choroidal thickness and acuity that is not accounted for by the shared variance between choroidal thickness and age and refractive error. Using the same logic, jumping off of the Empire State Building is no more risky than jumping off of a chair, corrected for height. It may be possible to include all of the variables if the sample size is large enough to overcome the effects of mutual confounding, as with the Beijing Eye Study, which evaluated 3233 subjects and found best corrected visual acuity was inversely correlated with subfoveal choroidal thickness even after including age and axial length [81].

In high myopia, we are often impressed by the minority of patients with retinal detachment or choroidal neovascularization, because they have sudden loss of large amounts of visual acuity. Many patients with high myopia have lesser amounts of acuity loss that individually may not seem all that important. However, the number of eyes involved is immense. By analogy in some areas of the world, people have deficient intake of iodine. A small minority of people in those areas develop cretinism. A much larger proportion of people have a small decrease in mental function. The cretinism cases are vivid examples; these few people have lost a lot. From a societal standpoint, the many people losing a smaller amount is also important.

10.13 Chorioretinal Atrophy in High Myopia

Regression analysis of choroidal thickness shows a linear trendline descending in proportion to the amount of myopia or age (Fig. 10.8). In general, this is a true representation, but there is a lower limit to how thin the choroid theoretically could be and still be functional. Red blood cells have a finite size and the vessels carrying these cells by necessity have to be larger. In OCT images of high myopes, the choroid can be as thin as 15 microns or less. Eyes with choroids this thin have marked alterations of pigmentation to include clumping

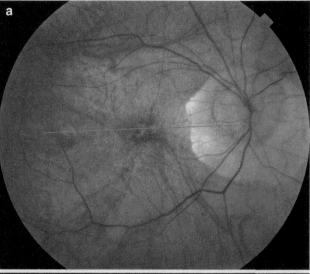

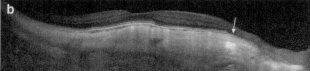

Fig. 10.8 A 70-year-old woman with high myopia. (**a**) The fundus picture shows attenuation of the choroidal vessels. Note in the central macular region there is a relative paucity of vessels. She is lightly pigmented and therefore doesn't show a prominent tessellated fundus. There is peripapillary atrophy. (**b**) The enhanced depth imaging (EDI) optical coherence tomography (OCT) shows a choroid that is quite thin (arrowheads); the subfoveal choroidal thickness is 14 µm. Note the choroid seems to come to an abrupt end at the border of the normal choroid and the peripapillary atrophy (arrow)

and rarefaction in adjacent areas. These areas of extreme attenuation of the choroid are seen adjacent to zones of what appears to be complete absence of the choroid. These areas are brilliantly white because there does not appear to be any extant RPE or choroid, and therefore the underlying sclera is readily visible (Figs. 10.9, 10.10, and 10.11). These areas have attenuation of the overlying retina and have been called patchy atrophy. (The term patchy atrophy is misleading in that in the surrounding areas the choroid is also atrophic.) At the border of the chorioretinal atrophy, the choroid does not necessarily gradually thin to non-existence, it often has a border where a very thin choroid abruptly terminates. This is probably secondary to the anatomic configuration of the remnants of choroid with vessels having either a quantum thickness or not being present at all. With loss of the choroid, there is a concomitant loss of the ability to supply oxygen and metabolites, so the remaining choroidal stroma and the overlying RPE and outer retina appears to wane. Another mechanism that can lead to complete loss is following lacquer crack formation. Each crack in Bruch's membrane causes a traumatic rupture of the choriocapillaris. The potential repair that takes place to the choriocapillaris is not known at present. However, repeated formation of lacquer cracks

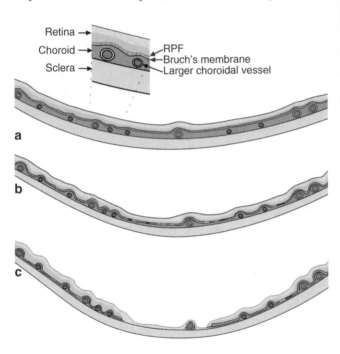

Fig. 10.9 Schematic drawing of choroidal thinning and atrophy. (**a**) In high myopes, the choroid is thinner, with what appears to be attenuation of the middle choroid in particular. The larger choroidal vessels may fill much of the thickness of the choroid. (**b**) With increasing thinning of the choroid, the larger choroidal blood vessels indent the overlying RPE monolayer. (**c**) The choroid appears to become so attenuated in older highly myopic patients that it no longer maintains the vitality of the overlying retina and retinal pigment epithelium or itself for that matter. Areas of absence of the outer retina, RPE, and choroid appear. The remaining tissue is essentially the inner retina. Since this is transparent and the underlying tissue is the sclera, these areas appear white

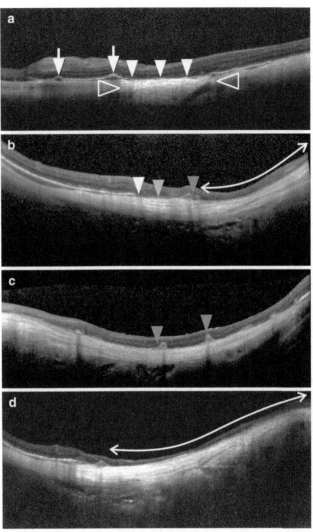

Fig. 10.10 OCT examples of advanced choroidal atrophy in high myopia. (**a**) The choroid is attenuated in this eye, and two larger choroidal vessels (arrows) are seen elevating the RPE. Some authors have called these elevations "choroidal microfolds," which is clearly incorrect since the choroid is not folded. In areas of loss of the RPE, there is increased light transmission to deeper layers (open arrowheads). Within this zone, what appears to be Bruch's membrane is seen (arrowheads). (**b**) With more profound loss of the choroid, the RPE terminates leaving a vestige of Bruch's membrane (white arrowhead) and remnants of Bruch's membrane (yellow arrowhead). Around a larger choroidal vessel, there appears to be residual portions of associated choroidal stroma (blue arrowhead). The double-ended white arrow shows a stretch of the posterior pole without any visible vascularized choroid. Note the loss of substance and laminations in the overlying retina. (**c**) This eye shows a nearly complete loss of the choroid in the region of the OCT scan. There are two remaining larger choroidal vessels with small vestiges of choroidal tissue (blue arrowheads). (**d**) In an eye with more chronic loss of the choroid, as shown by the extent of the double-ended white arrow, the overlying retina is remarkably thinned

likely takes a toll and decreases the integrity of the choriocapillaris in an affected area.

Okabe and associates analyzed three eyes with chorioretinal atrophy and pathologic myopia enucleated for various

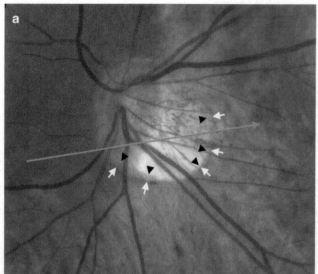

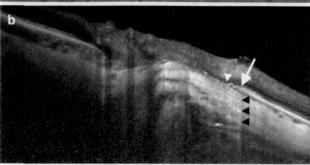

Fig. 10.11 Tilted disc and conus in a high myope. The infrared scanning laser image was projected onto the color picture to be able to accurately locate the scan line shown as the green arrow. (**a**) This eye shows a tilted disc and profound atrophy within a conus inferotemporal to the disc. At the outer border of the conus are two concentric curves. The outer one (white arrows) is where the orange color terminates, and the second is the continuation of a more subtle zone of shading prior to the intensely reflective inner zone of the conus. This boundary is shown by the black arrowheads. (**b**) The termination of the orange color corresponds to the white arrow. Note the increased penetration of light posterior to this zone, as demarcated by the black arrowheads. These signs are taken to mean the RPE stops, or at least becomes attenuated, at this juncture. There is a thinner curved structure that stops nasally (white arrowhead), and this structure appears to be the termination of Bruch's membrane. The termination of this layer corresponds to the line demarcated by the black arrowheads in the color photograph

reasons: herpetic keratitis and secondary glaucoma, intraocular hemorrhage, and painful filamentous keratitis [82]. One eye had -20D of myopia, and the amount of myopia was not defined for the two other eyes included. Histopathological observations have provided valuable information in high myopia: the choroid was thin with vessels present in some areas but completely absent in others [82]. The authors hypothesized that the choriocapillaris was obstructed and disappeared earlier than the other choroidal vessels under the conditions of excessive myopia and that the choriocapillaris obstruction occurs in a lobulated fashion. The associated conditions in these eyes probably influenced the ultrastructure of the analyzed tissue.

10.14 Intrachoroidal Cavitation

A yellowish-orange lesion typically located immediately inferior to optic nerve occurs in eyes with high myopia [83–89]. This lesion was originally termed peripapillary detachment in pathologic myopia1 because the defect was thought to represent an elevation of the retina and the retinal pigment epithelium (RPE). Peripapillary detachment in pathologic myopia was found in 4.9% of highly myopic eyes in a series reported by Shimada and coworkers [84]. A steep excavation of the inferior myopic conus was detected adjacent to the peripapillary detachment [85]. Revision of the concepts involving the lesion highlighted some aspects that were inconsistent with the known pathoanatomy of RPE detachments – the lesion appeared to be a cavity but appeared to be located in the choroid [86, 87]. Tateno and colleagues thought the RPE was not separated from the choroid; instead, there was a schisis within the choroid [86]. In their case description, Toranzo and colleagues stated "deep hyporeflectivity was present in the underlying choroid, resembling an intrachoroidal cavitation separating the retinal pigment epithelium from the sclera" [87]. As a consequence, they changed the name of the defect to peripapillary intrachoroidal cavitation (ICC) [87]. Wei and associates expanded on the concept of peripapillary ICC and proposed a complex of forces composed of "posterior expansion force, the vitreous traction force, and the vitreous fluid dynamics determine the size and shape of the lesion" [88]. Investigation of a series of 16 eyes with peripapillary ICC using EDI-OCT and SS-OCT showed an interesting anatomic configuration [89]. The sclera in the region of the conus was displaced posteriorly, and the backward deflection of the sclera continued into the region of the ICC. The overall curvature of the retina, RPE, and Bruch's membrane complex was seen to be relatively unaffected over the region of the ICC. The cavitation was created by the expansion of the distance between the inner wall of the sclera and the posterior surface of Bruch's membrane. There also appeared to be alterations of the anatomy around the optic nerve caused by the posterior displacement of the sclera (Fig. 10.12). A full-thickness defect in the retina was found in one quarter of the eyes at the border of the conus.

The eye ordinarily is inflated by its intraocular pressure with the wall of the eye acting as the outer barrier, resisting outward expansion. The ability of the wall of the eye to resist deformation is related to its inherent elasticity and its thickness. Over normal expanses, the wall of the eye is composed of the retina, RPE, Bruch's membrane, the choroid, and sclera. In the region of the conus, there is no choroid, RPE, Bruch's membrane, or outer retina. The inner retina can be very attenuated. The underlying sclera is thinned in eyes with high myopia, particularly in the region of the conus. The comparatively thin eye wall in the area of the conus is exposed to the same force per unit area from intraocular pressure as other areas in the eye and therefore is more likely

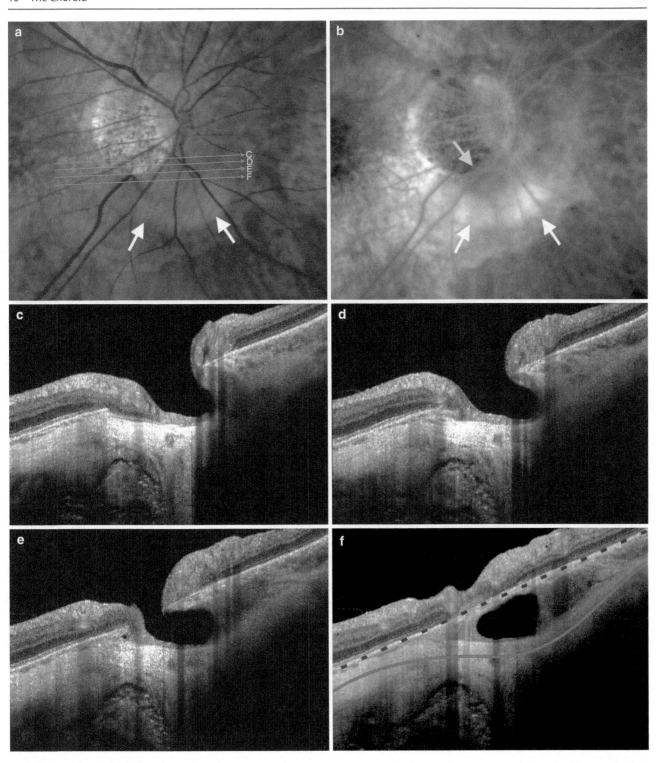

Fig. 10.12 (**a**) This color photograph shows the yellow orange region of the intrachoroidal cavitation (white arrows). The green arrows show the locations of subsequent optical coherence tomography (OCT) sections. (**b**) A fluorescein angiogram shows a modest late collection of dye within the cavity. Note the edge of the retinal defect is more clearly evident than in the color photograph. (**c–f**) Successive serial sections using swept source OCT showing the inner retinal defect and the exten-sion of the cavitation into the choroid. There is a veil of tissue extending through the thickness of the choroid at the border of the cavitation. In (**f**), note that the hyperreflective band corresponding to the retinal pigment epithelium is nearly straight, as illustrated by the blue dashed line overlay. The sclera shows an outbowing posteriorly with the red line at the center point thickness

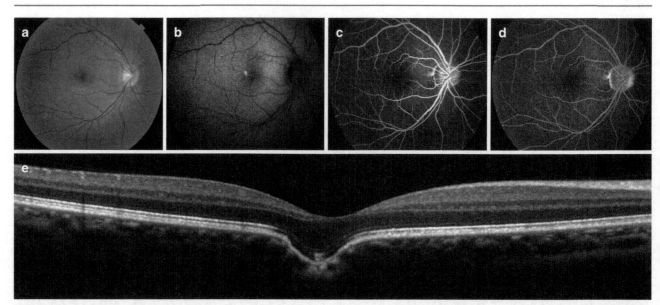

Fig. 10.13 A 33-year-old man with a conforming focal choroidal excavation. (**a**) Color photograph of the right eye reveals a perifoveal yellowish spot consistent with a small vitelliform lesion. (**b**) Fundus autofluorescent image of the right eye reveals a focal area of hyperautofluorescence corresponding to the vitelliform material. Late venous phase (**c**) and recirculation phase (**d**) fluorescein angiographic images reveal a focal hyperfluorescent spot supratemporal to the fovea. (**e**) Spectral-domain optical coherence tomographic scan through the fovea reveals a conforming focal choroidal excavation with a small area of outer retinal hyperreflectivity corresponding to the vitelliform lesion (**a**). (From Reference [97])

to experience deformation as compared with regions of the eye having all layers intact. Since the sclera has some stiffness, the posterior deformation continues into surrounding normal areas, thus causing the separation or cavitation in the choroid. There appears to be more staphylomatous expansion of these eyes at the inferotemporal portion of the disc, possibly explaining the frequent inferior location of peripapillary ICC [89].

This same mechanical defect potentially can exist in other regions and may offer explanation for similar cavitations in the macular region of high myopes. These cavitations occurred in the posterior pole of eyes with neighboring areas of loss of the choroid and overlying RPE [90]. The posterior displacement of the sclera continued into relatively normal surrounding areas which appears to be the cause of macular ICC. Almost one-fourth of eyes with ICC have a retinal defect located near the border between the attenuated retina and the surrounding normal retina. In some patient, fluid dissecting under the retina has resulted in a localized retinal detachment.

10.15 Focal Choroidal Excavation

Eyes with myopia generally have decreasing choroidal thickness in proportion with their amount of myopic refractive error. An unusual group of patients have what is termed focal choroidal cavitation and entity in which there is a localized loss of choroidal thickness within the macula [91–93]. These patients are generally myopic with some being highly myopic. Affected eyes have solitary localized areas that usually show pigmentary alterations, but the cavitation itself is difficult to see by biomicroscopy. The cavitations are readily visible using OCT (Fig. 10.13). These areas show hypofluorescence during both fluorescein and indocyanine green angiography and localized hypoautofluorescence. In a group of ten eyes, EDI-OCT was performed in six, and these showed a choroid that appeared to be abnormally thick in the regions surrounding the excavation [93]. The choroid was thin at the excavation, and the choroidal-scleral junction showed no abnormalities. The excavation was thought to represent a localized hypoplastic region. The same thinning can be seen following resolution of focal inflammation.

10.16 Future Trends for Research

There is much to be learned about the choroid in myopia. The process of emmetropization appears to be misdirected or abnormal in high myopes and is mediated in part by the choroid. Yet in high myopia, the choroid becomes increasingly abnormal. The influence these changes have on the progression of myopia is not known. The ability to image the thickness of the choroid using OCT is relatively recent, so there is an absence of any long-term data. Classification systems for the posterior pole changes in high myopia have relied on ophthalmoscopy alone. Integrating choroidal thickness into the classification system would introduce a variable that has biologic plausibility to both influence visual function and preserve associated tissue. Decreased choroidal perfusion also may be related to secondary abnormalities seen in high myopia such as choroidal neovascularization as discussed in a separate chapter in this text.

There are many research efforts aiming to reduce the progression of myopia, but reduction of the choroidal effects related to myopia would obviate many of the common reasons for visual loss in the first place. Thickening of the choroid is seen in inflammatory diseases [94] and in central serous chorioretinopathy [95]. It is possible that pharmacologic manipulation can influence choroidal thickness. Oral sildenafil caused an increase in choroidal thickness in normal volunteers [96, 97]. Corticosteroids are associated with central serous chorioretinopathy and may have an associated effect of increasing choroidal thickness. One older high myope was imaged and found to have a thickened choroid. Interestingly, she had a kidney transplant in the past and had been treated with oral prednisone for many years (Fig. 10.14).

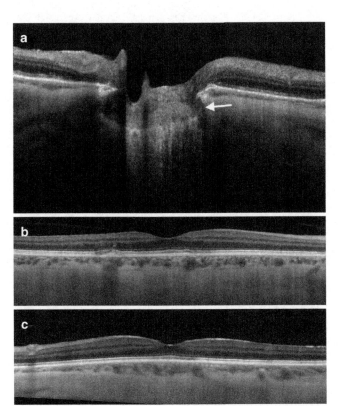

Fig. 10.14 (**a**) This highly myopic, 66-year-old woman had typical features of a high myope, including a dehiscence in the lamina cribrosa as seen in this swept source OCT scan, but her choroid was unexpectedly thick. (**b, c**) Given her age and axial length, she would be expected to have a subfoveal choroidal thickness of about 50 microns. Instead her choroid was nearly 200 microns thick. She had a kidney transplantation and was using oral prednisone for many years to prevent rejection

10.16.1 Potential Use of Choroidal Thickness in Grading Myopic Fundus Changes

Epidemiologic studies use grading systems to classify and quantitate incidence and severity of myopic changes in populations. There are key attributes required of any grading system to be useful. The grading system should be exhaustive of all possibilities of disease expression, the stages in the grading system should be relevant to important stages of the disease process and be based on objective information, and the results should be accurate and reproducible. Current classification systems grade myopia based on attributes such as tessellation, diffuse atrophy, patchy atrophy, lacquer cracks, and Fuch's spots. This list does not represent an exhaustive tabulation of possibilities, grading of any of these attributes is quite subjective, and the presence of these findings is dependent on the population being graded. For example, tessellation is the presence of a striped pattern caused by visualization of larger choroidal blood vessels contrasted by intervening pigment in the outer choroid. Eyes with the tessellated fundus appearance have thinner choroids than eyes with a normal fundus appearance. Thinning of the choroid is associated with loss of the middle layer, allowing visualization of deeper layers. The contrast between the vessels and the pigmented portions depends in part on how much pigment is present. A person with a highly pigmented choroid would have tessellation only if the choroid was thinned from myopia. A person who is of Northern European extraction with less pigmentation could easily have tessellation with a normal thickness choroid and no myopia. Thus, the utility of tessellation may be dependent on pigmentation. Efforts have been made to quantify tessellation based on image analysis [98]. The degree of tessellation was highly associated with choroidal thickness. Fuch's spots are pigmented scars left by choroidal neovascularization. It is common for patients with blonde fundi to not develop a pigmented scar after choroidal neovascularization and for eyes treated with anti-VEGF agents to not develop scars in the first place. In the case of either tessellation or Fuch's spots, the grading of presence or absence is highly subjective and not a consistent sign among various groups of people.

10.16.2 Optical Coherence Tomography Angiography

OCT angiography is useful in evaluating myopic choroidal neovascularization, and this use is covered in a separate chapter. OCT angiography can be used to evaluate the choriocapillaris flow. Earlier application of the technology analyzed areas in which the flow could not be detected in the choriocapillaris layer, and these are called flow voids [99–101]. Frame averaging of choriocapillaris images

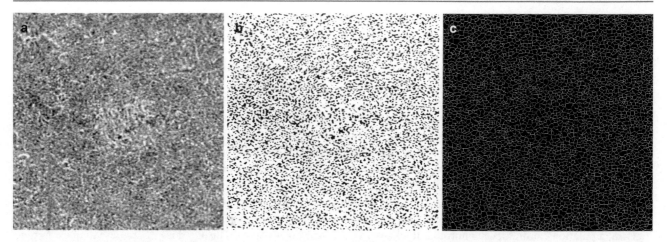

Fig. 10.15 Choriocapillaris imaging. (**a**) Frame averaged OCT angiography demonstrates the choriocapillaris structure in an emmetrope. (**b**) Binarized image of (**a**). (**c**) Skeletonized image created from (**b**). This image can be analyzed for branch length and number of branches per square millimeter. The choriocapillaris of a high myope. Although the choriocapillaris mesh is visible to a degree, the medium and large vessels of this subject are also visible in part

improves image quality by increasing the signal-to-noise ratio (Fig. 10.15) [102]. There are several problems with imaging the choriocapillaris in highly myopic eyes. The first area that can be imaged is somewhat limited because of the limited depth of imaging current commercial OCT instruments. Second, segmentation of highly myopic eyes can be error-prone, and so manual correction of the segmentation lines may be necessary. Third, the segmentation slab for the choriocapillaris can be 15 or 20 μm in thickness. This may represent a significant portion of a highly myopic choroid, which have only 30 μm in total thickness. Vessels below the level of the choriocapillaris are imaged as well. It can be difficult to subtract the deeper vessels from the more superficial in choroidal imaging. Without this removal, the vascular density and flow in the choroid may be overestimated. To gain an OCT angiographic image of the entirety of the choroid in high myopes, one interesting approach is to place the segmentation slab in the sclera and image the projection artifacts from the thickness of the choroid [103].

References

1. Parver LM, Auker C, Carpenter DO. Choroidal blood flow as a heat dissipating mechanism in the macula. Am J Ophthalmol. 1980;89(5):641–6.
2. Wangsa-Wirawan ND, Linsenmeier RA. Retinal oxygen: fundamental and clinical aspects. Arch Ophthalmol. 2003;121(4):547–57.
3. Parver LM, Auker C, Carpenter DO. Choroidal blood flow as a heat dissipating mechanism in the macula. Am J Ophthalmol. 1980;84:641–6.
4. Yuan X, Gu X, Crabb JS, et al. Quantitative proteomics: comparison of the macular Bruch membrane/choroid complex from age-related macular degeneration and normal eyes. Mol Cell Proteomics. 2010;9:1031–46.
5. Nickla DL, Wallman J. The multifunctional choroid. Prog Retin Eye Res. 2010 Mar;29(2):144–68.
6. Sellheyer K. Development of the choroid and related structures. Eye (Lond). 1990;4(Pt 2):255–61.
7. Mund ML, Rodrigues MM, Fine BS. Light and electron microscopic observations on the pigmented layers of the developing human eye. Am J Ophthalmol. 1972;73(2):167–82.
8. Meriney SD, Pilar G. Cholinergic innervation of the smooth muscle cells in the choroid coat of the chick eye and its development. J Neurosci. 1987;7(12):3827–39.
9. Schroedl F, Brehmer A, Neuhuber WL, et al. The normal human choroid is endowed with a significant number of lymphatic vessel endothelial hyaluronate receptor 1 (LYVE-1)-positive macrophages. Invest Ophthalmol Vis Sci. 2008;49(12):5222–9.
10. May CA. Non-vascular smooth muscle cells in the human choroid: distribution, development and further characterization. J Anat. 2005;207(4):381–90.
11. Poukens V, Glasgow BJ, Demer JL. Nonvascular contractile cells in sclera and choroid of humans and monkeys. Invest Ophthalmol Vis Sci. 1998;39(10):1765–74.
12. Flugel-Koch C, May CA, Lutjen-Drecoll E. Presence of a contractile cell network in the human choroid. Ophthalmologica. 1996;210(5):296–302.
13. Schrödl F, De Laet A, Tassignon MJ, Van Bogaert PP, Brehmer A, Neuhuber WL, Timmermans JP. Intrinsic choroidal neurons in the human eye: projections, targets, and basic electrophysiological data. Invest Ophthalmol Vis Sci. 2003;44(9):3705–12.
14. Spaide RF. Choroidal blood flow: review and potential explanation for the choroidal venous anatomy including the vortex vein system. Retina. 2020;40(10):1851–64.
15. Flower RW, Fryczkowski AW, McLeod DS. Variability in choriocapillaris blood flow distribution. Invest Ophthalmol Vis Sci. 1995;36:1247–58.
16. Saint-Geniez M, Kurihara T, Sekiyama E, et al. An essential role for RPE-derived soluble VEGF in the mainte-

nance of the choriocapillaris. Proc Natl Acad Sci U S A. 2009;106(44):18751–6.

17. Bernstein MH, Hollenberg MJ. Fine structure of the choriocapillaris and retinal capillaries. Investig Ophthalmol. 1965;4(6):1016–25.

18. Federman JL. The fenestrations of the choriocapillaris in the presence of choroidal melanoma. Trans Am Ophthalmol Soc. 1982;80:498–516.

19. Peters S, Heiduschka P, Julien S, et al. Ultrastructural findings in the primate eye after intravitreal injection of bevacizumab. Am J Ophthalmol. 2007;143(6):995–1002.

20. Hirata A, Negi A. Morphological changes of choriocapillaris in experimentally induced chick myopia. Graefes Arch Clin Exp Ophthalmol. 1998;236:132–7.

21. Rutnin U, Schepens CL. Fundus appearance in normal eyes. II. The standard peripheral fundus and developmental variations. Am J Ophthalmol. 1967;64(5):840–52.

22. Hayreh SS. In vivo choroidal circulation and its watershed zones. Eye (Lond). 1990;4(Pt 2):273–89.

23. Hayreh SS. Posterior ciliary artery circulation in health and disease: the Weisenfeld lecture. Invest Ophthalmol Vis Sci. 2004;45(3):749–8.

24. Chen JC, Fitzke FW, Pauleikhoff D, Bird AC. Functional loss in age-related Bruch's membrane change with choroidal perfusion defect. Invest Ophthalmol Vis Sci. 1992;33:334–40.

25. Reiner A, Fitzgerald MEC, Del Mar N, Li C. Neural control of choroidal blood flow. Prog Retin Eye Res. 2018;64:96–130.

26. Nilsson SF. Neuropeptide Y (NPY): a vasoconstrictor in the eye, brain and other tissues in the rabbit. Acta Physiol Scand. 1991;141(4):455–67.

27. Lütjen-Drecoll E. Choroidal innervation in primate eyes. Exp Eye Res. 2006;82(3):357–61.

28. Granstam E, Nilsson SF. Non-adrenergic sympathetic vasoconstriction in the eye and some other facial tissues in the rabbit. Eur J Pharmacol. 1990;175(2):175–86.

29. Li C, Fitzgerald ME, Del Mar N, et al. Disinhibition of neurons of the nucleus of solitary tract that project to the superior salivatory nucleus causes choroidal vasodilation: implications for mechanisms underlying choroidal baroregulation. Neurosci Lett. 2016;633:106–11.

30. Houssier M, Raoul W, Lavalette S, et al. CD36 deficiency leads to choroidal involution via COX2 down-regulation in rodents. PLoS Med. 2008;5(2):e39.

31. Geiser MH, Bonvin M, Quibel O. Corneal and retinal temperatures under various ambient conditions: a model and experimental approach. Klin Monatsbl Augenheilkd. 2004;221(5):311–4.

32. Biesemeier A, Schraermeyer U, Eibl O. Chemical composition of melanosomes, lipofuscin and melanolipofuscin granules of human RPE tissues. Exp Eye Res. 2011;93:29–39.

33. Ulshafer RJ, Allen CB, Rubin ML. Distributions of elements in the human retinal pigment epithelium. Arch Ophthalmol. 1990;108:113–7.

34. Biesemeier A, Julien S, Kokkinou D, Schraermeyer U, Eibl O. A low zinc diet leads to loss of Zn in melanosomes of the RPE but not in melanosomes of the choroidal melanocytes. Metallomics. 2012;4:323–32.

35. Geeraets WJ, Berry ER. Ocular spectral characteristics as related too hazards from lasers and other light sources. Am J Ophthalmol. 1968;66:15–20.

36. Ketterer SG, Wiegand BD. Hepatic clearance of indocyanine green. Clin Res. 1959;7:289.

37. Hayashi K, Hasegawa T, Tokoro T, Delaey JJ. Value of indocyanine green angiography in the diagnosis of occult choroidal neovascular membrane. Jpn J Ophthalmol. 1988;42:827–9.

38. Hewick SA, Fairhead AC, Culy JC, Atta HR. A comparison of 10 MHz and 20 MHz ultrasound probes in imaging the eye and orbit. Br J Ophthalmol. 2004;88(4):551–5.

39. Hoffer KJ. Ultrasound velocities for axial eye length measurement. J Cataract Refract Surg. 1994;20(5):554–62.

40. Spaide RF, Koizumi H, Pozzoni MC. Enhanced depth imaging spectral-domain optical coherence tomography. Am J Ophthalmol. 2008;146(4):496–500.

41. Chinn SR, Swanson EA, Fujimoto JG. Optical coherence tomography using a frequency-tunable optical source. Opt Lett. 1997;22(5):340–2.

42. Choma M, Sarunic M, Yang C, Izatt J. Sensitivity advantage of swept source and Fourier domain optical coherence tomography. Opt Express. 2003;11(18):2183–9.

43. Ohno-Matsui K, Akiba M, Moriyama M, et al. Imaging retrobulbar subarachnoid space around optic nerve by swept-source optical coherence tomography in eyes with pathologic myopia. Invest Ophthalmol Vis Sci. 2011;52(13):9644–50.

44. Branchini L, Regatieri CV, Flores-Moreno I, et al. Reproducibility of choroidal thickness measurements across three spectral domain optical coherence tomography systems. Ophthalmology. 2012;119:119–23.

45. Ikuno Y, Maruko I, Yasuno Y, et al. Reproducibility of retinal and choroidal thickness measurements in enhanced depth imaging and high-penetration optical coherence tomography. Invest Ophthalmol Vis Sci. 2011;52(8):5536–40.

46. Tan CS, Ouyang Y, Ruiz H, Sadda SR. Diurnal variation of choroidal thickness in normal, healthy subjects. Invest Ophthalmol Vis Sci. 2012;53(1):261–6.

47. Manjunath V, Taha M, Fujimoto JG, Duker JS. Choroidal thickness in normal eyes measured using Cirrus HD optical coherence tomography. Am J Ophthalmol. 2010;150(3):325–9.e1.

48. Hirata M, Tsujikawa A, Matsumoto A, et al. Macular choroidal thickness and volume in normal subjects measured by swept-source optical coherence tomography. Invest Ophthalmol Vis Sci. 2011;52(8):4971–8.

49. Margolis R, Spaide RF. A pilot study of enhanced depth imaging optical coherence tomography of the choroid in normal eyes. Am J Ophthalmol. 2009;147(5):811–5.

50. Ikuno Y, Kawaguchi K, Nouchi T, Yasuno Y. Choroidal thickness in healthy Japanese subjects. Invest Ophthalmol Vis Sci. 2010;51(4):2173–6.

51. Benavente-Perez A, Hosking SL, Logan NS, Bansal D. Reproducibility-repeatability of choroidal thickness calculation using optical coherence tomography. Optom Vis Sci. 2010;87(11):867–72.

52. Esmaeelpour M, Povazay B, Hermann B, et al. Three-dimensional 1060-nm OCT: choroidal thickness maps in normal subjects and improved posterior segment visualization in cataract patients. Invest Ophthalmol Vis Sci. 2010;51(10):5260–6.

53. Li XQ, Larsen M, Munch IC. Subfoveal choroidal thickness in relation to sex and axial length in 93 Danish university students. Invest Ophthalmol Vis Sci. 2011;52(11):8438–41.

54. Feeney-Burns L, Burns RP, Gao CL. Age-related macular changes in humans over 90 years old. Am J Ophthalmol. 1990;109(3):265–78.

55. Sarks SH. Ageing and degeneration in the macular region: a clinico-pathological study. Br J Ophthalmol. 1976;60(5):324–41.

56. Ramrattan RS, van der Schaft TL, Mooy CM, et al. Morphometric analysis of Bruch's membrane, the choriocapillaris, and the choroid in aging. Invest Ophthalmol Vis Sci. 1994;35(6):2857–64.

57. Read SA, Collins MJ, Sander BP. Human optical axial length and defocus. Invest Ophthalmol Vis Sci. 2010;51(12):6262–9.

58. Wallman J, Wildsoet C, Xu A, et al. Moving the retina: choroidal modulation of refractive state. Vis Res. 1995;35(1):37–50.

59. Wildsoet C, Wallman J. Choroidal and scleral mechanisms of compensation for spectacle lenses in chicks. Vis Res. 1995;35(9):1175–94.

60. Troilo D, Nickla DL, Wildsoet CF. Choroidal thickness changes during altered eye growth and refractive state in a primate. Invest Ophthalmol Vis Sci. 2000;41(6):1249–58.

61. Hung LF, Wallman J, Smith EL 3rd. Vision-dependent changes in the choroidal thickness of macaque monkeys. Invest Ophthalmol Vis Sci. 2000;41(6):1259–69.

62. Rohrer K, Frueh BE, Walti R, et al. Comparison and evaluation of ocular biometry using a new noncontact optical low-coherence reflectometer. Ophthalmology. 2009;116(11):2087–92.

63. Brown JS, Flitcroft DI, Ying GS, et al. In vivo human choroidal thickness measurements: evidence for diurnal fluctuations. Invest Ophthalmol Vis Sci. 2009;50(1):5–12.

64. Ho J, Branchini L, Regatieri C, et al. Analysis of normal peripapillary choroidal thickness via spectral domain optical coherence tomography. Ophthalmology. 2011;118(10):2001–7.

65. Tanabe H, Ito Y, Terasaki H. Choroid is thinner in inferior region of optic disks of normal eyes. Retina. 2012;32(1):134–9.

66. Fong AH, Li KK, Wong D. Choroidal evaluation using enhanced depth imaging spectral-domain optical coherence tomography in Vogt-Koyanagi-Harada disease. Retina. 2011;31(3):502–9.

67. Spaide RF, Fujimoto JG, Waheed NK, et al. Optical coherence tomography angiography. Prog Retin Eye Res. 2018;64:1–55.

68. Fujiwara T, Imamura Y, Margolis R, et al. Enhanced depth imaging optical coherence tomography of the choroid in highly myopic eyes. Am J Ophthalmol. 2009;148(3):445–50.

69. Chui TY, Song H, Burns SA. Individual variations in human cone photoreceptor packing density: variations with refractive error. Invest Ophthalmol Vis Sci. 2008;49(10):4679–87.

70. Spaide RF. Age-related choroidal atrophy. Am J Ophthalmol. 2009;147:801–10.

71. Mrejen S, Spaide RF. The relationship between pseudodrusen and choroidal thickness. Retina. 2014;34(8):1560–6.

72. Moriyama M, Ohno-Matsui K, Futagami S, et al. Morphology and long-term changes of choroidal vascular structure in highly myopic eyes with and without posterior staphyloma. Ophthalmology. 2007;114(9):1755–62.

73. Quaranta M, Arnold J, Coscas G, et al. Indocyanine green angiographic features of pathologic myopia. Am J Ophthalmol. 1996;122(5):663–71.

74. Akyol N, Kukner AS, Ozdemir T, Esmerligil S. Choroidal and retinal blood flow changes in degenerative myopia. Can J Ophthalmol. 1996;31(3):113–9.

75. Ikuno Y, Tano Y. Retinal and choroidal biometry in highly myopic eyes with spectral-domain optical coherence tomography. Invest Ophthalmol Vis Sci. 2009;50(8):3876–80.

76. Ohno-Matsui K, Akiba M, Moriyama M, et al. Intrachoroidal cavitation in macular area of eyes with pathologic myopia. Am J Ophthalmol. 2012;154(2):382–93.

77. Nishida Y, Fujiwara T, Imamura Y, et al. Choroidal thickness and visual acuity in highly myopic eyes. Retina. 2012;32(7):1229–36.

78. Flores-Moreno I, Ruiz-Medrano J, Duker JS, Ruiz-Moreno JM. The relationship between retinal and choroidal thickness and visual acuity in highly myopic eyes. Br J Ophthalmol. 2013;97(8):1010–3.

79. Chalam KV, Sambhav K. Choroidal thickness measured with swept source optical coherence tomography in posterior staphyloma strongly correlates with axial length and visual acuity. Int J Retina Vitreous. 2019;5:14.

80. Gupta P, Cheung CY, Saw SM, et al. Choroidal thickness does not predict visual acuity in young high myopes. Acta Ophthalmol. 2016;94(8):e709–15.

81. Wei WB, Xu L, Jonas JB, et al. Subfoveal choroidal thickness: the Beijing Eye Study. Ophthalmology. 2013;120(1):175–80.

82. Okabe S, Matsuo N, Okamoto S, Kataoka H. Electron microscopic studies on retinochoroidal atrophy in the human eye. Acta Med Okayama. 1982;36(1):11–21.

83. Freund KB, Ciardella AP, Yannuzzi LA, et al. Peripapillary detachment in pathologic myopia. Arch Ophthalmol. 2003;121:197–204.

84. Shimada N, Ohno-Matsui K, Nishimuta A, Tokoro T, Mochizuki M. Peripapillary changes detected by optical coherence tomography in eyes with high myopia. Ophthalmology. 2007;114:2070–6.

85. Shimada N, Ohno-Matsui K, Yoshida T, et al. Characteristics of peripapillary detachment in pathologic myopia. Arch Ophthalmol. 2006;124:46–52.

86. Tateno H, Takahashi K, Fukuchi T, Yamazaki Y, Sho K, Matsumura M. Choroidal schisis around the optic nerve in myopic eyes evaluated by optical coherence tomography. Jpn J Clin Ophthalmol. 2005;59:327–31.

87. Toranzo J, Cohen SY, Erginay A, Gaudric A. Peripapillary intrachoroidal cavitation in myopia. Am J Ophthalmol. 2005;140:731–2.

88. Wei YH, Yang CM, Chen MS, Shih YF, Ho TC. Peripapillary intrachoroidal cavitation in high myopia: reappraisal. Eye (Lond). 2009;23:141–4.

89. Spaide RF, Akiba M, Ohno-Matsui K. Evaluation of peripapillary intrachoroidal cavitation with swept source and enhanced depth imaging optical coherence tomography. Retina. 2012;32:1037–44.

90. Shimada N, Ohno-Matsui K, Iwanaga Y, Tokoro T, Mochizuki M. Macular retinal detachment associated with peripapillary detachment in pathologic myopia. Int Ophthalmol. 2009;29:99–102.

91. Jampol LM, Shankle J, Schroeder R, Tornambe P, Spaide RF, Hee MR. Diagnostic and therapeutic challenges. Retina. 2006;26(9):1072–6.

92. Wakabayashi Y, Nishimura A, Higashide T, Ijiri S, Sugiyama K. Unilateral choroidal excavation in the macula detected by spectral-domain optical coherence tomography. Acta Ophthalmol. 2010;88(3):e87–91.

93. Margolis R, Mukkamala SK, Jampol LM, Spaide RF, Ober MD, Sorenson JA, Gentile RC, Miller JA, Sherman J, Freund KB. The expanded spectrum of focal choroidal excavation. Arch Ophthalmol. 2011;129(10):1320–5.

94. Maruko I, Iida T, Sugano Y, Oyamada H, Sekiryu T, Fujiwara T, Spaide RF. Subfoveal choroidal thickness after treatment of Vogt-Koyanagi-Harada disease. Retina. 2011;31:510–7.

95. Imamura Y, Fujiwara T, Margolis R, Spaide RF. Enhanced depth imaging optical coherence tomography of the choroid in central serous chorioretinopathy. Retina. 2009;29:1469–73.

96. Harris A, Kagemann L, Ehrlich R, Ehrlich Y, López CR, Purvin VA. The effect of sildenafil on ocular blood flow. Br J Ophthalmol. 2008;92:469–73.

97. Vance SK, Imamura Y, Freund KB. The effects of sildenafil citrate on choroidal thickness as determined by enhanced depth imaging optical coherence tomography. Retina. 2011;31:332–5.

98. Yamashita T, Terasaki H, Tanaka M, et al. Relationship between peripapillary choroidal thickness and degree of tessellation in young healthy eyes. Graefes Arch Clin Exp Ophthalmol. 2020;258(8):1779–85.

99. Mastropasqua R, Viggiano P, Borrelli E, et al. In vivo mapping of the Choriocapillaris in high myopia: a Widefield swept source optical coherence tomography angiography. Sci Rep. 2019;9(1):18932.

100. Su L, Ji YS, Tong N, et al. Quantitative assessment of the retinal microvasculature and choriocapillaris in myopic patients using swept-source optical coherence tomography angiography. Graefes Arch Clin Exp Ophthalmol. 2020;258(6):1173–80.

101. Wong CW, Teo YCK, Tsai STA, et al. Characterization of the choroidal vasculature in myopic maculopathy with optical coherence tomographic angiography. Retina. 2019;39(9):1742–50.

102. Spaide RF, Ledesma-Gil G. Novel method for image averaging of optical coherence tomography angiography images. Retina. 2020;40(11):2099–105.

103. Maruko I, Spaide RF, Koizumi H, et al. Choroidal blood flow visualization in high myopia using a projection artifact method in optical coherence tomography angiography. Retina. 2017;37(3):460–5.

Theories of Myopization: Potential Role of a Posteriorly Expanding Bruch's Membrane

11

Jost B. Jonas, Kyoko Ohno-Matsui, and Songhomitra Panda-Jonas

11.1 Introduction

The process of emmetropization with myopization as an axial overshooting of this process has remained unclear so far. Based on the studies by Smith and colleagues and others, axial myopia may be the sequel of a failure of emmetropization secondary to the attempt to eliminate a hyperopic blur in the equatorial region of the globe [1, 2]. If the equatorial retina is the afferent arm in the feedback circuit controlling the axial elongation, it has remained elusive so far, which part of the eye is primarily responsible for effectively elongating the eye. While previous investigations have been centered on the choroid and sclera as the most promising candidates to elongate the eye, this review is focused on the potential role Bruch's membrane (BM) may play in the process of emmetropization and myopization [1–10].

Axial elongation is characterized by a thinning of the choroid, most marked in the subfoveal region [11–13]. This hallmark of axial elongation cannot be explained if the sclera was the primary structure elongating the globe. In that case, a widening of the choroidal space would have occurred. As a hypothesis, one may therefore consider BM to be the structure expanding posteriorly and elongating the globe. Such a posterior advancement of BM would lead to a compression and thinning of the choroid, most marked at the posterior pole, and the sclera would secondarily relent, similar to the development of dellen in a bone after prolonged local pressure [10]. This notion of BM as the primary structure elongating the eye is supported by anatomical and clinical findings.

11.2 Sclera

Histomorphometric investigations showed that the cross-sectional area and volume of the sclera were not correlated with age and axial length in persons with an age of 3+ years [13, 14]. It was concluded that the volume of the sclera did not change during the process of emmetropization and myopization and that the available scleral tissue was rearranged during axial elongation [13, 15]. In children up to an age of 2 years, the scleral cross-sectional area and volume increased with age. Other studies revealed that in primary axial myopia, the thickness of the sclera decreased only in the posterior half of the globe [15–18]. The scleral thinning was most marked at the posterior pole and least marked at the equator or at the ora serrata, while the scleral thickness anterior to the ora serrata and the corneal thickness and diameters was not related with axial length in eyes with primary myopia. One inferred that the process of emmetropization and myopization occurred in the posterior half of the eye, with the scleral changes taking place predominantly at the posterior pole. The finding that the scleral volume was not associated with axial length in individuals aged 3 + years pointed against the sclera having an active role in the process of emmetropization/myopization. In contrast, in eyes with secondary high myopia due to congenital glaucoma, thinning and elongation of the sclera was found in all regions of the eye. Parallel to this finding, the cornea enlarged lost in thickness in these eyes with secondary high myopia due to congenital glaucoma [19, 20].

J. B. Jonas (✉)
Department of Ophthalmology, Medical Faculty Mannheim of the Ruprecht-Karls-University of Heidelberg, Mannheim, Germany
e-mail: jost.jonas@medma.uni-heidelberg.de

K. Ohno-Matsui
Department of Ophthalmology and Visual Science, Tokyo Medical and Dental University, Bunkyo-Ku, Tokyo, Japan
e-mail: k.ohno.oph@tmd.ac.jp

S. Panda-Jonas
Department of Ophthalmology, Medical Faculty Mannheim of the Ruprecht-Karls-University of Heidelberg, Mannheim, Germany

Institute of Clinical and Scientific Ophthalmology and Acupuncture Jonas & Panda, Heidelberg, Germany

© Springer Nature Switzerland AG 2021
R. F. Spaide et al. (eds.), *Pathologic Myopia*, https://doi.org/10.1007/978-3-030-74334-5_11

11.3 Choroid

Parallel to the observations made on the sclera, the cross-sectional area and volume of the choroid in individuals aged 18+ years was not associated with axial length in histomorphometric studies. It suggested that the choroidal thinning, similar as the scleral thinning, was not due to a change in volume but presumably to a rearrangement of the available tissue [14]. It pointed against the choroid having an active role in the process of emmetropization/myopization.

11.4 Bruch's Membrane (BM)

In contrast to the sclera and choroid, the thickness of BM did not get thinner with longer axial length, so that highly myopic eyes and emmetropic eyes did have the same thickness of BM at the posterior pole and any other location in the globe [21, 22]. It indicated that the volume of BM increased with longer axial length, pointing toward an active growth of BM and thus an active role in the process of axial elongation [10]. Since the thickness of the choroid and of the sclera decreased with axial length, the ratio of posterior choroidal thickness to BM thickness and the ratio of posterior scleral thickness to BM thickness were reduced in axially elongated eyes at positions posterior to the equator.

In eyes with secondary high myopia due to congenital glaucoma as compared to eyes with primary myopia or emmetropic eyes, the thickness BM was significantly reduced, while the choroidal and scleral thickness did not vary significantly between the eyes with primary myopia and the eyes with secondary myopia [19]. It may indicate that the increased intraocular pressure in congenital glaucoma was the main factor for the expansion of the eye, so that all three layers, the sclera, choroid, and BM, became elongated and thinned in all regions of the eyes.

The physiological opening of BM at the optic nerve head is called the BM opening (BMO). In moderately myopic eyes, the BMO shifts into the temporal direction, leading to an overhanging of BM into the intrapapillary compartment at the nasal side of the optic disc and to a lack of BM (i.e., parapapillary gamma zone) in the temporal parapapillary region [23]. In eyes with an axial length exceeding 26.0 mm or 26.5 mm, the BMO enlarges with longer axial length, leading to a circular enlargement of gamma zone and appearance of gamma zone also in the nasal parapapillary region [23]. In eyes with an the axial length of ≥28.0 mm, the BMO size was significantly smaller in eyes with macular BM defects than in eyes without macular BM defects [23, 24]. It suggested that a large gamma zone was protective against the development of macular BM defects.

These macular BM defects can be detected upon light microscopical histology and upon optical coherence tomography (OCT)-based histology. Their prevalence and number increase with axial length beyond an axial length of about 26.5 mm [25–28]. They are characterized by the lack of BM, retinal pigment epithelium (RPE), and choriocapillaris and by the almost complete loss of the outer and middle retinal layers and of Haller's and Sattler's layer of the choroid [25]. In a cross-sectional study on highly myopic eyes, the number of BM defects increased after an enlargement of parapapillary gamma zone and delta zone [23, 28]. It suggested that during the process of axial elongation, first the BMO enlarged before secondary defects in BM in the posterior region developed. The macular BM defects correspond to the so-called patchy chorioretinal atrophies as part of the definition of myopic maculopathy [26, 29, 30]. In the patchy atrophy areas, the region with an RPE loss is larger than the region of the BM defect [30].

11.5 Macular BM Length and Density of Retinal Pigment Epithelium Cells and Retinal Thickness in the Macular Region and Fundus Periphery

The distance between the foveola and the optic disc increases with longer axial length [31, 32]. The enlargement of the disc-fovea distance is due to the development and enlargement of parapapillary gamma zone as BM-free zone. The distance between the peripheral border of gamma zone and the foveola is independent of the axial length in myopic eyes without BM defects [32, 33]. The length of BM in the macular region was thus not related with the axial length. In a parallel manner, the distance between the superior temporal arterial arcade and the inferior temporal arterial arcade in eyes without macular BM defects is independent of axial length, so that BM in the whole macular region does not enlarge and does not get stretched in axially elongated eyes without BM defects [31, 34]. Correspondingly, the thickness of BM does not get thinner with longer axial length. Since the disc-fovea increases with longer axial length and since the distance between the superior and inferior temporal vascular arcade is independent of axial length, the angle between the temporal vascular arcade decreases with longer axial length [34].

Corresponding to the finding that the macular BM does not enlarge with longer axial length, the density of the RPE cells and the thickness of the retina in the macular region are not correlated with axial length [35, 36]. It fits with the clinical observation that best corrected visual acuity is not correlated with axial length if eyes with myopic maculopathy are excluded [37]. In contrast to the macular region, the density of the RPE cells and the retinal thickness in the fundus periphery decreases with longer axial length [35, 36].

11.6 Optic Disc Size and Shape in Myopia

If the globe elongates, the optic disc shape changes from an almost circle to a vertically oval structure [38]. In parallel manner, parapapillary gamma zone develops and enlarges at the temporal disc border [24, 25, 28, 38, 39]. The width of gamma zone corresponds to the amount of overhanging of BM into the intrapapillary compartment on the opposite site [23]. Since BM overhanging is usually present on the nasal side of the optic disc, gamma zone is present in the temporal parapapillary region. One may infer that the development of gamma zone in medium myopic eyes is due to a shift of the BMO in direction to the macula, while the choroidal optic disc layer and the scleral optic disc layer (with the lamina cribrosa) stay behind. It may have also lead to the development of an oblique exit of the optic nerve fibers out of the eye, first in nasal anterior direction, before bending backward to the apex of the orbit. The shift of the BMO in direction to the macula fits with the notion of a production of BM in the equatorial region during the process of myopization.

Another reason for the vertical elongation of the optic disc shape upon ophthalmoscopy may be an ophthalmoscopically perspective artefact, since during axial elongation the ophthalmoscopical view onto the optic disc changes from a mostly perpendicular angle to an oblique angle [40]. It led to a perspectively relative shortening of the horizontal optic disc diameter.

A further mechanism potentially influencing the optic disc shape in highly myopic eyes is a potential backward pull of the optic nerve (dura mater) in adduction [41, 42]. The longer the axis of the eyes, the stronger may be the pull of the optic nerve dura mater on the sclera during extreme gaze position, since the optic nerve may be too short to allow a full adduction of a markedly elongated globe. Since the optic nerve originates in the nasal upper part of the orbit, adduction of a highly myopic globe will lead to a backward pull more marked on temporal optic nerve head border than on the nasal optic nerve head border. It may lead to an optic disc rotation around the vertical axis with the temporal optic disc border being drawn backward. It may also lead to a lengthening of the peripapillary scleral flange and thus enlargement of parapapillary gamma zone and delta zone. The potential optic nerve-related backward pull of the parapapillary sclera of highly myopic eyes may also explain the development of peripapillary suprachoroidal cavitations [10, 43, 44].

The size of the optic disc enlarges in highly myopic eyes, approximately beyond an axial length of about 26.5 mm or a myopic refractive error of approximately −8 diopters [45].

11.7 Process of Emmetropization

The process of emmetropization can be described as the adaptation of the length of the optical axis to the optical properties of the cornea and lens without compromise in the photoreceptor density and best corrected. It may consist of a feedback mechanism with an afferent and an efferent loop. Myopization could be regarded as an overshooting of the process of emmetropization. According to experimental investigations and clinical observations, the afferent part of the process of emmetropization may be located in the equatorial region of the globe [1, 46–48]. Based on the anatomical findings described above, one may discuss that the efferent loop of the feedback mechanism may also be located in the equatorial region and consist of a new production of BM by the local RPE cells, pushing the BM at the posterior pole backward. It would explain the thinning of the choroid at the posterior pole by a compression, and the scleral thinning at the posterior pole would occur secondarily. The increase in the area of BM in the equatorial region would also explain the decrease in the density of the RPE cells and in the retinal thickness in the equatorial region. Since BM in the macular region would remain untouched by the BM enlargement in the equatorial region, the hypothesis would be consistent with the histological findings that the thickness and length of BM, the RPE cell density, and the thickness of the choriocapillaris and retina in the macular region were independent of axial length. It would go along with the condicio sine qua non of the process of emmetropization not reducing the density of the macular photoreceptors, and it complies with the clinical finding that best corrected visual acuity is independent of axial length if eyes with maculopathies are excluded.

In the case that the image on the equatorial retina is out of focus in the sense of a hyperopic defocus, the mechanism would prolong the globe by introducing new BM area in the equatorial region. There are several reasons why the image in the equatorial region can be in hyperopic defocus while the central image is sharply focused onto the fovea [1]. These reasons include a discrepancy between the optical properties of the peripheral optical pathway as compared to the central pathway and others.

In the case of excessive equatorial enlargement of BM, mostly in the sagittal direction and to a minor degree into the horizontal and vertical directions, the tension or stress within BM in the posterior region may increase due to the enlargement of BM in the horizontal and vertical direction and/or due to an asymmetry in the BM enlargement between the meridians. It could lead to an enlargement of the BMO in the optic nerve head region and secondarily to the development of macular BM defects (as category III of the definition of myopic maculopathy).

The finding of recent experimental study agrees with the notion of BM playing a biomechanical role for size and shape of the eye. The average elastic moduli of BM at 0 and 5% strain were 1.60 ± 0.81 and 2.44 ± 1.02 MPa, respectively, and BM could withstand an intraocular pressure of 82 mmHg before rupture [49]. The notion of BM as biomechanically important structure may also give hints to the etiology of dome-shaped maculas and ridge-shaped maculas in highly myopic eyes [50, 51]. As described by Spaide and others, macular BM defects can occur also in non-highly myopic eyes, such as in globes with Stargardt's disease, in eyes with a toxoplasmotic retinochoroidal scar or in patients with pseudoxanthoma elasticum and peripapillary atrophy [52–54]. Future studies may assess the effect of such BM defects on the occurrence of local collateral scleral staphylomas.

Recent experimental studies did not contradict the notion of BM as a potentially driven structure in the process of axial elongation. In a study performed by Dong and colleagues, a study group of young guinea pigs underwent lens-induced axial elongation, while a control group of young guinea pigs did not have any intervention [55]. It revealed that the experimental axial elongation was associated with a thinning of the retina, choroid, and sclera and a decrease in density of the RPE cells, with the changes most marked at the posterior pole. In contrast, BM thickness was not related to axial elongation. It agreed with the findings obtained in aforementioned histomorphometric examination of human globes [21, 22]. In another investigation conducted by Dong and coworkers, amphiregulin antibody applied intravitreally was associated with a reduction in lens-induced axial elongation and with a reduction of the physiological eye growth, while amphiregulin itself increased the axial elongation in young guinea pigs with and without lens-induced axial elongation [56]. Eyes with lens-induced axial elongation as compared to eyes without lens-induced axial elongation revealed an increased visualization of amphiregulin upon immunohistochemistry and higher expression of mRNA of endogenous amphiregulin and EGF receptor, in particular in the outer part of the retinal inner nuclear layer and in the RPE [56]. Amphiregulin is a member of the epidermal growth factor (EGF) family, and the RPE possesses receptors for EGF including amphiregulin. In particular, EGF increases the proliferation of RPE cells in cell culture. The RPE produces BM, the inner layer of which is formed by the basal membrane of the RPE.

When discussing the findings presented above, one should take into account the limitations of this review. First, it has to be emphasized that this review was focused on the potential role of BM in the process of emmetropization and myopization and that it was not balanced with respect to other or complementing theories of the process of axial elongation. Neglecting in this review other hypotheses, such as those on the role of the choroid and sclera in myopization, does not indicate that these hypotheses are not valid [3–9]. Second, it has remained unclear whether anatomical differences between normal eyes and myopic eyes were the cause or the effect of the process of emmetropization and the process of axial elongation. The changes in the ocular structure may be just related to the mechanism of expansion, not to the causes of the phenomenon of axial elongation. Third, in particular, it has to be stressed that there may be many counterarguments against the hypothesis of BM as a driving structure in the process of axial elongation. It could be that the choroid has a tendency to mold itself to the supporting sclera, so that

there would be no reason for the development of a suprachoroidal cavitation in the case the scleral were the primary structure moving backward. It would even more hold true if in the process of axial elongation BM followed the choroid and brought the retina with it. It has also to be acknowledged that a proliferation of BM in the process of axial elongation has not directly been shown yet. Indeed, one of the characteristic features of myopia is the development of BM defects in the macular region, a finding what primarily may speak against a proliferation of BM. The notion is, however, that BM proliferates in the equatorial region leading to an increase in diameters of the globe, to a major part in the sagittal axis and to a minor part in the horizontal and vertical directions. The globe enlargement in the coronal direction may lead to a tension within BM at the posterior pole, resulting first in an enlargement of the BM opening of the optic nerve head and in a second step to the development of new BM defects in the macular region. From that point of view, a proliferation of BM in the equatorial region may be in agreement with BM defects at the posterior pole. Fourth, it should also be noted that although it may now generally be accepted that the peripheral retina has a regulatory role in the process of emmetropization, it may not mean that the central retina has no role, as has also been expressed in a recent report on animal models and myopia [9].

In conclusion, BM as a composite of five layers, i.e., the basal membrane of the RPE, a collagenous layer, an elastic layer, a collagenous layer, and the basal membrane of the choriocapillaris, may potentially play a biomechanical role in influencing size and shape of the eye and may thus be involved in the process of emmetropization and myopization.

Financial Disclosures Jost B. Jonas: Patent holder with Biocompatibles UK Ltd. (Farnham, Surrey, UK) (Title: Treatment of eye diseases using encapsulated cells encoding and secreting neuroprotective factor and/or anti-angiogenic factor; Patent number: 20120263794) and Europäische Patentanmeldung 16720043.5 and Patent application US 2019 0085065 A1 "Agents for use in the therapeutic or prophylactic treatment of myopia or hyperopia".

Songhomitra Panda-Jonas: Patent holder with Biocompatible UK Ltd. (Title: Treatment of eye diseases using encapsulated cells encoding and secreting neuroprotective factor and/or anti-angiogenic factor; Patent number: 20120263794) and patent application with university of Heidelberg (Title: Agents for use in the therapeutic or prophylactic treatment of myopia or hyperopia; Europäische Patentanmeldung 15000771.4).

References

1. Smith EL 3rd, Hung LF, Huang J, et al. Effects of optical defocus on refractive development in monkeys: evidence for local, regionally selective mechanisms. Invest Ophthalmol Vis Sci. 2010;51:3864–73.
2. Smith EL 3rd. Prentice award lecture 2010: a case for peripheral optical treatment strategies for myopia. Optom Vis Sci. 2011;88(9): 1029–44. https://doi.org/10.1097/OPX.0b013e3182279cfa.

3. Troilo D, Wallman J. The regulation of eye growth and refractive state: an experimental study of emmetropization. Vis Res. 1991;31:1237–50.

4. Nickla DL, Wallman J. The multifunctional choroid. Prog Retin Eye Res. 2010;29:144–68.

5. Guo L, Frost MR, Siegwart JT Jr, et al. Scleral gene expression during recovery from myopia compared with expression during myopia development in tree shrew. Mol Vis. 2014;20:1643–59.

6. Wang KK, Metlapally R, Wildsoet CF. Expression profile of the integrin receptor subunits in the Guinea pig sclera. Curr Eye Res. 2017;42:857–63.

7. Wang M, Schaeffel F, Jiang B, Feldkaemper M. Effects of light of different spectral composition on refractive development and retinal dopamine in chicks. Invest Ophthalmol Vis Sci. 2018;59:4413–24.

8. Hung LF, Arumugam B, She Z, Ostrin L, Smith EL 3rd. Narrow-band, long-wavelength lighting promotes hyperopia and retards vision-induced myopia in infant rhesus monkeys. Exp Eye Res. 2018;176:147–60.

9. Troilo D, Smith EL III, Nickla DL, et al. IMI – report on experimental models of emmetropization and myopia. Invest Ophthalmol Vis Sci. 2019;60:M31–88.

10. Jonas JB, Ohno-Matsui K, Jiang WJ, et al. Bruch's membrane and the mechanism of myopization. A new theory. Retina. 2017;37:1428–40.

11. Fujiwara T, Imamura Y, Margolis R, et al. Enhanced depth imaging optical coherence tomography of the choroid in highly myopic eyes. Am J Ophthalmol. 2009;148:445–50.

12. Wei WB, Xu L, Jonas JB, et al. Subfoveal choroidal thickness: the Beijing Eye Study. Ophthalmology. 2013;120:175–80.

13. Jonas JB, Holbach L, Panda-Jonas S. Scleral cross section area and volume and axial length. PLoS One. 2014;9:e93551.

14. Shen L, You QS, Xu X, et al. Scleral and choroidal volume in relation to axial length in infants with retinoblastoma versus adults with malignant melanomas or end-stage glaucoma. Graefes Arch Clin Exp Ophthalmol. 2016;254:1779–86.

15. Heine L. Beiträge zur Anatomie des myopischen Auges. Arch Augenheilk. 1899;38:277–90.

16. Olsen TW, Aaberg SY, Geroski DH, et al. Human sclera: thickness and surface area. Am J Ophthalmol. 1998;125:237–41.

17. Norman RE, Flanagan JG, Rausch SM, et al. Dimensions of the human sclera: thickness measurement and regional changes with axial length. Exp Eye Res. 2010;90:277–84.

18. Vurgese S, Panda-Jonas S, Jonas JB. Sclera thickness in human globes and its relations to age, axial length and glaucoma. PLoS One. 2012;7:e29692.

19. Jonas JB, Holbach L, Panda-Jonas S. Histologic differences between primary high myopia and secondary high myopia due to congenital glaucoma. Acta Ophthalmol. 2016;94:147–53.

20. Shen L, You QS, Xu X, et al. Scleral and choroidal thickness in secondary high axial myopia. Retina. 2016;36:1579–85.

21. Jonas JB, Holbach L, Panda-Jonas S. Bruch's membrane thickness in high myopia. Acta Ophthalmol. 2014;92:e470–4.

22. Bai HX, Mao Y, Shen L, et al. Bruch's membrane thickness in relationship to axial length. PLoS One. 2017;12:e0182080.

23. Zhang Q, Xu L, Wei WB, Wang YX, Jonas JB. Size and shape of Bruch's membrane opening in relationship to axial length, gamma zone and macular Bruch's membrane defects. Invest Ophthalmol Vis Sci. 2019;60:2591–8.

24. Jonas JB, Jonas SB, Jonas RA, et al. Parapapillary atrophy: histological gamma zone and delta zone. PLoS One. 2012;7:e47237.

25. Jonas JB, Ohno-Matsui K, Spaide RF, et al. Macular Bruch's membrane defects and axial length: association with gamma zone and delta zone in peripapillary region. Invest Ophthalmol Vis Sci. 2013;54:1295–302.

26. Ohno-Matsui K, Jonas JB, Spaide RF. Macular Bruch's membrane holes in highly myopic patchy chorioretinal atrophy. Am J Ophthalmol. 2016;166:22–8.

27. You QS, Peng XY, Xu L, et al. Macular Bruch's membrane defects in highly myopic eyes. The Beijing Eye Study. Retina. 2016;36:517–23.

28. Jonas JB, Fang Y, Weber P, et al. Parapapillary gamma zone and delta zone in high myopia. Retina. 2018;38:931–8.

29. Ohno-Matsui K, Kawasaki R, Jonas JB, et al. International classification and grading system for myopic maculopathy. Am J Ophthalmol. 2015;159:877–83.

30. Du R, Fang Y, Jonas JB, Yokoi T, Takahashi H, Uramoto K, Kamoi K, Yoshida T, Ohno-Matsui K. Clinical features of patchy chorioretinal atrophy in pathologic myopia. Retina. 2019; https://doi.org/10.1097/IAE.0000000000002575. [Epub ahead of print]

31. Jonas RA, Wang YX, Yang H, et al. Optic disc – fovea distance, axial length and parapapillary zones. The Beijing Eye Study 2011. PLoS One. 2015;10:e0138701.

32. Guo Y, Liu LJ, Tang P, et al. Optic disc-fovea distance and myopia progression in school children: the Beijing Children Eye Study. Acta Ophthalmol. 2018; https://doi.org/10.1111/aos.13728. [Epub ahead of print]

33. Jonas JB, Wang YX, Zhang Q, et al. Macular Bruch's membrane length and axial length. The Beijing Eye Study. PloS ONE. 2015;10:e0136833.

34. Jonas RA, Wang YX, Yang H, et al. Optic disc-fovea angle: the Beijing Eye Study. PLoS One. 2015;10:e0141771.

35. Jonas JB, Ohno-Matsui K, Holbach L, et al. Retinal pigment epithelium cell density in relationship to axial length in human eyes. Acta Ophthalmol. 2017;95:e22–8.

36. Jonas JB, Xu L, Wei WB, et al. Retinal thickness and axial length. Invest Ophthalmol Vis Sci. 2016;57:1791–7.

37. Shao L, Xu L, Wei WB, et al. Visual acuity and subfoveal choroidal thickness. The Beijing Eye Study. Am J Ophthalmol. 2014;158:702–9.

38. Guo Y, Liu LJ, Tang P, et al. Parapapillary gamma zone and progression of myopia in school children: the Beijing Children Eye Study. Invest Ophthalmol Vis Sci. 2018;59:1609–16.

39. Dai Y, Jonas JB, Huang H, et al. Microstructure of parapapillary atrophy: Beta zone and gamma zone. Invest Ophthalmol Vis Sci. 2013;54:2013–8.

40. Dai Y, Jonas JB, Ling Z, et al. Ophthalmoscopic-perspectively distorted optic disc diameters and real disc diameters. Invest Ophthalmol Vis Sci. 2015;56:7076–83.

41. Demer JL. Optic nerve sheath as a novel mechanical load on the globe in ocular ductionoptic nerve sheath constrains duction. Invest Ophthalmol Vis Sci. 2016;57:1826–38.

42. Wang X, Rumpel H, Lim WE, et al. Finite element analysis predicts large optic nerve head strains during horizontal eye movements. Invest Ophthalmol Vis Sci. 2016;57:2452–62.

43. Dai Y, Jonas JB, Ling Z, et al. Unilateral peripapillary intrachoroidal cavitation and optic disc rotation. Retina. 2015;35:655–9.

44. Jonas JB, Dai Y, Panda-Jonas S. Peripapillary suprachoroidal cavitation, parapapillary gamma zone and optic disc rotation due to the biomechanics of the optic nerve dura mater. Invest Ophthalmol Vis Sci. 2016;57:4373.

45. Jonas JB. Optic disc size correlated with refractive error. Am J Ophthalmol. 2005;139:346–8.

46. Benavente-Pérez A, Nour A, Troilo D. Axial eye growth and refractive error development can be modified by exposing the peripheral retina to relative myopic or hyperopic defocus. Invest Ophthalmol Vis Sci. 2014;55:6765–73.

47. Hasebe S, Jun J, Varnas SR. Myopia control with positively aspherized progressive addition lenses: a 2-year, multicenter, randomized, controlled trial. Invest Ophthalmol Vis Sci. 2014;55:7177–88.

48. Harder BC, von Baltz S, Schlichtenbrede FC, et al. Intravitreal bevacizumab for retinopathy of prematurity: refractive error results. Am J Ophthalmol. 2013;155:1119–24.

49. Wang X, Teoh CKG, Chan ASY, et al. Biomechanical properties of Bruch's membrane-choroid complex and their influence on optic nerve head biomechanics. Invest Ophthalmol Vis Sci. 2018;59:2808–17.

50. Fang Y, Jonas JB, Yokoi T, et al. Macular Bruch's membrane defect and dome-shaped macula in high myopia. PLoS One. 2017;12:e0178998.

51. Fang Y, Du R, Jonas JB, et al. Ridge-shaped macula progressing to Bruch membrane defects and macular suprachoroidal cavitation. Retina. 2018; https://doi.org/10.1097/IAE.0000000000002404. [Epub ahead of print]52

52. Park SP, Chang S, Allikmets R, et al. Disruption in Bruch membrane in patients with Stargardt disease. Ophthalmic Gen. 2012;33:49–52.

53. Spaide RF, Jonas JB. Peripapillary atrophy with large dehiscences in Bruch membrane in pseudoxanthoma elasticum. Retina. 2015;35:1507–10.

54. Jonas JB, Panda-Jonas S. Secondary Bruch's membrane defects and scleral staphyloma in toxoplasmosis. Acta Ophthalmol. 2016;94:e664–e66.

55. Dong L, Shi XH, Kang YK, Wei WB, Wang YX, Xu XL, Gao F, Jonas JB. Bruch's membrane thickness and retinal pigment epithelium cell density in experimental axial elongation. Sci Rep. 2019;9:6621.

56. Dong L, Shi XH, Kang YK, Wei WB, Wang YX, Xu XL, Gao F, Yuan LH, Zhen J, Jiang WJ, Jonas JB. Amphiregulin and ocular axial length. Acta Ophthalmol. 2019; https://doi.org/10.1111/aos.14080. [Epub ahead of print]

The Optic Nerve Head in High Myopia/ Abnormalities of the Intrapapillary and Parapapillary Region

12

Jost B. Jonas and Songhomitra Panda-Jonas

The optic nerve head (ONH) or "papilla nervi optici" is a defect in the wall of the posterior segment of the eye to allow the exit of the retinal nerve fibers and central retinal vein and the entrance of the central retinal artery. Simultaneously, it is part of the ocular wall and thus serves to keep up the difference between a higher pressure inside of the eye (so called intraocular pressure) and outside of the eye [1, 2]. The ONH can be regarded as a three-layered hole, with Bruch's membrane opening (BMO) forming the inner layer, the hole in the choroid forming the middle layer, and the scleral canal forming the outer layer of the ONH [3]. The ONH can be divided into the intrapapillary region as all area within the scleral and choroidal canal and the parapapillary region as the area surrounding the intrapapillary region. If the scleral canal, covered by the lamina cribrosa, is taken for the definition of the bottom of the intrapapillary region, the ophthalmoscopically visible boundary of the ONH is the peripapillary ring. The latter is the ophthalmoscopical equivalent of the peripapillary border tissue of the choroid (Jacoby) which merges with the end of Bruch's membrane (BM) on its inner side and which continues into the peripapillary border tissue of the scleral flange (Elschnig) on its outer side [3]. The peripapillary border tissue of the scleral flange itself is a continuation of the optic nerve pia mater.

12.1 Intrapapillary Region

12.1.1 Optic Disc

Ophthalmoscopically, the intrapapillary region is composed of the neuroretinal rim as the equivalent of the retinal nerve fibers and the central optic cup as the whole area not filled up by the optic nerve fibers [1, 2]. The optic disc is the sum of optic cup and neuroretinal rim. The area of the ONH shows a marked interindividual variability of about 1:7 within a normal non-highly myopic Caucasian population [1]. The ONH area additionally shows an inter-ethnic variability, with Caucasians having the smallest optic disc and Afro-Americans the largest discs [2]. As rule of thumb, the disc size increases with the decreasing distance to the equator. Within the non-highly myopic group, the disc size is slightly correlated with the refractive error and thus the size of the globe: the disc is smaller in hyperopic eyes, and it is slightly larger in medium myopic eyes. At a cutoff value of about −8 diopters of myopia or an axial length of 26.5 mm, the disc size increases more markedly with myopic refractive error and longer axial length. It leads to secondary or acquired macrodiscs in highly myopic eyes. These secondary macrodiscs have to be differentiated from primary macrodiscs in non-highly myopic eyes. Primary macrodiscs have a normal mostly circular shape, and their size is not markedly associated with refractive error or axial length. Primary macrodiscs are associated with large and relatively flat corneas and with large globe diameters in the horizontal and vertical direction, without much elongation of the sagittal globe diameter. Secondary macrodiscs in highly myopic eyes appear to have an elliptical or oval shape. This may at least partially be due to an ophthalmoscopical artifact, since the myopic elongation of the globe by the increase in the fovea-disc distance moves the ONH more to the nasal wall of the globe. By that, the ophthalmoscopic view onto the ONH is no longer en face or perpendicular, but it occurs in an oblique direction onto the ONH surface. This can lead to a seemingly oblique disc shape and an underestimation of the horizontal optic disc

J. B. Jonas (✉)
Department of Ophthalmology, Medical Faculty Mannheim of the Ruprecht-Karls-University of Heidelberg, Mannheim, Germany
e-mail: jost.jonas@medma.uni-heidelberg.de

S. Panda-Jonas
Department of Ophthalmology, Medical Faculty Mannheim of the Ruprecht-Karls-University of Heidelberg, Mannheim, Germany

Institute of Clinical and Scientific Ophthalmology and Acupuncture Jonas & Panda, Heidelberg, Germany

© Springer Nature Switzerland AG 2021
R. F. Spaide et al. (eds.), *Pathologic Myopia*, https://doi.org/10.1007/978-3-030-74334-5_12

diameter. In non-highly myopic eyes, the disc size is correlated with the number of cones and rods of the retinal photoreceptors, the number of retinal pigment epithelium (RPE) cells, the number of retinal nerve fibers (and presumably retinal ganglion cells), and the number of lamina cribrosa pores and the total pore area [4, 5]. Since high myopia is an acquired condition and since the number of retinal cells does presumably not increase after birth, the relationship between disc size and retinal cell number may not be valid in highly myopic eyes. The variability in optic disc size is pathogenically important since optic disc drusen, pseudopapilledema, and non-arteritic anterior ischemic optic neuropathy occur almost exclusively in small optic discs, while congenital pits of the optic disc are more common in large optic nerve heads [2]. The prevalence of arteritic anterior ischemic optic neuropathy and of central retinal artery occlusion or central retinal vein occlusion is independent of the disc size [2]. It may imply that the frequency of disc drusen, pseudopapilledema, and non-arteritic anterior ischemic optic neuropathy may be lower in ethnic groups with large optic disc than in Caucasians with relatively small ONHs and the prevalence of these diseases may be lower in highly myopic eyes than in emmetropic eyes.

Upon ophthalmoscopy, the optic disc has a slightly vertically oval form with the vertical diameter being about 7–10% larger than the horizontal one [1, 2]. The disc form is not correlated with age, gender, and body weight and height. Abnormal disc shapes may be divided into discs with a rotation around the vertical disc axis ("vertically rotated discs"), discs with a rotation around the horizontal disc axis ("horizontally rotated discs"), and discs with a rotation along the sagittal axis. In the case of vertically rotated optic discs, a passive movement of the ONH to the nasal ocular wall by the myopic enlargement of the posterior pole might play a role. It leads to an oblique view onto the ONH surface and a seemingly reduced horizontal disc diameter as an optical artifact in the two-dimensional ophthalmoscopical examination. Horizontally rotated discs were called "tilted discs." The prevalence of horizontally rotated discs is independent of the refractive error, while vertically rotated discs are associated with high myopia. Horizontally rotated discs are significantly correlated with an increased corneal astigmatism and amblyopia. In contrast, vertically rotated discs in highly myopic eyes are not associated with an increased corneal astigmatism, since the changes associated with the development of high myopia occur mostly behind the equator and leave the cornea unchanged. According to a recent study, a major factor shaping the disc form may be a misalignment of the three ONH layers [6]. If the BMO shifts during the process of emmetropization or myopization into the temporal direction, the overhanging of BM on the nasal disc side leads to a vertically oval disc shape upon ophthalmoscopy. If the BMO shifts into the inferior direction, an overhanging of

BM at the superior disc border occurs, leading to a horizontally oval disc shape upon ophthalmoscopy. If the BMO shifts into the nasal direction, a "situs inversus papillae" may develop, with a gamma zone on the nasal side and an exit of the retinal vessels first into the nasal direction before turning around into the temporal direction toward the macular region.

12.1.2 Neuroretinal Rim

The neuroretinal rim is the intrapapillary equivalent of the retinal nerve fibers and optic nerve fibers [1, 2]. As any biologic quantitative parameter, the neuroretinal rim size is not interindividually constant but shows, similar to the optic disc and cup, a high interindividual variability. The rim size is correlated with the optic disc area. The increase of rim area with enlarging disc area is most marked for eyes with no disc cupping, medium pronounced for eyes with a temporal flat sloping of the optic cup, and least marked in eyes with circular steep disc cupping. The correlation between rim area and disc area corresponds with the positive correlation between optic disc size and optic nerve fiber count. These associations are valid only for non-highly myopic eyes since high myopia develops after birth, while the number retinal nerve fibers do not increase after birth. Possible reasons for the interindividual size variability of the rim are differences in the nerve fiber count, ratio between formed and regressed retinal ganglion cell axons during embryogenesis, density of nerve fibers within the optic disc, lamina cribrosa architecture, diameters of retinal ganglion cell axons, proportion of glial cells on the whole intrapapillary tissue, and in other factors [2]. The nerve fibers within the neuroretinal rim are retinotopically arranged, with axons from ganglion cells close to the optic disc lying more centrally in the optic disc while axons from cells in the retinal periphery lie at the optic nerve head margin. It corresponds to the nerve fiber distribution in the retinal nerve fiber layer. Although not examined in highly myopic eyes, one may assume that the retinotopic arrangement of the retinal nerve fibers is preserved in highly myopic eyes.

The shape of the neuroretinal rim follows the ISNT (inferior-superior-nasal-temporal) rule: it is usually wider at the inferior disc pole, followed by the superior disc pole, the nasal disc region, and smallest in the temporal disc sector (Fig. 12.1). While many normal eyes can have a wider rim superiorly than inferiorly, and while the rim width in the nasal region is of minor clinical importance, the most important part of the ISNT rule is the "T" in that more than 95% of normal eyes have the smallest rim part in the temporal 60° of the ONH. The ISNT rule is of importance for the early detection of glaucomatous optic nerve damage, and it is valid also in highly myopic eyes.

In non-highly myopic eyes, the rim shape (ISNT rule) is associated with the diameter of the retinal arterioles which

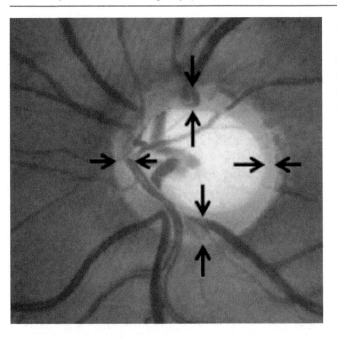

Fig. 12.1 Optic disc photograph of a primary macrodisc, illustrating the ISNT (inferior-superior-nasal-temporal) rule: the neuroretinal rim is wider at the inferior disc pole, followed by the superior disc pole, the nasal disc region, and smallest in the temporal disc sector

the size of the image of posterior fundus structures. Furthermore, the color contrast between the neuroretinal rim and the optic cup is decreased since the rim in highly myopic eyes is markedly less pink than in emmetropic eyes. It has remained unclear whether this effect is due to a thinner nerve tissue in the highly myopic neuroretinal rim so that the underlying collagenous tissue of the lamina cribrosa can better gleam through and/or whether it may reflect a decrease in the density of blood capillaries or blood supply into the neuroretinal rim. These problems in outlining the border between neuroretinal rim and optic cup are one of the reasons for the difficulty in detecting glaucomatous or glaucoma-like optic nerve damage in highly myopic eyes. Other reasons are that the assessment of the retinal nerve fiber layer is markedly hampered by the bright peripapillary fundus reflectance in highly myopic eyes and by myopia-associated changes in the retinal nerve fiber layer, such as a peripapillary retinoschisis; that the fundus changes associated with myopic retinopathy are sufficient reasons for perimetric defects so that the role of perimetry for the detection of glaucoma is reduced; and that the intraocular pressure in the highly myopic type of primary open-angle glaucoma is often within the normal range.

12.1.3 Optic Cup

Parallel to the optic disc and the neuroretinal rim, also the optic cup shows a high interindividual variability. Large optic cups (macrocups) can be differentiated into primary macrocups which occur in primary macrodiscs and secondary or acquired macrocups. The latter can further be subclassified into secondary, highly myopic macrocups in highly myopic eyes with secondary macrodiscs due to the myopic stretching of the optic nerve head and into secondary macrocups which developed due to the glaucomatous loss of neuroretinal rim. In non-glaucomatous eyes including non-glaucomatous highly myopic eyes, the areas of the optic cup and disc are correlated with each other: the larger is the optic disc, the larger is the optic cup. Due to the vertically oval optic disc and the horizontally oval optic cup, the cup/disc diameter ratios in normal eyes are horizontally significantly larger than vertically. In less than 7% of non-glaucomatous eyes, the horizontal cup/disc ratio is smaller than the vertical one. It indicates that the quotient of the horizontal-to-vertical-cup/disc ratios is usually higher than 1.0. It is important for the diagnosis of glaucoma, in which, in the early to medium advanced stages, the vertical cup/disc diameter ratio increases faster than the horizontal one. It leads to an increase of the quotient of horizontal-to-vertical-cup/disc ratios to values lower than 1.0. This holds true also for the detection of glaucomatous optic nerve damage in highly myopic eyes. As ratio of cup diameter-to-disc diameter, the cup/disc ratios depend on the size of the optic disc

are significantly wider in the inferotemporal arcade than in the superotemporal arcade; with the visibility and the thickness of the retinal nerve fiber layer which are significantly better detectable and thicker in the inferotemporal region than in the superotemporal region; with the location of the foveola about 0.5 inferior to the horizontal optic disc axis center; with the morphology of the lamina cribrosa with the largest pores and the least amount of inter-pore connective tissue in the inferior and superior regions as compared to the temporal and nasal sectors; and with the distribution of the thin and thick nerve fibers in the optic nerve just behind the ONH where the thin fibers from the foveal region are located in the temporal part of the nerve [2]. Although these relationships have not explicitly been examined in highly myopic eyes, one may assume that they prevail also in highly myopic eyes unless the position of the fovea has markedly changed during the process of axial elongation.

While the neuroretinal rim gets lost and changes its shape in glaucoma, rim size and shape remains mostly unchanged if non-glaucomatous optic nerve damage develops. These statements hold true for non-highly myopic eyes and for highly myopic eyes.

The delineation of the neuroretinal rim from the optic cup is more difficult in highly myopic eyes than in emmetropic eyes, since the spatial contrast between the height of the rim and the depth of the cup is reduced due to the myopic stretching of the ONH in high myopia; the spatial contrast additionally appears optically to be diminished due to the longer axis in the highly myopic eyes and the consequent reduction in

and cup. The high interindividual variability in the optic disc and cup diameters explains the high physiological interindividual variability in cup/disc ratios ranging in the nonglaucomatous population between 0.0 and almost 0.9. It includes the highly myopic group.

12.1.4 Histology of the Intrapapillary Region

The bottom of the intrapapillary region is formed by the lamina cribrosa which extends from the circular peripapillary scleral flange (Figs. 12.2 and 12.3) [7]. The peripapillary border tissue of the peripapillary scleral flange (Elschnig) is intertwined in a perpendicular manner with the scleral flange in its transition into the lamina cribrosa [3]. The lamina cribrosa may be compared with a multilayered structure of collagenous sheets with numerous pores. In the region of the neuroretinal rim, the retinal nerve fibers pierce through the lamina cribrosa pores, get myelinated just when leaving the lamina cribrosa and form the retrobulbar optic nerve. In the region of the optic cup, the lamina cribrosa pores appear to be sealed by connective tissue covering the lamina cribrosa. It has remained unclear whether this tissue sheet is watertight or whether it allows a leakage of intraocular fluid into the retrobulbar cerebrospinal fluid space. Clinical observations on accumulations of large pigmented particles at the bottom of the cup in eyes after pars plana vitrectomies may allow the speculation that the lamina cribrosa can function like a sieve allowing some leakage of fluid and keeping

larger particles back. If that is the case, it would mean an additional outflow pathway of aqueous humor and would indicate that the cerebrospinal fluid just behind the globe may have another composition than in the apex of the orbit.

In normal eyes, the lamina cribrosa has a hanging-mat-like shape. In eyes with advanced glaucomatous optic nerve damage, the lamina cribrosa gets condensed and thinned, and it changes its shape [6]. It develops a slight elevation in its central region, where the central retinal vessel trunk appears to stabilize the lamina cribrosa and a sectorial deepening in the inferior and superior peripheral regions. It leads to a W-shaped configuration.

The thickness of the lamina cribrosa was not significantly associated with the thickness of the cornea in a previous histologic study [8, 9]. In a parallel manner, corneal thickness was neither correlated with the thickness of the peripapillary scleral flange nor with the shortest distance between intraocular space and cerebrospinal fluid space. It suggested that an assumed relationship between central corneal thickness and glaucoma susceptibility could not be explained by a cor-

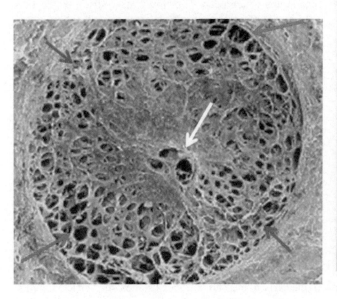

Fig. 12.2 Electron micrograph of the inner surface of the lamina cribrosa after digestion of the retinal nerve fibers. White arrow, central retinal vessel trunk; red arrows, large lamina cribrosa pores in the inferior and superior disc region; blue arrows, small lamina cribrosa pores in the temporal and nasal disc region; the pores are generally larger closer to the optic disc margin; green stars, retrobulbar cerebrospinal fluid space

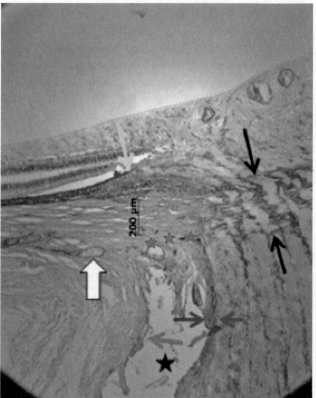

Fig. 12.3 Photomicrograph of a normal optic nerve head in a medium myopic eye. Black arrows, lamina cribrosa of normal thickness; yellow arrow, end of Bruch's membrane, leaving a parapapillary region free of Bruch's membrane ("gamma zone"); red arrows, peripapillary scleral flange of normal thickness and length; blue arrows, pia mater of the optic nerve; green arrow, dura mater of the optic nerve; black star, retrobulbar cerebrospinal fluid space; white arrow, arterial circle of Zinn-Haller

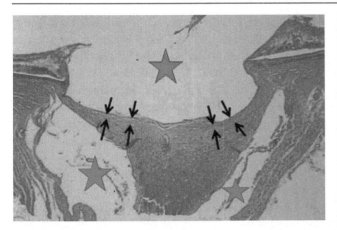

Fig. 12.4 Histophotograph showing the optic nerve head of a highly myopic eye; black arrows, thinned lamina cribrosa; red star, intraocular compartment; green stars, retrobulbar cerebrospinal fluid space

responding anatomy between corneal thickness and the histomorphometry of the optic nerve head [9, 10].

In highly myopic eyes, the lamina cribrosa is markedly thinned and elongated (Fig. 12.4) [10]. It has been speculated that these myopia-associated lamina cribrosa changes may be some of the reasons for the increased glaucoma susceptibility in highly myopic eyes [11]. The thinning of the lamina cribrosa leads to a shortening of the distance between the intraocular space with the intraocular pressure and the retrobulbar space with the orbital cerebrospinal fluid pressure. A decrease in the distance is geometrically associated with a steepening of the translamina cribrosa pressure gradient. Recent studies have discussed that the translamina cribrosa pressure difference (and gradient) more than the transcorneal pressure difference (so called intraocular pressure) is important for the physiology of the optic nerve head and may potentially play a role in the pathogenesis of glaucomatous optic neuropathy [12].

Studies by Anderson and later by Hernandez and coworkers and Quigley and colleagues assessed the elastic fibers in the lamina cribrosa and their replacement or augmentation by collagen fibers with increasing age or the development of glaucoma [13, 14]. Investigations by Burgoyne and coworkers addressed the remodeling of the lamina cribrosa in glaucomatous ONHs [15]. It has remained unclear so far whether the lamina cribrosa changes in high myopia are comparable to the age-related and glaucoma-associated changes in the connective tissue of the lamina.

12.2 Parapapillary Region

12.2.1 Parapapillary Atrophy

Conventionally, the parapapillary region was divided into an alpha zone and beta zone (Fig. 12.5) [16, 17]. Alpha zone

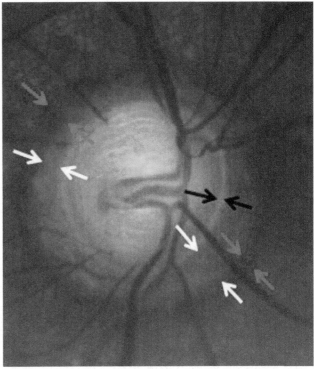

Fig. 12.5 Optic nerve head photograph of a glaucomatous, non-highly myopic optic nerve head. White arrows, parapapillary beta zone; red arrows, parapapillary alpha zone; black arrows, peripapillary ring

was defined by an irregular pigmentation and was detected in almost all eyes. On its outer side, alpha zone was adjacent to the retina, and on its inner side it was in touch with beta zone or, if beta zone was not present, with the peripapillary ring. Beta zone was ophthalmoscopically characterized by a visible large choroidal vessels and visible sclera and was found in about 25% of normal eyes and in a significantly higher proportion of glaucomatous eyes. In cross-sectional and in longitudinal studies, beta zone, not alpha zone, was associated with an increasing glaucomatous loss in neuroretinal rim and an increasing glaucomatous visual field loss. All highly myopic eyes had the (old) beta zone due to the myopic crescent surrounding highly myopic ONHs, independently whether there was glaucomatous optic nerve damage (Fig. 12.6) [18]. In contrast to glaucomatous optic neuropathy, non-glaucomatous optic nerve damage was not associated with an enlargement of beta zone.

In recent clinical and histological studies, however, the concept of (old) beta zone has been challenged [19–21]. In a histological study, it was differentiated between alpha zone characterized by the presence of BM with irregularly structured and pigmented RPE, beta zone defined as the presence of BM without RPE, gamma zone characterized by the lack of BM and normal thickness of the peripapillary scleral flange, and delta zone characterized by the lack of BM and a markedly elongated and thinned peripapillary scleral flange

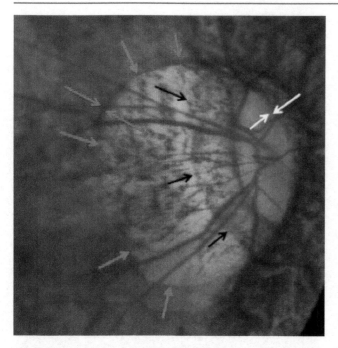

Fig. 12.6 Optic nerve head photograph of a highly myopic optic nerve head. Green arrows, parapapillary alpha zone; red arrows, parapapillary beta zone; black arrows, potentially the insertion line of the dura mater of the optic nerve into the posterior sclera; central to this line would be the peripapillary scleral flange; white arrows, peripapillary ring

(Figs. 12.7 and 12.8). It was shown that beta zone (BM without RPE) was correlated with glaucoma but not markedly with globe elongation; that gamma zone (peripapillary sclera without overlying choroid, BM and deep retinal layers) was related with axial globe elongation and that it was mostly independent of glaucoma; and that delta zone was present only in highly axially elongated globes. Since the old beta zone definition included the histological new beta zone, gamma zone, and delta zone, and since gamma zone was not related with glaucoma, one may infer that a clinical differentiation between the new beta zone and gamma zone may increase the clinical diagnostic value of the redefined clinical beta zone (without gamma zone) for the diagnosis of glaucoma. The finding that beta zone was associated with glaucoma and that it was not profoundly associated with myopia suggested that the histological changes observed in histological beta zone, i.e., loss of RPE cells and photoreceptors and a closure of the choriocapillaris, may be related to the glaucomatous optic neuropathy. A recent study suggested that the beta zone may develop due to an intraocular pressure elevation-associated shifting of the parapapillary RPE on BM [22]. Interestingly, the region of BM with the underlying choriocapillaris occluded was significantly smaller than beta zone (defined as BM without RPE cells). One discussed that a complete loss of RPE cells may occur earlier than a complete closure of the choriocapillaris. It could indicate that a loss of RPE cells would lead to the closure of the choriocap-

illaris since an intact choriocapillaris depends on an intact RPE layer. One has to clearly keep in mind, however, that disturbances in the blood perfusion of the choriocapillaris may have first led to a damage and loss of the RPE, which could then lead to the complete choriocapillaris closure.

Interestingly, gamma zone was strongly associated with axial length with a steep increase beyond an axial length of 26.5 mm. The cutoff value of an axial length of 26.5 mm was similar to the cutoff values of about −8 diopters for the differentiation between medium myopia and high myopia as suggested in clinical studies. Parapapillary gamma zone has been discussed to develop in two steps. The first step consists of a temporal shift of the BMO during the process of moderate myopization, leading to an overhanging of BM into the intrapapillary compartment at the nasal side of the optic disc and to a lack of BM (i.e., gamma zone) in the temporal parapapillary region. In a second step, if the axial length exceeds 26.0 mm or 26.5 mm, the BMO enlarges, leading to a circular enlargement of gamma zone and appearance of gamma zone also in the nasal parapapillary region [6]. The basis for the notion of a temporal shift of the BMO, leading to a misalignment between the scleral canal and the BMO in eyes with moderate myopia, is the hypothesis that axial elongation occurs by new production of BM in the equatorial region and the sliding BM theory. Since BM is not firmly fixed with the sclera but separated from the sclera by the spongy choroid and the suprachoroidal cleft, one may assume that the spongy choroid allows a sliding or movement of BM in spatial relationship to the sclera. The "supertraction" of the retina and choroid to the temporal side with an overhanging of BM into the open area of the scleral opening of the ONH at the nasal disc side and a region on the temporal ONH side with no BM has already been described by Heine in 1899 [23]. Former ophthalmologists used to call Bruch's membrane pushing into the nasal intrapapillary region a "supertraction" and a BM-free temporal parapapillary region a "distraction crescent." The sliding of BM has also been observed in eyes after a marked reduction of IOP [24].

The parapapillary zones gamma and delta are associated with changes in the deep layers of the macula in highly myopic eyes [25]. Highly myopic eyes can show defects in BM in the macular region as demonstrated in recent histologic and clinical studies [25–28]. These defects in BM are associated with a complete lack of RPE and choriocapillaris and a marked reduction of photoreceptors and large choroidal vessels. The existence of such macular BM holes is strongly associated with axial length and with the parapapillary gamma zone and delta zones. In a recent study, a larger size of the papillary BMO was associated with a lower prevalence of macular BM defects [6].

The parapapillary zones alpha, beta, gamma, and delta as defined and described in histological studies can also be

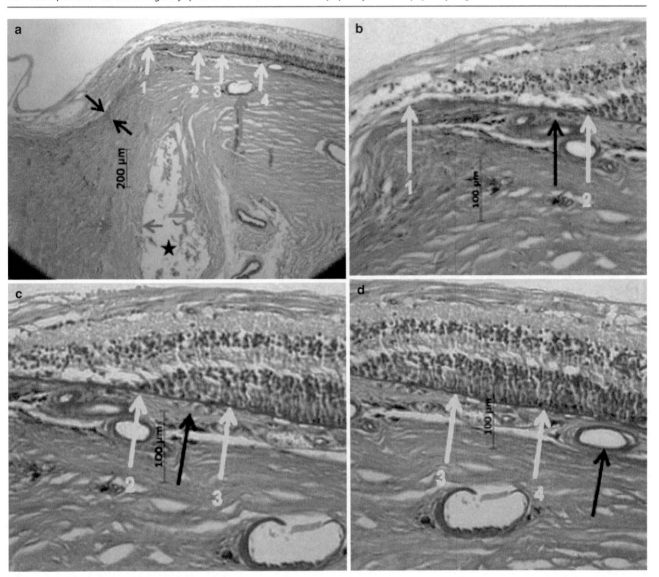

Fig. 12.7 (**a**) Photomicrograph of a glaucomatous optic nerve head in a non-highly myopic eye. Black arrows, condensed thinned lamina cribrosa; blue arrows, pia mater of the optic nerve; red arrow, arterial circle of Zinn-Haller; yellow arrows, (1) end of Bruch's membrane at the optic nerve head border, (2) end of photoreceptors; (3) end of retinal pigment epithelium layer, (4) end of regularly structured layer of the retinal pigment epithelium; black star, retrobulbar cerebrospinal fluid space. (**b**) Photomicrograph of a glaucomatous optic nerve head in a non-highly myopic eye (same eye as in Fig. 12.7a; higher magnification). Yellow arrows, (1) end of Bruch's membrane at the optic nerve head border, (2) end of photoreceptors; black arrow, end of open choriocapillaris. (**c**) Photomicrograph of a glaucomatous optic nerve head in a non-highly myopic eye (same eye as in Fig. a; higher magnification). Yellow arrows, (2) end of photoreceptors, (3) end of retinal pigment epithelium layer; black arrow, open choriocapillaris. (**d**) Photomicrograph of a glaucomatous optic nerve head in a non-highly myopic eye (same eye as in Fig. a; higher magnification). Yellow arrows, (3) end of retinal pigment epithelium layer, (4) start of regularly structured retinal pigment epithelium; black arrow, large choroidal vessel

visualized and analyzed clinically by using enhanced depth imaging of optical coherence tomography [21]. In a recent clinical study, gamma zone was significantly associated with longer axial length, longer vertical disc diameter, older age, and absence of glaucoma, while beta zone was associated with longer axial length and presence of glaucoma. It shows that gamma zone and beta zone can clinically be differentiated from each other and that the differentiation is clinically useful [21, 29].

12.2.2 Peripapillary Border Tissue of the Choroid and Peripapillary Scleral Flange

The choroid and the peripapillary scleral flange are separated from the intrapapillary compartment and the lamina cribrosa by the peripapillary border tissue of the choroid (Jacoby) and the peripapillary border tissue of the scleral flange (Elschnig), respectively [3]. In a histomorphometric study, a thicker choroidal border tissue (mean: 68.8 ± 35.7 µm) was correlated with shorter axial length, and a longer choroidal border tissue (mean: 531 ± 802 µm) was associated with longer axial length. Correspondingly, the cross-sectional area of the choroidal border tissue was not related with axial length. A thicker scleral flange border tissue (mean: 83 ± 21 µm) was associated with the presence of glaucoma as was the thickness of the optic nerve pia mater [3]. Since the border tissues connect BM with the lamina cribrosa, these findings may be of interest for the biomechanics of the optic nerve head in general and in particular in high myopia.

12.2.3 Peripapillary Scleral Flange

The peripapillary scleral flange originates in the inner half of the posterior sclera and continues into the lamina cribrosa, the thickness of which is almost identical with the thickness of the peripapillary scleral flange (Figs. 12.3, 12.8, and 12.9) [19, 20]. While the inner 50% of the posterior sclera form the peripapillary scleral flange, the outer 50% of the sclera merge with the dura mater of the retrobulbar optic nerve. The peripapillary scleral flange is the part of the sclera between the optic nerve border (defined as optic nerve head scleral canal or the anterior continuation of the pia mater) and the point where the optic nerve dura mater merges with the sclera. The peripapillary scleral flange thus forms the anterior roof of the orbital cerebrospinal fluid space. The peripapillary scleral flange may also serve for functional dynamic purposes: the pulse wave in the orbital cerebrospinal fluid space and the pulse wave in the eye ("ocular pulse") may have their maxima at slightly different time points. This would lead to a fluctuating change in the translamina cribrosa pressure difference and consequently to an undulating movement of the lamina cribrosa in sagittal direction. The peripapillary scleral flange could function here as a flange similar to the flange or a hinge in a door swinging in and out.

The length of the scleral flange increases with axial length and decreases with the thickness of the flange [17, 18]. The increased length of the flange in highly myopic eyes leads to an extension of the orbital cerebrospinal fluid space into the retrobulbar peripapillary region. At this location, the cerebrospinal fluid is separated from the vitreous cavity just by a thin peripapillary scleral flange (as thin as 50 µm), retinal nerve fibers, and the retinal inner limiting membrane. It has remained unclear, whether, and if yes, in which layer, a watertight shed exists between the intraocular compartment and the compartment of the extended peripapillary cerebrospinal fluid space. Considering that the highly myopic scleral flange is not covered on its inner side by Bruch membrane and RPE, one may speculate whether there may be some leakage of fluid through the retinal nerve fiber layer and the

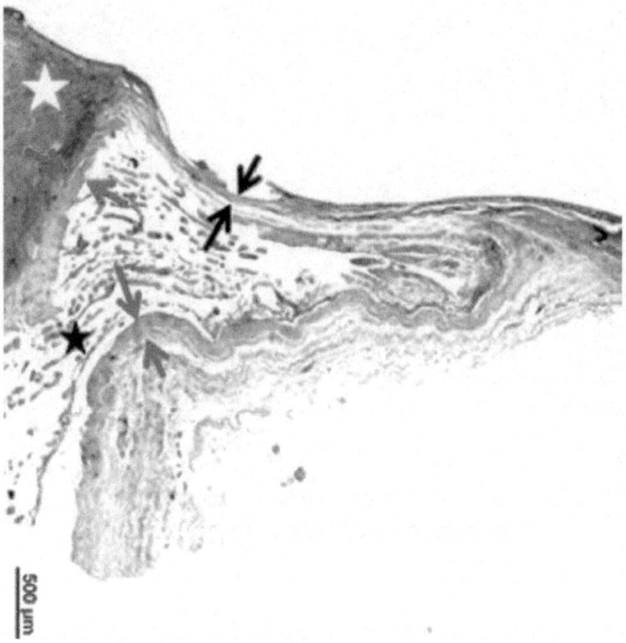

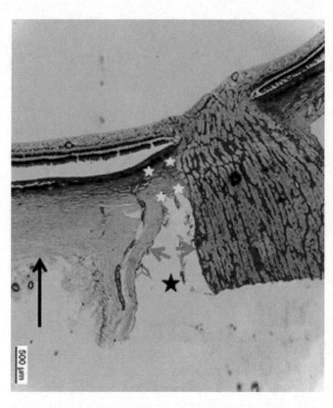

Fig. 12.8 Photomicrograph of a highly myopic eye. Black arrows, elongated peripapillary scleral flange ("delta zone"); green arrows, dura mater of the optic nerve; red arrows, pia mater of the optic nerve; black star, retrobulbar cerebrospinal fluid space; white arrow, optic nerve

Fig. 12.9 Photomicrograph of a normal eye. Black arrow, posterior full-thickness sclera; yellow stars, peripapillary scleral flange; green arrows, dura mater of the optic nerve; red arrows, pia mater of the optic nerve; black star, retrobulbar cerebrospinal fluid space

water permeable scleral tissue. This fluid leakage would reduce the intraocular pressure and lead to a different composition of the cerebrospinal fluid in the retrobulbar region as compared to the apex of the orbit. It has also remained unclear so far, whether the extension of the retrobulbar cerebrospinal spinal fluid space into the parapapillary region has pathophysiological consequences. One may speculate whether the very thin peripapillary scleral flange in highly myopic eyes may act in a similar manner as open fontanelles do in babies. The scleral flange may undulate as consequence of the ocular pulse and may thus lead to a change in the ocular pulse.

In highly myopic eyes, the peripapillary scleral flange elongates from about 500 μm to 5 mm by a factor of 10. Simultaneously, the flange thins from about 500 μm to 50 μm by a factor of 1/10. Considering the peripapillary scleral flange as biomechanical anchor for the lamina cribrosa, the myopia-associated stretching and thinning of the flange may be one of the reasons for the increased glaucoma susceptibility in highly myopic eyes. The biomechanical consequence of a thin parapapillary sclera in the highly myopic eyes may further be aggravated by the finding that the highly myopic eyes did not have the normal composition of the parapapillary anatomy. In the highly myopic eyes as in contrast to the non-highly myopic eyes, the parapapillary retina is composed of retinal nerve fiber layer (or its remnants) only, without elements of any other retinal layer, without parapapillary Bruch membrane or choroid. The implications of a missing Bruch membrane as stable element in the whole architecture of the retina-choroid complex and the consequence of missing choroidal vessels at the border of highly myopic optic nerve head have remained unknown so far.

The elongation of the peripapillary scleral flange in delta zone of highly myopic eyes is associated with an increased distance between the peripapillary arterial circle of Zinn-Haller and the optic disc border. The arterial circle of Zinn-Haller is usually located close to the merging point of the dura mater with the posterior sclera [30]. Since the arterial circle of Zinn-Haller supports the blood vessels in the optic nerve head, in particular in the lamina cribrosa, one may speculate whether the tenfold increase in the distance between the arterial circle and the lamina cribrosa may lead to a malperfusion of the lamina cribrosa. Anatomical studies which specifically examined the communicating vessels between the arterial circle of Zinn-Haller and the tissue of the lamina cribrosa in highly myopic eyes have been missing so far.

The thinning of the scleral flange in highly myopic eyes is paralleled by myopia-associated changes of the sclera in other fundus regions. Examining formalin-fixed human globes, a recent histomorphometric study showed that in non-axially elongated eyes with an axial length of ≤26 mm, the sclera was thickest at the posterior pole (0.94 ± 0.18 mm),

followed by the perioptic nerve region (0.86 ± 0.21 mm), the midpoint between posterior pole and equator (0.65 ± 0.15 mm), the limbus (0.50 ± 0.11 mm), the ora serrata (0.43 ± 0.14 mm), the equator (0.42 ± 0.15 mm), and finally the peripapillary scleral flange (0.39 ± 0.09 mm) [31]. In axially elongated eyes, scleral thinning occurred at and posterior to the equator, being more marked closer to the posterior pole and the longer the axial length was. Scleral thickness anterior to the equator did not markedly differ between the highly myopic eyes and the non-highly myopic eyes. Within the anterior and posterior segment, respectively, scleral thickness measurements were correlated with each other. Posterior scleral thickness was correlated with the lamina cribrosa thickness. Scleral thickness measurements at any location of examination were not significantly correlated with corneal thickness or with age, gender, and presence of absolute secondary angle-closure glaucoma [31].

References (Further References Are Found in These Citations)

1. Jonas JB, Gusek GC, Naumann GO. Optic disc, cup and neuroretinal rim size, configuration and correlations in normal eyes. Invest Ophthalmol Vis Sci. 1988;29:1151–8.
2. Jonas JB, Budde WM, Panda-Jonas S. Ophthalmoscopic evaluation of the optic nerve head. Surv Ophthalmol. 1999;43:293–320.
3. Jonas RA, Holbach L. Peripapillary border tissue of the choroid and peripapillary scleral flange in human eyes. Acta Ophthalmol. 2020;98:e43–e9.
4. Jonas JB, Schmidt AM, Müller-Bergh JA, Schlötzer-Schrehardt UM, Naumann GOH. Human optic nerve fiber count and optic disc size. Invest Ophthalmol Vis Sci. 1992;33:2012–8.
5. Panda-Jonas S, Jonas JB, Jakobczyk M, Schneider U. Retinal photoreceptor count, retinal surface area, and optic disc size in normal human eyes. Ophthalmology. 1994;101:519–23.
6. Zhang Q, Xu L, Wei WB, Wang YX, Jonas JB. Size and shape of Bruch's membrane opening in relationship to axial length, gamma zone and macular Bruch's membrane defects. Invest Ophthalmol Vis Sci. 2019;60:2591–8.
7. Jonas JB, Mardin CY, Schlötzer-Schrehardt U, Naumann GOH. Morphometry of the human lamina cribrosa surface. Invest Ophthalmol Vis Sci. 1991;32:401–5.
8. Jonas JB, Berenshtein E, Holbach L. Anatomic relationship between lamina cribrosa, intraocular space, and cerebrospinal fluid space. Invest Ophthalmol Vis Sci. 2003;44:5189–95.
9. Jonas JB, Holbach L. Central corneal thickness and thickness of the lamina cribrosa in human eyes. Invest Ophthalmol Vis Sci. 2005;46:1275–9.
10. Jonas JB, Berenshtein E, Holbach L. Lamina cribrosa thickness and spatial relationships between intraocular space and cerebrospinal fluid space in highly myopic eyes. Invest Ophthalmol Vis Sci. 2004;45:2660–5.
11. Xu L, Wang Y, Wang S, Wang Y, Jonas JB. High myopia and glaucoma susceptibility. The Beijing Eye Study. Ophthalmology. 2007;114:216–20.
12. Ren R, Jonas JB, Tian G, Zhen Y, Ma K, Li S, Wang H, Li B, Zhang X, Wang N. Cerebrospinal fluid pressure in glaucoma. A prospective study. Ophthalmology. 2010;117:259–66.

13. Hernandez MR. Ultrastructural immunocytochemical analysis of elastin in the human lamina cribrosa. Changes in elastic fibers in primary open-angle glaucoma. Invest Ophthalmol Vis Sci. 1992;33:2891–903.

14. Quigley EN, Quigley HA, Pease ME, Kerrigan LA. Quantitative studies of elastin in the optic nerve heads of persons with primary open-angle glaucoma. Ophthalmology. 1996;103:1680–5.

15. Roberts MD, Grau V, Grimm J, Reynaud J, Bellezza AJ, Burgoyne CF, Downs JC. Remodeling of the connective tissue microarchitecture of the lamina cribrosa in early experimental glaucoma. Invest Ophthalmol Vis Sci. 2009;50:681–90.

16. Jonas JB, Nguyen XN, Gusek GC, Naumann GO. Parapapillary chorioretinal atrophy in normal and glaucoma eyes. I. Morphometric data. Invest Ophthalmol Vis Sci. 1989;30:908–18.

17. Jonas JB, Naumann GOH. Parapapillary chorio-retinal atrophy in normal and glaucoma eyes. II. Correlations. Invest Ophthalmol Vis Sci. 1989;30:919–26.

18. Jonas JB, Gusek GC, Naumann GOH. Optic disk morphometry in high myopia. Graefes Arch Clin Exp Ophthalmol. 1988;226:587–90.

19. Jonas JB, Jonas SB, Jonas RA, Holbach L, Panda-Jonas S. Histology of the parapapillary region in high myopia. Am J Ophthalmol. 2011;152:1021–9.

20. Jonas JB, Jonas SB, Jonas RA, Holbach L, Dai Y, Sun X, Panda-Jonas S. Parapapillary atrophy: Histological gamma zone and delta zone. PLoS One. 2012;7:e47237.

21. Dai Y, Jonas JB, Huang H, Wang M, Sun X. Microstructure of parapapillary atrophy: Beta zone and gamma zone. Invest Ophthalmol Vis Sci. 2013;54:2013–8.

22. Wang YX, Jiang R, Wang NL, Xu L, Jonas JB. Acute peripapillary retinal pigment epithelium changes associated with acute intraocular pressure elevation. Ophthalmology. 2015;122:2022–8.

23. Heine L. Beiträge zur Anatomie des myopischen Auges. Arch Augenheilkd. 1899;38:277–90.

24. Panda-Jonas S, Xu L, Yang H, Wang YX, Jonas SB, Jonas JB. Optic disc morphology in young patients after antiglaucomatous filtering surgery. Acta Ophthalmol. 2014;92:59–64.

25. Jonas JB, Ohno-Matsui K, Spaide RF, Holbach L, Panda-Jonas S. Macular Bruch's membrane holes in high myopia: associated with gamma zone and delta zone of parapapillary region. Invest Ophthalmol Vis Sci. 2013;54:1295–30.

26. Ohno-Matsui K, Jonas JB, Spaide RF. Macular Bruch membrane holes in highly myopic patchy chorioretinal atrophy. Am J Ophthalmol. 2016;166:22–8.

27. Ohno-Matsui K, Jonas JB, Spaide RF. Macular Bruch membrane holes in choroidal neovascularization-related myopic macular atrophy by swept-source optical coherence tomography. Am J Ophthalmol. 2016;162:133–9.

28. Fang Y, Jonas JB, Yokoi T, Cao K, Shinohara K, Ohno-Matsui K. Macular Bruch's membrane defect and dome-shaped macula in high myopia. PLoS One. 2017;12:e0178998.

29. Manalastas PIC, Belghith A, Weinreb RN, Jonas JB, Suh MH, Yarmohammadi A, Medeiros FA, Girkin CA, Liebmann JM, Zangwill LM. Automated beta zone parapapillary area measurement to differentiate between healthy and glaucoma eyes. Am J Ophthalmol. 2018;191:140–8.

30. Jonas JB, Jonas SB. Histomorphometry of the circular arterial ring of Zinn-Haller in normal and glaucomatous eyes. Acta Ophthalmol. 2010;88:e317–22.

31. Vurgese S, Panda-Jonas S, Jonas JB. Sclera thickness in human globes and its relations to age, axial length and glaucoma. PLoS One. 2012;7:e29692.

Vitreous Changes in Myopia

13

Shoji Kishi

13.1 Introduction

The vitreous has a transparent gel-like structure with 4 ml of volume. The vitreous gel is covered by the vitreous cortex which consists of densely packed collagen. The Cloquet's canal arises from Martegiani space at the optic disc and traverses the central vitreous to retrolental space known as Berger's space. Although the vitreous appears inert, it plays a major role in various fundus diseases including rhegmatogenous retinal detachment, macular hole, epiretinal membrane, and progression of proliferative diabetic retinopathy. Recently vitreous surgery expands its indication in vitreoretinal diseases such as diabetic macular edema and myopic foveoschisis [1, 2]. The vitreous is not a homogeneous tissue which is the subject for resection in vitrectomy. The vitreous has its own structure which has been elucidated by biomicroscopy of postmortem eyes. Recent advance of optical coherent tomography greatly improved our understanding on vitreous anatomy and vitreoretinal interface diseases.

In myopic eyes, vitreous liquefaction develops at an early age which results in earlier posterior vitreous detachment (PVD). There is a strong statistical relation between axial myopia and rhegmatogenous retinal detachment [3]. Vitreous surgeons frequently encounter a membranous structure on the retina in eyes with myopic foveoschisis despite the apparent PVD with Weiss ring. In this chapter, the vitreous anatomy and its age-related change are described in normal eyes as well as vitreous changes in myopic eyes.

13.2 Anatomy of the Vitreous

13.2.1 Embryology of the Vitreous [4]

13.2.1.1 Formation of Primary Vitreous (Fourth to Sixth Week; 4–13 mm Stage)

The primary vitreous first appears in the narrow space between the surface and neural ectoderm during the fourth week of gestation, when the embryo is 4–5 mm in length. It derived mostly from the surface and neural ectoderm and partly from the mesoderm invaded through the embryonic choroidal fissure. The condensed fibrils of the primary vitreous form the *capsula perilenticularis fibrosa* around the lens. At the 5–7 mm stage, the hyaloid artery enters the distal part of optic stalk through the fetal fissure. It reaches the *capsula perilenticularis fibrosa* at 7 mm stage. The *capsula* is then vascularized by hyaloid artery and develops the *tunica vasculosa lentis* by the 13 mm stage.

13.2.1.2 Formation of Secondary Vitreous (Sixth Week to Third Month; 13–70 mm Stage)

The secondary vitreous is the major component of the adult vitreous body which is derived from the neural ectoderm. At the end of the sixth week or 13 mm stage, the secondary vitreous emerges between the developing retina and the primary vitreous. It grows around the primary vitreous and crowds it axially. An intravitreal limiting membrane develops as a condensation layer between the primary and secondary vitreous; it becomes the wall of Cloquet's canal. By the third month, the secondary vitreous fills two-thirds of the volume of the optic cup. After the 16 mm stage, hyaloid artery forms the *vasa hyaloidea propria*, which reaches maximum at the 40–60 mm stage. During the second month to the fifth month, a cone-shaped cellular mass called Bergmeister's papilla develops. Lens *zonule of Zinn* develops during 70–110 mm stage.

S. Kishi (✉)
Department of Ophthalmology, Gunma University School of Medicine, Gunma University Hospital, Maebashi, Gunma, Japan
e-mail: shojikishi@gunma-u.ac.jp

© Springer Nature Switzerland AG 2021
R. F. Spaide et al. (eds.), *Pathologic Myopia*, https://doi.org/10.1007/978-3-030-74334-5_13

13.2.1.3 Late Fetal Development

During the fourth to ninth month, or between the 110 and 300 mm stage, the globe undergoes rapid growth. The vitreous body enlarges as a result of growth of the secondary vitreous. Hyaloid vascular system atrophies, leaving a few filamentous structures in Cloquet's canal. Between the 110 and 150 mm stage, or during the fifth month, the *tunica vasculosa lentis* regresses.

13.2.2 Vitreous Development After Birth

At birth, vitreous gel appears homogeneous with no liquefaction. Cloquet's canal runs a straight course from the lens to the optic disc. Thereafter, it sags until its superior portion hangs behind the posterior lens surface. The vitreous gel shows pattern of radial fibers at newborn. At adolescent, lamellar structure which is called "tractus vitreales" is formed in anterior part of the vitreous [5]. Tractus vitreales traverse the whole vitreous in adult. In the macular area, early sign of vitreous liquefaction is seen at newborn [6]. The premacular bursa, sometimes called the posterior precortical vitreous pocket [7] develops by the age of 5 years.

13.2.3 Microscopic Anatomy

13.2.3.1 The Vitreous Body

The vitreous consists of 98% water and 2% protein which include collagen, hyaluronan, chondroitin sulfate, and other non-collagenous proteins. Collagen builds up three-dimensional meshwork of the vitreous gel. Type II collagen comprises 75% of the total collagen content [8], and type IX accounts for 15% [9]. Hyaluronan is a large polyanion which entangles to the vitreous collagen fibrils and attracts a large amount of water in the vitreous gel. The vitreous base is a circumferential zone with 2–6 mm width from peripheral retina to pars plana of the ciliary body. Vitreous fibers splay out from the vitreous base to the ciliary body, central vitreous, and posterior pole. The vitreous cortex is a shell of the vitreous gel which has higher density of collagen than inner vitreous. The vitreous cortex is 100–200 um thick. Hyalocytes are embedded in the vitreous cortex with highest density in the vitreous base followed by the posterior pole. Its role in metabolism is controversial. Hyalocytes appear to act as tissue macrophage [10]. The anterior vitreous cortex attaches to the posterior lens capsule in a circular zone about 8 mm in diameter (Weiger's ligament).

13.2.4 Vitreoretinal Interface

In the outermost layer of the vitreous cortex, vitreous collagen merges with the internal limiting membrane (ILM) of the retina and the basement membrane of the ciliary epithelium. The ILM consists of type IV collagen, associated with glycoprotein, type VI collagen which may contribute to vitreoretinal adhesion, and type XVIII, which binds opticin. Opticin binds to heparin sulfate, contributing to vitreoretinal adhesion [11]. The posterior vitreous cortex has lamellar structure [12], which may attribute the splitting of vitreous cortex in partial vitreous detachment. The strength of vitreous attachment to the surrounding tissue differs on the location. The vitreous base has the firmest attachment. The vitreous collagen fibrils are radially oriented and inserted in the basement membrane or cell processes of adjacent retinal and ciliary epithelial cells in the vitreous base. A second firm area of attachment is along the peripheral margin of the optic nerve head. The relatively firm vitreoretinal attachment is present at the margin and the center of the fovea, which cause perifoveal vitreous detachment. Vitreoretinal adhesion is occasionally observed along the retinal vessels. The ILM is the basement membrane of Müller cells. The ILM is uniformly thin (51 nm) within the vitreous base but progressively and irregularly thickened in the equatorial zone (sixfold) and posterior zone (37-fold) [13]. The ILM is extremely thin at the vitreous base, optic disc, and fovea. The ILM is also very thin over major retinal vessels where defect allows glial cells to extend on to the inner retina [14]. The location of firm vitreoretinal attachment corresponds to the area of thinner ILM.

13.2.5 Biomicroscopic Anatomy

The anatomy of the vitreous has been studied using dark-field slit microscopy on postmortem eyes by carefully separating the sclera, choroid, and retina from the vitreous and immersed in physiological solution to preserve its three-dimensional structure. Eisner [5] observed vitreous veils which he labeled *tracts hyaloideus* (inner wall of Cloquet's canal), *tractus coronarius*, *tractus medianus, and tractus preretinalis*. These vitreous veils are not observed in newborn but only developed in adult (Fig. 13.1).

Worst studied the vitreous by selective colored India ink injection after removal of the sclera, choroid, and retina from vitreous body. He showed a cistern system in the adult eyes [15, 16] (Fig. 13.2). The cistern system comprises 72 cisterns around the vitreous core at the level of posterior margin of the ciliary body, 36 cisterns at the level of the equator, and 12 large cisterns in the posterior vitreous. The central posterior vitreous consists of the *cistern preoptica* (prepapillary area of Martegiani), the *bursa premacularis*, and the *circum-papillo-macular cisterns*. The *bursa premacularis* is the posterior extension of the *canalis ciliobursale* which runs in an incomplete spiral from the ciliary body region toward the macular area. The posterior wall of the *bursa* was very thin, the fibers consisted of fine radiating lines, and there

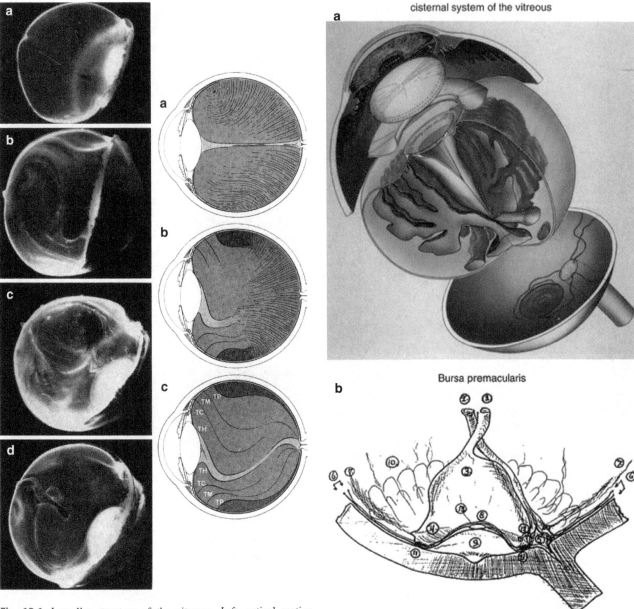

Fig. 13.1 Lamellar structure of the vitreous. *Left*: optical section through the vitreous body from the papilla toward the middle of the posterior surface of the lens. (**a**) 7-month-old child, (**b**) 40-year-old man, (**c**) 35-year-old man, (**d**) 60-year-old man. *Right*: schematic drawing of development of vitreous structure. (**a**) Newborn, (**b**) adolescent, (**c**) adult. *TC* tractus coronarius, *TH* tractus hyaloideus, *TM* tractus medianus, *TP* tractus preretinalis. (Reprint from Eisner [5], p106 (*right*) and p107 (*left*))

Fig. 13.2 *Top*: cisternal system of the vitreous according to worst. (Reprint from Sebag [35], p163. *Bottom*: bursa premacularis. Enlarged schematic: *1* canal of Cloquet, *2* superior branching channel, *3* capula of bursa premacularis, *4* fornix of bursa, *5* area of Martegiani, *6* vitreo-retinal limiting membrane (Gärtner), *7* tractus preretinalis (Eisner), *8* pars patelliformis membranae vitrealis, *9* spatium subbursale premacu-lare, *10* corona petaliformis, *11* perimacular bonding ring, *12* lower branching channel, *13* ocellus prefovealis. (Reprint from Worst [16])

were three concentric rings at the posterior portion that provided strong adhesion between the vitreous of the posterior wall of the bursa to the macula. The *bursa premacularis* is situated on the convexly detached vitreous cortex which forms *subbursal space*. In his early publication [16], Worst stated that a separation was present between the prefoveal part of the *bursa premacularis* and the fovea, which he named the "subbursal space." This space could be viewed through the center of the base of the *bursa premacularis* named the "ocellus prefovealis." From his point of view, the

posterior wall of the bursa is anatomically detached from the retina, which makes impossible the posterior wall to exert the anterior traction to the macula. In later specimens, Worst noted that this was a postmortem artifact. He revised that the posterior wall of the *bursa* is a thin vitreous cortex itself [17].

Sebag et al. [18] observed two holes in the vitreous cortex which corresponded to prepapillary hole and premacular hole. Vitreous fibers extruded posteriorly through the premacular hole (Fig. 13.3 top).

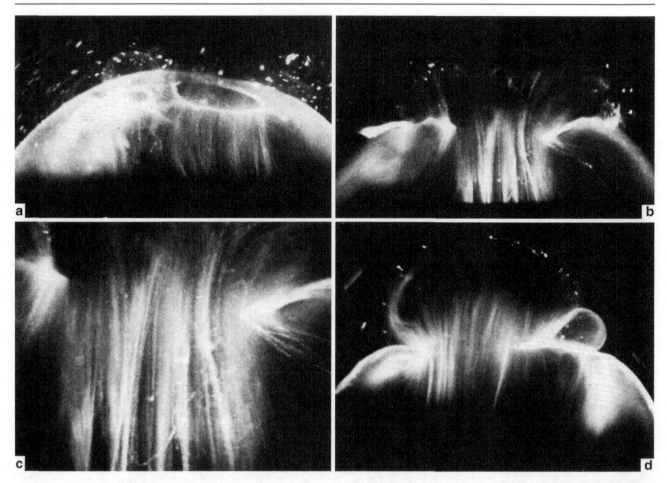

Fig. 13.3 (**a**) Posterior vitreous in the left eye of a 52-year-old male. The vitreous is enclosed by the vitreous cortex. There are two holes in the prepapillary (small, to the *left*) and premacular (large, to the *right*) vitreous cortex. Vitreous fibers are oriented toward the premacular region. (**b**) Posterior vitreous in a 57-year-old male. A large bundle of prominent fibers is seen coursing anteroposteriorly and entering the ret-rohyaloid space via the premacular hole in the vitreous cortex. (**c**) Same as (**b**) at higher magnification. (**d**) Posterior vitreous in the right eye of a 53-year-old female. There is posterior extrusion of the vitreous out the prepapillary hole (to the *right*) and premacular (large extrusion to the *left*) vitreous cortex. Fibers course anteroposteriorly out into the retro-hyaloid space (Reprint from Sebag [35])

13.2.6 Posterior Precortical Vitreous Pocket (PPVP)

13.2.6.1 Biomicroscopy of Posterior Precortical Vitreous Pocket

Kishi et al. studied the vitreous structure and the vitreoretinal interface (by preserving the retina in a bisected eyeball specimen) by staining its gel component with fluorescein [7]. The vitreous lacuna anterior to the posterior pole was always present in adult eyes. The posterior wall of the lacuna was a thin vitreous cortex, and the anterior extent was delineated by vitreous gel (Fig. 13.4). This physiological vitreous lacuna was defined as "posterior precortical vitreous pocket" (PPVP). This is seemingly the same structure as observed by Worst (*bursa permacularis*) [16]. The presence of the premacular bursa or PPVP differs from older concepts of vitreomacular traction where it was believed that anteroposteriorly oriented vitreous fiber exerts the direct traction to the fovea. Because vitreous gel and posterior vitreous cortex is separated by PPVP, the vitreous traction to fovea should be transmitted through the posterior vitreous cortex. The posterior wall of PPVP is the posterior vitreous cortex attached to the retina. There is no subbursal space between the bursa and the retina. While its posterior wall of PPVP is a thin vitreous cortex itself, the anterior border is a vitreous gel. The anterior extent of the PPVP becomes larger and ill-defined in the eyes with vitreous liquefaction. It is difficult to observe the entire structure of transparent PPVP by slit-lamp biomicroscopy in living eyes. Triamcinolone-assisted vitreous surgery clearly demonstrates the PPVP [19].

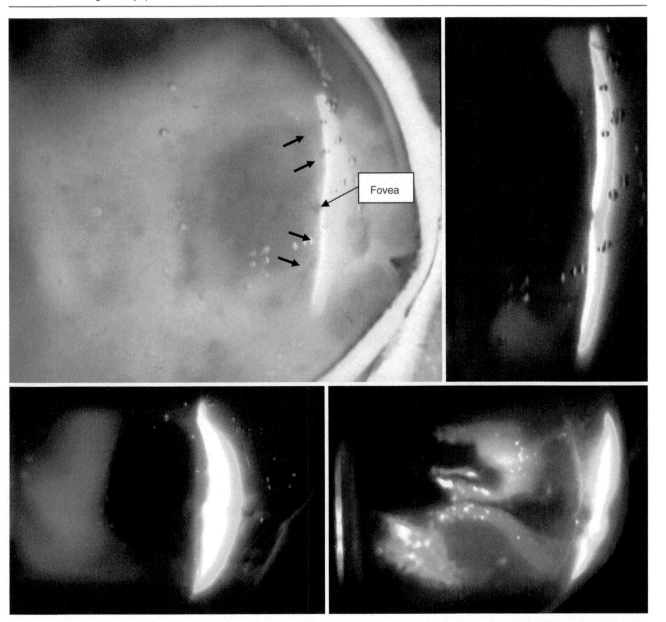

Fig. 13.4 Posterior precortical vitreous pocket (PPVP). *Top*: (*left*) bisected senile eye with background illumination. *Arrows* indicate the posterior wall of the PPVP. Optical section of PPVP in the same specimen. Posterior wall of the PPVP is a thin vitreous cortex. *Bottom*: optical section of PPVP in an eye of a 28-year-old adult (*left*) with no liquefied lacuna in the inner vitreous and senile eye (*right*) with liquefied lacunae in the inner vitreous. (Reproduced from Kishi and Shimizu [7])

13.2.6.2   Optical Coherence Tomography of Posterior Precortical Vitreous Pocket

Spectral domain optical coherence tomography (SD-OCT) and its noise-reduced version enabled the first visualizations of the PPVP in vivo [20, 21]. Recently introduced swept source OCT (SS-OCT) enabled further clear demonstration of entire structure of PPVP (Fig. 13.5). PPVP is a boat-shaped vitreous lacuna in front of the posterior pole [22]. The superior bow of the boat is elevated interiorly in sitting position. The posterior wall is a thin vitreous cortex which is thinnest at the fovea. The anterior extent of PPVP is delineated by the vitreous gel. In eyes with little liquefaction, the anterior border of PPVP is sharply demarcated. There is a septum between the Martegiani space in Cloquet's canal and PPVP. A channel over the anterior border of the septum connects the two spaces. In the vitreous gel surrounding the PPVP, a vitreous fiber is perpendicularly inserted in the vitreous cortex. The configuration of the PPVP was almost symmetrical in both eyes of each subject. Fully developed PPVP is seen even in children older than 5 years. Yokoi et al. recently reported precursor stage of PPVP in newborn babies using SS-OCT [6].

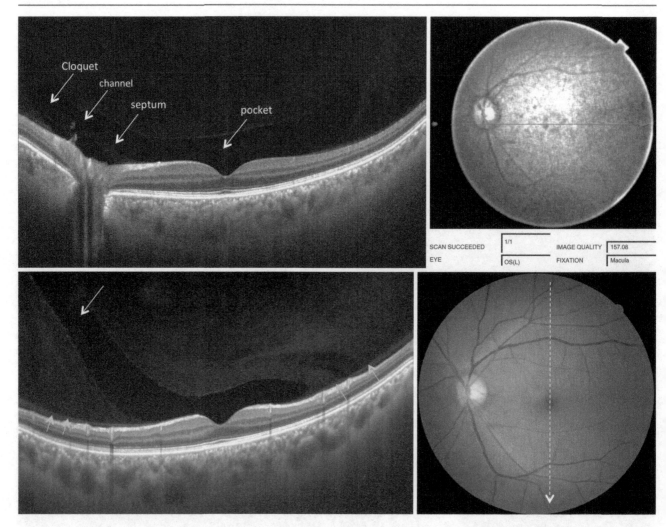

Fig. 13.5 Normal posterior precortical vitreous pocket (PPVP) with little vitreous liquefaction observed by SS-OCT. Left eye of a 46-year-old man with moderate myopia of −5.0D. *Top*: in horizontal section, PPVP is boat shaped, which is sharply demarcated by vitreous gel. There is a connecting channel between Cloquet's canal and the pocket over the septum. *Bottom*: in vertical section, superior portion of PPVP is usually elevated (*arrows*). In the vitreous gel outer to the PPVP, vitreous fiber perpendicularly inserted in the vitreous cortex

13.2.6.3 Clinical Implication of Posterior Precortical Vitreous Pocket

Pseudo PVD

Because of PPVP, vitreous gel is always separated from the retina. The vitreous cortex, which serves as a posterior wall of PPVP, is invisible on slit-lamp biomicroscopy as long as it is attached to the retina. This condition is often misdiagnosed as PVD. Balazs [23] termed "vitreoschisis" to denote severe liquefaction in the posterior vitreous but persistent attachment of the outermost layer of posterior vitreous cortex on the retina. Vitreoschisis can be interpreted as a large PPVP which often develops in axial myopia.

Perifoveal PVD

The posterior wall of the PPVP exists as a membrane separated from the gel. The premacular cortex is spared from direct traction of vitreous gel but tends to develop trampoline-like detachment. However, there is a strong attachment at the fovea, which modifies the trampoline PVD to perifoveal PVD. In perifoveal PVD, the vitreous cortex is inwardly detached in the perifoveal area, which suggests elastic nature of premacular cortex. Persistent vitreous traction by perifoveal PVD may cause macular hole [24, 25] or vitreomacular traction syndrome. Perifoveal PVD physiologically occurs in the precursor stage of complete PVD [26, 27] (Fig. 13.6).

Residual Vitreous Cortex

Because the premacular vitreous cortex is separated from the gel before initiation of PVD, it occasionally remains attached to the retina during PVD [28]. The residual cortex becomes the main source of epiretinal membrane. In eyes with ERM, oval defect of premacular hyaloid is often observed in detached posterior hyaloid [29].

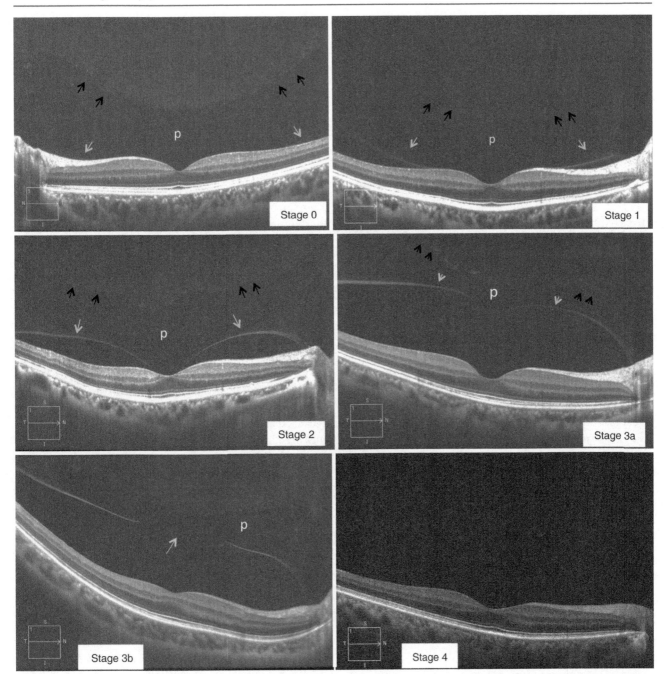

Fig. 13.6 *Top left*: Stage 0: no PVD. Posterior precortical vitreous pocket (PPVP) (p) is present anterior to the macula. Posterior wall of the PPVP is thin vitreous cortex (*yellow arrows*) and anterior border is vitreous gel (*black arrows*). *Top right*: Stage 1, vitreous cortex is detached in paramacular area (*yellow arrows*). *Black arrows* are the anterior border of the PPVP (p). *Middle left*: Stage 2, perifoveal PVD (*yellow arrows*). *Black arrows* indicate the anterior border of the PPVP

(p). *Middle right*: Stage 3a, macular PVD with intact vitreous cortex or the posterior wall (*yellow arrows*) of the PPVP (p). *Black arrows* indicate the anterior border of the PPVP. *Bottom left*: Stage 3b, macular PVD with disrupted posterior wall (*yellow arrow*) of the PPVP (p). *Bottom right*: Stage 4, complete PVD with Weiss ring. No vitreous structure is observed

Diabetic Retinopathy

In diabetic retinopathy, fibrovascular proliferation tends to develop around the PPVP which results in ring-shaped fibrovascular proliferation [30]. Vitreous detachment tends to occur outer to the PPVP, but not in the area of PPVP. Outer to the PPVP, vitreous fibers insert into the vitreous cortex; thus, the gel and the cortex detach together. However, premacular vitreous cortex is spared from direct traction of vitreous gel because of PPVP. The posterior wall of the pocket develops trampoline-like PVD or perifoveal PVD which may cause cystoids macular edema [31].

Vitreoretinal Adhesion at the Fovea

Kishi et al. examined 59 human postmortem eyes with complete PVD by scanning electron microscope [28]. They found vitreous cortex remnants at the fovea in 26 out of 58 (44%) eyes. One half of the 26 eyes had 500 μm diameter disc of remnant cortex at the fovea, which was occasionally surrounded by another 1500 μm diameter ring of remnant cortex (Fig. 13.7a top). A 500 μm diameter ring of cortical remnant was adherent to the outer margin of the fovea in 30% of the eyes (Fig. 13.7b left bottom). Twenty percent of the eyes showed a pseudocyst formation where a 200–300 μm diameter disc of vitreous cortex bridged over the foveal pit (Fig. 13.7b right bottom). These findings suggest strong adhesion of vitreous cortex at the fovea and the outer margin of the foveal pit. These cortical remnants were membranes with no overlying vitreous gel because vitreous cortex is separated from gel by intervening PPVP. Spaide et al. observed the foveal anatomy in patients with perifoveal PVD (mainly patients with macular holes and those with early macular hole states) using OCT [32]. They reported that the diameter of the vitreous attachment in eyes with perifoveal PVD correlated with induced changes in foveal anatomy. Normal foveal depression is seen in eyes with vitreous attachment of 1828 μm diameter, whereas loss of foveal depression is seen in vitreous attachment with 840 μm diameter and foveal cavitation in 281 μm of vitreous attachment.

13.3 Age-Related Change of the Vitreous

13.3.1 Liquefaction

Balazs measured the volumes of vitreous liquefaction and gel in 610 human eyes [33]. Liquid vitreous appears by the age of five and increases throughout life until it constitutes more than 50% of volume of the vitreous during the tenth decade (Fig. 13.8). Gel vitreous volume increases during the first decade while the eye is growing in size. The volume of gel vitreous remains stable till about the age of 40, when it begins to decrease in equivalent to the increase in liquid vitreous. Foos studied the relationship between synchysis (liquefaction) senilis of vitreous and posterior vitreous detachment (PVD) in 2246 autopsied eyes using the technique of suspension in air [34]. They showed that with age, liquefaction and incidence of PVD increases. There was a significant increase in PVD associated with grade 3 (50% destruction) and grade 4 (67%) synchysis. Using dark-field slit illumination, Eisner [5] and Sebag [18, 35] showed age-related changes of the vitreous. The vitreous is composed of homogeneous gel with Cloquet's canal in a 7-month-old child [5]. There is no liquefied lacuna in the eyes of 4- and 8-year-old children. Vitreous extruded into retrohyaloid space through the premacular vitreous cortex. There is no liquefaction or fibers in the vitreous. In the eyes of a 57-year-old male, a large bundle of prominent fibers is seen coursing anteroposteriorly and entering the retrohyaloid space via the premacular hole in the vitreous cortex [35] (Fig. 13.3b bottom). In the eyes of an 88-year-old woman, the fibrous structure of the vitreous was degenerated with fibers being thickened and tortuous [35]. The entire inner vitreous undergoes dissolution with empty spaces adjacent to the thickened fibers. It is believed that dissolution of the HA-collagen complex results in the simultaneous formation of liquid vitreous and aggregation of collagen into bundle of parallel fibrils and seen as large fibers. Slit-lamp biomicroscopy shows that vitreous liquefaction is associated with aggregation of collagen fibers (Fig. 13.9). In the vitreous samples obtained during vitrectomy, vitreous hyaluronan level was significantly decreased with aging [36].

13.3.2 Posterior Vitreous Detachment (PVD)

PVD occurs when liquefied vitreous passes through a break of vitreous cortex to retrohyaloid space. Vitreous cortex detaches from internal limiting membrane of the retina during PVD. Incidence of PVD increases markedly between ages 50 and 70 years [33, 34]. As shown by Sebag in autopsy eyes, vitreous gel extrudes to retrohyaloid space through premacular hole in living eyes (Fig. 13.10). Premacular hole seems to correspond to the defect or break of the posterior wall of the PPVP. Since vitreoretinal adhesion is the strongest

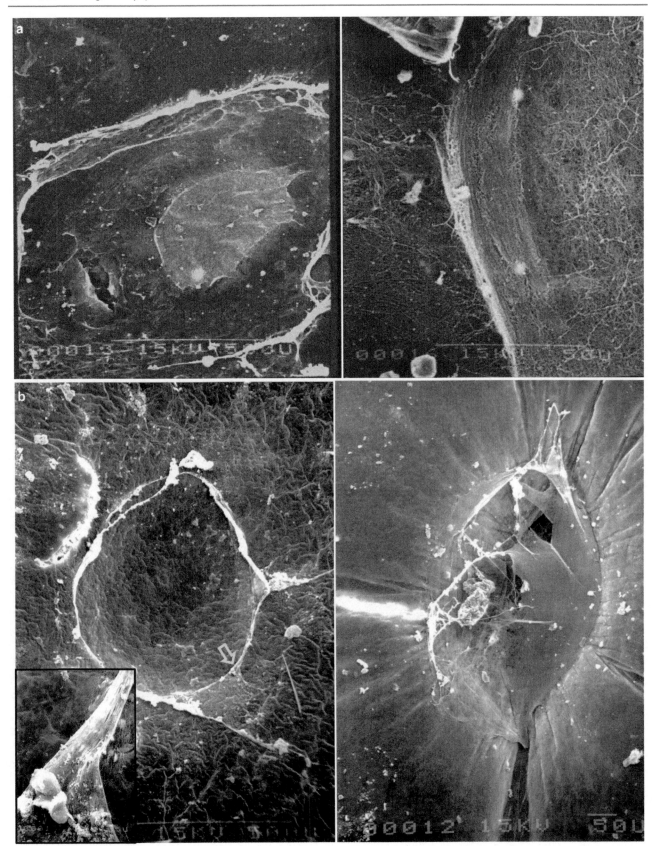

Fig. 13.7 Scanning electron microscopy of vitreous cortex remnant at the fovea (Reproduced from Kishi et al. [28]). *Top*: (*left*) 500 μm diameter disc of remnant cortex at the fovea, which was surrounded by another 1500 μm diameter ring of remnant cortex. (*Right*) high magnification of residual vitreous cortex. *Bottom*: (*left*) ring-shaped remnant at the outer margin of foveal pit. *Inset* shows high magnification of the site of yellow arrow. (*Right*) vitreous cortex bridging the foveal pit

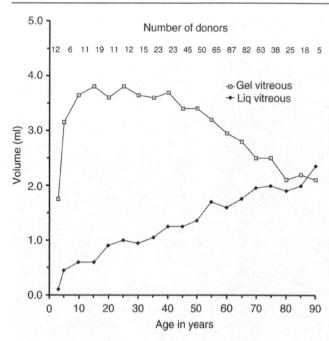

Fig. 13.8 The volumes of vitreous liquefaction and gel in 610 human eyes. (Reprint from Balazs and Flood [33])

at the optic nerve head, presence of prepapillary ring called Weiss ring in the detached vitreous cortex signifies completion of PVD (Fig. 13.11).

13.3.3 Evolution of Vitreomacular Detachment

PVD had been believed to be an acute event. However, OCT has revealed a precursor stage of complete PVD [26, 27]. Because of PPVP, the premacular vitreous cortex is spared from direct traction of the vitreous gel. Premacular vitreous cortex or posterior wall of PPVP tends to develop trampoline-like detachment. Tangential contraction of the premacular cortex may generate anterior vector which promotes trampoline-like PVD. Strong vitreous retinal adhesion at fovea may modify trampoline to perifoveal PVD. In our prospective study in normal non-myopic eyes (Fig. 13.6) [27], PVD first occurs in paramacular area (stage 1) and progresses to a perifoveal PVD (stage 2). Then vitreous cortex detaches at the fovea (stage 3). In vitreo-foveal separation (stage 3), some individuals may have an intact cortex, and some may have a break in the cortex. Finally

Fig. 13.9 Vitreous liquefaction in slit-lamp biomicroscopy. (*Left*) non-myopic eye with posterior vitreous detachment (PVD). (*Right*) myopic eye with large lacuna (*L*) which mimics PVD

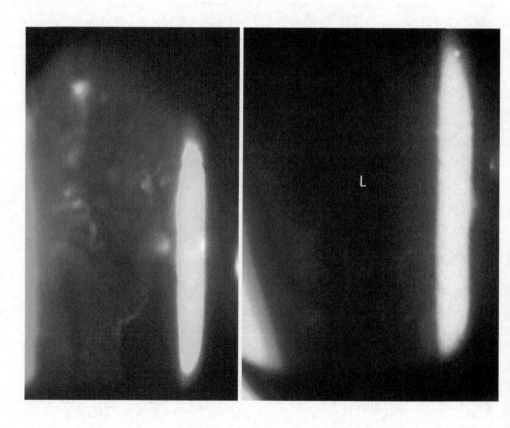

Fig. 13.10 Slit-lamp biomicroscopy of posterior vitreous detachment. (*Left*) posterior vitreous cortex (*yellow arrows*) is seen anterior to the macula. (*Right*) vitreous gel (*yellow arrow*) extruded posteriorly through the premacular defect of the vitreous cortex

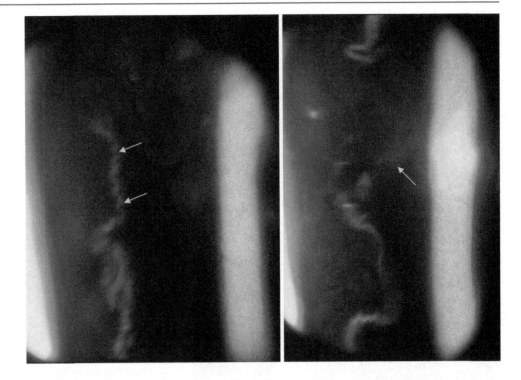

vitreous detachment at the disc results in complete PVD with Weiss ring (stage 4). Figure 13.12 shows the incidence of each stage in different decades in normal non-myopic population [27].

13.3.4 Splitting of Vitreous Cortex

Because of lamellar structure of the vitreous cortex, splitting of vitreous cortex may occur especially at the posterior wall of the PPVP. In our study of normal human eyes with spectral domain OCT [20], splitting of the vitreous cortex was seen in 22% of the eyes aged over 51 years (Fig. 13.13). In case of persistent vitreous traction such as vitreomacular traction syndrome, vitreous cortex splitting is more likely to occur [37] (Fig. 13.14). This suggests the possibility that outer layer of vitreous cortex may remain on the retina after PVD even with detachment of intact posterior wall of the PPVP. Sebag called the splitting of vitreous cortex as "vitreoschisis" and formed a basis to explain vitreoretinal interface diseases [12, 38].

13.4 Vitreous Changes in Myopic Eyes

13.4.1 Formation of Large Lacuna

Axial myopia is associated with vitreous liquefaction and PVD occurring at a younger age as compared to non-myopic eyes [39–41]. Highly myopic eyes have a large liquefied lacuna which may mimic PVD (Fig. 13.9 right). Because poockets of liquefied vitreous is a source of subretinal fluid in rhegmatogenous retinal detachment without PVD, retinal detachment is more likely to develop in myopic eyes. During PVD, a large amount of liquefied vitreous escapes to retrohyaloid space resulting in vitreous collapse. Retinal detachment tends to be severe in high myopic eyes.

It is not well understood why highly myopic eyes develop a large lacuna. In chick model of form-deprivation myopia, axial elongation is associated with an elongation of the vitreous chamber depth and an increase of the vitreous volume [42, 43]. An increase in the vitreous in myopic eyes was attributed on changes in the volume of the liquid vitreous, but not of the

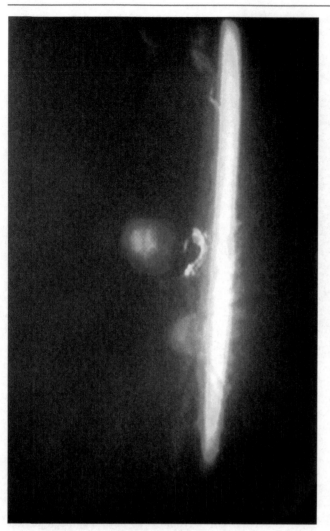

Fig. 13.11 Weiss ring in detached vitreous cortex

gel vitreous [42]. Using this chick model, Seko et al. found the disturbance of electrolyte balance in the vitreous [44]. The concentration of potassium and phosphate were decreased in liquefied vitreous, whereas chloride was increased. Potassium is released from the retina into the vitreous to maintain the homeostatic condition of the retina, and Müller cell plays an important role to regulate the extracellular potassium [45]. Visual deprivation may cause reduction of phototransduction and metabolic activity in the retina, particularly Müller cells.

Since the vitreous gel seems to be generated from retina or Müller cells, reduced metabolic activity of the retina or Müller cell in axial myopia may cause formation of large lacuna.

OCT reveals that posterior aspect of PPVP is preserved despite the vitreous liquefaction. Liquefied lacuna may be formed early in central part of the vitreous. In such case, PPVP maintains normal configuration with sharply demarcated anterior border. Liquefied lacuna presents anterior to PPVP with intervening vitreous gel (Fig. 13.15). There is a significant correlation between the PPVP height and myopic refractive error [22]. In myopic eye, PPVP is enlarged and its anterior border becomes irregular, even though the posterior wall of PPVP and the septum adjacent to Cloquet's canal are preserved (Fig. 13.16). In case of large PPVP, perifoveal PVD may occur at a young age (Figs. 13.16 and 13.17). If PPVP is markedly large, its anterior border is out of the scope of SS-OCT (Figs. 13.17 and 13.18). Even in such condition, posterior wall of PPVP and the connecting channel are preserved, and perifoveal PVD is common (Figs. 13.16, 13.17, and 13.18). The configuration of the PPVP is almost symmetrical in both eyes of each subject. However, if refractive error differs in both eyes of the subject, the configuration and size of PPVP differs in both eyes (Fig. 13.19).

13.4.2 Incomplete PVD

The features of incomplete PVD in high myopia were first demonstrated by SS-OCT. If Weiss ring is not detected despite anterior displacement of vitreous gel by slit-lamp biomicroscopy, we should consider it a large PPVP or extensive liquefaction. SS-OCT can better detect the vitreous cortex or posterior wall of PPVP attached on the retina or partially detached. Perifoveal PVD is common in myopic eyes as in non-myopic eyes. In case of no PVD on slit-lamp biomicroscopy, SS-OCT well visualized the posterior vitreous cortex detached at the macula but attached to optic disc (Fig. 13.20 top). In case of vitreomacular separation, posterior wall of the PPVP may attach on the retina which acts as epiretinal membrane (Fig. 13.20 bottom). SS-OCT demonstrates the flatten PPVP in case of PVD in the macular area (Fig. 13.21). PPVP may have an intact posterior wall or a disrupted wall (Fig. 13.6 bottom).

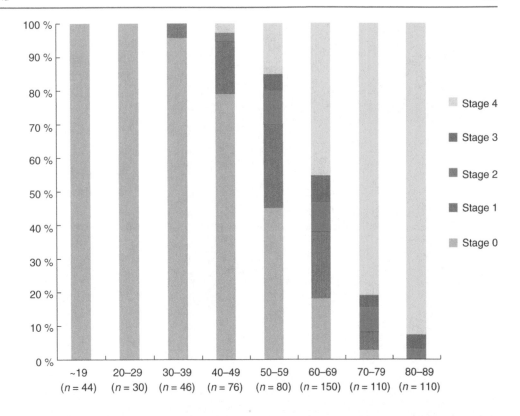

Fig. 13.12 The incidence of each stage in different decades in normal non-myopic population. Stage 4 is complete PVD and stage 0 is no PVD (Reproduced from Itakura and Kishi [27])

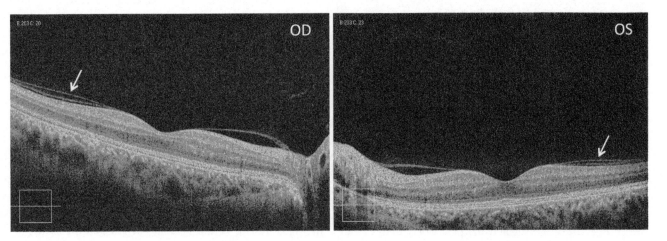

Fig. 13.13 Splitting of vitreous cortex (*arrow*) in both eyes of a 58-year-old female. Horizontal sections of SD-OCT. (Reprint from Itakura and Kishi [20])

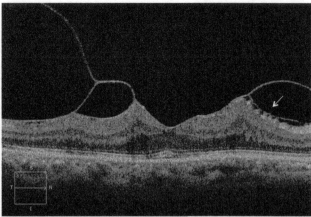

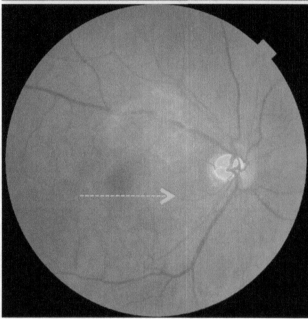

Fig. 13.14 Vitreous cortex splitting (*arrow*) in vitreomacular traction syndrome. (Reprint from Itakura and Kishi [37])

13.4.3 Early PVD

We prospectively investigated the posterior vitreous using SD-OCT or SS-OCT in non-myopic eyes (control) and high myopia of more than −8.0D. We defined complete PVD as detached vitreous cortex with Weiss ring. In ages from 20 to 39 years, control eyes had only 8.3% partial PVD, while high myopic eyes had already 27.8% of complete PVD and 16.7%

of partial PVD (Fig. 13.22). In the ages of 40–59 years, high myopics had 43.2% of complete PVD and 35.1% of partial PVD, while control eyes had only 8.2% of complete PVD and 38.8% of partial PVD (Fig. 13.23). In ages between 60 and 79 years, high myopics had 91.4% of complete PVD and 8.6% of partial PVD, while control eyes had 60.6% of complete PVD and 29.4% of partial PVD (Fig. 13.24).

13.4.4 Residual Vitreous Cortex in Eyes with Complete PVD

Residual vitreous cortex attached on the retina is only detected by SS-OCT. In our prospective study, residual cortex was seen in 6.7% of 105 non-myopic eyes with PVD and 37.7% of 53 highly myopic eyes (Fig. 13.25). Residual vitreous on the surface of the retina are commonly found during vitrectomy surgery.

It is difficult to evaluate the vitreous by slit-lamp biomicroscopy in myopic eyes. If we observe anterior displacement of vitreous gel with extensive liquefaction but no Weiss ring, we assume no PVD. SS-OCT gives more concrete answer demonstrating the posterior wall of the PPVP and the septum adjacent to Martegiani space (Fig. 13.26 top). Vitreous surgeons frequently note the residual vitreous cortex in posterior staphyloma despite the apparent PVD with Weiss ring during surgery in myopic foveoschisis eyes [46]. SS-OCT demonstrates the residual vitreous cortex in the eyes of myopic foveoschisis with PVD with Weiss ring (Fig. 13.26 bottom).

During vitreous surgery for myopic foveoschisis with complete PVD, we occasionally encounter the case with no residual vitreous cortex. In such case, we only remove ILM in the posterior pole. SS-OCT clearly demonstrates no vitreous cortex on the retina preoperatively (Fig. 13.27 top). Despite the apparent PVD with Weiss ring, very thin vitreous cortex may remain on the retina in highly myopic eyes (Figs. 13.27 bottom and 13.28). The residual cortex can be interpreted as the remnants of posterior wall of PPVP or outermost layer of the split vitreous cortex. It may be not a residual cortex but a newly formed epiretinal membrane by proliferated glial cells or pigment epithelial cells. Another possibility is regenerated vitreous cortex after PVD which yet to be proved.

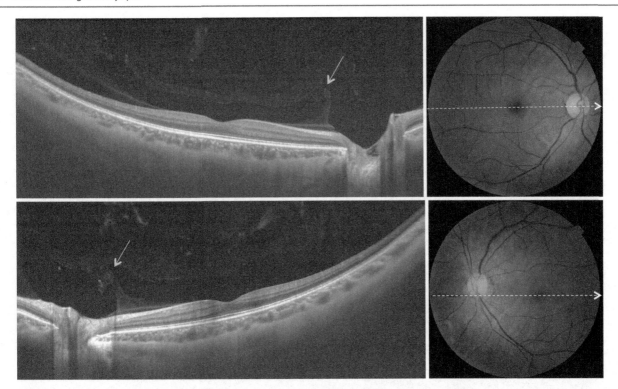

Fig. 13.15 A 46-year-old female. Her vision was 1.2 × −5.5D in the right and 1.2 × −8.5D in the left eye. There is a similarity in the configuration of posterior precortical vitreous pocket (PPVP) in both eyes. PPVP is a flat boat shaped. Connecting channel (*arrow*) between PPVP and Martegiani space of Cloquet's canal. There are liquefied spaces superior to the PPVP in both eyes

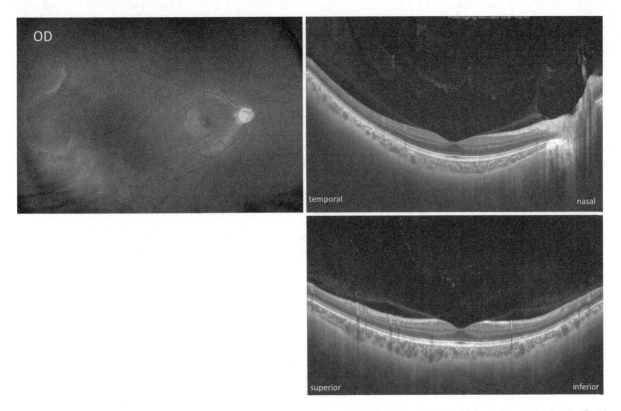

Fig. 13.16 Right eye of a 24-year-old male with moderate myopia. He had focal retinal detachment in the temporal periphery of the right eye. His vision was 1.2 × −5.0D in the right and 1.2 × −5.5D in the left eye. No PVD was noted biomicroscopically in the right eye. SS-OCT showed relatively large PPVP with irregular anterior border. Perifoveal PVD is noted in horizontal (*right top*) and vertical (*right bottom*) sections. Septum between PPVP and Martegiani space of Cloquet's canal is seen in the horizontal section

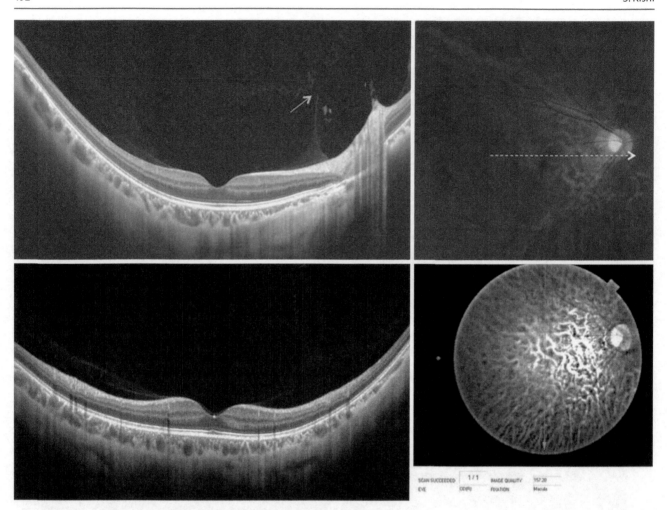

Fig. 13.17 A 21-year-old male. His vision was 1.2 × −11.0D in the right eye which showed liquefaction but no PVD in slit-lamp biomicroscopy. His fellow eye underwent retinal detachment surgery. *Top*: SS-OCT shows large PPVP; the connecting channel (*arrow*) is seen at the top of the septum. *Bottom*: large PPVP and perifoveal PVD is seen

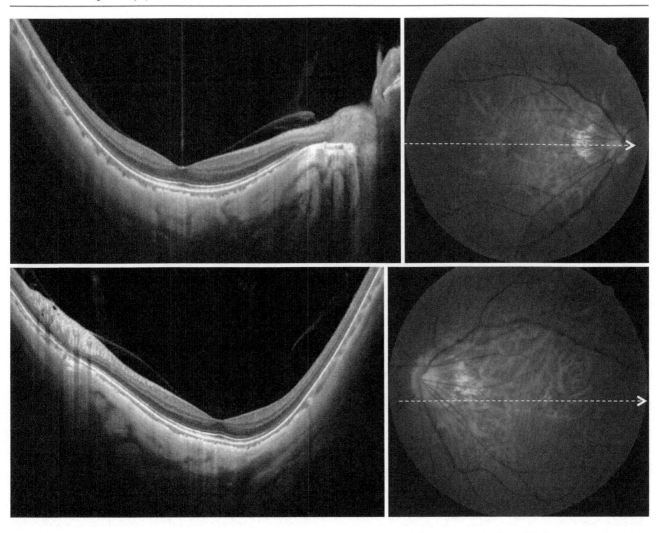

Fig. 13.18 A 48-year-old female. Her vision was $1.2 \times -11.5D$ in the right and $1.2 \times -12.5D$. Both eyes had large PPVP whose anterior border was not detected. Focal PVD was seen in paramacular area in both eyes

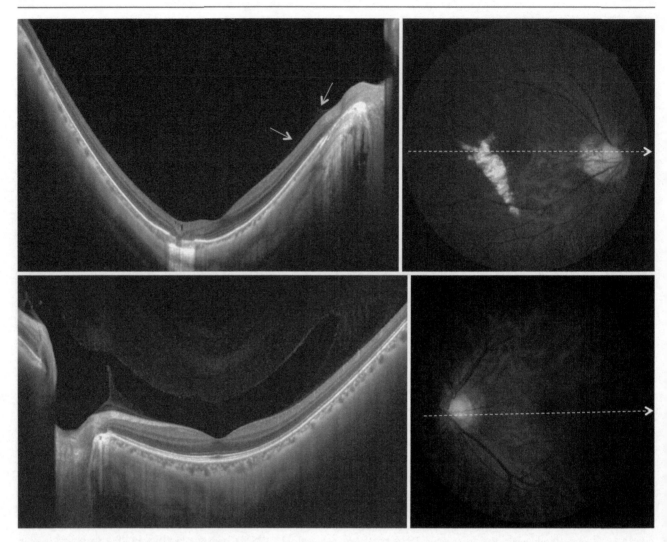

Fig. 13.19 A 44-year-old man with enlarged lacquer crack in his right eye. His vision is 1.0 × −12.0D in the right and 1.2 × −6.0D in the left eye. No PVD was detected in both eyes. *Top*: SS-OCT showed extensive liquefaction, and anterior border of PPVP was not detected in the right eye. Slightly detached vitreous cortex and the septum at temporal border of Cloquet's canal were seen (*arrows*). *Bottom*: the left eye showed boat-shaped PPVP. There is a liquefied lacuna anterior to the PPVP

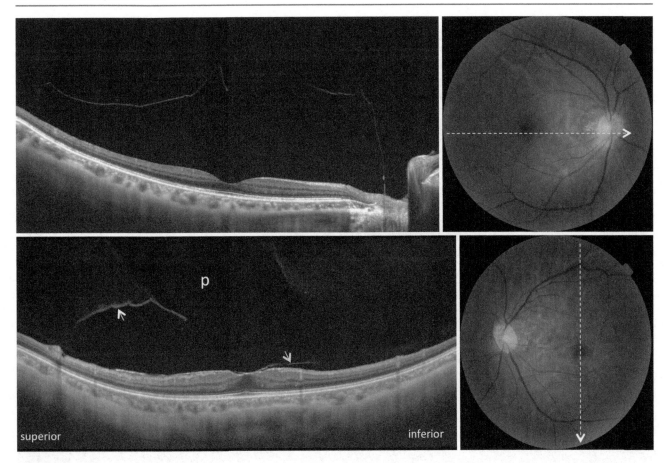

Fig. 13.20 A 59-year-old woman with epiretinal membrane in the left eye. Her vision was $1.2 \times -10D$ in the right and $1.2 \times -7.0D$ in the left eye. *Top*: the right eye had PVD in the macular area but vitreous cortex attached to the optic disc. The detached posterior wall of the PPVP which is a premacular vitreous cortex was disrupted. *Bottom*: in the vertical section of the left eye, vitreous cortex was detached in the superior to the fovea (*white arrow*) but attached on the inferior to the fovea. Epiretinal membrane (*yellow arrow*) appears to correspond to the posterior wall of the PPVP which is seen as an empty space (*p*)

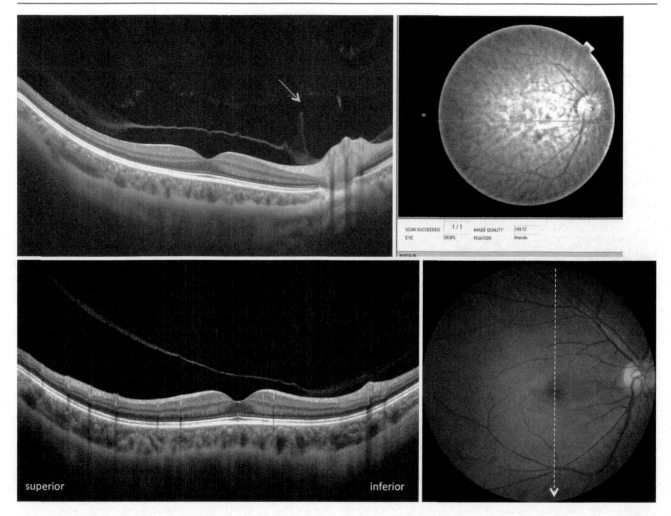

Fig. 13.21 A 43-year-old female. Her vision is 1.2 × −6.0D in the right eye. SS-OCT showed PVD in the macular area but vitreous attached at optic disc. Premacular vitreous cortex which is a posterior wall of the PPVP was intact (*top* and *bottom*). There is a connecting channel (*arrow*) between PPVP and Martegiani space of Cloquet's canal in horizontal section (*top*). Her left eye had retinal detachment

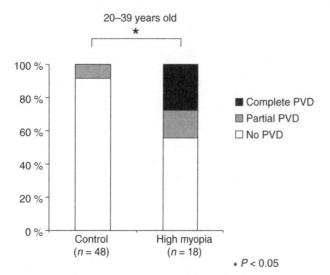

Fig. 13.22 The incidence of PVD in non-myopic control and high myopia of more than −8.0D in the population of 20–39 years old

13.5 Conclusion

The pathological condition of the vitreous in posterior staphyloma has been unclear because of invisible structure by slit-lamp biomicroscopy. Using time-domain OCT, we first reported myopic foveoschisis [1] in 1999. At that time, time-domain OCT could not depict the vitreous structure. Recently developed SS-OCT sheds light on the manifestation of vitreous cortex in high myopia. The posterior wall of PPVP plays an important role in vitreoretinal interface diseases in high myopia and in non-myopic eyes.

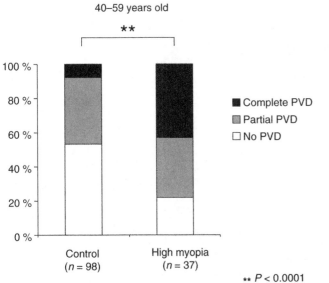

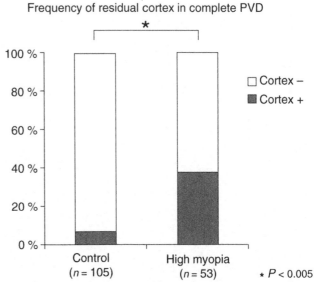

Fig. 13.23 The incidence of PVD in non-myopic control and high myopia of more than −8.0D in the population of 40–59 years old

Fig. 13.25 Frequency of residual cortex with complete PVD detected by SS-OCT in non-myopic control and high myopia more than −8.0D

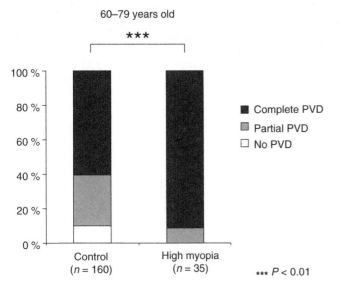

Fig. 13.24 The incidence of PVD in non-myopic control and high myopia of more than −8.0D in the population of 60–79 years old

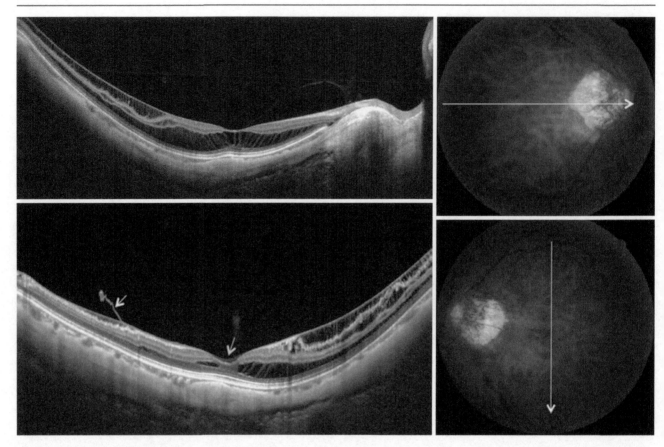

Fig. 13.26 A 58-year-old woman has myopic foveoschisis in both eyes. Her vision is 1.2 × −14.0D in both eyes. Slit-lamp biomicroscopy showed no PVD in the right and PVD with Weiss ring in the left eye. *Top*: SS-OCT showed partially detached vitreous cortex nasal to the fovea in the right eye. Anterior border of PPVP is not seen. *Bottom*: partially detached epiretinal membrane (*white arrow*) is seen superior to the fovea, from which the membrane attached on the retina to the fovea (*yellow arrow*)

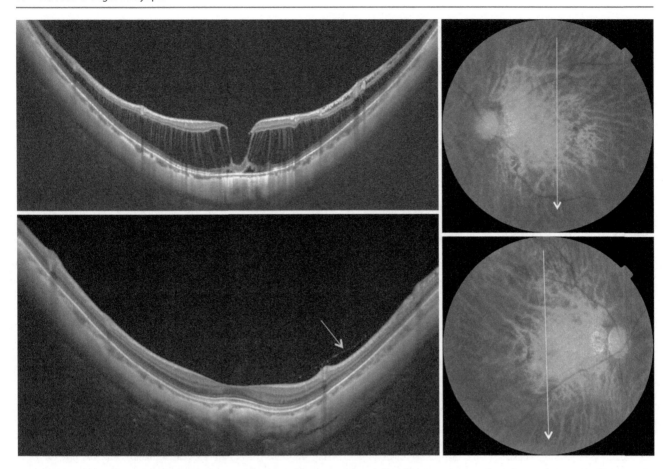

Fig. 13.27 A 70-year-old female with myopic foveoschisis in the right eye. Her vision was 0.8p × −10.5D in the right and 1.2 × −9.0D in the left eye. Both eyes had PVD with Weiss ring. There was no residual vitreous cortex on the retina in the right eye (*top*), which was later con- firmed by vitrectomy for foveoschisis. There is a slightly detached vit- reous cortex (*arrow*) inferior to the macula in the left eye despite PVD (*bottom*)

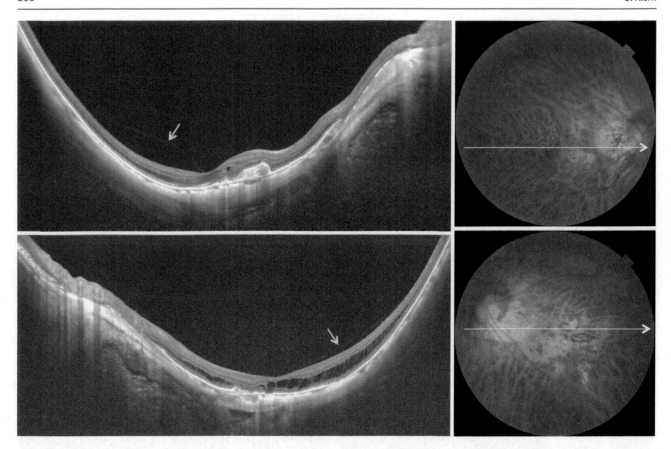

Fig. 13.28 A 73-year-old woman. She has myopic choroidal neovascularization which was treated by intravitreal bevacizumab in the right eye. The left eye has myopic foveoschisis. Her vision is 0.5 × −15.0D in the right and 0.1 × −15.0D in the left eye. Although PVD with Weiss ring was observed in both eyes on slit-lamp biomicroscopy, SS-OCT revealed slightly detached thin possibly vitreous cortex (*arrow*) temporal to the fovea in both eyes (*top* and *bottom*)

References

1. Takano M, Kishi S. Foveal retinoschisis and retinal detachment in severely myopic eyes with posterior staphyloma. Am J Ophthalmol. 1999;128(4):472–6.

2. Kobayashi H, Kishi S. Vitreous surgery for highly myopic eyes with foveal detachment and retinoschisis. Ophthalmology. 2003;110(9):1702–7.

3. Schepens CL, Marden D. Data on the natural history of retinal detachment. Further characterization of certain unilateral nontraumatic cases. Am J Ophthalmol. 1966;61(2):213–26.

4. Tolentino FI, Schepens CL, Freeman HM. Vitreoretinal disorders. Philadelphia: W.B. Sanders Co.; 1976. p. 1–12.

5. Eisner G. Biomicroscopy of the peripheral fundus. New York: Springer; 1979. p. 20, 21, 106, 107.

6. Yokoi T, Toriyama N, Yamane T, Nakayama Y, Nishina S, Azuma N. Development of a premacular vitreous pocket. JAMA Ophthalmol. 2013;131(8):1095–6.

7. Kishi S, Shimizu K. Posterior precortical vitreous pocket. Arch Ophthalmol. 1990;108(7):979–82.

8. Schmut O, Mallinger R, Paschke E. Studies on a distinct fraction of bovine vitreous body collagen. Graefes Arch Clin Exp Ophthalmol. 1984;221(6):286–9.

9. Bishop PN, Crossman MV, McLeod D, Ayad S. Extraction and characterization of the tissue forms of collagen types II and IX from bovine vitreous. Biochem J. 1994;299(Pt 2):497–505.

10. Sakamoto T, Ishibashi T. Hyalocytes: essential cells of the vitreous cavity in vitreoretinal pathophysiology? Retina. 2011;31(2):222–8.

11. Ramesh S, Bonshek RE, Bishop PN. Immunolocalisation of opticin in the human eye. Br J Ophthalmol. 2004;88(5):697–702.

12. Gupta P, Yee KM, Garcia P, Rosen RB, Parikh J, Hageman GS, Sadun AA, Sebag J. Vitreoschisis in macular diseases. Br J Ophthalmol. 2011;95(3):376–80.

13. Foos RY. Vitreoretinal juncture; topographical variations. Investig Ophthalmol. 1972;11(10):801–8.

14. Kishi S, Numaga T, Yoneya S, Yamazaki S. Epivascular glia and paravascular holes in normal human retina. Graefes Arch Clin Exp Ophthalmol. 1986;224(2):124–30.

15. Worst JG. Cisternal systems of the fully developed vitreous body in the young adult. Trans Ophthalmol Soc U K. 1977;97(4):550–4.

16. Worst J. Extracapsular surgery in lens implantation (Binkhorst lecture). Part IV. Some anatomical and pathophysiological implications. J Am Intraocul Implant Soc. 1978;4:7–14.

17. Worst J, Los L. Cisternal anatomy of the vitreous. Amsterdam: Kugler Publications; 1995. p. 28.

18. Sebag J, Balazs EA. Human vitreous fibers and vitreoretinal disease. Trans Ophthalmol Soc U K. 1985;104:123–8.

19. Fine HF, Spaide RF. Visualization of the posterior precortical vitreous pocket in vivo with triamcinolone. Arch Ophthalmol. 2006;124(11):1663.

20. Itakura H, Kishi S. Aging changes of vitreomacular interface. Retina. 2011;31(7):1400–4.

21. Itakura H, Kishi S. Alterations of posterior precortical vitreous pockets with positional changes. Retina. 2013;33(7):1417–20.

22. Itakura H, Kishi S, Li D, Akiyama H. Observation of posterior precortical vitreous pocket using swept-source optical coherence tomography. Invest Ophthalmol Vis Sci. 2013;54(5):3102–7.

23. Balazs EA. The vitreous. In: Zinn K, editor. Ocular fine structure for the clinician, vol. 15. Boston: Little, Brown; 1973. p. 53–63.

24. Kishi S, Hagimura N, Shimizu K. The role of the premacular liquefied pocket and premacular vitreous cortex in idiopathic macular hole development. Am J Ophthalmol. 1996;122(5):622–8.

25. Johnson MW, Van Newkirk MR, Meyer KA. Perifoveal vitreous detachment is the primary pathogenic event in idiopathic macular hole formation. Arch Ophthalmol. 2001;119(2):215–22.

26. Uchino E, Uemura A, Ohba N. Initial stages of posterior vitreous detachment in healthy eyes of older persons evaluated by optical coherence tomography. Arch Ophthalmol. 2001;119(10):1475–9.

27. Itakura H, Kishi S. Evolution of vitreomacular detachment in healthy subjects. Arch Ophthalmol. 2013;131(10):1348–52.

28. Kishi S, Demaria C, Shimizu K. Vitreous cortex remnants at the fovea after spontaneous vitreous detachment. Int Ophthalmol. 1986;9(4):253–60.

29. Kishi S, Shimizu K. Oval defect in detached posterior hyaloid membrane in idiopathic preretinal macular fibrosis. Am J Ophthalmol. 1994;118(4):451–6.

30. Kishi S, Shimizu K. Clinical manifestations of posterior precortical vitreous pocket in proliferative diabetic retinopathy. Ophthalmology. 1993;100(2):225–9.

31. Imai M, Iijima H, Hanada N. Optical coherence tomography of tractional macular elevations in eyes with proliferative diabetic retinopathy. Am J Ophthalmol. 2001;132:81–4.

32. Spaide RF, Wong D, Fisher Y, Goldbaum M. Correlation of vitreous attachment and foveal deformation in early macular hole states. Am J Ophthalmol. 2002;133(2):226–9.

33. Balazs EA, Flood MT. Data first presented at 3rd International Congress for Eye Research, Osaka, Japan. In: Sebag J, editor. The vitreous. New York: Springer; 1989. p. 81.

34. Foos RY, Wheeler NC. Vitreoretinal juncture. Synchysis senilis and posterior vitreous detachment. Ophthalmology. 1982;89(12):1502–12.

35. Sebag J. The vitreous. New York: Springer; 1989. p. 41, 76, 78, 79, 85.

36. Itakura H, Kishi S, Kotajima N, Murakami M. Decreased vitreal hyaluronan levels with aging. Ophthalmologica. 2009;223(1):32–5.

37. Itakura H, Kishi S. Vitreous cortex splitting in cases of vitreomacular traction syndrome. Ophthalmic Surg Lasers Imaging. 2012;43:e27–9.

38. Sebag J. Anomalous posterior vitreous detachment: a unifying concept in vitreo-retinal disease. Graefes Arch Clin Exp Ophthalmol. 2004;242(8):690–8.

39. Sanna G, Nervi I. Statistical research on vitreal changes in relation to age and refraction defects. Ann Ottalmol Clin Ocul. 1965;91(5):322–35.

40. Novak MA, Welch RB. Complications of acute symptomatic posterior vitreous detachment. Am J Ophthalmol. 1984;97(3):308–14.

41. Akiba J. Prevalence of posterior vitreous detachment in high myopia. Ophthalmology. 1993;100(9):1384–8.

42. Pickett-Seltner RL, Doughty MJ, Pasternak JJ, Sivak JG. Proteins of the vitreous humor during experimentally induced myopia. Invest Ophthalmol Vis Sci. 1992;33(12):3424–9.

43. Wallman J, Adams JI. Developmental aspects of experimental myopia in chicks: susceptibility, recovery and relation to emmetropization. Vis Res. 1987;27(7):1139–63.

44. Seko Y, Shimokawa H, Pang J, Tokoro T. Disturbance of electrolyte balance in vitreous of chicks with form-deprivation myopia. Jpn J Ophthalmol. 2000;44(1):15–9.

45. Newman EA. Regional specialization of retinal glial cell membrane. Nature. 1984;309(5964):155–7.

46. Spaide RF, Fisher Y. Removal of adherent cortical vitreous plaques without removing the internal limiting membrane in the repair of macular detachments in highly myopic eyes. Retina. 2005;25(3):290–5.

Ultra-widefield Imaging of Vitreous in Pathologic Myopia

14

Hiroyuki Takahashi and Kyoko Ohno-Matsui

14.1 Introduction: 'In Vivo' Widefield Vitreous Imaging

14.1.1 Ultrasonography

B-mode ultrasonography (US) can demonstrate structural changes in vitreous humor. The vitreous compartment appears as a uniformly sonolucent cavity with no internal sound reflections. The vitreoretinal interface forms a smooth, concave curvature. Ultrasonography provides information of vitreous which is unhindered by opaque media with advantage of the penetration [1, 2]. Also, US imaging allows real-time visualization of vitreal motion in response to saccades. Recent studies address quantitative analysis of vitreous echodensities for diagnostics and clinical decision-making [3].

14.1.2 Optical Coherence Tomography

Optical coherence tomography (OCT) has revolutionized clinical observation of the vitreoretinal disorders since its introduction by Huang et al. in 1991 [4]. The clinically available spectral-domain (SD) or swept source OCT instruments provide three-dimensional (3D) image of posterior vitreous of approximately 30 degrees with high resolution [5–7]. On the other hand, this modality has been used infrequently in the peripheral retina because of limited quality of the images.

Previous investigators obtained widefield OCT images using photo-editing software to montage together individual OCT images [8–10]. Tsukahara et al. reported age-dependent development of posterior vitreous detachment (PVD) using this technique [9]. In these studies, a montage approach is able to produce a single OCT image from equator to equator.

Choudhry et al. reported OCT images of far periphery fundus including vitreous base steering SD-OCT instrument. Although this technique is limited by poor gaze fixation and pupil dilation, and media opacities, the detailed anatomic information of the peripheral retina and vitreous is well depicted [11].

14.1.3 Prototype Widefield Optical Coherence Tomography Instrument

To overcome limited image quality and increased image editing time, widefield OCT systems have been developed and applied in previous studies [12–14]. McNabb et al. obtained a retinal image at macular and peripheral area within a single volume acquisition using swept source OCT systems. The authors suggested that swept source OCT has advantage to gain a large number of A scan for widefield view, compared to SD-OCT [14].

Takahashi et al. examined the posterior vitreous using ultra-widefield swept source OCT (UWF-OCT) which light source is a tunable laser (Canon Corp., Tokyo, Japan) [15]. The A scan repetition rate was 100,000 Hz. With the range of 23 mm and the depth of 5 mm, the posterior vitreous was clearly visualized on UWF-OCT images, unless its adhesion to the retinal surface is released completely (Fig. 14.1).

14.2 Ultra-widefield OCT Imaging of Vitreous in Pathologic Myopia

14.2.1 Early Posterior Vitreous Detachment

Itakura et al. evaluated the presence of partial or complete PVD in 151 highly myopic (HM) eyes and 363 healthy control eyes and reported that HM eyes with partial or complete PVD were younger than control subjects with partial or complete PVD [16]. These results were supported by the recent study in which UWF-OCT examination revealed that

H. Takahashi · K. Ohno-Matsui (✉)
Department of Ophthalmology and Visual Science, Tokyo Medical and Dental University Graduate School of Medical and Dental Sciences, Bunkyo-Ku, Tokyo, Japan
e-mail: k.ohno.oph@tmd.ac.jp

© Springer Nature Switzerland AG 2021
R. F. Spaide et al. (eds.), *Pathologic Myopia*, https://doi.org/10.1007/978-3-030-74334-5_14

Fig. 14.1 Ultra-widefield optical coherence tomographic (UWF-OCT) images of a non-highly myopic eye. Right eye of a 37-year-old woman without retinal disease. Horizontal scan image with a length of 23 mm shows paramacular posterior vitreous detachment. Premacular bursa (white arrows) and Martegiani space of Cloquet's canal (open white star) are identified on UWF-OCT image

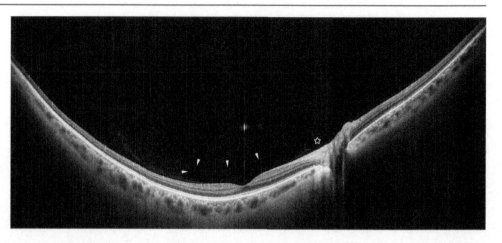

advanced forms of partial PVDs were found more frequently in HM eyes than in non-HM eyes, even though HM subjects were significantly younger than the non-HM subjects [15].

14.2.2 Asymmetrical Posterior Vitreous Detachment

Takahashi et al. investigated 9 non-HM eyes and 94 HM eyes with vitreofoveal adhesion and reported that the PVD was symmetrical in 5 eyes (56%) of the 9 non-HM eyes which was significantly higher than the 6 eyes (6%) of 94 HM eyes [15]. Thus, 88 eyes (94%) of the HM eyes had an asymmetrical PVD. Of these eyes, perifoveal PVDs were detected more frequently temporal and inferior to the fovea, and the locations of the asymmetrical PVDs corresponded to the site where the sclera was displaced most posteriorly, i.e., the regions of outpouching. These observations suggest that the asymmetrical PVDs in HM eyes may have occurred in parallel with the changes of scleral curvature.

14.2.3 Multiple and Multi-layered Posterior Vitreous Detachment

Multiple PVDs with the posterior vitreous adhered to the inner retinal surface at multiple points were observed in 15 HM eyes (9.0%) of 167 eyes (Figs. 14.2 and 14.3). The borders of the multiple PVDs corresponded to the sites of vitreous adhesions onto the retinal vessels in 11 eyes (73%) of 15 eyes. These observations suggested that the posterior vitreous moved during eye movements which would result in changing degrees of tractional force on the retinal vessels along with that on the surrounding inner retinal tissues.

In addition to the multiple PVDs, multi-layered PVDs were also observed in 12 eyes (7.2%) of 167 HM eyes. In these 12 eyes, 11 eyes had sites where the retinal vessels were lifted by the posterior vitreous cortex (Figs. 14.4 and

14.5). The pathogenesis of the multi-layered PVDs in HM still remains unclear. Considering the fact that asymmetrical PVDs were detected frequently in HM eyes, it is possible that the multi-layered PVDs were caused by anomalous PVDs. The multi-layered PVDs might be a split of the posterior vitreous cortex, described as vitreoschisis in non-HM eyes by Sebag [17].

14.2.4 Long Strands of Posterior Vitreous

In 32 eyes (19%) of 167 HM eyes, long strands of posterior vitreous were observed. These strands adhered to retinal vessels and ran a long distance anteriorly without attaching any other structures on UWF-OCT images (Fig. 14.6). Thus, these strands appeared to be floating from retinal vessels perpendicularly (Figs. 14.7 and 14.8). In 14 eyes (48%) of these 32 eyes with long strands, the retinal vessels and the retinal tissue were lifted by these strands. It seems possible that the traction on the retinal vessels by such long strand was very intense.

14.3 Relationship Between Posterior Vitreous and Retinal Vessels in Pathologic Myopia

14.3.1 Histology; Vitreo-vascular Interface

After the foetal development of the primary vitreous terminates with the formation of the lens capsule, the secondary vitreous is formed in intimate contact with retinal glial cells. As hyaloid vessels stop growing and begin to atrophy, avascular vitreous continued to be formed by retina. After birth, vitreous body and retina is divided by delicate membranes, cortical vitreous, and internal limiting membrane (ILM) of retina.

On the outer surface and within the superficial cortical layers of the vitreous, large, flat cells are observed especially

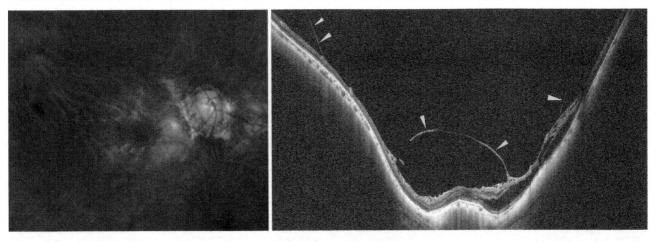

Fig. 14.2 A 58-year-old woman with pathologic myopia. Her axial length is 30.14 mm in the right eye. Colour fundus photograph shows diffuse chorioretinal atrophy in the posterior fundus, and macular involving posterior staphyloma is present. The vertical scan image of ultra-widefield optical coherence tomography shows multiple posterior vitreous detachment (yellow arrowheads). Retinal vessels are lifted up by the posterior vitreous

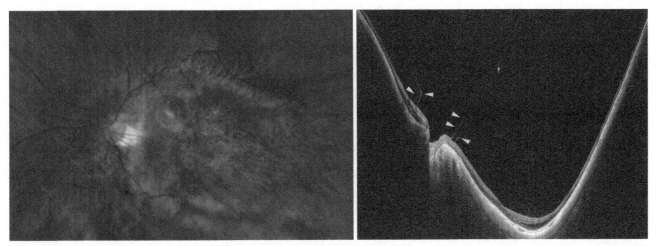

Fig. 14.3 A 76-year-old man with pathologic myopia. His axial length is 30.65 mm in the left eye. Colour fundus photograph shows tessellated fundus, and macular involving staphyloma is present. Ultra-widefield optical coherence tomography scans across the optic disc and shows multiple posterior vitreous detachment. Posterior vitreous adheres to the retina around the optic disc at multiple points (yellow arrowheads)

along the peripheral retina and near retinal vessels. On the other hand, where the retinal vessels approach the surface, the ILM is thinner than that of the other surrounding retina. These characteristics may suggest the presence of physiological and metabolic interactions between vitreous and retinal vessels [18].

14.3.2 Vitreal Adhesion to Retinal Vessels

A thickened vitreous cortex was observed in the UWF-OCT images as a hyperreflective membranous tissue. The posterior surface of the vitreous cortex was seen to be adhered to

the retinal vessels in 84 (50%) of the 167 HM eyes and in only 1 (9.1%) of 11 non-HM eyes [15]. The retinal vessels were lifted anteriorly by the posterior vitreous cortex at the sites of the adhesions. The posterior vitreous was adherent to the inner retinal surface not only at the fovea but also several points that corresponded to the retinal vessels (Fig. 14.9). The presence of strong adhesion of vitreous to retinal vessels was reported in previous studies [19–21]. Kishi et al. examined the retinal surface of autopsy eyes by scanning electron microscopy and found that glialike cells were often observed along retinal vessels [21]. Spencer et al. reported paravascular retinal rarefaction which was associated with an attached posterior vitreous [19].

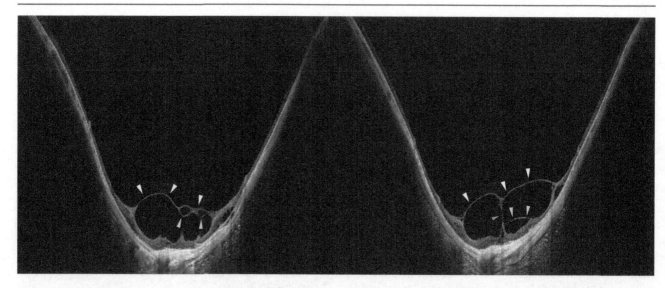

Fig. 14.4 Series of radial scan image of ultra-widefield optical coherence tomography of the right eye of a 71-year-old man with axial length of 31.88 mm. Thickened vitreous cortex is adherent to the inner retinal surface at multiple points (white arrowheads). Posterior to one layer of vitreous cortex, another layer is also seen separated from the retinal surface (yellow arrowheads). Between vitreous cortex and inner retinal surface, column-like tissue is present (light blue arrowhead)

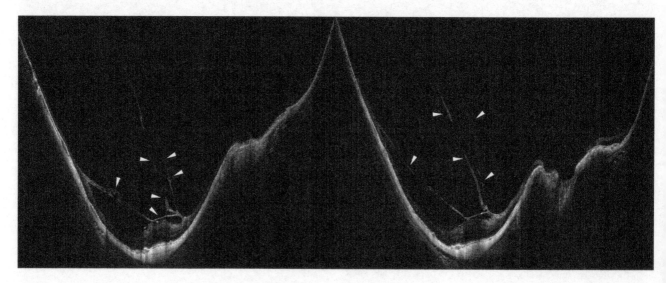

Fig. 14.5 Series of radial scan image of ultra-widefield optical coherence tomography of the right eye of a 54-year-old woman with axial length of 34.15 mm. Thickened vitreous cortex with non-uniform thickness (white arrowheads) is adherent inner surface of retina at multiple points. Vitreous cortex splits to multi-layers and separated from each other

14.3.3 Paravascular Cystic Lesion, Paravascular Lamellar Hole, and Vascular Microfold

Vascular microfolds and paravascular retinal cysts were observed in 114 (68%) and 80 (48%) in the 167 HM eyes, respectively. Paravascular lamellar holes were present in 20 (12%) of the 167 HM eyes. In some cases, a retinoschisis was observed around the lifted retinal vessels (Fig. 14.10). These results suggested that strong tractional force due to vitreoretinal adhesion on the retinal vessels may be one of the causes of paravascular abnormalities.

14.3.4 Relationship Between Posterior Vitreous and Macular Retinoschisis

Takahashi et al. investigated 54 HM eyes with macular retinoschisis (MRS) and 113 HM eyes without MRS and reported that the frequency of eyes with an adherence of the posterior vitreous to retinal vessels was higher in eyes with an MRS than without an MRS [15]. At the paravascular area, cystic lesions, lamellar holes, and retinoschisis were more commonly observed in eyes with an MRS than without an MRS (Fig. 14.11). Shimada et al. reported similar findings that paravascular lamellar holes and paravascular retinal

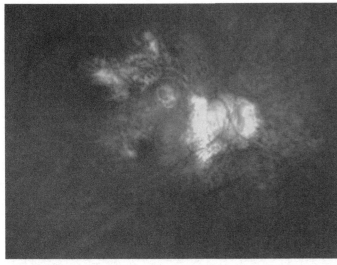

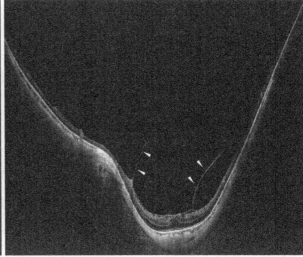

Fig. 14.6 A 55-year-old woman with severely elongated axial length. Her axial length is 32.26 mm in the right eye. Colour fundus image shows fibrous-like vitreal opacity, and chorioretinal atrophic lesions present at the paravascular and peripapillary areas. Ultra-widefield opti- cal coherence tomography shows long strands of posterior vitreous cor- tex. The strands adhere to the retinal surface and appear to be floating (white arrowheads)

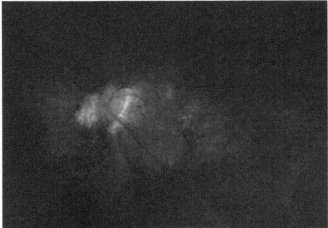

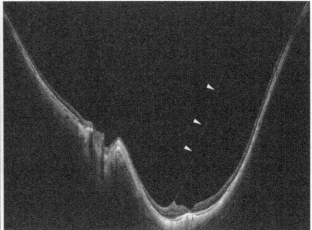

Fig. 14.7 A 55-year-old woman with pathologic myopia. Her axial length is 32.41 mm in the left eye. Colour fundus image shows diffuse chorioretinal atrophy in the posterior fundus. Ultra-widefield optical coherence tomography scans across the optic disc and shows long strand of posterior vitreous cortex. The strand appears to be floating without adhering peripheral fundus (white arrowheads)

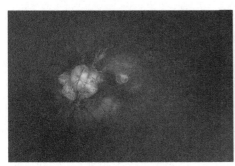

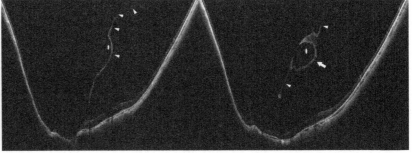

Fig. 14.8 A 53-year-old woman with pathologic myopia. Her axial length is 30.17 mm in the left eye. Colour fundus image shows enlarged optic disc and diffuse chorioretinal atrophy in the posterior fundus. Series of ultra-widefield optical coherence tomographic images shows long strand of posterior vitreous cortex floating running anteriorly from the retinal surface (white arrowheads). Ring-like structure is identified within vitreous cortex (white arrow)

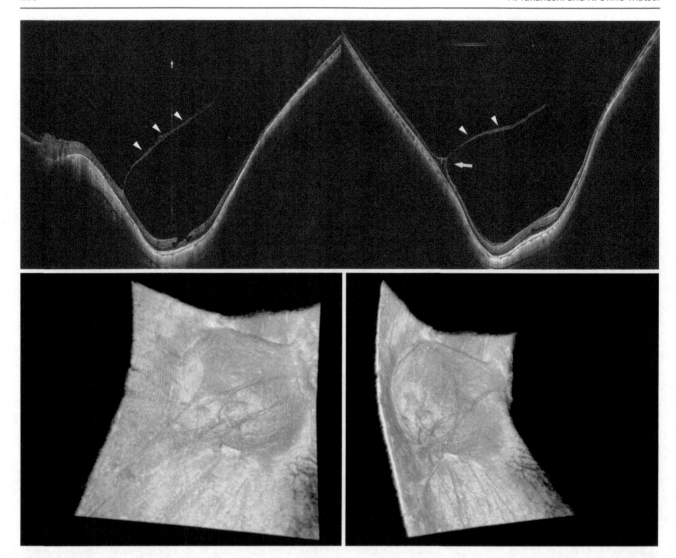

Fig. 14.9 (Top row) The horizontal scan and the vertical scan images of left eye of a 51-year-old woman with pathologic myopia. Her axial length is 30.29 mm posterior vitreous which expands above the retinal surface (white arrowheads) and adheres to retinal vessel which lifted up due to traction (yellow arrow). (Bottom row) Three-dimensional images of posterior fundus and vitreous of the patient. Posterior vitreous, which is coloured with bright purple, expands above the posterior fundus and macular staphyloma. Posterior vitreous adheres to the retinal surface at multiple points with foot-like process

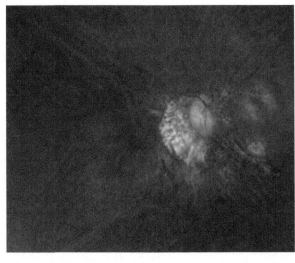
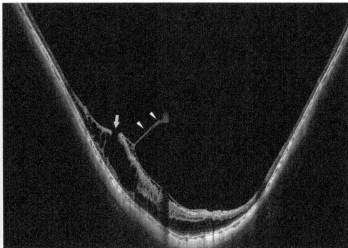

Fig. 14.10 A 63-year-old woman with myopic macular retinoschisis. Her axial length is 30.93 mm in the right eye. Colour fundus image shows tessellated fundus and tilted optic disc. Ultra-widefield OCT image shows that posterior vitreous adheres to the retinal surface (white arrowheads). Beside the site of adhesion, paravascular lamellar hole is present and accompanied with outer retinoschisis (yellow arrow)

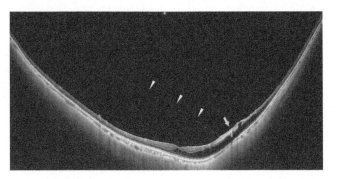

Fig. 14.11 Ultra-widefield optical coherence tomographic image of a 65-year-old man with myopic macular retinoschisis. His axial length is 28.65 mm. Myopic macular retinoschisis expands from foveal retina to the out of the macular area. Posterior vitreous (white arrowheads) detaches from the foveal retina but not from retinal vessel (yellow arrow)

cysts were found more often in eyes with MRS [22]. These studies showed that pathological vitreous changes and persistent adhesion of vitreous to retinal vessels might be the cause of intense traction on the retinal vessels which eventually results in the development of MRS.

References

1. Coleman DJ. Reliability of ocular and orbital diagnosis with B-scan ultrasound; 1. Ocular diagnosis. Am J Ophthalmol. 1972;73(4):501–16.
2. Jack RL, Hutton WL, Machemer R. Ultrasonography and vitrectomy. Am J Ophthalmol. 1974;78(2):265–74.
3. Sebag J, Silverman RH, Coleman DJ. To see the invisible: the quest of imaging vitreous. In: Sebag J, editor. Vitreous in health and disease. New York: Springer; 2014. p. 193–219.
4. Huang D, Swanson EA, Lin CP, et al. Optical coherence tomography. Science. 1991;254:1178–81.
5. Liu JJ, Witkin AJ, Adhi M, et al. Enhanced vitreous imaging in healthy eyes using swept source optical coherence tomography. PLoS One. 2014;9(7):e102950.
6. Stanga PE, Sala-Puigdollers A, Caputo S, et al. In vivo imaging of cortical vitreous using 1050-nm swept-source deep range imaging optical coherence tomography. Am J Ophthalmol. 2014;157:397–404.
7. Spaide RF. Visualization of the posterior vitreous with dynamic focusing and window averaging swept source optical coherence tomography. Am J Ophthalmol. 2014;158:1267–74.
8. Mori K, Kanno J, Gehlbach PL, et al. Montage images of spectral-domain optical coherence tomography in eyes with idiopathic macular holes. Ophthalmology. 2012;119:2600–8.
9. Tsukahara M, Mori K, Gehlbach PL, et al. Posterior vitreous detachment as observed by wide-angle OCT imaging. Ophthalmology. 2018;125(9):1372–83.
10. Gregori NZ, Lam BL, Gregori G, et al. Wide-field spectral-domain optical coherence tomography in patients and carriers of X-linked retinoschisis. Ophthalmology. 2013;120:169–74.
11. Choundhry N, Golding J, Manry MW, et al. Ultra-widefield steering-based spectral-domain optical coherence tomography imaging of the retinal periphery. Ophthalmology. 2016;123:1368–74.
12. Reznicek L, Klein T, Wieser W, et al. Megahertz ultra-wide-field swept-source retina optical coherence tomography compared to current existing imaging devices. Graefes Arch Clin Exp Ophthalmol. 2014;252:1009–16.
13. Uji A, Yoshimura N. Application of extended field imaging to optical coherence tomography. Ophthalmology. 2015;122:1272–4.
14. McNabb RP, Grewal DS, Mehta R, et al. Wide field of view swept-source optical coherence tomography for peripheral retinal disease. Br J Ophthalmol. 2016;100:1377–82.
15. Takahashi H, Tanaka N, Shinohara K, et al. Ultra-widefield optical coherence tomographic imaging of posterior vitreous in eyes with high myopia. Am J Ophthalmol. 2019;206:102–12.
16. Itakura H, Kishi S, Li D, et al. Vitreous changes in high myopia observed by enhanced vitreous imaging of spectral domain optical coherence tomography. Invest Ophthalmol Vis Sci. 2014;55(3):1447–52.

17. Sebag J. Vitreoschisis. Graefes Arch Clin Exp Ophthalmol. 2008;246:329–32.
18. Fine BS, Yanoff M. The retina. In: Ocular histology: text and atlas. 2nd ed. Hagerstown, MD: Harper & Row; 1979. p. 61–127.
19. Spencer LM, Foos RY. Paravascular vitreoretinal attachments. Role in retinal tears. Arch Ophthalmol. 1970;84:557–64.
20. Foos RY. Vitreoretinal juncture over retinal vessels. Albrecht Von Graefes Arch Klin Exp Ophthalmol. 1977;204:223–34.
21. Kishi S, Numaga T, Yoneya S, et al. Epivascular glia and paravascular holes in normal human retina. Graefes Arch Clin Exp Ophthalmol. 1986;224:124–30.
22. Shimada N, Ohno-Matsui K, Nishimuta A, et al. Detection of paravascular lamellar holes and other paravascular abnormalities by optical coherence tomography in eyes with high myopia. Ophthalmology. 2008;115:708–17.

Part III

Sequella of Pathologic Myopia and Their Potential Treatments

Staphyloma I

15

Richard F. Spaide

15.1 Historical Development of Ideas

The first description of a staphyloma was made by Antonio Scarpa, a skilled anatomist who in 1801 described two eyes from a cadaver in which the posterior portion of each eye had pronounced outward bulges [1] (Fig. 15.1). Staphylomas of the anterior segment were a recognized complication of inflammation or tumors at that time, but the posterior staphyloma seemed to be different than the anterior types. In 1830, Ammon described two eyes that had expansion of the eye in the region of the fetal fissure [2]. Similar abnormalities were described in later years occurring in the context of colobomas of the iris and lens, so the fluid-filled space, referred to as posterior staphyloma of Ammon, was probably a coloboma. Arlt made the connection between the posterior staphyloma of Scarpa and myopia [3, 4]. He noted myopic eyes had a conus, an area of absent choroid and retinal pigment epithelium. For the most part, a conus was only seen in eyes with myopia, although it was known that emmetropic and even hyperopic eyes could have a conus. Following the discovery by Arlt, myopia and staphyloma were thought to be synonymous, with myopia being secondary to the staphyloma. The presence of a staphyloma was inferred to be present in myopic eyes by seeing the presence of a conus. (This was at a time when there was not widespread use of binocular ophthalmoscopy.) Arlt reasoned the conus was the result of atrophy of the choroid but seemed to have a harder time trying to determine the retinal abnormalities that accompanied the conus. Arlt knew that eyes with a conus had a larger blind spot and therefore must have had a localized absence of light-sensitive cells. Other competing ideas were a conus was due to inflammation or was congenital.

Through extensive analysis of myopic eyes, Tscherning in 1883 determined many eyes with myopia that did not have a staphyloma [5]. In 1898, Schnabel [6] reviewed the published cases and added additional new information. He found staphylomas only in eyes with greater than 8 diopters of myopic refractive error. These eyes nearly always had a conus, although a conus could frequently be found in eyes with less than 8 diopters of myopic refractive error. Schnabel thought the conus was present from early in life, but with ocular expansion due to growth and myopia became increasingly evident. The divergence in the early ideas about the conus carried through to ideas of how staphyloma formed. One was that atrophy of the choroid along with "the strain of near work" produced a staphyloma in an otherwise normal eye [7]. A second line of reasoning was the sclera was abnormal due to defective development and later stretched to cause a staphyloma. Another hypothesis was localized inflammation caused anterior staphyloma as well. However, Knowles discredited this idea by noting a lack of objective signs of inflammation in most of these eyes [8]. The definition of a staphyloma was codified over time. An ectasia was an outpouching of the wall of the eye without uveal tissue. A staphyloma was an outpouching of an eye with associated uveal tissue. These definitions continue to have weaknesses in that in advanced stages of myopic degeneration, the choroid within the region of the staphyloma can appear to completely regress leaving what is called chorioretinal atrophy. Despite the absence of uveal tissue, the area is still called a staphyloma.

15.2 Classification

Curtin greatly expanded the clinical understanding of staphyloma formation in myopes [9, 10]. Curtin divided the ophthalmoscopic appearance of a group of 250 patients with staphylomas into 10 different patterns (Fig. 15.2). The first five were posterior outpouchings, which Curtin called simple staphylomas, and involved the macula and optic nerve region or were centered on the macula, directly over the optic disc, nasal to the optic disc, or inferior to the optic disc

R. F. Spaide (✉)
Vitreous, Retina, Macula Consultants of New York, New York, NY, USA

R. F. Spaide et al. (eds.), *Pathologic Myopia*, https://doi.org/10.1007/978-3-030-74334-5_15

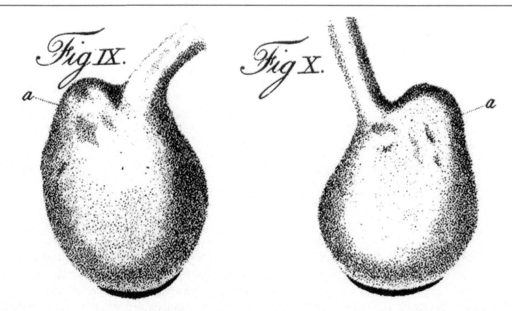

Fig. 15.1 From Scarpa [1]: "…I have twice happened to meet with the staphyloma of the sclerotic coat in its posterior hemisphere, in the dead subject, where I do not know that it has been seen or described by any other. The first time was in an eye taken from the body of a woman 40 years old, for another purpose. [In reference to Figure IX.] This eye was of an oval figure, and upon the whole, larger than the found one of the opposite eye. On the posterior hemisphere of this eye, and on the external side of the entrance of the optic nerve, or on the part corresponding to the temple of that side, the sclerotic was elevated in the form of an oblong tumor of the size of a small nut. [In reference to Figure IX, a.] When the posterior hemisphere of the eye was immersed in spirit of wine, with a few drops of nitrous acid added to it, in order to give the retina consistence and opacity, I could perceive distinctly that there was a deficiency of the nervous expansion of the retina within the cavity of the staphyloma; that the choroid coat was very thin and discolored at this part and wanted its usual vascular plexus; and that the sclerotic, particularly at the apex of the staphyloma, was rendered so thin as scarcely to equal the thickness of writing paper. I knew that the woman from whom the eye had been taken had lost the faculty of seeing on the side some years before, during an obstinate ophthalmia, attended with a most acute and almost habitual pain in the head." Figure X in the same text was from an eye contributed to Scarpa

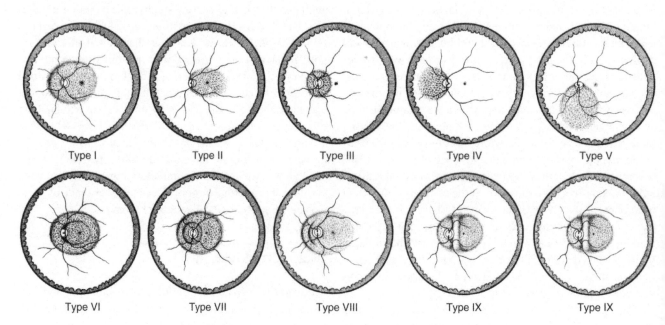

Fig. 15.2 Curtin classified the staphylomas he found in myopes into ten categories. The first five were simpler configurations, while the last five were either more intricate in their configuration

[10]. Curtin showed the inferior staphyloma to be associated with a tilted optic disc, a condition that will be described in greater detail. However, other staphyloma types may also be associated with a tilted disc appearance. The remaining five were termed compound staphylomas, and these appeared to be composites of more than one type of staphyloma or were an elaboration from simple staphylomas. For example, a Type VI staphyloma is a combination of a Type I, a staphyloma over the posterior pole along with a Type II staphyloma, which is one centered on the macula. This creates a two-tiered depression. A Type IX staphyloma are two adjacent staphylomas, one principally involving the disc and the second the macula. Many of these types of staphyloma can be associated with a tilted disc, although this was not mentioned. The Curtin classification is not exhaustive of all types of staphyloma. Many of the eyes imaged by Moriyama and associates with high-resolution magnetic resonance imaging (MRI) and 3D rendering had staphyloma configurations not anticipated by Curtin [11]. The classification scheme a landmark though, because it implicitly considered a staphyloma to be a particular anatomic configuration in the context of the overall structure of the eye. Whereas Arlt considered the staphyloma to be myopia, and vice versa, Curtin's classification highlighted the specific structural abnormalities that sometimes could be seen in eyes with increasing amounts of myopia.

The distinction of a staphyloma as being a separate sequela of myopia as opposed to being an integral part of myopia is not universally accepted. It is still common for authors to refer to abnormalities in the posterior pole of myopic eyes, even ones that do not involve outpouching, as being staphylomas [12]. The curvature of the posterior pole of the eye in high myopes has been called a posterior staphyloma without evidence being shown that there was an alteration in the generalized curvature of the eye or any semblance of an outpouching [13]. Part of the confusion is related to how the axial length of the eye may increase as a consequence of a staphyloma. In that case, the incremental exaggeration in the refractive error of the eye is due to the increase in axial length caused by the staphyloma. Much of the confusion concerning staphylomas is due to the lack of an unambiguous and detailed definition for staphyloma beyond the rather nebulous concept of a "posterior outpouching" of the eye.

Curtin used ophthalmoscopy and fundus drawings to classify the staphyloma types, while other studies employed color fundus photographs or a combination of ultrasonography and indirect ophthalmoscopy. Curtin found that the most common type of staphyloma involved the posterior pole in general, causing an outpouching of the region encompassing the nerve and macula. This staphyloma type accounted for approximately one-half of all staphylomas seen in a series of 250 affected patients [10]. Curtin's Type II staphyloma, which is centered on the macula, was the second most com-

mon type seen in patients aged 3–19 years but became less common in older individuals. More complex forms of staphyloma seen in older patients were Type VIII through Type X. Type VIII is a combination of a Type I and a Type II. It is possible that the peculiar anatomy of the scleral collagen fibers affects the configuration observed. In the posterior portion of the eye, some of the scleral fibers form annular rings around the scleral opening for the nerve. It is possible that selective alteration of the scleral fibers could allow some of the annular fibers to remain relatively unaffected, thus producing a septum in the middle of what would have been a larger Type II staphyloma to produce a Type IX staphyloma. A Type X staphyloma is a modification of a Type II, but with a shallow temporal border and an incomplete border around the optic nerve.

The staphylomatous process results in a localized thinning of structures in the posterior pole and potentially increases the likelihood of ocular abnormalities. In reality, the abnormalities seen in high myopes is highly correlated with axial length but may be exaggerated in posterior staphylomas. There are some types of staphyloma that confer special risk for ocular abnormalities, and these will be discussed later.

15.3 Prevalence of Staphyloma

The prevalence of staphylomas in highly myopic eyes could be expected to vary based on the composition of the group being evaluated in regard to axial length and method of patient recruitment. Patients being randomly selected from a pool of high myopes may have a different proportion of staphylomas than a group attending an eye clinic. The method of detecting staphylomas highly influences what is considered a staphyloma. Curtin and Karlin used ophthalmoscopy to examine eyes, but did not state what they considered a staphyloma to be [10]. Hsiang et al. used ultrasonography to evaluate eyes; they measured the depth of the eye posterior to the optic nerve [14]. This method axiomatically considers eyes with staphylomas only involving the optic nerve to have no staphyloma, since in these eyes the optic nerve is the most posterior part of the eye. In an eye with a spherical shape and the fovea in the optic axis, the fovea would by default be posterior to the optic nerve. Therefore, a normal eye would be considered to have a staphyloma, albeit small, using this methodology.

Estimates of staphyloma prevalence therefore are more of a guide than an absolute. Curtin and Karlin found the prevalence increased dramatically with elongated axial length. Curtin and Karlin determined the prevalence of posterior staphyloma increased from 1.4% in eyes 26.5–27.4 mm to 71.4% in eyes having an axial length from 33.5 to 36.6 mm. The mix of the type of staphyloma varied with age. Younger eyes had a predominance of simple forms, with staphylomas involving either the entire posterior pole or just the macular region accounting for nearly all staphylomas seen. In older eyes the proportion of more complex staphylomas increased. Hsiang et al. using ultrasonography determined staphylomas were present in 90% of a group of 209 eyes with high myopia. They too found the complexity of staphylomas increased with advancing patient age [14].

15.4 Proposed Nomenclature

A highly myopic eye may have shape distortion where the curvature of the eye deviates from the flattened sphere seen in emmetropes without having a staphyloma. The barrel-type shape as described by Moriyama and coauthors based on 3D MRI is an example of a shape distortion that does not necessarily have staphyloma formation. A staphyloma can be given a formal definition of an outpouching of the wall of the eye that has a radius of less than the surrounding curvature of the wall of the eye (Fig. 15.3). A simple staphyloma is a region that has only one radius of curvature. A complex staphyloma is an expansion that has two distinct radii of curvature with a total or partial overlap in the curves. A compound staphyloma is present when there are two or more separate outpouchings that are not concentric. Thus, what Curtin called a Type VII coloboma, which is a staphyloma around the optic nerve embedded in a staphyloma involving the posterior pole, would be considered a complex staphyloma. The Type IX, which is two staphylomas side by side, would be a compound staphyloma. As shown in Fig. 15.4, it is relatively easy to find staphylomas

that don't fit into Curtin's classification system. As such, a description of the staphylomas using this proposed nomenclature would prove to be more accurate. Many of the eyes shown by Moriyama et al. appear to have compound staphylomas in arrangements not anticipated by the Curtin classification. This proposed nomenclature avoids the problem of merging the idea of pathologic myopia with that of a staphyloma.

15.5 Etiology

The enigma of the staphyloma is wrapped in the mystery of myopia. The ocular shape experiments in animal models of emmetropization show the eye is capable of local reaction to defocus [15–24]. An error signal appears to be created, and the eye is capable of responding by regional growth changes to minimize the error signal [17, 24]. The defocus induced can arbitrarily be selected by using eyeglass lenses to induce a compensatory hyperopia or myopia. This implies that the amount and direction of the error signal are correctly interpreted in the response by the eye [24]. Removing the lens inducing a refractive shift from the eye of a chick results in a recovery of the eye with reduction or elimination of the induced refractive error. Obscuring vision in the growing eye sets off a related series of events that leads to myopia formation. In this situation, the emmetropization process seems to be clamped into producing one of the two potential extremes, myopia.

In animal models, there appear to be two main modalities at play in ocular adaptation to defocus. In bird, there can be a large change in the thickness of the choroid. The increase in thickness is accomplished with the aid of the lymphatic

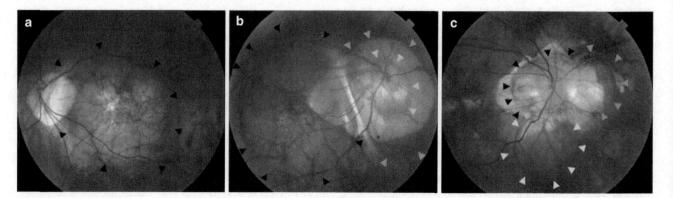

Fig. 15.3 Three different configurations of staphyloma are shown (**a**) A staphyloma involving the macula region with its nasal border abutting the optic nerve. This would probably be close to what Curtin called a Type II staphyloma, but note that the optic nerve is tilted in this case. The posterior pole shows generic effects of the staphyloma; there is thinning of the choroid that is more pronounced in the staphyloma with overlying pigmentary changes. (**b**) The patient appears to have two staphylomas adjacent to each other (black and green arrowheads) and therefore would be most similar to a Type IX staphyloma as described by Curtin. However, close inspection reveals another staphyloma (light blue arrowheads) contained in the staphyloma around the nerve (green arrowheads). (**c**) This patient has three adjacent staphylomas (black, green, and yellow arrowheads) and therefore does not resemble any of the staphyloma types described by Curtin

Fig. 15.4 Proposed nomenclature for staphylomas. (**a**) Normal eye shape. (**b**) Axial expansion occurring in the equatorial region that does not induce any altered curvature in the posterior aspect of the eye. The eye would have axial myopia and no staphyloma. (**c**) A second curvature of the eye occurs in the posterior portion of the eye, and this second curvature (r_2) has a smaller radius of curvature than the surrounding eye wall (r_1). This additional curvature is a staphyloma because there is only one; it is considered to be a simple staphyloma. (**d**) Some eyes have a second staphyloma in the first and are considered to have a complex staphyloma. Note the two secondary radii, r_2 and r_3. (**e**) Other eyes have more than one non-associated secondary curvatures and are considered to have a compound staphyloma

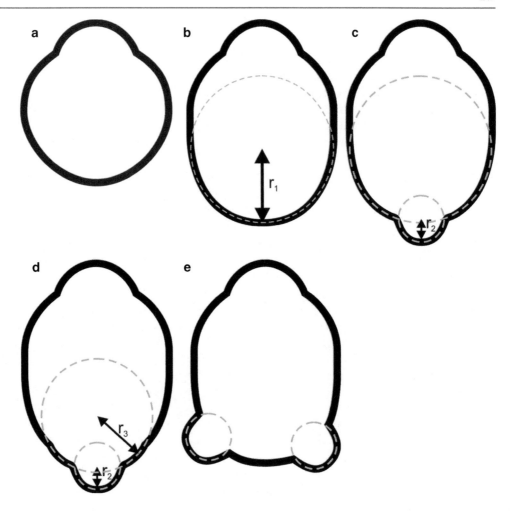

system found in bird eyes [25]. Myopization is associated with decreased choroidal blood flow and potential for choriocapillaris changes even in the short term [26, 27]. Humans, of course, have no lymphatic system, but defocus can induce a small change in the thickness of the choroid as determined by optical low-coherence reflectometry [28]. Longer-term alterations in emmetropization are related to increase in axial length caused by expansion of the eye. The sclera undergoes remodeling and thinning and develops increased elasticity. Animal models with optically imposed defocus in one hemifield produced alteration in the size of that hemifield in particular [29, 30]. This suggests there are mechanisms that afford local and selective control of eye growth and refractive development. Subsequently the role of the entire retina in producing axial lengthening was studied. Interestingly, foveal ablation in the monkey followed by form deprivation still causes myopia with increased axial length [31]. Relative peripheral hyperopic defocus causes axial length changes, leading to the suggestion that peripheral optical approaches may be a potential strategy in the prevention and treatment of myopia [18, 32].

The major component of the sclera is Type I collagen. These form fibrils that provide structural strength of the eye. There is a gradient in scleral fibril size from the inner to outer sclera, and this gradient follows the development of the sclera, which progresses from the inner side to the outer surface. In high myopes, there is a decrease in the dry weight of collagen as compared with emmetropes, and the fibril diameter is decreased as well. The sclera of high myopes does not show the typical gradient of fibril diameters, as all of the fibrils are small in diameter. This change is most evident in the posterior portion of the eye, even in the absence of a staphyloma [33, 34]. There are decreased glycosaminoglycans as compared with emmetropic eyes as well. In animal models of myopia, the changes in the sclera, manifested by scleral thinning, is the result of a loss of tissue and stretching. The thinning of the sclera, along with some increase in elasticity, [35] results in increased stretching (strain) for any given stretch (stress). By La Place's law, the stress on the sclera can be estimated by $\delta = PR/2\ T$, where δ is the stress, P the intraocular pressure, R the radius, and T the wall thickness. In high myopes, the wall stress increases with expansion of the eye and decreased wall thickness.

In most adults, the refractive error and axial length remain stable over time. In high myopes, a subset of the population, both axial length and refractive error, can increase over time, even in adults [36, 37]. While there may be some weak genetic influence for the development of high myopia, for the most part, this disorder appears to be inducible in susceptible populations. This is evidenced by epidemiologic studies showing near work and lack of outdoor activities being the strongest risk factors, by the appearance of myopia in agrarian and hunting populations that began schooling, and by animal experimentation [38–48]. This implies there is a change in highly myopic eyes that confers increased risk for progressive changes in the architecture of the sclera, not only during phases of rapid growth, such as in late childhood, but much later in life. Given that emmetropization appears to involve local control, it is possible that regional defocus of images could cause regional alterations in scleral growth and mechanical properties. Outdoor activities involve distances that are generally greater than 1 meter from the observer. That means a range of refractive differences that at most can be 1 diopter. In the bright illumination of sunlight, small pupil sizes lead to an increased depth of field, reducing the defocus of images even more. On the other hand, the range of distances from the eye varies substantially indoors; some objects may be centimeters away, while others are meters away. These distances range across a large breadth of diopters. Illumination levels are lower indoors, and the spectral composition of light may be more myopigenic [49]. In this case, it is easily possible that regions of the eye can be in focus, while other areas are defocused. Indeed, one of the strongest factors related to global expansion is the amount of peripheral, not central, refractive error. Results of animal models strongly implicate image defocus in the response of regional adaptive mechanisms in the eye. The influence that prolonged defocus of images has on the development of staphylomas in humans is not known. However, in animals, defocus is a commonly used method to cause myopia. If this same pathogenic mechanism exists in humans, localized defocus could cause regional expansion of the eye. It is possible that various regions of the eye wall have varying susceptibility to ocular expansion in the adult human eye leading to nonuniform expansion.

A second but related possibility is that choroidal abnormalities may play a role in the development of nonuniform expansion of the eye [50]. This intriguing possibility is suggested by the observation of rapid and profound ocular expansion with the development of high myopia in an adult following resolution of Vogt-Kayanagi-Harada disease in which there was marked thinning of the choroid seen. The scleral composition and shape has been theorized to be controlled in part by the choroid. In the development of high myopia, the choroid becomes quite thin and in some

regions disappears altogether. Any potential mechanisms involved in maintenance of ocular shape and size could potentially be altered.

15.6 Special Problems in High Myopes That Can Be Attributed to Staphylomas

The stretching of the ocular layers in a staphyloma is locally exaggerated within a staphyloma. The adverse effects of any stretching may therefore be worsened within the confines of the staphyloma. The change in contour of the eye wall may also cause potential abnormalities if the inflection point is somewhere near the macula. This is exactly what happens in a Type V staphyloma, also known as an inferior staphyloma or as tilted-optic disc syndrome.

Type V staphylomas are unusual in that the center of the macula can be bisected by the change in curvature of the upper edge of the staphyloma. The superior half is less distended than the inferior portion. The nerve is usually at the border of the staphyloma and has a tilted appearance. This has led to two different names for this structural configuration: inferior staphyloma or tilted optic disc syndrome, which was the first term used to describe the disorder [51–63]. There are numerous abnormalities described in association with this particular staphyloma. The inflection of the curve of the eye wall to the staphyloma has been associated with a band of decreased pigmentation extending in an arcuate manner along the upper edge of the staphyloma [61]. Some eyes show more complicated pigmentary patterns. The underlying choroid is thin and the sclera under that is thickened as compared with nearby areas. It is not uncommon for these eyes to have subretinal fluid 54. There are numerous potential theories as to the origin of the fluid: the atrophy of the retinal pigment epithelium may decrease its pumping function, or the scleral thickness may impede the uveal-scleral outflow there [63]. Some patients seem to have leaks seen during fluorescein angiography consistent with central serous chorioretinopathy, which is distinctly uncommon in high myopes. Some authors have proposed that the subretinal fluid caused the observed retinal pigment epithelial changes [63]. Tilted disc syndrome has been associated with an uneven distribution of drusen in which the superior portion had more drusen than the inferior more myopic aspect [58]. Polypoidal choroidal vasculopathy has been described in several eyes with tilted disc syndrome [56, 57]. Typical choroidal neovascularization, including cases with many foci, has been reported in these eyes [53]. It is possible that the region of the change of curvature has numerous microbreaks of Bruch's membrane, vascular stresses induced by the curvature, and scleral thickening and permeability changes. Eyes with tilted disc syndrome commonly have superior visual field defects, which can be ameliorated by changing the refraction used while measuring the visual field [59]. This appears to be related to the disparity in axial length, although there may be neurogenic or retinal contributions to the field defect in some patients.

15.7 Localized Retinal Detachment Over a Staphyloma

The exaggerated effects of thinning and curvature of the eye can induce local effects in the staphyloma (see Fig. 15.3a). The more subtle effects of decreasing choroidal thickness on visual acuity may come into play within a staphyloma if the choroidal thickness is severely compromised. The outpouching of the eye also causes the surface area occupied within that region to be greater than what it would have been for structures lining the wall of the eye. For example, the retina is stretched over a larger area increasing the stress on the retina, which is elastic to a certain extent. Because of the curvature of the eye, and of the staphyloma, the forces generated by the retina can be resolved into vectors acting in the plane of the retina and perpendicularly inward from the retina (Fig. 15.4). This second vector has the propensity to lift the retina from the back wall of the eye. Any local traction on the retina through the epiretinal membrane or remnants of attached vitreous would increase this vector. Counteracting this vector would be the normal forces maintaining attachment. These include the pumping by the RPE and the normal vector of flow from the vitreous to the choroid [64]. The vector of forces directed perpendicularly inward can begin to exceed the tensile strength of the retina or the force of retinal attachment. This can lead to retinoschisis or retinal detachment, respectively. Surgical repair of the induced problems can include vitrectomy with removal of the plaque of vitreous alone or with removal of the internal limiting membrane (Figs. 15.5 and 15.6) [64].

15.8 Ocular Alignment Problems

Ocular alignment is related to precise interrelationships between the action of the extraocular muscles, the eye, and neural control. In conventional analysis of the eye motion, the contractile forces of the extraocular muscles are assumed to act on a spherical eyeball. The highly myopic eye often is not spherical because of nonuniform expansion. More complete coverage of strabismus in highly myopic patients occurs in another chapter, but germane to this chapter is the interaction between staphylomas and ocular motion. High-resolution magnetic resonance imaging of 21 consecutive myopic patients in a study by Demer has defined some of the factors that may be involved in problems with ocular alignment [65]. Most of the eyes were not spherical and demonstrated diffuse posterior, equatorial, or combined posterior and equatorial staphylomata. The staphylomata had the potential to act as cams during eye motion in which the effective lever arm moving the eye varied with gaze and staphyloma characteristic. The staphylomas could cause large displacements of the extraocular muscle paths.

15.9 Visual Field Abnormalities

Nonuniform ocular enlargement can lead to defocus of images in staphylomatous regions. The light encountered during a visual field test would be spread out over a larger area, decreasing the likelihood of detection [66]. The regions inside or along the edge of the a staphyloma may have marked thinning of the choroid, which may also affect threshold sensitivity [67]. Abnormalities in visual field testing may occur because of schisis, detachment, or potentially from the Stiles Crawford effect within a staphyloma. A patient with binasal staphylomas presented with bitemporal visual field defects [68].

15.10 Dome-Shaped Macula and Allied Disorders

Gaucher and colleagues described a new entity in eyes with high myopia [12]. The central portion of the macula appeared to bow inward, unlike typical staphylomas in high myopia in which staphylomas bow outward. They called the disorder dome-shaped macula in eyes with myopic staphyloma. The authors proposed that there was localized thickening of the choroid as a possible explanation. They did not demonstrate any outpouching of the eye, an axiomatic finding required to make the diagnosis of a staphyloma. Later in a letter to the editor, two additional possibilities were suggested, the first was the dome shape was due to vitreous traction and the second was there really was collapse of the posterior portion of the eye such that the sclera bowed inward [69]. The hypothesis that there was vitreous traction was not borne out by any of the OCTs, and the eyes with dome-shaped macula have normal intraocular pressure, making eye collapse highly implausible. Imamura and associates examined a group of 15 patients (23 eyes) with dome-shaped macula with EDI OCT. [70] The mean age of the patients was 59.3 years, and the mean refractive error was −13.6 diopters. The mean subfoveal scleral thickness in 23 eyes with dome-shaped macula was 570 μm and that in 25 eyes of myopic patients with staphyloma but without dome-shaped macula was 281 μm ($P < 0.001$) even though both groups had similar refractive error. The scleral thickness 3000 μm temporal to the fovea was not different in the eyes with dome-shaped macula, 337 μm as compared to the eyes without dome-shaped macula, 320 μm. Dome-shaped macula appears to be the result of regional thickness differences of the sclera in highly myopic

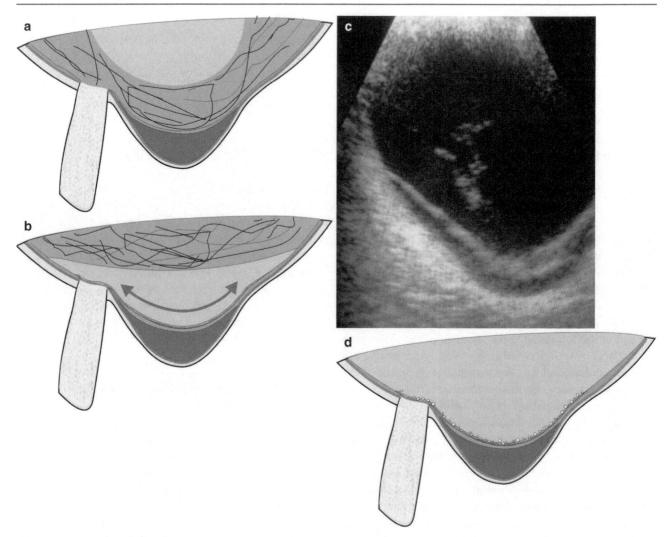

Fig. 15.5 The posterior extent of the sclera and choroid bulge backwards in a staphyloma. The forces leading to attachment include the net vector of flow that goes from the vitreous to the choroid and the pumping effect by the retinal pigment epithelium. The forces that lead to detachment include traction by the attached vitreous (**a**) or even adherent plaques of vitreous (**b**) after posterior vitreous detachment. The natural elasticity of the retina also is an important factor. The retina is usually taut across the staphyloma with the apparent forces in the plane of the retina (double arrow in b). This force can be resolved into 2 vectors, including one that is perpendicular to the retina leading to the center of the eye. (**c**) An illustrative contact B-scan ultrasound is shown of an eye with a localized detachment in a staphyloma. (**d**) Removal of vitreous traction can include using triamcinolone (shown as white crystals on the surface of the vitreous) and possible removal of the internal limiting membrane as well

eyes, and it does not corespond to any of the known types of staphyloma described (Fig. 15.6). As part of emmetropization and myopization, there are alterations in scleral and choroidal thickness. Regional variations in defocus can lead to compensatory changes in axial length and inverse changes in the thickness of the choroid and sclera. It is possible that during activities such as reading images, the central macula are relatively sharp, while the more peripheral areas are defocused. It is possible that the regional focus in the central macula and defocus in the areas outside of the macula could lead to adaptive effects that create the dome-shaped macula phenotype [70].

Additional reports of dome-shaped macula expanded the understanding of the phenotype and led to discovery of other related configurations. Errera and coworkers [71] reported

that DSM was associated with many inherited retinal disorders. In their series, 81% of eyes with DSM had myopia. The authors stated that their findings in highly myopic eyes supported the theory that DSM formation may be an adaptive mechanism to minimize defocus in the macula, much the same as proposed by Imamura and associates. In their series, a central serous-like phenotype was seen in 32.7% of the eyes, and these eyes did not have increased choroidal thickness as compared with what is typically seen in eyes with central serous chorioretinopathy. Viola and associates [72] reviewed longitudinal imaging results of 52 highly myopic eyes with DSM. Although serous detachment was seen in 44% of the cases without macular neovascularization, these eyes did not show hyperpermeability with indocyanine green

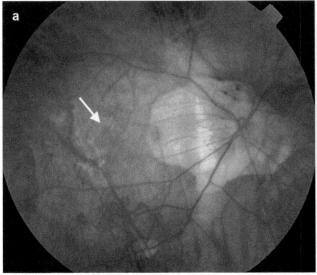
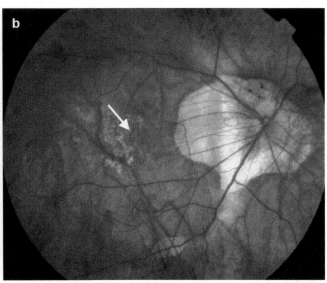

Fig. 15.6 (**a**) This patient has a shallow detachment of the retina over a staphyloma. Note the lack of visibility of the underlying choroidal details

(arrow). (**b**) After vitrectomy and flattening of the retina, the visual acuity improved. Note the increased visibility of the underlying details (arrow)

angiography, which is the hallmark of central serous chorioretinopathy. The eyes did have hyperfluorescent punctate spots during ICG angiography. Close examination of the OCT scans in the paper suggest some, but not all of these patients had macular neovascularization.

Alterations in the contour of the macula, along with the potential to have either subretinal fluid accumulation or the development of neovascularization, include more than just inferior staphyloma and DSM. There are eyes that seem to have a melding of inferior staphyloma and DSM. Other eyes may show varying amounts of inward protrusion of the macula as compared with the surrounding sclera according to the meridian evaluated [73]. In vertical DSM, the alteration in curvature appears to be greater than in the horizontal meridian. In less common circumstances, the opposite may be observed in which the horizontal meridian shows a larger amount of curvature variation than does the vertical meridian. Some eyes appear to have one or more ridges that course in a horizontal meridian [74, 75].

There has been variation in reports concerning the appearance of subretinal fluid in eyes with DSM. García-Ben and coworkers [76] evaluated 40 highly myopic eyes of 21 patients in Spain with vertical DSM and found 11 (27.5%) had subretinal fluid. The significant variables associated with the appearance of fluid were macular bulge height and reduced choroidal thickness. Ohno-Matsui and colleagues [77] evaluated 91 highly myopic eyes in 67 consecutive patients and found serous detachment in 5 (5.5%). Macula bulge height and subfoveal choroidal thickness were not associated with subretinal fluid. Errera et al. [71] found subretinal fluid in 19 (32.8%) of 58 eyes in 36 patients with DSM. They found that the subfoveal choroidal thickness in eyes with subretinal fluid was significantly greater than in

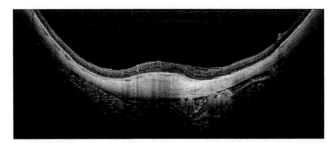

Fig. 15.7 This is a 12 mm scan obtained with a swept source optical coherence tomography instrument of a patient with a domeshaped macula. Note that lack of any 'outpouching' of the eye, meaning there was no demonstrated staphyloma. However the posterior sclera was thicker than the more peripheral portions, although both the subfoveal and peripheral wall were thinner than an emmetrope

eyes with no fluid. Hocaoglu and colleagues [73] examined 167 eyes with DSM in 90 patients in Turkey and found serous retinal detachment in 7.8% of eyes. Serous detachment was found to be associated with increased choroidal thickness and increased macular bulge height. These disparate results suggest there may be other variables to consider, such as race, amount of myopia or axial expansion, coexistent medical diagnoses, the configuration of the dome, integrity of Bruch's membrane, and thickness of the scleral under the dome (Fig. 15.7).

The inward bulging of the sclera may cause secondary changes in the overlying structures that may have pathologic consequences. The choroid is sandwiched between the sclera and Bruch's membrane. The scleral shows capability in remodeling. Less is known about the ability for Bruch's membrane to change in short-term or longer-term alterations in stress. Short-term increases in stress from trauma in any eye may cause breaks in Bruch's membrane, called angioid streaks. With ocular expansion during childhood, Bruch's membrane appears to expand without damage. However, with the ocular expansion of Bruch's membrane later in life with the development of pathologic myopia, it seems to show a propensity to form breaks, called lacquer cracks. These seem to be the result of increased tensile stress. The curious aspect is that the cracks may for years or decades after the expansion of the globe during the development of myopia. This suggests in adulthood, Bruch's membrane may not be remodeled and, in fact, may become more brittle. The lack of remodeling means that alterations in the underlying sclera may occur with less of a change in contour of Bruch's membrane. With development of a DSM, the intervening choroid may be squeezed between the dome of the thickened sclera and the taut overlying Bruch's membrane. At the base of the dome, the choroid may appear to be slightly thicker. The undue strains on Bruch's membrane may lead to cracks or fissures, which has the potential to alter the forces favoring elevation of the dome and overlying thickness of the choroid or to allow the ingrowth of neovascularization.

15.11 Potential Mechanisms of Serous Detachment in Staphyloma and Dome-Shaped Macula

The appearance of fluid in any one layer or region in the eye is a function of the amount of fluid inflow, production, and outflow [78]. Earlier in this chapter, the effects of traction to produce a detachment were discussed. In serous detach-

ments, the model expands to include additional features. In tissues throughout the body, fluid leaves capillaries by filtration across the capillary wall as influenced by the hydrostatic and oncotic pressure in the capillary and the hydrostatic and oncotic pressure in the interstitium around the capillary. The net fluid flux is dependent on the net driving pressure and the permeability of the vessel wall. The hydrostatic pressure drops along the course of the capillary. With fluid leaving the capillary, the oncotic forces driving fluid into the capillary increase. There is a net fluid outflow from the proximal portions of the capillary and net inflow in the distal portions and postcapillary venules. Excess fluid from any net difference the amount of fluid released and resorbed by the vessel is removed by the lymphatics. The eye has interesting variations on this theme. The capillaries of the choriocapillaris have fenestrae, which augments the permeability of the vessels. In addition, the choroid has no lymphatic system. Excess fluid produced in the choroid ordinarily exist the eye through the sclera (Fig. 15.8). If there is an excessive production of fluid in the choroid, such as in central serous chorioretinopathy, the choroid expands, fluid becomes loculated in the choroid, and the barrier function of the RPE can be breached in the form of leaks. Eyes with central serous are usually hyperopic and have thick scleras. It is possible that in these eyes, any amount of fluid production by the choroid has a more difficult time leaving the posterior portion of the eye.

Although the posterior portion of the staphyloma shows thinning of the choroid and sclera, the border of the staphyloma, the sclera, can appear to be regionally thickened (Fig. 15.9). The vessels (and the RPE) traversing the inflec-

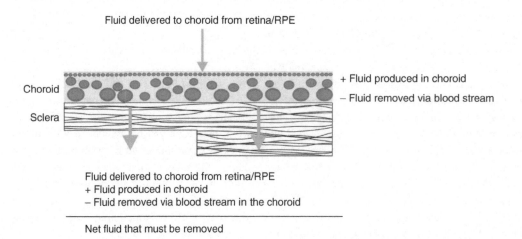

Fig. 15.8 Schematic of ocular fluid physiology. (**a**) Fluid is delivered to the choroid from the retina via the RPE. The choriocapillaris is highly permeable and also appears to be able to participate in fluid resorption. Fluid may also leave the choroid through the sclera. Areas of thin sclera would be expected to have a higher permeability than thicker areas. (**b**) The net fluid that needs to leave the eye, such as through the sclera, is the amount delivered by the RPE plus the amount produced in the choroid minus the amount leaving the eye in the blood stream. Increasing the production of fluid would increase the net amount needing to leave. The facility of outflow of the sclera represents the chief hindrance to fluid leaving through the sclera

a

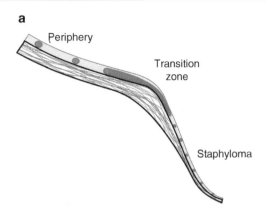

Periphery

Transition zone

Staphyloma

b

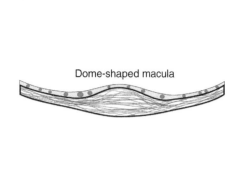

Dome-shaped macula

Fig. 15.9 Accumulation of fluid in high myopia related to scleral abnormalities. Only the choroid and sclera are shown in these schematics. (**a**) At the border of a staphyloma, the sclera is thickened, which likely reduces the permeability in that region. In addition, there may be various stress placed on the choroidal circulation in this zone, which may affect the amount of fluid produced. (**b**) In an analogous fashion, dome-shaped macula has a region of scleral thickening that may reduce the local facility of fluid outflow. The vessels at the borders of the elevation may also experience stress because of the change in contour

tion point in the ocular curvature may be put under additional stress. Any choroidal fluid would have more difficulty leaving posteriorly and may possibly contribute to subretinal fluid accumulation as has been seen in some of these eyes [79]. An extension of this theory can be used to analyze DSM. The outflow of fluid through the thickened sclera under the dome is likely to be reduced. The alteration of forces acting on the choroid through the sclera/Bruch's membrane mismatch may contribute to fluid leakage from choroidal vessels. These factors may play a role in the accumulation of fluid in the subretinal space. These factors may also influence the propensity for fluid accumulation associated with neovascularization. Ordinarily, myopic neovascularization has minimal amounts of subretinal fluid as compared with what typically would be seen in age-related macular degeneration. In DSM, the ability to remove fluid from the subretinal space may be compromised, and even minimal leakage from macular neovascularization could lead to fluid accumulation.

Treatment of eyes with fluid related to DSM is vexing. The fluid can wax and wane without treatment. There may be some rationale to treat cases with choroidal vascular hyperpermeability, a minority of cases, with photodynamic therapy to try to reduce choroidal leakage. In the absence of hyperpermeability, it is possible that photodynamic therapy [80] could have some marginal effect, but only by damaging the choriocapillaris. While this may lead to a short-term improvement in fluid, it does so at the risk of long-term atrophy. There are reports that carbonic anhydrase inhibitors [81] or grid laser photocoagulation [80] may appear to help resolve fluid, without improving visual acuity, in some patients, but there is no proven reliable treatment for subretinal fluid in DSM.

References

1. Scarpa A. Chapter 17. Dello Stafiloma. Practical observations on the principal diseases of the eyes. Pravia: Presso Baldassare Comino; 1801. p. 215–28.
2. Lawrence W. Section III. Staphyloma scleroticae, in a treatise of the diseases of the eye. 3rd ed. London: Henry G. Bohn; 1844. p. 337–9.
3. Arlt F. Die Krankenheiten des Auges fur praktische Artze. Prague: F.A. Credner; 1859.
4. Arlt F. Über die Ursachen und die Entstehung der Kurzsichtigkeit. Vienna: Wilhelm Braumueller; 1876.
5. Tscherning M. Studien über die Aetiologie der Myopie. Graefes Arch Clin Exp Ophthalmol. 1883;29:201–72.
6. Schnabel I. The anatomy of staphyloma posticum, and the relationship of the condition to myopia. In: Norris WF, Oliver CA, editors. System of diseases of the eye. Vol 3. Local diseases, glaucoma, wounds and injuries, operations. Philadelphia: J.B. Lippincott Co; 1898. p. 395–411.
7. Souter WN. Posterior staphyloma in the refraction and motility of the eye. For students and practitioners. Philadelphia: Lea Brothers & Co; 1903. p. 249–55.
8. Knowles RH. An encyclopedia-dictionary and reference handbook of the ophthalmic sciences. New York: The Jewelers Circular Publishing Company; 1903.
9. Curtin BJ, Karlin DB. Axial length measurements and fundus changes of the myopic eye. Part 1. The posterior fundus. Trans Am Opthalmal Soc. 1970;68:312–34.
10. Curtin BJ, Karlin DB. Axial length measurements and fundus changes of the myopic eye. I. The posterior fundus. Trans Am Ophthalmol Soc. 1970;68:312–34.
11. Moriyama M, Ohno-Matsui K, Modegi T, et al. Quantitative analyses of high-resolution 3D MR images of highly myopic eyes to determine their shapes. Invest Ophthalmol Vis Sci. 2012;53(8):4510–8.
12. Gaucher D, Erginay A, Lecleire-Collet A, et al. Dome-shaped macula in eyes with myopic posterior staphyloma. Am J Ophthalmol. 2008;145:909–14.
13. Ikuno Y, Tano Y. Retinal and choroidal biometry in highly myopic eyes with spectral-domain optical coherence tomography. Invest Ophthalmol Vis Sci. 2009;50(8):3876–80.

14. Hsiang HW, Ohno-Matsui K, Shimada N, Hayashi K, Moriyama M, Yoshida T, Tokoro T, Mochizuki M. Clinical characteristics of posterior staphyloma in eyes with pathologic myopia. Am J Ophthalmol. 2008;146(1):102–10.

15. Young FA. The effect of nearwork illumination level on monkey refraction. Am J Optom Arch Am Acad Optom. 1962;39:60–7.

16. Shen W, Vijayan M, Sivak JG. Inducing form-deprivation myopia in fish. Invest Ophthalmol Vis Sci. 2005;46(5):1797–803.

17. Wallman J, Gottlieb MD, Rajaram V, Fugate-Wentzek LA. Local retinal regions control local eye growth and myopia. Science. 1987;237(4810):73–7.

18. Smith EL 3rd, Hung LF, Huang J. Relative peripheral hyperopic defocus alters central refractive development in infant monkeys. Vis Res. 2009;49(19):2386–92.

19. Schaeffel F, Glasser A, Howland HC. Accommodation, refractive error, and eye growth in chickens. Vis Res. 1988;28:639–57.

20. Smith EL 3rd., Hung LF. The role of optical defocus in regulating refractive development in infant monkeys. Vis Res. 1999;39:1415–35.

21. Graham B, Judge SJ. The effects of spectacle wear in infancy on eye growth and refractive error in the marmoset (Callithrix jacchus). Vis Res. 1999;39:189–206.

22. Norton TT, Siegwart JT, Amedo AO. Effectiveness of hyperopic defocus, minimal defocus, or myopic defocus in competition with a myopiagenic stimulus in tree shrew eyes. Invest Ophthalmol Vis Sci. 2006;47:4687–99.

23. Shen W, Sivak JG. Eyes of a lower vertebrate are susceptible to the visual environment. Invest Ophthalmol Vis Sci. 2007;48:4829–37.

24. Zhu X, Park TW, Winawer J, Wallman J. In a matter of minutes, the eye can know which way to grow. Invest Ophthalmol Vis Sci. 2005;46(7):2238–41.

25. Nickla DL, Wallman J. The multifunctional choroid. Prog Retin Eye Res. 2010;29(2):144–68.

26. Fitzgerald ME, Wildsoet CF, Reiner A. Temporal relationship of choroidal blood flow and thickness changes during recovery from form deprivation myopia in chicks. Exp Eye Res. 2002;74(5):561–70.

27. Hirata A, Negi A. Morphological changes of choriocapillaris in experimentally induced chick myopia. Graefes Arch Clin Exp Ophthalmol. 1998;236(2):132–7.

28. Read SA, Collins MJ, Sander BP. Human optical axial length and defocus. Invest Ophthalmol Vis Sci. 2010;51:6262–9.

29. Smith EL 3rd, Huang J, Hung LF, Blasdel TL, Humbird TL, Bockhorst KH. Hemiretinal form deprivation: evidence for local control of eye growth and refractive development in infant monkeys. Invest Ophthalmol Vis Sci. 2009;50(11):5057–69.

30. Smith EL 3rd, Hung LF, Huang J, Blasdel TL, Humbird TL, Bockhorst KH. Effects of optical defocus on refractive development in monkeys: evidence for local, regionally selective mechanisms. Invest Ophthalmol Vis Sci. 2010;51(8):3864–73.

31. Smith EL 3rd, Ramamirtham R, Qiao-Grider Y, Hung LF, Huang J, Kee CS, Coats D, Paysse E. Effects of foveal ablation on emmetropization and form-deprivation myopia. Invest Ophthalmol Vis Sci. 2007;48(9):3914–22.

32. Smith EL 3rd. Prentice award lecture 2010: a case for peripheral optical treatment strategies for myopia. Optom Vis Sci. 2011;88(9):1029–44.

33. Phillips JR, McBrien NA. Form deprivation myopia: elastic properties of sclera. Ophthalmic Physiol Opt. 1995;15:357–62.

34. McBrien NA, Gentle A. Role of the sclera in the development and pathological complications of myopia. Prog Retin Eye Res. 2003;22(3):307–38.

35. McBrien NA, Cornell LM, Gentle A. Structural and ultrastructural changes to the sclera in a mammalian model of high myopia. Invest Ophthalmol Vis Sci. 2001;42(10):2179–87.

36. McBrien NA, Adams DW. A longitudinal investigation of adult-onset and adult-progression of myopia in an occupational group. Refractive and biometric findings. Invest Ophthalmol Vis Sci. 1997;38(2):321–33.

37. Saka N, Ohno-Matsui K, Shimada N, Sueyoshi S, Nagaoka N, Hayashi W, Hayashi K, Moriyama M, Kojima A, Yasuzumi K, Yoshida T, Tokoro T, Mochizuki M. Long-term changes in axial length in adult eyes with pathologic myopia. Am J Ophthalmol. 2010;150(4):562–8, e1.

38. Rose KA, Morgan IG, Smith W, Burlutsky G, Mitchell P, Saw SM. Myopia, lifestyle, and schooling in students of Chinese ethnicity in Singapore and Sydney. Arch Ophthalmol. 2008;126(4):527–30.

39. Jones LA, Sinnott LT, Mutti DO, Mitchell GL, Moeschberger ML, Zadnik K. Parental history of myopia, sports and outdoor activities, and future myopia. Invest Ophthalmol Vis Sci. 2007;48(8):3524–32.

40. Dirani M, Tong L, Gazzard G, Zhang X, Chia A, Young TL, Rose KA, Mitchell P, Saw SM. Outdoor activity and myopia in Singapore teenage children. Br J Ophthalmol. 2009;93(8):997–1000.

41. Morgan RW, Speakman JS, Grimshaw SE. Inuit myopia: an environmentally induced "epidemic"? Can Med Assoc J. 1975;112(5):575–7.

42. Alward WL, Bender TR, Demske JA, Hall DB. High prevalence of myopia among young adult Yupik Eskimos. Can J Ophthalmol. 1985;20(7):241–5.

43. Lv L, Zhang Z. Pattern of myopia progression in Chinese medical students: a two-year follow-up study. Graefes Arch Clin Exp Ophthalmol. 2012;251(1):163–8.

44. Mutti DO, Mitchell GL, Moeschberger ML, Jones LA, Zadnik K. Parental myopia, near work, school achievement, and children's refractive error. Invest Ophthalmol Vis Sci. 2002;43:3633–40.

45. Zylbermann R, Landau D, Berson D. The influence of study habits on myopia in Jewish teenagers. J Pediatr Ophthalmol Strabismus. 1993;30:319–22.

46. Hepsen IF, Evereklioglu C, Bayramlar H. The effect of reading and near-work on the development of myopia in emmetropic boys: a prospective, controlled, three-year follow-up study. Vis Res. 2001;41:2511–20.

47. Kinge B, Midelfart A, Jacobsen G, Rystad J. The influence of near-work on development of myopia among university students: a three-year longitudinal study among engineering students in Norway. Acta Ophthalmol Scand. 2000;78:26–9.

48. Rose KA, Morgan IG, Ip J, et al. Outdoor activity reduces the prevalence of myopia in children. Ophthalmology. 2008;115:1279–85.

49. Rucker FJ, Wallman J. Chick eyes compensate for chromatic simulations of hyperopic and myopic defocus: evidence that the eye uses longitudinal chromatic aberration to guide eye-growth. Vis Res. 2009;49(14):1775–83.

50. Kyoko patient.

51. Young SE, Walsh FB, Knox DL. The tilted disk syndrome. Am J Ophthalmol. 1976;82:16–23.

52. Prost M, De Laey JJ. Choroidal neovascularization in tilted disc syndrome. Int Ophthalmol. 1988;12(2):131–5.

53. Quaranta M, Brindeau C, Coscas G, Soubrane G. Multiple choroidal neovascularizations at the border of a myopic posterior macular staphyloma. Graefes Arch Clin Exp Ophthalmol. 2000;238:101–3.

54. Cohen SY, Quentel G, Guiberteau B, Delahaye-Mazza C, Gaudric A. Macular serous retinal detachment caused by subretinal leakage in tilted disc syndrome. Ophthalmology. 1998;105:1831–4.

55. Cohen SY, Quentel G. Chorioretinal folds as a consequence of inferior staphyloma associated with tilted disc syndrome. Graefes Arch Clin Exp Ophthalmol. 2006;244:1536–8.

56. Becquet F, Ducournau D, Ducournau Y, Goffart Y, Spencer WH. Juxtapapillary subretinal pigment epithelial polypoid pseudocysts associated with unilateral tilted optic disc: case report with clinicopathologic correlation. Ophthalmology. 2001;108(9):1657–62.

57. Mauget-Faÿsse M, Cornut PL, Quaranta El-Maftouhi M, Leys A. Polypoidal choroidal vasculopathy in tilted disk syndrome and high myopia with staphyloma. Am J Ophthalmol. 2006;142(6):970–5.

58. Cohen SY, Quentel G. Uneven distribution of drusen in tilted disc syndrome. Retina. 2008;28(9):1361–2.

59. Vuori ML, Mäntyjärvi M. Tilted disc syndrome may mimic false visual field deterioration. Acta Ophthalmol. 2008;86(6):622–5.

60. Nakanishi H, Tsujikawa A, Gotoh N, et al. Macular complications on the border of an inferior staphyloma associated with tilted disc syndrome. Retina. 2008;28(10):1493–501.

61. Cohen SY, Dubois L, Ayrault S, Quentel G. T-shaped pigmentary changes in tilted disk syndrome. Eur J Ophthalmol. 2009;19(5):876–9.

62. Ohno-Matsui K, Shimada N, Nagaoka N, Tokoro T, Mochizuki M. Choroidal folds radiating from the edge of an inferior staphyloma in an eye with tilted disc syndrome. Jpn J Ophthalmol. 2011;55(2):171–3.

63. Maruko I, Iida T, Sugano Y, Oyamada H, Sekiryu T. Morphologic choroidal and scleral changes at the macula in tilted disc syndrome with staphyloma using optical coherence tomography. Invest Ophthalmol Vis Sci. 2011;52(12):8763–8.

64. Spaide RF, Fisher Y. Removal of adherent cortical vitreous plaques without removing the internal limiting membrane in the repair of macular detachments in highly myopic eyes. Retina. 2005;25(3):290–5.

65. Demer JL. Knobby eye syndrome. Strabismus. 2018;26(1):33–41.

66. Fledelius HC, Goldschmidt E. Eye shape and peripheral visual field recording in high myopia at approximately 54 years of age, as based on ultrasonography and Goldmann kinetic perimetry. Acta Ophthalmol. 2010;88(5):521–6.

67. Tanaka Y, Shimada N, Ohno-Matsui K. Extreme thinning or loss of inner neural retina along the staphyloma edge in eyes with pathologic myopia. Am J Ophthalmol. 2015;159(4):677–82.

68. Gupta A, Smith JM. Bitemporal hemianopia secondary to nasal staphylomata. J Neuroophthalmol. 2015;35(1):99–101.

69. Mehdizadeh M, Nowroozzadeh MH. Dome-shaped macula in eyes with myopic posterior staphyloma. Am J Ophthalmol. 2008;146:478; author reply -9

70. Imamura Y, Iida T, Maruko I, et al. Enhanced depth imaging optical coherence tomography of the sclera in dome-shaped macula. Am J Ophthalmol. 2011;151:297–302.

71. Errera MH, Michaelides M, Keane PA, et al. The extended clinical phenotype of dome-shaped macula. Graefes Arch Clin Exp Ophthalmol. 2014;252(3):499–508.

72. Viola F, Dell'Arti L, Benatti E, et al. Choroidal findings in dome-shaped macula in highly myopic eyes: a longitudinal study. Am J Ophthalmol. 2015;159(1):44–52.

73. Hocaoglu M, Ersoz MG, Sayman Muslubas I, et al. Factors associated with macular complications in highly myopic eyes with dome-shaped macular configuration. Graefes Arch Clin Exp Ophthalmol. 2019;257(11):2357–65.

74. Liang IC. Horizontal ridge as a posterior pole finding in a highly myopic eye with dome-shaped macula. Retina. 2017;37(7):1261–2.

75. Fang Y, Du R, Jonas JB, et al. Ridge-shaped macula progressing parallel to bruch membrane defects and macular suprachoroidal cavitation. Retina. 2020;40(3):456–60.

76. García-Ben A, Sanchez MJM, Gómez AG, et al. Factors associated with serous retinal detachment in highly myopic eyes with vertical oval-shaped dome. Retina. 2019;39(3):587–93.

77. Ohno-Matsui K, Fang Y, Uramoto K, et al. Peri-dome choroidal deepening in highly myopic eyes with dome-shaped maculas. Am J Ophthalmol. 2017;183:134–40.

78. Spaide RF, Yannuzzi LA. Mechanisms maintaining retinal and pigment epithelial attachment: a theoretical framework with practical considerations. In: Marmor MF, Wolfensberger TJ, editors. The retinal pigment epithelium. New York: Oxford Press; 1998.

79. Ishida T, Moriyama M, Tanaka Y, et al. Radial tracts emanating from staphyloma edge in eyes with pathologic myopia. Ophthalmology. 2015;122(1):215–6.

80. Chinskey ND, Johnson MW. Treatment of subretinal fluid associated with dome-shaped macula. Ophthalmic Surg Lasers Imaging Retina. 2013;44(6):593–5.

81. Chen NN, Chen CL, Lai CH. Resolution of unilateral dome-shaped macula with serous detachment after treatment of topical carbonic anhydrase inhibitors. Ophthalmic Surg Lasers Imaging Retina. 2019;50(8):e218–21.

Staphyloma II: Morphological Features of Posterior Staphyloma in Pathologic Myopia – Analysis Using 3D MRI and Ultra-widefield OCT

Kyoko Ohno-Matsui, Muka Moriyama, and Kosei Shinohara

16.1 Introduction

A posterior staphyloma is an outpouching of a circumscribed region of the posterior fundus and has been considered a hallmark of pathologic myopia [1, 2]. In 1977, Curtin [1] classified a posterior staphyloma in eyes with pathologic myopia into ten different types. Types I to V are considered a primary staphyloma, and Types VI to X are considered a combined staphyloma (see Chap. 15 for details).

Moriyama et al. used three-dimensional magnetic resonance imaging (3D MRI) to analyze the entire shape of the eye [3, 4]. Ohno-Matsui et al. [5] used a combination of 3D MRI and ultra-widefield fundus imaging to classify posterior staphylomas into six different types, based on the size, shape, and location of the staphylomas. 3D MRI is considered suitable to analyze the eye shape of wide region like posterior staphyloma in a 3D way from any angle. However, 3D MRI is not feasible as a screening technique. Because the 3D-MRI technique uses T2-weighted images showing intraocular fluid, 3D MRI demonstrates the vitreoretinal interface or the inner surface of the retina and does not show the scleral curvature.

Most of the staphyloma involves a wide area of the fundus; thus, the entire extent of staphyloma often does not fit within the 50° angle of the conventional fundus photos. Optical coherence tomography (OCT) is a useful tool for analyzing the curvature of the eye; however, the maximum scan length of commercially available OCT is not long enough to cover the entire extent of a wide staphyloma.

A new prototype of an ultra-widefield swept source OCT (UWF-OCT) system uses not only one but multiple scan lines and generates scan maps allowing the 3D reconstruction of posterior staphylomas in a region of interest of 23 × 20 mm and a depth of 5 mm [6, 7]. By using this UWF-OCT, a visualization of wide staphylomas in their full 3D extent became possible. The detectability of staphylomas on the UWF-OCT images versus 3D MRI revealed no significant difference, suggesting UWF-OCT may replace 3D MRI in assessing posterior staphylomas [6].

Thus, in this chapter, we propose a simple classification and examined the morphological features of staphylomas based on 3D MRI images and UWF-OCT images.

Principles for Classification of Staphyloma

1. *Only the contour of the outermost border of posterior staphyloma was analyzed.*
   - Combined staphylomas in Curtin's classification [1] are characterized by the presence of irregularities within the staphylomatous area. However, recent enhanced-depth imaging OCT (EDI-OCT) [8] and swept source OCT have shown that there are more numerous and more complicated irregularities of the sclera within a staphyloma than expected earlier, such as dome-shaped macula [9–13], peripapillary intrachoroidal cavitation (ICC) [14], macular ICC [15], scleral dehiscence within patchy atrophy or at the emissary openings [16], change of scleral curvature at the dura attachment site [17], and posterior protrusion of peripapillary sclera exposed onto the dilated subarachnoid space [17]. Thus, it is difficult to include many different kinds of scleral irregularities into the classification of staphyloma. From the reasons above, we analyzed the outermost border only. That is, Types VI to X are included under the same category with Type I (Fig. 16.1).
2. *Staphyloma type is renamed according to its location and distribution (Fig. 16.2).*
   - Type I → wide, macular staphyloma
   - Type II → narrow, macular staphyloma
   - Type III → peripapillary
   - Type IV → nasal

K. Ohno-Matsui (✉) · M. Moriyama · K. Shinohara
Department of Ophthalmology and Visual Science, Tokyo Medical and Dental University, Tokyo, Japan
e-mail: k.ohno.oph@tmd.ac.jp

© Springer Nature Switzerland AG 2021
R. F. Spaide et al. (eds.), *Pathologic Myopia*, https://doi.org/10.1007/978-3-030-74334-5_16

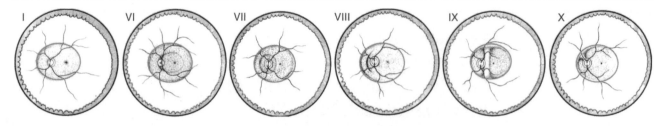

Fig. 16.1 The curvature of the outermost line of staphyloma is considered for a classification. The outermost line of staphyloma is depicted in red line. In such case, Types VI through X fit into the same category of Type I (in Curtin's classification)

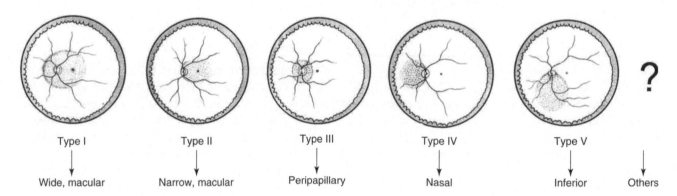

Fig. 16.2 Renaming of staphyloma according to its distribution

- Type V → inferior
- Staphyloma other than Type I through Type V → others

16.2 Detection of Staphyloma Edges by Ultra-widefield OCT

Different from 3D MRI with a relatively low spatial resolution, UWF-OCT can detect even shallow staphylomas because of its high resolution. The detection of staphylomas by using UWF-OCT can be made accurately by detecting OCT features of "staphyloma edges" in addition to posterior bowing of a limited area of posterior sclera (Fig. 16.3).

Morphological hallmarks of the posterior staphylomas as examined by UWF-OCT were a smoothly configured border with a gradual thinning of the choroid from the periphery toward the edge of the staphyloma and a gradual re-thickening of the choroid in direction toward the posterior pole (Fig. 16.3). Additionally, there was a gradual thickening and inward protrusion of the sclera at the staphyloma edge.

UWF-OCT showed that early signs of staphylomas can be seen even in children and adolescents [18].

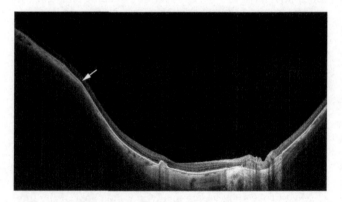

Fig. 16.3 Ultra-widefield OCT image of posterior staphyloma (cited with permission from the Ref. [6]). In addition to posterior bowing of the sclera in staphylomatous area, staphyloma edge (arrow) shows two distinct features: (1) a gradual thinning of the choroid from the periphery toward the edge of the staphyloma and a gradual re-thickening of the choroid in direction toward the posterior pole and (2) a gradual thickening and inward protrusion of the sclera at the staphyloma edge

16.2.1 Highly Myopic Eyes Without Evident Staphyloma (Fig. 16.4)

Staphyloma edges can be seen as pigmentary abnormalities especially when the edges are steep. In Optos images of highly myopic eyes without evident staphyloma, no clear abnormalities suggesting the staphyloma edge are found both in color images and fundus autofluorescence (FAF)

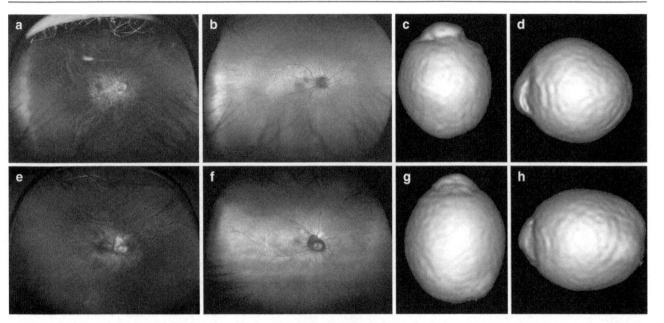

Fig. 16.4 Optos images and three-dimensional magnetic resonance imaging (3D MRI) of highly myopic eyes without evident staphyloma. (**a**) Right fundus shows yellowish chorioretinal atrophy in the posterior fundus. Pigmentary abnormalities suggesting the border of staphyloma are not obvious. (**b**) Fundus autofluorescence (FAF) image shows no abnormal autofluorescence suggestive of border of staphyloma. (**c, d**) 3D MRI images of this patient. 3D MRI images of the right eye viewed inferiorly (**c**) and the image viewed nasally (**d**) show that the globe is elongated into an ellipsoid shape. No notch suggestive of an abrupt change of the curvature of the globe is found. (**e**) Right fundus shows yellowish chorioretinal atrophy in the posterior fundus. Pigmentary abnormalities suggesting the border of staphyloma are not obvious. (**f**) Fundus autofluorescence (FAF) image shows no abnormal autofluorescence suggestive of border of staphyloma. (**g, h**) 3D MRI images of this patient. 3D MRI images of the right eye viewed inferiorly (**g**) and the image viewed nasally (**h**) show that the globe is elongated anterior-posteriorly and the globe shows a barrel-shaped appearance

images, although posterior fundus shows characteristic findings to pathologic myopia, such as myopic chorioretinal atrophy and myopic conus (Fig. 16.4a, e). 3D MRI images show an elliptical shape (Fig. 16.4c, d) or barrel shape (Fig. 16.4g, h) both in horizontal and vertical sections. Highly myopic eyes with longer axial length (especially >30.0 mm) tend to have barrel-shaped globe than elliptical shape when they do not have evident staphyloma. In UWF-OCT image (Fig. 16.5) of highly myopic eyes without evident staphyloma, no OCT features suggesting staphyloma edges were detected, and the choroidal thickness was uniformly distributed in the posterior fundus.

16.3   Highly Myopic Eyes with Evident Staphyloma (Figs. 16.6, 16.7, 16.8, 16.9, 16.10, 16.11, and 16.12)

Although the detecting methodologies were different, the results on the prevalence of each type of staphylomas were similar among studies. Wide macular staphyloma (equivalent to Type I staphyloma by Curtin) is by far the most prevalent type (74% of eyes with staphyloma [5]). The second most common type was narrow macular staphyloma (equiva-

lent to Type II staphyloma by Curtin), which was seen in 14% of eyes with staphyloma [5].

16.4   Macular Staphyloma

Macular staphyloma is further divided into wide and narrow, mainly due to a location of nasal edge of staphyloma. When the nasal edge of macular staphyloma is along the nasal edge of the optic disc, the eye is regarded as having a narrow, macular staphyloma. On the other hand, when the nasal edge of macular staphyloma exists more nasally to the nasal edge of the optic disc, the eye is considered as having a wide, macular staphyloma.

16.5   Wide, Macular Staphyloma (Fig. 16.6)

In the Optos images, the border of the staphyloma is observed as pigmented or depigmented lines in color images and as hypoautofluorescent lines in FAF images in most cases. Generally, the upper and temporal border of the staphyloma is more clearly observed than the lower or nasal border. In some cases, band-shaped or tongue-shaped hypoautofluores-

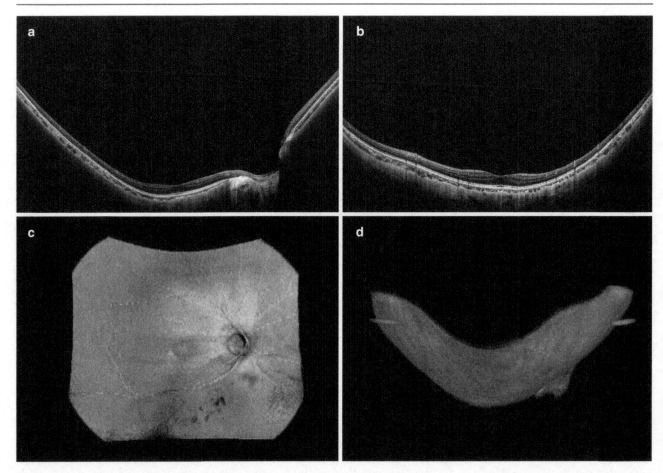

Fig. 16.5 An eye classified by widefield optical coherence tomography (WF-OCT) as having no staphyloma (also confirmed by 3D MRI). (**a**, **b**) Cross-sectional WF-OCT images. (**d**) Horizontal scan. (**e**) Vertical scan. Scleral curvature is generally steep; however, no OCT features indicating a staphyloma edge are seen. (**c**, **d**) Three-dimensional WF-OCT images viewed from anterior (**c**) and from the inferior side (**d**) without showing any staphyloma edge

cent lesions surrounded by irregular hyperautofluorescence seem to radiate outward from the border of staphyloma (arrows, Fig. 16.6b, j, n) in FAF images. This lesion shows pigmentation in color fundus (Fig. 16.6m); however, this lesion is more clearly seen in FAF images than the color images.

3D MRI images show a protrusion of wide area of the posterior segment both in the images viewed from the inferior and nasal to the eye. Corresponding to the Optos images, the upper or temporal border is more abrupt than the lower or nasal border in the images viewed nasally in most cases. Thus, there is a notch-like dent along the upper border of protrusion (arrows, Fig. 16.6d, p) or along the temporal border of the protrusion (Fig. 16.6c, k, o) in most cases. However, some cases have a notch along the lower border (Fig. 16.6l) or do not have obvious notch (Fig. 16.6h). Although all of the 3D MRI images viewed inferiorly show a wide area of pro-

trusion, in the 3D MRI images viewed nasally, however, the size of protruded area is not wide in some eyes (Fig. 16.6l). This suggests that the staphyloma is horizontally wide in some of the eyes with wide macular staphyloma.

In UWF-OCT images of eyes with wide macular staphylomas, a posterior displacement of scleral curvature is seen in a large extent with clearly detected staphyloma edges. Macroscopic image of a highly myopic eye with very wide staphyloma is shown in Fig. 16.7.

16.6 Narrow, Macular Staphyloma (Fig. 16.8)

In the Optos images, the area of protrusion is restricted to a narrow area from the nasal edge of the optic disc and temporal to the central fovea. Sometimes another small, shal-

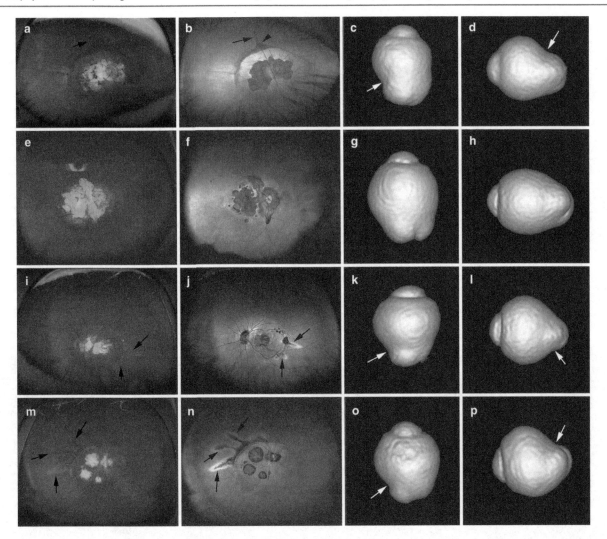

Fig. 16.6 Optos images and three-dimensional magnetic resonance imaging (3D MRI) of highly myopic eyes with wide, macular staphyloma. (**a**) Right fundus shows a macular chorioretinal atrophy merged with myopic conus. The upper border of staphyloma is recognized as pigmented lines. (**b**) Fundus autofluorescence (FAF) image shows a hypoautofluorescence along the upper edge of staphyloma. A band-shaped linear hypoautofluorescent lesion is seen to course from the upper edge of staphyloma (arrow). An area with intense hypoautofluorescence (arrowhead) is observed at the root of this band-shaped lesion. (**c, d**) 3D MRI images of this patient. 3D MRI image of the right eye viewed inferiorly (**c**) shows that a wide area of posterior segment is protruded posteriorly. The temporal border of protrusion is more abrupt than the nasal border. Thus, a notch (arrow) is observed along the temporal border of protrusion. Protrusion of wide area of posterior segment is also seen in the 3D MRI image viewed nasally (**d**). The upper border (arrow) seems to be more abrupt than the lower border. (**e**) Right fundus shows a macular chorioretinal atrophy merged with myopic conus. The border of staphyloma is slightly pigmented; however, the staphyloma edge is not as evident as the previous case. (**f**) FAF image shows no evident abnormalities along the border of staphyloma. (**g** and **h**) 3D MRI images of this patient. 3D MRI image of the right eye viewed inferiorly (**g**) shows that a wide area of posterior segment is protruded posteriorly. Neither temporal nor nasal border of protrusion is abrupt. 3D MRI image of the right eye viewed nasally (**h**) shows that a wide area of posterior segment is protruded posteriorly. Neither upper nor lower border of protrusion is abrupt. A ridge is observed within a protruded area in both images. (**i**) Left fundus shows a macular atrophy in the posterior fundus. The border of staphyloma is observed as pigmented line especially along the temporal border. Two linear lesions radiating from the temporal edge of staphyloma are seen (arrows). (**j**) FAF image shows hypoautofluorescence along the border of staphyloma (especially along the temporal border). Two hypoautofluorescent linear lesions surrounded by irregular hyperautofluorescence are shown to emanate from the temporal border of staphyloma (arrows). (**k** and **l**) 3D MRI images of this patient. 3D MRI image of the right eye viewed inferiorly (**k**) shows that a wide area of posterior segment is protruded posteriorly. Temporal border is more abrupt than the nasal border; thus, a notch is observed along the temporal border of protrusion. 3D MRI image viewed nasally (**l**) shows that protruded area is not as wide as that seen in the image viewed inferiorly, suggesting a protrusion in this patient is horizontally wide. The lower edge seems to be more abrupt than the upper edge, and a notch is found along the lower edge (arrow). (**m**) Right fundus shows areas of chorioretinal atrophic patches in the posterior fundus. The border (especially upper border) of staphyloma shows pigmentation. Three pigmented linear lesions (arrows) are seen to radiate from the upper-temporal edge of staphyloma. A ridge formation temporal to the optic disc is observed. (**n**) FAF image shows hypoautofluorescence along the border of staphyloma (especially along the upper border). Three hypoautofluorescent linear lesions surrounded by irregular hyperautofluorescence are seen to emanate from the upper-temporal border of staphyloma (arrows). (**o** and **p**) 3D MRI images of this patient. 3D MRI image of the right eye viewed inferiorly (**o**) and the image viewed nasally (**p**) show that a wide area of posterior segment is protruded posteriorly. Temporal border is more abrupt than the nasal border; thus, a notch is observed along the temporal border of protrusion in (**o**). Also, the upper edge seems to be more abrupt than the lower edge, and a notch is found along the upper edge (arrow). A ridge formation is observed as a linear groove within a protrusion

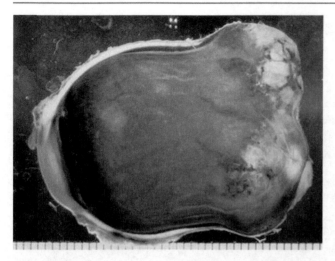

Fig. 16.7 Macroscopic view of a highly myopic eye with big multiple protrusions in wide, macular staphyloma. Both peripapillary and macular regions are posteriorly protruded (arrows). An extensive chorioretinal atrophy is seen in the entire posterior fundus. (Courtesy of Emeritus Professor Shigekuni Okisaka in National Defense Medical College)

low staphyloma is observed nasal to the optic disc (Fig. 16.8e, f). The border of staphyloma, especially upper and temporal border, shows pigmented abnormalities (Fig. 16.8a, e). FAF abnormalities along the border of staphyloma are not as remarkable as those seen in eyes with wide macular staphyloma, although FAF sometimes shows slight hyperautofluorescence. In some cases, band-shaped abnormal FAF lesions radiating from the upper border of staphyloma are seen (Fig. 16.8f). However, this lesion is much less frequent and less evident than in eyes with wide, macular staphyloma.

3D MRI images show a "cylinder shape" which we previously reported [3]. Protruded area is narrow in the images viewed both nasally and inferiorly, and the protrusion of posterior segment seems to be pointed as a triangle, which is different from a broad and blunt protrusion seen in eyes with wide, macular staphyloma. In most of the eyes, the upper border is more acute than the lower border in the images viewed nasally (Fig. 16.8d, h). However, the abruptness is

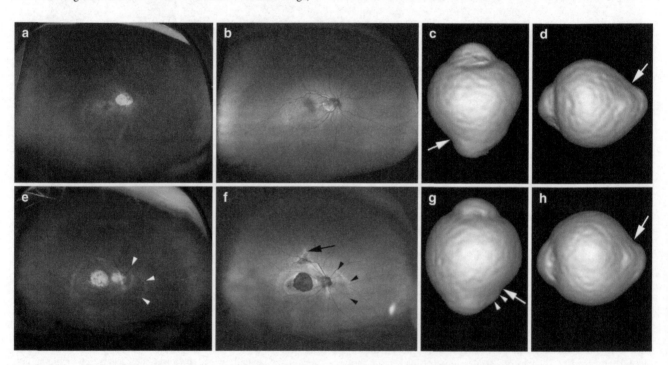

Fig. 16.8 Optos images and three-dimensional magnetic resonance imaging (3D MRI) of highly myopic eyes with narrow, macular staphyloma. (**a**) Right fundus shows a narrow area of staphyloma. The upper and temporal border of staphyloma shows a slight depigmentation. Nasal edge of the staphyloma is along the nasal edge of the optic disc, and the optic disc shows a tilted appearance. (**b**) Fundus autofluorescence (FAF) imaging shows no abnormal autofluorescence suggestive of border of staphyloma. (**c**, **d**) 3D MRI images of this patient. 3D MRI image of the right eye viewed inferiorly (**c**) and the image viewed nasally (**d**) show that a protruded area is narrow and the protrusion of posterior segment seems to be pointed as a triangle. The temporal border is more abrupt than the nasal border (**c**, arrow), and the upper border is more acute than the lower border (**d**, arrow). The most protruded point exists along the central axis in all of the eyes in the images viewed nasally. (**e**) Right fundus shows a narrow area of staphyloma. The upper and temporal border of staphyloma shows a slight depigmentation.

Nasal edge of the staphyloma is along the nasal edge of the optic disc, and the optic disc shows a tilted appearance. In this patient, another small staphyloma is also seen nasal to the optic disc (arrowheads). (**f**) FAF image shows slight hyperautofluorescence along the border of staphyloma. A short linear hypoautofluorescent lesion surrounded by hyperautofluorescence is seen to emanate from the upper border of staphyloma (arrow). (**g** and **h**) 3D MRI images of this patient. 3D MRI image of the right eye viewed inferiorly (**g**) and the image viewed nasally (**h**) show that a protruded area is narrow and the protrusion of posterior segment seems to be rather pointed. The nasal border is more abrupt than the temporal border (**g**, arrow) in the image viewed inferiorly. Small additional staphyloma nasal to the optic disc is also identified (arrowheads). The upper border is more acute than the lower border (**h**, arrow). The most protruded point exists along the central axis in all of the eyes in the images viewed nasally

milder than that in eyes with wild, macular staphyloma in general. And in the images viewed inferiorly, the temporal border is more evident than the nasal border in most of the eyes (Fig. 16.8c); however, in some eyes, the nasal border is more evident (Fig. 16.8g). The most protruded point exists along the central axis in all of the eyes in the images viewed nasally.

Macroscopic image of a narrow macular staphyloma is shown in Fig. 16.9.

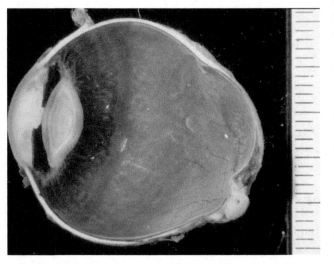

Fig. 16.9 Macroscopic view of a highly myopic eye with narrow, macular staphyloma. Macular area is posteriorly protruded, and the sclera is extremely thinned in the protruded area. (Courtesy of Emeritus Professor Shigekuni Okisaka in National Defense Medical College)

16.7   Inferior Staphyloma (Fig. 16.10)

In the Optos images, the staphyloma exists in a wide area of lower fundus accompanying myopic chorioretinal atrophy within a staphyloma. Optos images show that the upper border is clearly observed as pigmented line in color fundus images and hyper- or hypoautofluorescent lines in FAF images (Fig. 16.10a, b). Some areas of the border of staphyloma show patchy areas of clear hypoautofluorescence which suggests an atrophy of retinal pigmented epithelium. Band-shaped or tongue-shaped hypoautofluorescent lesions surrounded by irregular hyperautofluorescence are sometimes seen to radiate from the upper or temporal border of staphyloma (Fig. 16.10b). 3D MRI images of the eye with inferior staphyloma show a protrusion of lower segment of the eye. Because an area of protrusion affects as widely as the entire lower half of the globe (Fig. 16.10d), the lower boundary of protrusion is not obvious, and the curvature of the protrusion is gradually continuous to the curvature of the other parts of the lower half of the globe. The most protruded pointed exists lower to the central axis in the images viewed nasally.

In UWF-OCT image, the entire extent of inferior staphyloma is clearly seen.

16.8   Peripapillary Staphyloma (Fig. 16.11)

In the Optos images, the boundary of peripapillary staphyloma is usually not obvious in color fundus images and FAF images, probably because the change of eye curvature is not

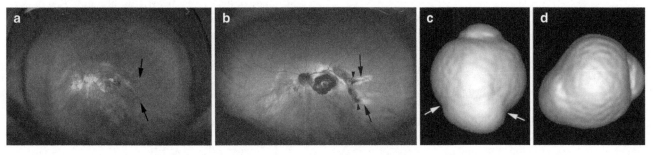

Fig. 16.10 Optos images and three-dimensional magnetic resonance imaging (3D MRI) of a highly myopic eye with inferior staphyloma. (**a**) Left fundus shows an inferior staphyloma. The optic disc is tilted inferiorly, and the inferior conus is seen. Macular atrophy is also seen. The upper border of inferior staphyloma shows pigmentation especially at the upper-temporal to temporal edge. Two linear lesions emanating from the temporal edge of staphyloma are observed (arrows). (**b**) Fundus autofluorescence image shows a hypoautofluorescence corresponding to the pigmentation along the upper-temporal to temporal edge of staphyloma. Other parts of the upper border of staphyloma show slight hyperfluorescence. Two linear lesions are seen to emanate

from the temporal border of staphyloma (arrows). The upper one has hyperautofluorescence in the center of the line, and the outside is surrounded by hyperautofluorescence. The lower lesion shows hyperautofluorescence. At the bottom of these linear lesions, an intense hypoautofluorescence is observed (arrowheads). (**c, d**) 3D MRI images of this patient. 3D MRI image viewed inferiorly (**c**) shows a protrusion of wide area. A notch is observed both along the temporal and nasal edge of protrusion (arrows). In the image viewed nasally (**d**), the protrusion is decentered toward inferiorly. The lower border of protrusion is gradually continuous to the other parts of the eye; thus, the border between the protrusion and the other parts of the eye is not obvious

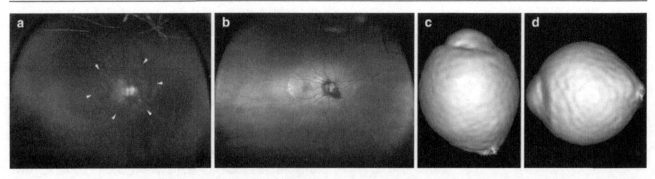

Fig. 16.11 Optos images and three-dimensional magnetic resonance imaging (3D MRI) of a highly myopic eye with peripapillary staphyloma. (**a**) Right fundus shows a border of peripapillary staphyloma as slight depigmentation (arrowheads). (**b**) Fundus autofluorescence image shows a slight hyperautofluorescence corresponding to the pigmentation along the temporal edge of staphyloma. (**c**, **d**) 3D MRI images of this patient. 3D MRI image viewed inferiorly (**c**) shows a protrusion of a limited area around the optic nerve attachment site. In the image viewed nasally (**d**), the eye shape is similar to cylinder type; however, the area of protrusion tends to be more restricted. The change of eye curvature toward the protrusion is relatively linear, and the posterior pole of the eye seems to be protruded like a triangle

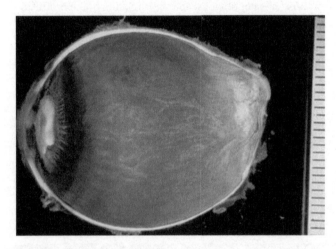

Fig. 16.12 Macroscopic view of a highly myopic eye with peripapillary staphyloma. The peripapillary region is posteriorly protruded, and the optic nerve is situated at the bottom of the protruded area. The sclera is extremely thinned in the protruded area. (Courtesy of Emeritus Professor Shigekuni Okisaka in National Defense Medical College)

abrupt. However, yellowish diffuse atrophy is seen especially around the optic disc (Fig. 16.8a), and we can see the depigmented demarcation line around the optic disc along the border of peripapillary staphyloma in some cases. The 3D MRI analyses show a protrusion of a limited area around the optic nerve attachment site in an image viewed inferiorly. In the image viewed nasally, the eye shape is similar to cylinder type which is observed in eyes with narrow, macular staphyloma; however, the area of protrusion tends to be more restricted around the optic nerve. The change of eye curvature toward the protrusion is relatively linear, and the posterior pole of the eye seems to be protruded like a triangle (Fig. 16.11c).

Macroscopic view of an eye with peripapillary staphyloma is shown in Fig. 16.12. Note that the area around the

optic nerve is specifically protruded, and the subsequent atrophy of retina-choroid is seen in the peripapillary region.

16.9 Nasal Staphyloma (Fig. 16.13)

In the Optos images, the boundary of nasal staphyloma is usually not obvious in most cases. However, yellowish diffuse atrophy is seen nasal to the optic disc, together with the nasal tilting of the optic disc and nasal conus. In some cases, the band-shaped line with abnormal autofluorescence is seen to course in parallel to the orientation of eye expansion away from the staphyloma border (Fig. 16.13b). Although the overall shape of the eye by 3D MRI is similar to that of peripapillary staphyloma, the protruded area is wider, and the change of curvature is more gradual. Thus, the curvature of the posterior pole of the eye is more curvilinear than triangular.

16.10 Others

16.10.1 Peripapillary, Wide

Peripapillary staphyloma is generally seen just around the optic nerve. However, peripapillary staphyloma sometimes becomes wide and includes the central fovea. In Optos images, different from typical peripapillary staphyloma, the staphyloma is sometimes not concentrically around the optic disc. The temporal edge of the staphyloma is obliquely across the central fovea. 3D MRI images show similar features to those of peripapillary staphyloma; however, a protrusion is wider than typical peripapillary staphyloma. In UWF-OCT images, the entire extent of staphylomas is clearly seen. This type of staphyloma is also seen in non-

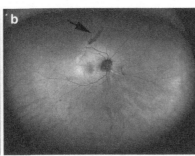 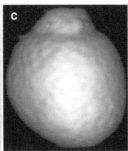 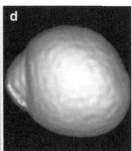

Fig. 16.13 Optos images and three-dimensional magnetic resonance imaging (3D MRI) of a highly myopic eye with nasal staphyloma. (**a**) Right fundus shows an ectasia of nasal fundus. The optic disc is tilted nasally and accompanies with nasal conus. Yellowish diffuse atrophy is seen nasal to the optic disc. No obvious findings suggestive of a border of staphyloma are observed. (**b**) Fundus autofluorescence image shows no obvious abnormalities suggestive of staphyloma. A linear hypoauto-fluorescent lesion surrounded by a margin of hyperfluorescence (arrow) is seen in the upper fundus away from the nasal staphyloma. The orien-tation of this linear lesion seems parallel to the nasal tilting. (**c**, **d**) 3D MRI images of this patient. 3D MRI image viewed inferiorly (**c**) shows a protrusion of nasal part of the eye, and the image viewed nasally (**d**) shows a protrusion of the lower part of the eye. Although the overall shape of the eye by 3D MRI is similar to that of peripapillary staphy-loma, the protruded area is wider, and the change of curvature is more gradual. Thus, the curvature of the posterior pole of the eye is more curvilinear than triangular

highly myopic eyes with staphyloma as reported by Wang et al. [19] because the fovea is on the edge of staphylomas.

16.10.2 Comments

In addition to a combination of Optos and 3D MRI, UWF-OCT is useful to delineate the entire extent of posterior staphyloma in a 3D way. 3D MRI images show various distinct features according to the types of staphyloma identified by Optos. In Optos images, the border of staphyloma is more clearly seen as pigmentary abnormalities in eyes with wide, macular staphyloma or inferior staphyloma, than the other types of staphyloma. UWF-OCT enables the clear visualiza-tion of posterior staphylomas in their full extent. Because of its feasibility and high-resolution images, UWF-OCT is expected to be the most powerful tool to objectively and quantitatively determine posterior staphylomas.

Different from 3D MRI, UWF-OCT can visualize the ner-vous tissues simultaneously with scleral changes represented by staphylomas [7, 20]. This enables the clear understanding how staphylomas contribute to the development of various fundus complications due to pathologic myopia and enables the establishment of the most suitable surgical approaches to treating staphyloma-related fundus complications. Finally, as shown in the chapter "sclera-targeted therapy," the thera-pies to treat and prevent staphylomas themselves are expected to be available. The detection of presence and degree of staphylomas by UWF-OCT can become a powerful tool for that purpose as well.

References

1. Curtin BJ. The posterior staphyloma of pathologic myopia. Trans Am Ophthalmol Soc. 1977;75:67–86.

2. Ohno-Matsui K, Jonas JB. Posterior staphyloma in pathologic myopia. Prog Retin Eye Res. 2018;70:99–109.

3. Moriyama M, Ohno-Matsui K, Hayashi K, et al. Topographical analyses of shape of eyes with pathologic myopia by high-resolution three dimensional magnetic resonance imaging. Ophthalmology. 2011;118(8):1626–37.

4. Moriyama M, Ohno-Matsui K, Modegi T, et al. Quantitative analyses of high-resolution 3D MR images of highly myo-pic eyes to determine their shapes. Invest Ophthalmol Vis Sci. 2012;53(8):4510–8.

5. Ohno-Matsui K. Proposed classification of posterior staph-ylomas based on analyses of eye shape by three-dimen-sional magnetic resonance imaging. Ophthalmology. 2014;121(9):1798–809.

6. Shinohara K, Shimada N, Moriyama M, et al. Posterior staphylomas in pathologic myopia imaged by widefield optical coherence tomography. Invest Ophthalmol Vis Sci. 2017;58(9):3750–8.

7. Shinohara K, Tanaka N, Jonas JB, et al. Ultra-widefield optical coherence tomography to investigate relationships between myopic macular retinoschisis and posterior staphyloma. Ophthalmology. 2018;125(10):1575–86.

8. Margolis R, Spaide RF. A pilot study of enhanced depth imaging optical coherence tomography of the choroid in normal eyes. Am J Ophthalmol. 2009;147(5):811–5.

9. Gaucher D, Erginay A, Lecleire-Collet A, et al. Dome-shaped mac-ula in eyes with myopic posterior staphyloma. Am J Ophthalmol. 2008;145(5):909–14.

10. Imamura Y, Iida T, Maruko I, et al. Enhanced depth imaging optical coherence tomography of the sclera in dome-shaped macula. Am J Ophthalmol. 2011;151(2):297–302.

11. Pardo-Lopez D, Gallego-Pinazo R, Mateo C, et al. Serous macular detachment associated with dome-shaped macula and tilted disc. Case Rep Ophthalmol. 2011;2(1):111–5.

12. Coco RM, Sanabria MR, Alegria J. Pathology associated with optical coherence tomography macular bending due to either dome-shaped macula or inferior staphyloma in myopic patients. Ophthalmologica. 2012;228(1):7–12.

13. Jonas JB, Jonas SB, Jonas RA, et al. Parapapillary atro-phy: histological gamma zone and delta zone. PLoS One. 2012;7(10):e47237.

14. Spaide RF, Akiba M, Ohno-Matsui K. Evaluation of peri-papillary intrachoroidal cavitation with swept source and

enhanced depth imaging optical coherence tomography. Retina. 2012;32(6):1037–44.

15. Ohno-Matsui K, Akiba M, Moriyama M, et al. Intrachoroidal cavitation in macular area of eyes with pathologic myopia. Am J Ophthalmol. 2012;154(2):382–93.

16. Ohno-Matsui K, Akiba M, Moriyama M, et al. Acquired optic nerve and peripapillary pits in pathologic myopia. Ophthalmology. 2012;119(8):1685–92.

17. Ohno-Matsui K, Akiba M, Moriyama M, et al. Imaging the retrobulbar subarachnoid space around the optic nerve by swept source optical coherence tomography in eyes with pathologic myopia. Invest Ophthalmol Vis Sci. 2011;52:9644–50.

18. Tanaka N, Shinohara K, Yokoi T, et al. Posterior staphylomas and scleral curvature in highly myopic children and adolescents investigated by ultra-widefield optical coherence tomography. PLOS One. 2019;14(6):e0218107.

19. Wang NK, Wu YM, Wang JP, et al. Clinical characteristics of posterior staphylomas in myopic eyes with axial length shorter than 26.5 mm. Am J Ophthalmol. 2016;162:180–90.

20. Takahashi H, Tanaka N, Shinohara K, et al. Ultra-widefield optical coherence tomographic imaging of posterior vitreous in eyes with high myopia. Am J Ophthalmol. 2019;206:102–12.

Myopic Maculopathy

17

Yuxin Fang and Kyoko Ohno-Matsui

17.1 Introduction

The development of myopic macular lesions is characteristic to pathologic myopia (Figs. 17.1 and 17.2), and various lesions of myopic maculopathy have been well-known since a long time ago (see Chap. 1 for details). Thus, Schweizer (1890) examined 2910 myopes and found the changes at the macula in 6.3% of all myopes, in 14% of myopes above 3 diopters (D), and in 100% above 20D. Myopic macular complications described by Schweizer (1890) and later Sattler (1907) include macular hemorrhages, white spots of atrophy, and an atrophic sclerosis of the small vessels, although later studies have revealed that the choroidal vessels were not truly sclerotic. They also described that eventually large areas of atrophy may appear, until the choroid and retina may have disappeared over a wide area of the central region. A central circular dark spot (the Förster-Fuchs spot), which is now considered a proliferation of retinal pigment epithelium (RPE) around myopic choroidal neovascularization (CNV), was first clinically described by Forster (1862), first anatomically examined by Lehmus (1875), and extensively studied by Fuchs (1901). Lacquer cracks were found by Salzmann in 1902 as cleft-shaped or branched defects in the lamina vitrea (an ancient name for Bruch's membrane) [1, 2].

Curtin did outstanding observations of various kinds of lesions of myopic maculopathy [3]. He analyzed the development of myopic maculopathy in association with posterior staphyloma and also according to the patients' age (birth to age 30, ages 30 to 60, and age 60 or above). Grossniklaus and Green [4] performed histological analyses of the eyes with myopic maculopathy and provided important insights in understanding the pathologies of myopic maculopathy. Avila [5] graded myopic maculopathy on a scale of increasing severity.

Later Tokoro updated and organized the lesions of myopic maculopathy in his atlas [6]. Tokoro [6] classified myopic macular lesions into four kinds of categories based on ophthalmoscopic findings: (1) tessellated fundus (Fig. 17.2a), (2) diffuse chorioretinal atrophy (Fig. 17.2b), (3) patchy chorioretinal atrophy (Fig. 17.2c), and (4) macular hemorrhage (Fig. 17.2d). Macular hemorrhage was subclassified into two types of lesions—myopic CNV and simple macular hemorrhage. Later, Hayashi et al. [7] made some modifications and considered lacquer cracks as an independent lesion from diffuse atrophy (Table 17.1). Each of these lesions is explained in detail in this chapter.

Myopic maculopathy is important because it is often bilateral and irreversible, and it frequently affects individuals during their productive years. Because the definition of myopic maculopathy is different among studies, it is impossible to simply compare the results of different studies. However, myopic maculopathy is the leading cause (22%) of blindness in Japanese adults aged 40 years or older [8], the third cause (6.6%) of blindness in Chinese adults 50 years and older in urban southern China [9], and the third cause (6.7%) of visual impairment in the ethnic Indians aged more than 40 years living in Singapore [10]. A survey of 2263 Japanese adults aged 40–79 years showed that the OR of visual impairment for myopic adults was 2.9 (95% CI 1.4, 6.0) [11]. Besides East Asian countries, myopic maculopathy is currently the third cause of blindness in the adult Latinos aged 40 years or older in the USA [12], the second cause of bilateral blindness in an elderly urban Danish population [13], the fourth common cause of visual impairment in the elderly in UK [14], and the third most common cause of blindness in the working age population in Ireland [15] and Israel [16]. A recent study of

Y. Fang · K. Ohno-Matsui (✉)
Department of Ophthalmology and Visual Science, Tokyo Medical and Dental University, Bunkyo-Ku, Tokyo, Japan
e-mail: k.ohno.oph@tmd.ac.jp

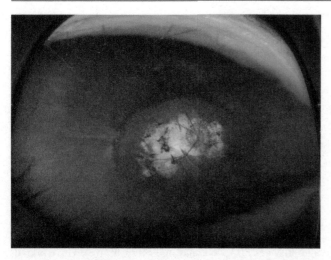

Fig. 17.1 Ultra-wide fundus photograph of an eye with pathologic myopia. An extensive chorioretinal atrophy fused with a large myopic conus is seen within the area of posterior staphyloma

4582 Chinese-American adults aged 50+ years revealed that the most common cause of blindness was myopic retinopathy [17]. Actually, the visual prognosis for highly myopic patients with myopic maculopathy was poorer than for those without maculopathy [18]. Earlier population-based studies showed a correlation between worse corrected visual acuity and a presence of myopic maculopathy [19, 20].

Recent advance in ocular imaging, especially optical coherence tomography (OCT), has provided novel and important information in the interpretation of myopic maculopathy. Thus, in this chapter, we will overview the features of each lesion of myopic maculopathy with the latest knowledge obtained by the latest technologies.

17.2 Features of Each Lesion of Myopic Maculopathy

17.2.1 Tessellated (or Tigroid) Fundus

In eyes with high myopia, hypoplasia of the retinal pigment epithelium (RPE) following axial elongation reduces the pigment, allowing the choroidal vessels to be seen (Fig. 17.2a). Tessellated fundus is one of the earliest visible signs in eyes with high myopia, like the myopic conus around the optic disc. Tessellation begins to develop around the optic disc, especially in the area between the optic disc and the central fovea. Although it is rare to detect other myopic fundus lesions (e.g., myopic chorioretinal atrophy or CNV) in the children and young patients with high myopia [21], tessellated fundus is often observed in children with high myopia. Highly myopic patients with tessellated fundus are significantly younger than the patients with other lesions of myopic maculopathy [7,

22]. Wang et al. [22] reported that the highly myopic patients with tessellated fundus alone had less myopia, shorter axial length, and less staphyloma than the highly myopic patients with diffuse chorioretinal atrophy. Tokoro [6] reported that about 90% of eyes with only tessellated fundus and no chorioretinal atrophy had an axial length less than 26 mm. This percentage decreases linearly in eyes with longer axial length and becomes 0 when the axial length is longer than 31 mm. Actually, a 1-mm elongation in axial length will lead to about a 13% increase of chorioretinal atrophy from eyes with only tessellated fundus and no chorioretinal atrophy.

What causes the tessellation of the fundus is not clear. The RPE cells become thinned due to a stretching and expansion of the posterior globe in the studies using animal models of experimental myopia [23, 24]. Also, the earlier studies using vitreous fluorophotometry showed that retinal blood barrier was damaged in myopic subjects already under the age 40 [25] and also in animal models of experimental myopia [26–28]. Tessellation can also be seen in other conditions as well, e.g., the fundus of the elderly or in chronic stages of Vogt-Koyanagi-Harada disease (as sunset glow fundus). Spaide [29] analyzed the features of the patients with age-related choroidal atrophy (choroidal thickness was less than 125 [m) and reported that all eyes had a tessellated fundus appearance. The mean (or median) choroidal thickness at subfovea in eyes with tessellated fundus in high myopia varies from 80 to 166 μm [22, 30–32], and choroidal thickness at all locations reduced almost by one-half compared to those with no myopic maculopathy in high myopia [30, 31]. These suggest that an attenuation of choroid occurs and RPE abnormalities could then develop.

Tessellation alone does not usually cause a decreased visual acuity, although it has been reported there are reduced amplitude and a delayed latency of multifocal ERG in highly myopic eyes with tessellated fundus alone [33–36].

In the study investigating the natural course of 806 eyes of 429 consecutive patients with high myopia (myopic refractive error >8 D or axial length ε 26.5 mm) for 5 to 32 years [7], only 13.4% of eyes with a tessellated fundus showed a progression; 10.1% developed diffuse chorioretinal atrophy, 2.9% developed lacquer cracks, and 0.4% developed a CNV. Progression was also observed in 19% in 10-year follow-up in Beijing Eye Study [37]. Another large series of 810 highly myopic eyes who followed more than 10 years (a mean follow-up of 18 years) showed 27% of eyes with tessellated fundus progressed in which 74.3% progressed to diffuse atrophy, 21.6% progressed to patchy atrophy, 10.8% developed new lacquer cracks, and 6.8% developed myopic CNV [38]. Since the eyes with other myopic fundus lesions showed a higher progression rate to the more advanced lesions than the eyes with tessellated

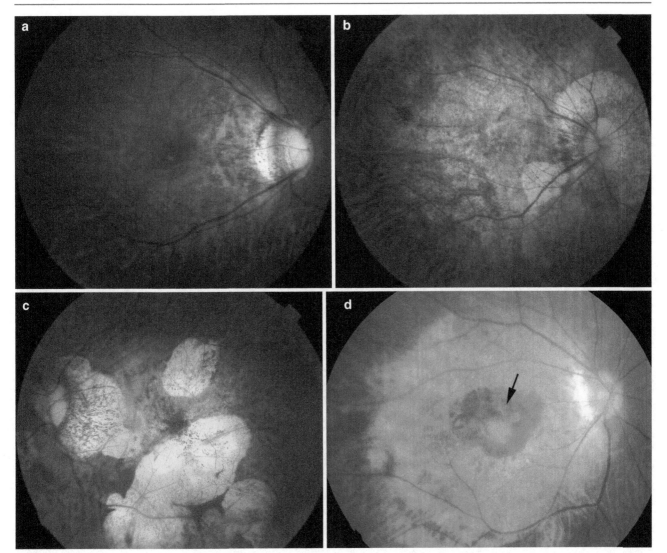

Fig. 17.2 Fundus lesions according to a classification of myopic maculopathy by Tokoro in 1998. (**a**) Tessellated fundus. Large choroidal vessels can be seen in the posterior fundus as a relief. (**b**) Diffuse chorioretinal atrophy. Yellowish, ill-defined atrophy is seen in the posterior fundus. (**c**) Patchy chorioretinal atrophy. Multiple lesions of well-defined whitish atrophy (as white as myopic conus) exist within the area of diffuse atrophy. (**d**) Macular hemorrhage. The fibrovascular membrane suggesting choroidal neovascular membrane (arrow) is also noted in this case

Table 17.1 Lesions of myopic maculopathy based on the natural progression (Hayashi et al. 2010)

Tessellated fundus
Diffuse chorioretinal atrophy
Lacquer cracks
Patchy chorioretinal atrophy
Myopic choroidal neovascularization

fundus, it is suggested that myopic maculopathy tends to progress more quickly after the myopic maculopathy has advanced past the tessellated fundus stage. A tessellated fundus might be a relatively stable condition, and highly myopic eyes might stay in this condition for a relatively long period.

17.2.2 Lacquer Cracks

Lacquer cracks are fine, irregular, yellow lines, often branching and crisscrossing, seen in the posterior fundus of highly myopic eyes (Fig. 17.3). Stereoscopic observation using magnified lens (e.g., +90D or +75D lens) shows that lacquer cracks are somewhat depressed compared to the surrounding retina. Larger choroidal vessels frequently traverse the lesions posteriorly. In rare occasions, lacquer cracks are also observed in the mid-periphery [39] or nasal to the optic disc [40]. Pruett et al. [41] analyzed the pattern of break formation in eyes with lacquer cracks, angioid streaks, or traumatic tears in Bruch's membrane. Lacquer cracks were found in a reticular distribution within a posterior staphyloma; angioid

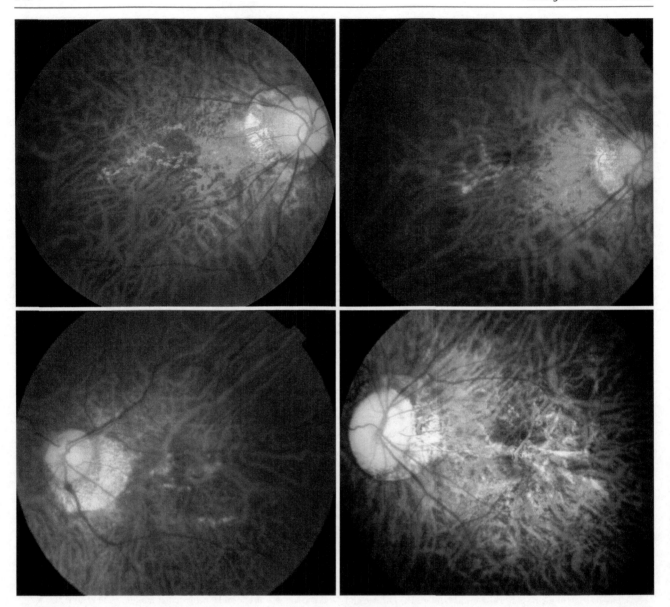

Fig. 17.3 Lacquer cracks. Lacquer cracks are observed as yellowish linear lesions which run in parallel or in crisscross pattern. Large choroidal vessels are observed to course posteriorly

streaks occurred in a spider-web configuration centered on the optic nerve; traumatic tears were characteristically curved, perineural, and eccentric temporally. Curtin and Karlin [42] reported that lacquer cracks were found in 4.3% of highly myopic eyes. Histologically, the lacquer cracks represent healed mechanical fissures in the RPE-Bruch's membrane-choriocapillaris complex [4].

Lacquer cracks can develop at a relatively early age in highly myopic patients (e.g., in the 30s). The greatest incidence of lacquer cracks was noted in the age groups of 20 to 39 years. Klein and Curtin [43] reported that the mean age of the patients with lacquer cracks was 32 years with a range of 14 to 52 years. Tokoro [6] reported that the frequency of lacquer cracks was low in patients younger than age 20 and in

the elderly but increases around ages 40 and 60 years. The frequency distribution of lacquer cracks showed two peaks in the age between 35 and 39 years and the age between 55 and 59 years.

The diagnosis of lacquer cracks has been mainly based on ophthalmoscopic identification. Fluorescein angiography (FA) has been an additional standard method to detect lacquer cracks [43]. Lacquer cracks show a consistent linear hyperfluorescence during the entire angiographic phase (Fig. 17.4), a window defect due to RPE atrophy overlying the defects of Bruch's membrane in the early angiographic phase and a staining of healed scar tissue filling the Bruch's membrane defect in the late phase. However, especially in the eyes with diffuse chorioretinal atrophy, it is sometimes difficult to observe yellowish lacquer cracks within the area of yellowish diffuse atrophy and also difficult to detect linear hyperfluorescence of lacquer cracks within mildly stained diffuse atrophy. The usefulness of indocyanine green angiography (ICGA) has also been reported [44–49]. Lacquer cracks are observed as linear hypofluorescence during the entire angiographic phase of ICGA. The hypofluorescence in ICGA is more easily recognized in late angiographic phase, because an intense fluorescence of retrobulbar blood vessels or large choroidal vessels impairs the observation of narrow linear hypofluorescence of lacquer cracks in the early angiographic phase. In some cases, lacquer cracks observed by ICGA are more numerous and longer than those observed by FA. Also, ICGA can detect the lacquer cracks even at the onset of rupture of Bruch's membrane as linear hypofluorescence beneath the subretinal bleeding [46]. Lacquer cracks also show linear hypo-autofluorescence by fundus autofluorescence (Fig. 17.4). It is difficult to detect lacquer cracks by using OCT, because it is such a narrow lesion. However, in some cases, the discontinuities of the RPE (and probably Bruch's membrane as well) and an increased penetrance into the deeper tissue

beyond the RPE are observed at the site of the lacquer cracks (Fig. 17.4). Once detected, OCT is considered to be the most accurate diagnostic tool, because only OCT can visualize the discontinuity of Bruch's membrane, which is an integral feature of lacquer cracks.

When the mechanical rupture of Bruch's membrane occurs, subretinal macular hemorrhage without CNV develops (Fig. 17.5) [50–52]. This subretinal bleeding is absorbed spontaneously, and after absorption we can observe lacquer cracks as yellowish linear lesion at the corresponding area of previous bleeding. Most of the patients with subretinal bleeding without CNV have a good visual recovery after absorption of hemorrhage. However, in the eyes whose bleeding was thick and penetrated into the inner retina beyond the external limiting membrane, the IS/OS defect seen at the onset by using OCT remains after absorption of hemorrhage, leaving the permanent vision loss [53].

Lacquer cracks might be a unique lesion among the various lesions of myopic maculopathy, because they seem to be caused almost purely by mechanical expansion of the globe and are not much influenced by aging. This is supported by the fact that chick models of experimental myopia which can

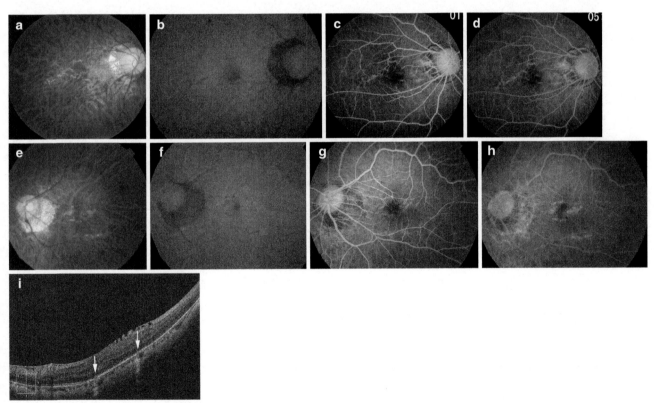

Fig. 17.4 Angiographic and optical coherence tomographic (OCT) findings of lacquer cracks. (**a**) Right fundus shows multiple lacquer cracks as fine, irregular, yellow lines, branching and crisscrossing in the posterior fundus. Larger choroidal vessels frequently traverse the lesions posteriorly. (**b**) Fundus autofluorescence (FAF) shows lacquer cracks as linear hypo-autofluorescence. (**c**, **d**) Fluorescein angiographic (FA) findings. Lacquer cracks show linear hyperfluorescence from the early angiographic phase (**c**) to the late phase (**d**). (**e**) Left fundus shows multiple lacquer cracks which run in parallel. (**f**) FAF shows linear hypo-autofluorescence corresponding to lacquer cracks. (**g**, **h**) Lacquer cracks show linear hyperfluorescence from the early angiographic phase (**g**) to the late phase (**h**) by FA. (**i**) OCT findings show the discontinuities of retinal pigment epithelium and deep penetrance of the light signal at the corresponding site of lacquer cracks

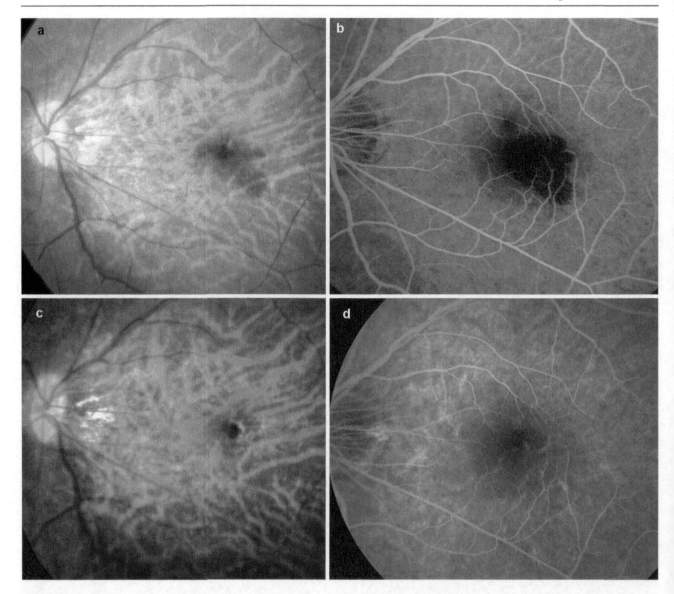

Fig. 17.5 Subretinal bleeding without choroidal neovascularization as a sign of new lacquer crack formation. (**a**) Left fundus shows subretinal bleeding in the macula. (**b**) Fluorescein angiogram (FA) shows a blocked fluorescence due to bleeding. (**c**) Two months later, the bleed-ing is absorbed spontaneously. Lacquer cracks are observed at the site of the previous bleeding. (**d**) FA shows lacquer cracks as linear hyperfluorescence

develop axial myopia in 2 weeks of visual deprivation can develop lacquer cracks [54]. Actually, lacquer cracks and subretinal bleeding caused by a new lacquer crack formation have been the only macular pathologies which reportedly develop in animal models of experimental myopia. This is also supported that lacquer cracks develop after LASIK surgery [55–59] or after laser photocoagulation [60].

Once lacquer cracks develop in the eye, it tends to develop one after another in the same eye. Thus, the patients with lacquer cracks tend to have multiple lacquer cracks in both eyes. It seems that there might be a genetic predisposition

toward lacquer crack formation among individuals with pathologic myopia.

There is no obvious correlation between the axial length and lacquer cracks in eyes with pathologic myopia. Klein and Curtin [43] reported that the mean axial length of the eyes with lacquer cracks was 31.8 mm (range, 29.8–34.7 mm). Tokoro [6] reported that the largest number of eyes with lacquer cracks appears between 29.0 and 29.4 mm.

It is uncommon for lacquer cracks to develop across the central fovea. Thus, lacquer cracks themselves do not usually impair the central vision; however, the subretinal bleeding which develops at the onset of the rupture of Bruch's membrane could cause the impairment of central vision even after absorption of the hemorrhage.

The Blue Mountains Eye Study (BMES) reported that 8.7% had new or increased numbers of lacquer cracks in 5 years [61]. In the follow-up study of 66 eyes with lacquer cracks for an average of 72.8 months (range, 7 to 243 months) [62], lacquer cracks progressed in 37 eyes (56.1%). Of these 37 eyes, the number of lacquer cracks increased in 14 eyes and turned into other myopic fundus changes in 25 eyes. These changes included patchy atrophy, diffuse atrophy, and CNV. In another study [7], 75 eyes with lacquer cracks were followed for more than 5 years and found that 32 eyes (42.7%) showed an increase in the width of the cracks and these eyes progressed to patchy chorioretinal atrophy (Fig. 17.6), 10 eyes (13.3%) developed CNV, and 10 eyes (13.3%) had an increase in number of lacquer cracks. The patchy atrophy that progressed from lacquer cracks is usually longitudinally oriented oval or rectangular (Fig. 17.6). The progression toward the patchy atrophy from lacquer cracks represents an increased area of rupture of Bruch's membrane. Thus, this progression is an increased area of macular Bruch's membrane defect (or opening). Xu [63] showed that the progression from lacquer cracks to patchy atrophy was not a uniform widening of the preexisting lacquer cracks but small circular areas of patchy atrophy that developed first along the lines of lacquer cracks, and then these circular areas enlarged and fused with each other. So, perhaps when the Bruch's membrane ruptures, the overlying RPE may remain continuous because the Bruch's membrane

rupture is narrow. Later with increasing mechanical tension, the overlying RPE ruptures, and RPE hole develops. This suggests that the RPE-Bruch's membrane complex does not disrupt simultaneously during lacquer crack formation.

Although lacquer cracks are often observed in the vicinity of CNV [5], it is unexpectedly uncommon for CNV to develop from the existing lacquer cracks. This suggests that the lacquer cracks which are observed as yellowish linear lesions are already-healed scar tissue and CNV could rarely develop once after the Bruch's rupture is healed completely by the scar tissue. When CNV develops in relation to lacquer cracks, new vessels might penetrate through Bruch's membrane defects just after the rupture occurs and before the rupture is sealed by the scar tissue. Cases which develop CNV shortly after the subretinal bleeding without CNV support this hypothesis.

Differential Diagnosis Myopic stretch lines

Myopic stretch lines were first reported by Dr. Yannuzzi [64] as hyper-autofluorescent linear lesions in the posterior fundus of highly myopic eyes (Fig. 17.7). Myopic stretch lines are observed as pigmented, brown lines alongside the large choroidal vessels (Fig. 17.7); however, it is sometimes difficult to observe this lesion funduscopically, and in that case only FA provides a clue of this lesion. Myopic stretch lines almost always develop in eyes with severe diffuse atrophy with a posterior staphyloma. Although ICGA showed similar findings (linear hypofluorescence) in two types of linear lesions in the posterior fundus of highly myopic eyes

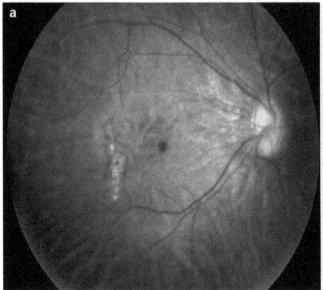
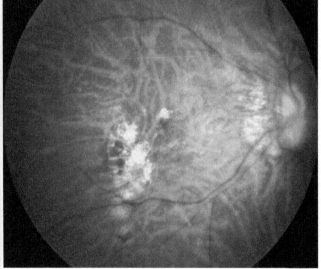

Fig. 17.6 Progression to patchy chorioretinal atrophy from lacquer cracks. (**a**) Right fundus of a 28-year-old woman shows a lacquer crack temporal to the central fovea. (**b**) Five years later, the width of the lac-

quer crack increased and progressed to patchy atrophy. New lacquer cracks are formed upper and lower to the fovea, and subretinal bleeding related to new lacquer crack formation is observed lower to the fovea

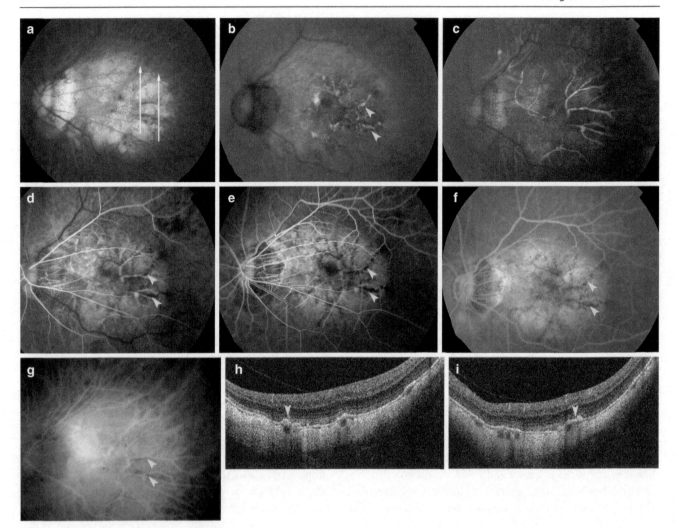

Fig. 17.7 Myopic stretch lines. (**a**) Left fundus shows brownish, pigmented lines along the large choroidal vessels temporal to the macula. White lines show the scanned lines by OCT in (**h**) and (**i**). (**b**) Fundus autofluorescence (FAF) shows multiple lines with hyper-autofluorescence radiated around the central fovea. Arrowheads show the same point of the stretch lines between (**b**), (**d**), (**e**), and (**f**). (**c**) Choroidal phase of fluorescein angiography (FA) shows large choroidal arteries. Some parts of large choroidal arteries show hypofluorescent spots by blocked fluorescence of overlying stretch lines. (**d**) Retinal arterial phase of FA. Myopic stretch lines appear as hypofluorescent linear lesions. (**e**) Retinal venous laminar flow phase of FA. Myopic stretch lines are clearly observed as multiple hypofluorescent lines around the central fovea and within the slightly stained diffuse atrophy. (**f**) Late phase of FA clearly shows myopic stretch lines as multiple hypofluorescent lines within the slightly stained diffuse atrophy. (**g**) Late phase of indocyanine green angiography shows a mild hypofluorescence corresponding to the stretch lines. (**h**, **i**) OCT shows that the almost entire thickness of the choroid is absent and only large choroidal vessels are sporadically present. Large choroidal vessels seem to protrude toward the vitreous, and clumps and proliferation of retinal pigmented epithelium are seen on and around the choroidal vessels (arrowheads)

(lacquer cracks and myopic stretch lines), the features obtained funduscopically, angiographically, and by OCT were different between these two types of linear lesions. Contrary to lacquer cracks, fundus autofluorescence (FAF) showed linear hyper-autofluorescence in myopic stretch lines (Fig. 17.7). OCT images show the clumps of RPE or RPE proliferation on and around the large choroidal vessels (which are protruded toward the vitreous subsequent to a disappearance of most of the choroidal layers) (Fig. 17.7). These suggest that myopic stretch lines might represent the RPE proliferation on and around the remaining large choroi-

dal vessels [65]. Because ICGA findings of myopic stretch lines are same with those of lacquer cracks and the diagnosis of lacquer cracks are sometimes based solely on ICGA in many studies, a caution is necessary for differentiating myopic stretch lines from lacquer cracks.

17.2.3 Diffuse Choroidal Atrophy

Diffuse choroidal atrophy is observed as ill-defined yellowish lesion in the posterior fundus of highly myopic eyes

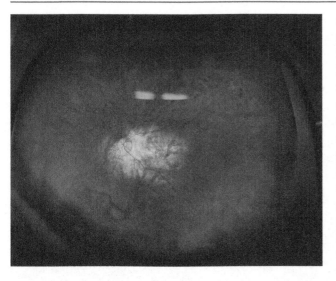

Fig. 17.8 Ultra-wide fundus photograph of diffuse choroidal atrophy. A yellowish, ill-defined lesion is seen in the posterior fundus

(Figs. 17.8 and 17.9). This lesion begins to appear around the optic disc and increases with age and finally covers the entire area within the staphyloma (Fig. 17.9). When diffuse atrophy is observed only around the optic disc, it needs to be differentiated from peripapillary intrachoroidal cavitation (peripapillary ICC) [66–70], because ICC also shows similar ophthalmoscopic appearance regardless of the difference in OCT images (see Chap. 9 for ICC).

The frequency of diffuse atrophy increases with aging as well as an increased axial length [6]. Diffuse atrophy begins to appear in the posterior fundus at around the age 40 and is observed in about 30–40% after age 40 [6]. The increasing rate of diffuse atrophy is about 10.5% per 10 years [6]. When the axial length is within the range of 27 to 33 mm, the increase in the percentage of eye with diffuse atrophy can be calculated using a simple regression equation. The increased percentage is 13.3%/mm in the total number of myopic eyes, 9.4%/mm in eyes under age 40, and 12.2%/mm in eyes over age 40 [6].

FA shows the mild hyperfluorescence due to tissue staining in the late angiographic phase (Fig. 17.10). On ICGA, diffuse atrophy itself does not show clear abnormalities; however, a marked decrease of the choroidal capillary, the medium- and large-sized choroidal vessels, is seen in the area of diffuse atrophy, and the blood vessels in the back of the eye are sometimes seen through the sclera in the posterior pole (Fig. 17.10). Because the penetrating site of short posterior ciliary arteries moves to the edge of posterior staphyloma, the choroidal blood vessels in the posterior pole become less dense (Fig. 17.10). In accordance with a marked decrease of choroidal vessels by ICGA, OCT shows a marked thinning of the choroid in the area of diffuse atrophy (Fig. 17.10). In most of the cases, the choroid is almost absent except sporadically present large choroidal vessels

(Fig. 17.10). The remaining large choroidal vessels appear to protrude toward the vitreous. It is interesting to know, even in the area where most of the choroidal layer is absent, the RPE layer and outer retina are present in the eyes with diffuse atrophy (Fig. 17.10). A presence of outer retina and RPE even in the area where most of the choroid is gone might explain a relatively preserved vision in eyes with diffuse atrophy. Okisaka [71] reported that the choroidal changes in pathologic myopia began from the obliteration of precapillary arterioles or postcapillary venules, then followed by an occlusion of choriocapillaris. Finally, large choroidal vessels are also obliterated, and the choroid seems to be absent. In parallel to the vascular changes in the choroid, choroidal melanocytes disappear as well. Although a choroid becomes thinned in eyes with tessellated fundus, the degree of choroidal thinning is much more serious in eyes with diffuse atrophy. And such disproportionate thinning of choroid compared to the surrounding tissue (RPE, outer retina, and sclera) might be a key phenomenon in diffuse atrophy.

Why diffuse atrophy shows yellow color is not clear. Diffuse atrophy is not uniformly yellow but shows granular yellow appearance (Fig. 17.10).

17.2.4 Patchy Chorioretinal Atrophy

Patchy chorioretinal atrophy is observed as a grayish-white, well-defined atrophy (Figs. 17.11 and 17.12) [6]. Due to an absence of RPE and most of the choroid, the sclera can be observed through transparent retinal tissue, which is considered to show white color. This lesion is also referred to as focal chorioretinal atrophy [3]. Large choroidal vessels seem to course within the area of patchy atrophy. In some cases, retrobulbar blood vessels are observed through the patchy atrophy with moving according to the gaze shift. Stereoscopic fundus examination shows that the area of patchy atrophy is somewhat excavated compared to surrounding diffuse atrophy. Pigment clumping is observed within the area of patchy atrophy especially along the margin of the atrophy or along the large choroidal vessels. FA as well as ICGA shows a choroidal filling defect in the area of patchy atrophy (Fig. 17.11), suggesting that this lesion is a complete closure of choriocapillaris [6].

Due to a subsequent loss of RPE in the area of patchy atrophy, the lesion shows a lack of fundus autofluorescence (Fig. 17.11). Using OCT, patchy atrophy is observed as a loss of most of the thickness of choroid, RPE, and outer retina (Fig. 17.11). Thus, the inner retina is directly on the sclera within the area of patchy atrophy. Swept-source OCT also showed the discontinuities of Bruch's membrane in the area of patchy atrophy [72, 73]. The RPE stopped outside of the margin of the macular Bruch's membrane defect. The edges of the macular Bruch's membrane defects showed an

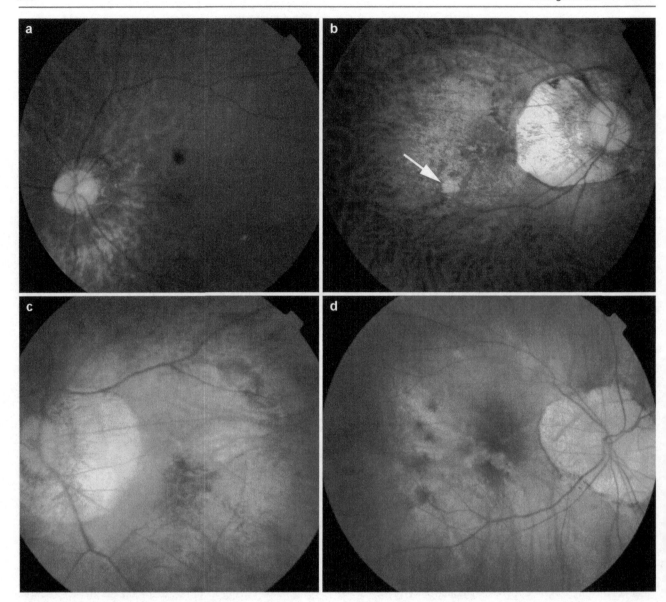

Fig. 17.9 Diffuse choroidal atrophy. (**a**) Early stage of diffuse atrophy. Yellowish, ill-defined lesions are observed lower to the optic disc. (**b**) Advanced stage of diffuse atrophy. Yellowish, ill-defined atrophy covers the entire macular area. A small lesion of patchy chorioretinal atrophy (arrow) is also seen within the area of diffuse atrophy. (**c**) Advanced stage of diffuse atrophy. The posterior fundus within a staphyloma is replaced by diffuse atrophy. The images in (**a**) to (**d**) are Asians' eyes. (**d**) Diffuse atrophy in a Caucasian patient. Diffuse atrophy is seen evident especially in the lower fundus. Diffuse atrophy tends to be more obvious in the pigmented eyes

abrupt termination and often an upturned edge. This is contrary to the fact that the RPE, Bruch's membrane, and outer retina are preserved in most of the eyes with diffuse atrophy, although it is not certain if the remaining photoreceptors and RPE function normally in those eyes.

Patchy atrophy is subclassified into three types (Fig. 17.12): patchy atrophy which develops from lacquer cracks, P(Lc); patchy atrophy which develops within the area of an advanced diffuse chorioretinal atrophy, P(D); and patchy atrophy which can be seen along the border of the posterior staphyloma, P(St) [7]. P(D) is often circular or elliptical, and P(Lc) is longitudinally oval in its shape. P(Lc)

is considered an enlargement of Bruch's membrane defect due to lacquer cracks, and P(D) might also represent a Bruch's membrane hole [74] developing within the area of advanced stage of diffuse atrophy. Jonas [74] recently reported that macular Bruch's membrane defects were found in 30.8% of highly myopic eyes whose axial length was ε 26.5 mm histologically. A lack of Bruch's membrane defects might be related to the development of macular ICC. Due to a lack of tensile Bruch's membrane in addition to a lack of choroid on the thin sclera, the area of patchy atrophy is very fragile against the inner pressure load. The sclera can be bowed posteriorly in the area of the patchy atrophy

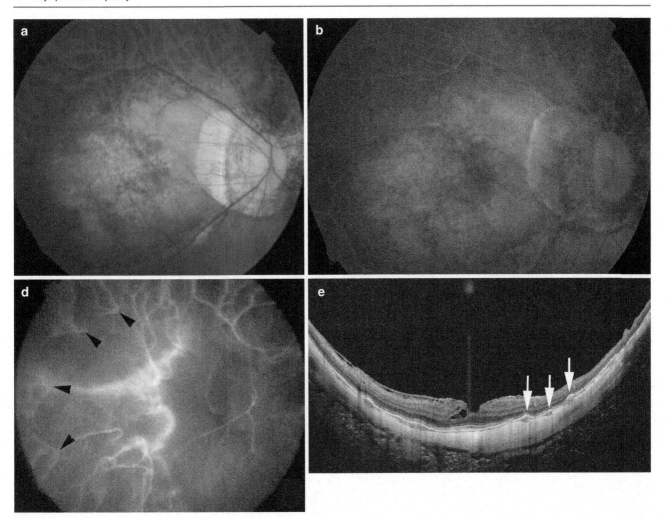

Fig. 17.10 Angiographic and optical coherence tomographic (OCT) findings of diffuse choroidal atrophy. (**a**) Left fundus shows the diffuse choroidal atrophy in the posterior fundus. (**b**) Late angiographic phase of fluorescein angiogram shows slight hyperfluorescence in the area of diffuse atrophy. (**c**) Indocyanine green angiography shows that the penetrating site of short posterior ciliary arteries into the choroid is shifted toward the edge of posterior staphyloma. There are few large- and medium-sized choroidal vessels in the macular area, and instead retrobulbar blood vessels show an intense fluorescence. (**d**) OCT examination shows that most of the choroidal thickness is absent and only large choroidal vessels are sporadically present. Large choroidal vessels are observed to protrude toward the retina (arrows)

(Fig. 17.14), which resembles the intrachoroidal cavitation that develops adjacent to a myopic conus in highly myopic eyes (peripapillary intrachoroidal cavitations; peripapillary ICC). Thus, the posterior displacement of sclera can be called as macular ICC [75]. Macular retinoschisis is significantly more frequently observed in the eyes with macular ICC than those without macular ICC [75]. This is because the mechanical dissociation attributable to the scleral bowing and the caving in of the retina might facilitate the development of retinoschisis in and around the patchy atrophy.

Patchy atrophy is reportedly present in 0.4% of general population aged ≥ 40 years in the Hisayama Study in Japan [76]. The percentage of patchy atrophy increases linearly with axial length of the eye and reaches 32.5% after age 60 years [6]. The percentage of patchy atrophy is 3.3% in the eyes whose axial length is from 27 to 27.9 mm, which exceeds 25% if the axial length is longer than 31 mm, and it exceeds 50% if the axial length is longer than 32 mm [6].

With increasing age, the patchy atrophy enlarges and coalesces with each other [3, 7, 38]. In the follow-up study of 74 eyes with patchy atrophy for ε 5 years, 52 eyes (70.3%) showed a progression [7]. Fifty eyes (67.6%) showed an enlargement of the patchy areas, ten eyes (13.5%) showed a fusion with P(D) or P(St), and two eyes (2.7%) developed a CNV [7]. In the eyes with advanced enlargement and fusion of patchy atrophy, the posterior fundus shows a "bare sclera" appearance (Fig. 17.13). Almost all eyes (95%) with patchy atrophy progressed after a mean follow-up of 18 years, in which an enlargement of the original patchy atrophy was found predominantly in 98% and new patchy atrophy was found in 47% followed by development of myopic CNV in 21.7% and patchy-related macular atrophy in 8.3% [38].

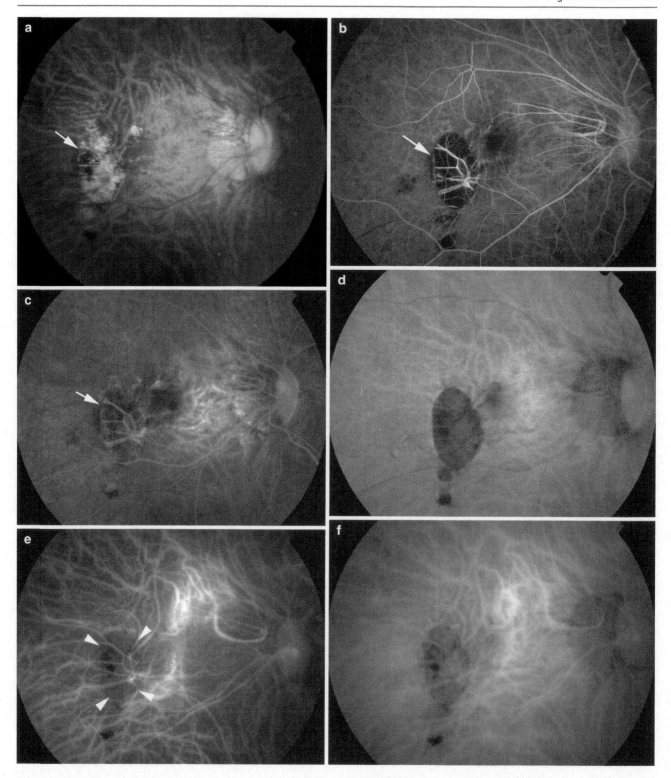

Fig. 17.11 Patchy chorioretinal atrophy. (**a**) Right fundus shows a patchy atrophy (arrow) temporal to the central fovea. According to the subclassification of patchy atrophy, this case has P(Lc). (**b**) Early phase of fluorescein angiogram (FA) shows a hypofluorescence due to the choroidal filling defects (arrow). (**c**) In the late phase of FA, the margin of the lesion becomes slightly hyperfluorescent (arrow). (**d**) Fundus autofluorescence shows a distinct hypo-autofluorescence corresponding to the patchy atrophy. (**e, f**) Indocyanine green angiogram shows hypofluorescence due to choroidal filling defect from early angiographic phase (**e**; arrowheads) to late phase (**f**). (**g**) Optical coherence tomography examinations show that in addition to the absence of the entire thickness of the choroid, the retinal pigment epithelium as well as outer retina is absent (between arrowheads). The hyper-reflectivity in deep tissue due to an increased light penetration is noted in the area of patchy atrophy

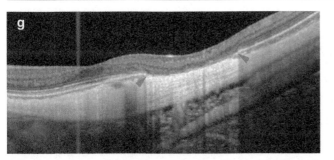

Fig. 18.11 (continued)

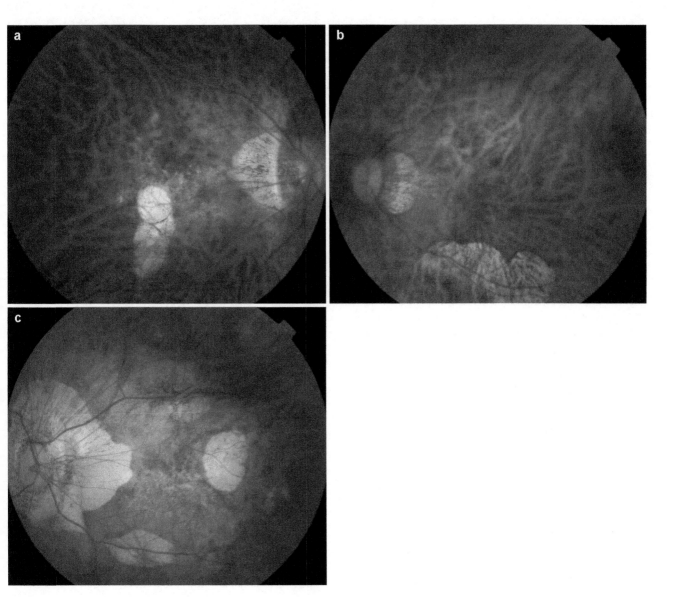

Fig. 17.12 Three types of patchy chorioretinal atrophy. (**a**) P(Lc), patchy atrophy progressed from lacquer cracks. Longitudinal atrophy is seen lower to the central fovea. Lacquer cracks are also found in and around the central fovea, and the degree of background diffuse atrophy is mild. (**b**) P(St), patchy atrophy which develops along the edge of posterior staphyloma. (**c**) P(D), patchy atrophy which develops within the advanced stage of diffuse atrophy. An oval atrophy is observed temporal to the fovea. P(St) is also found along the lower edge of staphyloma

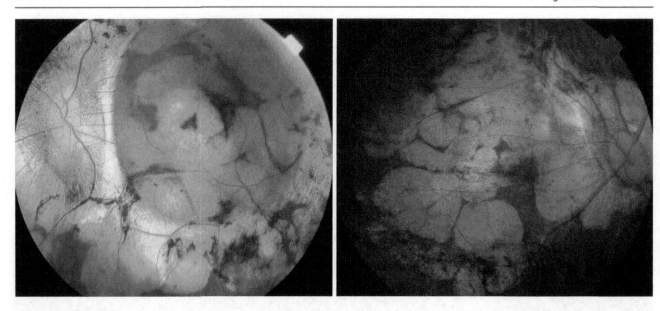

Fig. 17.13 "Bare sclera" appearance due to an enlargement of patchy chorioretinal atrophy. The entire area of posterior fundus is replaced by an enlarged patchy atrophy

Such high percentages of progression of eyes with patchy atrophy could be explained by the biomechanical properties of Bruch's membrane so that as soon as a defect is created, the Bruch's membrane defect would enlarge over time with ongoing axial elongation. The BMES showed that 5.2% of the participants had new or expanded areas of patchy chorioretinal atrophy in 5 years [61]. Ito-Ohara et al. [77] examined the direction of enlargement of patchy atrophy and found that the patchy atrophy in marginal lesions of a staphyloma enlarged toward the macula and the patchy atrophy in the macula enlarged in all directions [77]. However, it is uncommon for extrafoveal patchy atrophy later to involve the central fovea. This means that it is rare for patchy atrophy to cause the central vision loss although this lesion causes a paracentral absolute scotoma due to a loss of photoreceptors within the atrophic area.

Various kinds of vitreoretinal complications can develop in and around the patchy atrophy. Probably due to a weak adhesion between the inner retina and sclera in the area of patchy atrophy, the macular retinoschisis tends to occur preferably in the area of patchy atrophy [78]. In the area of extensive chorioretinal atrophy, the diagnosis of retinoschisis needs caution because the retinoschisis shows less column-like structures [79]. It is also reported that posterior paravascular linear retinal breaks occur over areas of patchy atrophy as a cause of retinal detachment in the patients with pathologic myopia [80].

Although the patchy atrophy itself does not impair the central vision, the development of CNV along the foveal margin of patchy atrophy impairs the central vision significantly (Fig. 17.14) [81]. The CNV develops especially in eyes with P(Lc), probably because lacquer cracks tend to

develop near the fovea and thus the P(Lc) occurs in the vicinity of the central fovea. Also, different from P(D) which develops within the area of advanced diffuse atrophy with a loss of most of the choroidal thickness, P(Lc) tends to develop in the eyes with less degree of choroidal atrophy. Once the CNV develops along the edge of patchy atrophy, the chorioretinal atrophy enlarges around the CNV and fuses with P(Lc), and the posterior fundus is eventually replaced by a large area of patchy atrophy (Fig. 17.14).

Differential Diagnosis

- *The atrophic phase of myopic CNV*

A well-defined chorioretinal atrophy develops around the scarred CNV and enlarges gradually (Fig. 17.15; see Chap. 19 for details), and the atrophic stage of myopic CNV is important to differentiate from patchy atrophy. Fundus features, angiographic findings, FAF findings, and OCT findings are all the same between the atrophic stage of myopic CNV and patchy atrophy. Especially long after the regression of myopic CNV, it becomes difficult to detect fibrovascular tissue remnants within the chorioretinal atrophy. The main difference between patchy atrophy and atrophic stage of myopic CNV is its location relative to the central fovea. The chorioretinal atrophy around the myopic CNV is almost always centered on the fovea and enlarges circumferentially around the fovea. In contrary, the patchy atrophy usually does not involve the fovea.

- *Multifocal Choroiditis (MFC) or Punctate Inner Choroidopathy (PIC)*

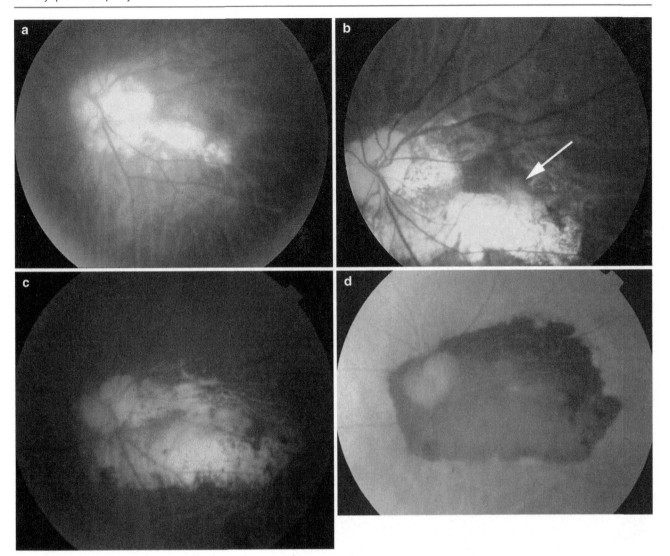

Fig. 17.14 A fusion with P(Lc) and an atrophy around the myopic choroidal neovascularization (CNV). (**a**) At the initial visit, horizontally longitudinal P(Lc) is observed lower to the central fovea. (**b**) Two years later, the CNV has developed along the foveal edge of an enlarged P(Lc). (**c**) Ten years after the CNV regression, an atrophy developed around the scarred CNV has enlarged and fused with P(Lc). (**d**) Fundus autofluorescence shows a large area of hypo-autofluorescence in the posterior fundus

MFC and PIC tend to affect young females (~75%) who are often myopic. These patients develop focal areas of inflammation in the deep retina and choroid that progress into atrophic and pigmentary chorioretinal scars. The acute lesions are typically multiple, bilateral, and yellow-white or grayish in appearance. When we observe the lesions similar to patchy atrophy in highly myopic eyes without diffuse chorioretinal atrophy (especially in young female), we need to consider the possibility of MFC/PIC.

MFC and PIC often develop CNV; thus, the differential diagnosis is necessary between myopic CNV and CNV caused by MFC/PIC.

17.2.5 Others

17.2.5.1 Macular Lesions in Dome-Shaped Macula

Dome-shaped macula (DSM) was originally described by Gaucher and associates [82] as a convex protrusion of macula within a staphyloma in highly myopic patients. By using enhanced depth imaging OCT (EDI-OCT), Imamura and Spaide [83] showed that a DSM is a result of a relative localized thickness variation of the sclera under the macula in highly myopic patients. OCT examination is indispensable for the diagnosis of DSM. DSM is not always

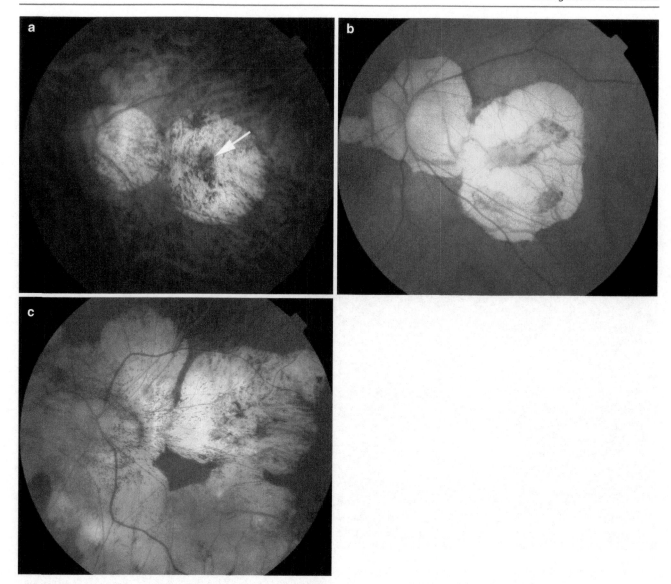

Fig. 17.15 Atrophic stage of myopic choroidal neovascularization (CNV). (**a**) Ten years after the onset of myopic CNV. Fibrovascular scar tissue is observed within the atrophy (arrow). (**b**) Eleven years after the onset of myopic CNV in an albino patient. Well-demarcated atrophy is observed around the scarred CNV. Atrophy is fused with myopic conus. (**c**) Twenty years after the onset of myopic CNV. The enlarged atrophy around the CNV is fused with P(St) as well as myopic conus

visible in all OCT scans, and it can be classified into three morphologic patterns, round dome and horizontally or vertically oval-shaped domes [84]. According to the following expanded definition, DSM can be diagnosed quantitatively as macular bulge height of >50 μm in the most convex scan in either vertical or horizontal scan [85]. The prevalence of serous RD is markedly variable from 2% to 67% depending on the series which is very rare in Asian [85–87] and much higher in Europe [82, 88]. As a mechanism of serous RD without CNV in eyes with DSM, Imamura and Spaide [83] suggested the possible obstruction of outflow of choroidal fluid by a thick sclera. Ellabban and associates [89] reported that CNV was frequently observed in eyes with DSM, in 41.2%. Gaucher et al. [82] also reported that 10 out of 15 eyes with DSM had a history of CNV. Although extrafoveal schisis was found in 17.6%, foveal schisis was uncommon in eyes with DSM, suggesting that the DSM might work in a protective fashion against the development of foveal schisis.

It is difficult to suspect the DSM solely from ophthalmoscopic findings; however, macular pigmentation and horizontal ridges connecting the optic disc and the fovea are often found in eyes with DSM and especially in the eyes whose DSM is evident only along the vertical section across the fovea [89]. Also, in the eyes with DSM along the vertical section across the fovea, the optic disc tends to be horizontally long oval. Because most of the myopic disc shows vertical or vertically oblique tilting except TDS, the horizontally long oval disc appearance might provide a clue to suspect the presence of DSM.

It is noted that DSM also can be detected in 9% of highly myopic children and young adults [90]. Compared with DSM in elderly patients, the domes in children are detected only in the vertical OCT scans and have a wider basis and smoother slope of the elevation without presence of macular Bruch's membrane defect and any type of staphyloma.

17.2.6 Macular Lesions Along the Edge of Tilted Disc Syndrome

Macular lesions observed in eyes with DSM appear somewhat similar to the lesions observed along the upper edge of staphyloma in eyes with tilted disc syndrome (TDS), such as serous RD due to subretinal leakage [91] or CNV [92]. Maruko and Iida [93] reported that serous RD was found in 7 of 24 eyes (29%) with TDS. By using EDI-OCT and swept-source OCT, they [93] also showed that the subfoveal choroid was relatively thin and the subfoveal sclera thickened in TDS with a staphyloma edge at the macula. From these findings, they suggested that the characteristic anatomic subfoveal scleral alterations might lead to a thinner choroid and inhibit chorioscleral outflow. Nakanishi and associates [92] reported that macular complications were found on the upper border of inferior staphyloma in 25 of the 32 eyes (78%) with TDSMyopic maculopathy. Macular complications included the polypoidal choroidal vasculopathy (PCV) in 22%, classic CNV in 3%, focal serous RD without PCV or CNV in 41%, and RPE atrophy in 13%. It is interesting to consider the similarities between DSM and TDS.

17.3 Frequency of Myopic Maculopathy

In the Blue Mountains Eye Study (BMES) [61], myopic retinopathy was defined to include the following specific signs: staphyloma, lacquer cracks, Fuchs spot, and myopic chorioretinal thinning or atrophy. Based on this definition, signs of myopic retinopathy were found in 1.2% of the eligible residents aged ≥ 49 years ($n = 3654$) who attended the BMES; staphyloma in 26 participants (0.7%), lacquer cracks in 8 participants (0.2%), Fuchs spot in 3 (0.1%), and chorioretinal atrophy in 7 (0.2%).

Using Tokoro's classification, Chen et al. [94] reported that myopic maculopathy was found in 443 of 604 eyes (73%) with high myopia (refractive error δ −6.0 D). Lacquer cracks were found to be the most prevalent type (29.1%) followed by CNV (20.7%), tessellated fundus (9.3%), patchy

chorioretinal atrophy (5.8%), diffuse chorioretinal atrophy (4.6%), and macular atrophy (3.8%). Asakuma et al. [76] used Hayashi's classification [7] and reported that myopic maculopathy was found in 1.7% of 1969 Japanese residents aged ε 40 years in the Hisayama Study. Asakuma et al. [76] reported that diffuse atrophy, patchy atrophy, lacquer cracks, and macular atrophy were present in 1.7%, 0.4%, 0.2%, and 0.4% of the subjects. A worse visual acuity was associated with lacquer cracks, macular atrophy, and CNV, while better visual acuity was associated with tessellated fundus and diffuse atrophy [19]. The use of inconsistent definitions of myopic maculopathy has led to limited comparability. The META-PM classification is now consistently used by many studies for investigation of the prevalence of myopic maculopathy [95–98].

From a population-based Singapore Epidemiology of Eye Diseases (SEED) study [96] including 8716 phakic adult ≥ aged 40 years, the age-standardized prevalence of myopic maculopathy (defined as Meta-PM category 2, 3, 4, or any "plus" lesion) was 3.8% in all and varied in races, i.e., 2.3% in Indians, 3.7% in Malays, and 4.6% in Chinese. The risk of myopic maculopathy is present not only in high myopia (−8.0 D < SE ≤−5 D; 17.1%) and severe myopia (SE ≤ −8 D; 53.3%) but also in low(−3.0 D < SE ≤ 0.5 D; 7.0%) and moderate (−5.0 D < SE ≤ -3 D; 10.4%) myopia. Using the same definitions, another population-based study in Japan (the Hisayama Study) investigated the trend in the prevalence of myopic maculopathy at three time points from 1.6% in 2005, 3.0% in 2012, to 3.6% in 2017, suggesting that the prevalence of myopic maculopathy increased significantly over 12 years [97]. However, the prevalence of myopic maculopathy in rural southern China showed that the prevalence of myopic maculopathy was low as 1.4% even though staphyloma was also included into the definition of myopic maculopathy [98].

17.4 Progression of Myopic Maculopathy

Figure 17.16 is a scheme showing a progressive pattern of various lesions of myopic maculopathy, which is modified from the study following 806 highly myopic eyes for a mean period of 12.7 years [7]. In this study, 40.6% of the eyes showed a progression. The first sign that a highly myopic eye has progressed to the myopic maculopathy stage is the appearance of a tessellated fundus. The CNV develops from various lesions of myopic maculopathy, and the lesions eventually resulted in a formation of macular atrophy. The representative cases which showed a progression are shown in Figs. 17.17, 17.18, and 17.19. Liu et al. [20] in the Beijing Eye Study reported that at the 5-year follow-up examination, enlargement of the chorioretinal atrophy at the posterior fundus was observed in 9% of the eyes. Vongphanit et al. [61]

reported that after a mean period of 61 months, a significant progression of myopic retinopathy was observed in 17.4% (an enlargement of peripapillary atrophy and the development of patchy chorioretinal atrophy).

Based on META-PM classification, a retrospective case series study including 810 eyes of 432 highly myopic patients who had been followed for ≥10 years was conducted. After the mean follow-up of 18 years, the progression of myopic

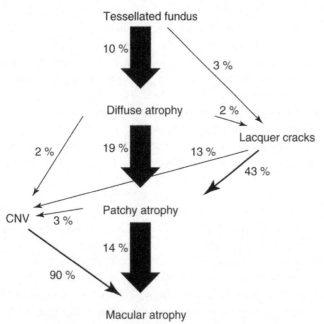

Fig. 17.16 A scheme of progression of myopic maculopathy suggested by a long-term follow-up study (Hayashi et al. 2010). The wide arrows in the center show the most prevalent pattern of progression in highly myopic patients. The number beside the arrows indicates the rate of each progression

maculopathy was observed in 58.6% for all in which 74.3% in eyes with pathologic myopia at baseline. The most frequent progression patterns were an extension of peripapillary diffuse atrophy to macular diffuse atrophy in diffuse atrophy, enlargement of the original atrophic lesion in patchy atrophy, and development of patchy atrophy in lacquer cracks. From two Chinese population-based longitudinal studies, the 10-year progression rate of myopic maculopathy was 35.5% in elderly Chinese (aged 40+) (Beijing Eye study) [37], and the 5-year progression rate was also 35.3% in rural Chinese adult population (aged 30+) (Handan Eye Study) [99]. In a large highly myopic Chinese cohort (Zhongshan Ophthalmic Center-Brien Holden Vision Institute High Myopia Cohort Study), the myopic maculopathy progressed in approximately 15% of 657 highly myopic eyes over 2 years [100].

17.5 Factors Correlating with the Development of Myopic Maculopathy

Age, axial length, and posterior staphyloma are the main factors affecting the development and progression of myopic maculopathy. Higher myopic retinopathy prevalence was associated with older age [3, 42, 101]. Young patients or children tend not to develop myopic maculopathy even though the axial length is very long [21, 102, 103]. This is especially true for the atrophic lesions of myopic maculopathy, because diffuse or patchy chorioretinal atrophy usually develops in aged patients. Lacquer cracks are exceptional, and they can develop in children [102] and young patients. Chen et al. [94] analyzed the risk factors associated with myopic macu-

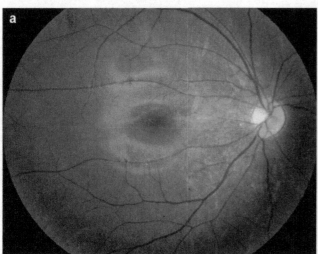

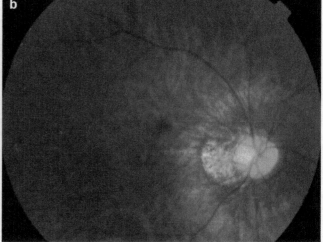

Fig. 17.17 Progression from tessellated fundus to diffuse chorioretinal atrophy. (**a**) Right fundus at the age of 5 years shows a tessellated fundus. Axial length is 26.8 mm. (**b**) Twenty years later, diffuse chorioreti-

nal atrophy has developed around the optic disc. Axial length has increased to 31.4 mm

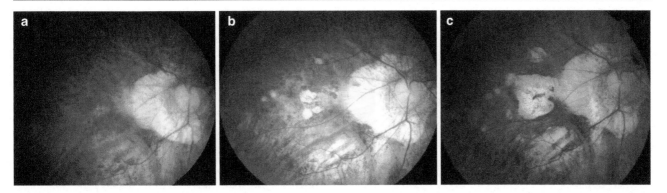

Fig. 17.18 Progression from diffuse chorioretinal atrophy to patchy chorioretinal atrophy. (**a**) Right fundus at the age 50 years shows diffuse chorioretinal atrophy especially in the lower fundus. Axial length is 29.5 mm. (**b**) Six years later, multiple, circular lesions of patchy atrophy have developed within the area of diffuse atrophy. Axial length is 30.2 mm. (**c**) Five more years later, the lesions are enlarged and are fused with each other. Axial length is 30.6 mm

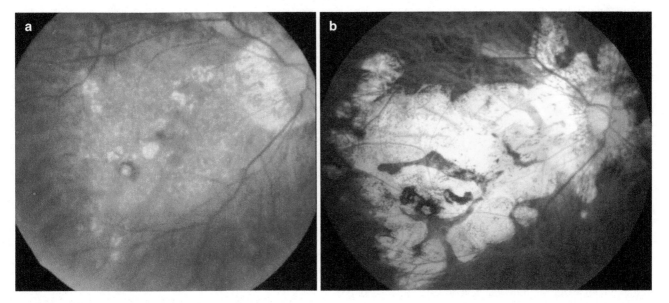

Fig. 17.19 Enlargement and fusion of the lesions of chorioretinal atrophy. (**a**) Right fundus at the age 55 years shows multiple lesions of patchy atrophy within the area of diffuse atrophy. Axial length is 30.3 mm. (**b**) Ten years later, multiple lesions of patchy atrophy are enlarged and have progressed to macular atrophy. Axial length is 31.1 mm

lopathy using general estimating equation (GEE) models. They reported that the older age was significantly associated with diffuse chorioretinal atrophy ($P = 0.024$), patchy chorioretinal atrophy ($P < 0.001$), CNV ($P < 0.001$), and macular atrophy ($P = 0.002$). Younger age was associated with lacquer cracks ($P < 0.001$).

A marked and highly non-linear relationship has been reported between refraction and the prevalence of myopic maculopathy [61, 101]. The prevalence of myopic retinopathy increased significantly ($P < 0.001$) with increasing myopic refractive error, from 3.8% in eyes with a myopic refractive error of < -4.0 diopters to 89.6% in eyes with a myopic refractive error of at least -10.0 diopters [20]. Myopes less than 5D had a myopic maculopathy prevalence of 0.42% as compared to 25.3% for myopes with greater

than 5 D of myopia, i.e., a 60-fold increase in risk in high myopes. A higher degree of myopia was a risk factor for almost all kinds of maculopathy, tessellated fundus, lacquer cracks, diffuse chorioretinal atrophy, patchy chorioretinal atrophy, and macular atrophy, whereas a lower degree of myopia was associated with CNV [94]. Steidl and Pruett [104, 105] reported that a linear relationship was observed between staphyloma grade and lacquer cracks and chorioretinal atrophy. However, there was an unexpected high frequency of myopic CNV in the lower staphyloma categories.

Regarding axial length, Curtin [3, 42] reported that myopic chorioretinal degeneration was found in more than 60% of the eyes whose axial length is ε 29.5 mm, whereas it was found in less than 40% in the eyes whose axial length is <29.5 mm. Lai et al. [106] reported that the eyes with axial length of ε29 mm were more likely to have posterior pole chorioretinal lesion including chorioretinal atrophy and lacquer cracks compared with eyes with axial length of <29 mm [106].

Age and the axial length affect the development of myopic maculopathy in a combined fashion. Lai et al. [106] reported that the eyes with myopic maculopathy had significantly older age (45.0 vs 34.8 years), longer axial length (28.84 vs 26.59 mm), and higher degree of mean spherical equivalent refractive error (−16.8 vs −9.4 D) ($P < 0.001$ for all three variables).

In the study analyzing the relationship between the scleral contour and myopic chorioretinal lesions by using swept-source OCT [107], myopic fundus lesions (myopic CNV, myopic chorioretinal atrophy, and myopic traction maculopathy) were present significantly more frequently in the eyes with irregular curvature.

Reduction of retinal blood flow in highly myopic eyes measured by laser Doppler velocimetry [108] and reduced blood flow of posterior ciliary artery as well as central retinal artery measured by color Doppler ultrasonography [109] might relate to the development of myopic chorioretinal atrophy. Benavente-Perez et al. [110] reported that the compromised pulsatile and hemodynamics of central retinal artery observed in young healthy myopes are an early feature of the decrease in ocular blood flow reported in pathological myopia. Li et al. [111] reported that myopic retinopathy was associated with attenuation of retinal vessels.

Recent OCT examinations (EDI-OCT and swept-source OCT) showed that the choroid remarkably thins in highly myopic eyes different from the retinal thickness [112–114]. Nishida and Spaide [115] reported that the subfoveal choroidal thickness was inversely correlated with logarithm of the minimum angle of resolution visual acuity. Actually, the only significant predictor in the pooled data for logarithm of the minimum angle of resolution visual acuity was subfoveal choroidal thickness ($P \leq 0.001$). Wang et al. [22] reported that the BCVA correlated significantly with macular choroidal thickness in the highly myopic patients with diffuse chorioretinal atrophy. Multiple linear regression analysis showed that age and macular choroidal thickness were the variables that associated most strongly with BCVA in the patients with diffuse atrophy, whereas neither refractive error nor axial length was a significant predictor of BCVA. However, Fujiwara et al. [112] showed that there were no correlations between logMAR visual acuity and subfoveal choroidal thickness in eyes without CNV and surgery. Pang et al. [116] also found that 70% of highly myopic eyes with extremely thin choroid (mean choroidal thickness, 14 μm) still had good BCVA (20/40 or better).

Also, the decrease of neurotrophic factor, pigment epithelium-derived factor (PEDF), in the aqueous humor has been reported in highly myopic eyes [117, 118]. However, it is not certain if this is a result due to degenerative changes of RPE cells, which is a main cell producing PEDF, or due to a dilation of PEDF because of a big volume of myopic eye, or a cause of developing myopic chorioretinal atrophy.

Myopic retinopathy was not associated significantly ($P > 0.20$) with body height and weight, gender, rural versus urban region of residence, level of education, intraocular pressure, or central corneal thickness [20]. Chen et al. [19] reported a relationship between myopic maculopathy and higher systolic blood pressure after adjustment for age, sex, smoking, body mass index, diastolic blood pressure, educational levels, alcohol drinking, and histories of diabetes or taking anti-hypertension medication.

17.6 Future Perspective

Mainly due to a recent advance of imaging technique, much has been clarified about the characteristics of each lesion of myopic maculopathy. However, the main concern would be that the classification and definition of myopic maculopathy have not been standardized worldwide. Also, the fundus color is largely affected by the original degree of pigmentation among races. The difference between tessellated fundus and diffuse atrophy might be due to a difference in how much choroid remains. In that case, the classification based on OCT findings might become an important and powerful tool.

References

1. Salzmann M. The choroidal changes in high myopia. Arch Ophthalmol. 1902;31:41–2.
2. Salzmann M. Die Atrophie der Aderhaut im kurzsichtigen Auge. Albrecht von Graefes Archiv fur Ophthalmologie. 1902;54:384.
3. Curtin BJ. Basic science and clinical management. In: Curtin BJ, editor. The myopias. New York: Harper and Row; 1985. p. 177.
4. Grossniklaus HE, Green WR. Pathologic findings in pathologic myopia. Retina (Philadelphia, Pa). 1992;12:127–33.
5. Avila MP, Weiter JJ, Jalkh AE, Trempe CL, Pruett RC, Schepens CL. Natural history of choroidal neovascularization in degenerative myopia. Ophthalmology. 1984;91:1573–81.
6. Tokoro T, editor. Atlas of posterior fundus changes in pathologic myopia. Tokyo: Springer-Verlag; 1998. p. 5–22.
7. Hayashi K, Ohno-Matsui K, Shimada N, et al. Long-term pattern of progression of myopic maculopathy: a natural history study. Ophthalmology. 2010;117:1595-611–1611 e1-4.
8. Iwase A, Araie M, Tomidokoro A, et al. Prevalence and causes of low vision and blindness in a Japanese adult population: the Tajimi Study. Ophthalmology. 2006;113:1354–62.
9. Huang S, Zheng Y, Foster PJ, Huang W, He M. Prevalence and causes of visual impairment in Chinese adults in urban southern China. Arch Ophthalmol. 2009;127:1362–7.
10. Zheng Y, Lavanya R, Wu R, et al. Prevalence and causes of visual impairment and blindness in an urban Indian population: the Singapore Indian Eye Study. Ophthalmology. 2011;118:1798–804.
11. Iwano M, Nomura H, Ando F, Niino N, Miyake Y, Shimokata H. Visual acuity in a community-dwelling Japanese population

and factors associated with visual impairment. Jpn J Ophthalmol. 2004;48:37–43.

12. Cotter SA, Varma R, Ying-Lai M, Azen SP, Klein R, Los Angeles Latino Eye Study G. Causes of low vision and blindness in adult Latinos: the Los Angeles Latino Eye Study. Ophthalmology. 2006;113:1574–82.

13. Buch H, Vinding T, La Cour M, Appleyard M, Jensen GB, Nielsen NV. Prevalence and causes of visual impairment and blindness among 9980 Scandinavian adults: the Copenhagen City Eye Study. Ophthalmology. 2004;111:53–61.

14. Evans JR, Fletcher AE, Wormald RP. Causes of visual impairment in people aged 75 years and older in Britain: an add-on study to the MRC trial of assessment and management of older people in the community. Br J Ophthalmol. 2004;88:365–70.

15. Kelliher C, Kenny D, O'Brien C. Trends in blind registration in the adult population of the Republic of Ireland 1996-2003. Br J Ophthalmol. 2006;90:367–71.

16. Avisar R, Friling R, Snir M, Avisar I, Weinberger D. Estimation of prevalence and incidence rates and causes of blindness in Israel, 1998-2003. Isr Med Assoc J. 2006;8:880–1.

17. Varma R, Kim JS, Burkemper BS, et al. Prevalence and causes of visual impairment and blindness in Chinese American adults: the Chinese American Eye Study. JAMA Ophthalmol. 2016;134:785–93.

18. Shih YF, Ho TC, Hsiao CK, Lin LL. Visual outcomes for high myopic patients with or without myopic maculopathy: a 10 year follow up study. Br J Ophthalmol. 2006;90:546–50.

19. Chen SJ, Cheng CY, Li AF, et al. Prevalence and associated risk factors of myopic maculopathy in elderly Chinese: the Shihpai Eye Study. Invest Ophthalmol Vis Sci. 2012;28:28.

20. Liu HH, Xu L, Wang YX, Wang S, You QS, Jonas JB. Prevalence and progression of myopic retinopathy in Chinese adults: the Beijing Eye Study. Ophthalmology. 2010;117:1763–8.

21. Kobayashi K, Ohno-Matsui K, Kojima A, et al. Fundus characteristics of high myopia in children. Jpn J Ophthalmol. 2005;49:306–11.

22. Wang NK, Lai CC, Chu HY, et al. Classification of early dry-type myopic maculopathy with macular choroidal thickness. Am J Ophthalmol. 2012;153:669-77–677 e1-2.

23. Lin T, Grimes PA, Stone RA. Expansion of the retinal pigment epithelium in experimental myopia. Vis Res. 1993;33:1881–5.

24. Harman AM, Hoskins R, Beazley LD. Experimental eye enlargement in mature animals changes the retinal pigment epithelium. Vis Neurosci. 1999;16:619–28.

25. Hosaka A. Permeability of the blood-retinal barrier in myopia. An analysis employing vitreous fluorophotometry and computer simulation. Acta Ophthalmol Suppl. 1988;185:95–9.

26. Yoshida A, Ishiko S, Kojima M, Hosaka A. Blood-ocular barrier permeability in experimental myopia. J Fr Ophtalmol. 1990;13:481–8.

27. Yoshida A, Ishiko S, Kojima M. Inward and outward permeability of the blood-retinal barrier in experimental myopia. Graefes Arch Clin Exp Ophthalmol. 1996;234:S239–42.

28. Kitaya N, Ishiko S, Abiko T, et al. Changes in blood-retinal barrier permeability in form deprivation myopia in tree shrews. Vis Res. 2000;40:2369–77.

29. Spaide RF. Age-related choroidal atrophy. Am J Ophthalmol. 2009;147:801–10.

30. Fang Y, Du R, Nagaoka N, et al. OCT-based diagnostic criteria for different stages of myopic maculopathy. Ophthalmology. 2019;126:1018–32.

31. Zhao X, Ding X, Lyu C, et al. Morphological characteristics and visual acuity of highly myopic eyes with different severities of myopic maculopathy. Retina (Philadelphia, Pa). 2018;40:461.

32. Zhou Y, Song M, Zhou M, Liu Y, Wang F, Sun X. Choroidal and retinal thickness of highly myopic eyes with early stage of myopic chorioretinopathy: tessellation. J Ophthalmol. 2018;2018:2181602.

33. Kawabata H, Adachi-Usami E. Multifocal electroretinogram in myopia. Invest Ophthalmol Vis Sci. 1997;38:2844–51.

34. Chen JC, Brown B, Schmid KL. Delayed mfERG responses in myopia. Vis Res. 2006;46:1221–9.

35. Luu CD, Lau AM, Lee SY. Multifocal electroretinogram in adults and children with myopia. Arch Ophthalmol. 2006;124:328–34.

36. Chan HL, Mohidin N. Variation of multifocal electroretinogram with axial length. Ophthalmic Physiol Opt. 2003;23:133–40.

37. Yan YN, Wang YX, Yang Y, et al. Ten-year progression of myopic maculopathy: the Beijing eye study 2001-2011. Ophthalmology. 2018;125:1253–63.

38. Fang Y, Yokoi T, Nagaoka N, et al. Progression of myopic maculopathy during 18-year follow-up. Ophthalmology. 2018;125:863–77.

39. Malagola R, Pecorella I, Teodori C, Santi G, Mannino G. Peripheral lacquer cracks as an early finding in pathological myopia. Arch Ophthalmol. 2006;124:1783–4.

40. Bottoni FG, Eggink CA, Cruysberg JR, Verbeek AM. Dominant inherited tilted disc syndrome and lacquer cracks. Eye. 1990;4:504–9.

41. Pruett RC, Weiter JJ, Goldstein RB. Myopic cracks, angioid streaks, and traumatic tears in Bruch's membrane. Am J Ophthalmol. 1987;103:537–43.

42. Curtin BJ, Karlin DB. Axial length measurements and fundus changes of the myopic eye. I. The posterior fundus. Trans Am Ophthalmol Soc. 1970;68:312–34.

43. Klein RM, Curtin BJ. Lacquer crack lesions in pathologic myopia. Am J Ophthalmol. 1975;79:386–92.

44. Brancato R, Trabucchi G, Introini U, Avanza P, Pece A. Indocyanine green angiography (ICGA) in pathological myopia. Eur J Ophthalmol. 1996;6:39–43.

45. Quaranta M, Arnold J, Coscas G, et al. Indocyanine green angiographic features of pathologic myopia. Am J Ophthalmol. 1996;122:663–71.

46. Ohno-Matsui K, Morishima N, Ito M, Tokoro T. Indocyanine green angiographic findings of lacquer cracks in pathologic myopia. Jpn J Ophthalmol. 1998;42:293–9.

47. Ikuno Y, Sayanagi K, Soga K, et al. Lacquer crack formation and choroidal neovascularization in pathologic myopia. Retina. 2008;28:1124–31.

48. Kim YM, Yoon JU, Koh HJ. The analysis of lacquer crack in the assessment of myopic choroidal neovascularization. Eye. 2011;25:937–46.

49. Wang NK, Lai CC, Chou CL, et al. Choroidal thickness and biometric markers for the screening of lacquer cracks in patients with high myopia. PLoS One. 2013;8:22.

50. Klein RM, Green S. The development of lacquer cracks in pathologic myopia. Am J Ophthalmol. 1988;106:282–5.

51. Ohno-Matsui K, Ito M, Tokoro T. Subretinal bleeding without choroidal neovascularization in pathologic myopia. A sign of new lacquer crack formation. Retina. 1996;16:196–202.

52. Yip LW, Au Eong KG. Recurrent subretinal haemorrhages and progressive lacquer cracks in a high myope. Acta Ophthalmol Scand. 2003;81:646–7.

53. Moriyama M, Ohno-Matsui K, Shimada N, et al. Correlation between visual prognosis and fundus autofluorescence and optical coherence tomographic findings in highly myopic eyes with submacular hemorrhage and without choroidal neovascularization. Retina. 2011;31:74–80.

54. Hirata A, Negi A. Lacquer crack lesions in experimental chick myopia. Graefes Arch Clin Exp Ophthalmol. 1998;236:138–45.

55. Ellies P, Pietrini D, Lumbroso L, Lebuisson DA. Macular hemorrhage after laser in situ keratomileusis for high myopia. J Cataract Refract Surg. 2000;26:922–4.

56. Loewenstein A, Lipshitz I, Varssano D, Lazar M. Macular hemorrhage after excimer laser photorefractive keratectomy. J Cataract Refract Surg. 1997;23:808–10.

57. Luna JD, Reviglio VE, Juarez CP. Bilateral macular hemorrhage after laser in situ keratomileusis. Graefes Arch Clin Exp Ophthalmol. 1999;237:611–3.

58. Principe AH, Lin DY, Small KW, Aldave AJ. Macular hemorrhage after laser in situ keratomileusis (LASIK) with femtosecond laser flap creation. Am J Ophthalmol. 2004;138:657–9.

59. Loewenstein A, Goldstein M, Lazar M. Retinal pathology occurring after excimer laser surgery or phakic intraocular lens implantation: evaluation of possible relationship. Surv Ophthalmol. 2002;47:125–35.

60. Johnson DA, Yannuzzi LA, Shakin JL, Lightman DA. Lacquer cracks following laser treatment of choroidal neovascularization in pathologic myopia. Retina. 1998;18:118–24.

61. Vongphanit J, Mitchell P, Wang JJ. Prevalence and progression of myopic retinopathy in an older population. Ophthalmology. 2002;109:704–11.

62. Ohno-Matsui K, Tokoro T. The progression of lacquer cracks in pathologic myopia. Retina (Philadelphia, Pa). 1996;16:29–37.

63. Xu X, Fang Y, Uramoto K, et al. Clinical features of Lacquer Cracks in eyes with pathologic myopia. Retina (Philadelphia, Pa). 2019;39:1265–77.

64. Yannuzzi LA. The retinal atlas. New York: Elsevier; 2010. p. 526–43.

65. Shinohara K, Moriyama M, Shimada N, Tanaka Y, Ohno-Matsui K. Myopic stretch lines: linear lesions in fundus of eyes with pathologic myopia that differ from lacquer cracks. Retina. 2014;34(3):461–9.

66. Freund KB, Ciardella AP, Yannuzzi LA, et al. Peripapillary detachment in pathologic myopia. Arch Ophthalmol. 2003;121:197–204.

67. Freund KB, Mukkamala SK, Cooney MJ. Peripapillary choroidal thickening and cavitation. Arch Ophthalmol. 2011;129:1096–7.

68. Shimada N, Ohno-Matsui K, Yoshida T, et al. Characteristics of peripapillary detachment in pathologic myopia. Arch Ophthalmol. 2006;124:46–52.

69. Spaide RF, Akiba M, Ohno-Matsui K. Evaluation of peripapillary intrachoroidal cavitation with swept source and enhanced depth imaging optical coherence tomography. Retina. 2012;32:1037–44.

70. Toranzo J, Cohen SY, Erginay A, Gaudric A. Peripapillary intrachoroidal cavitation in myopia. Am J Ophthalmol. 2005;140:731–2.

71. Shin JY, Yu HG. Visual prognosis and spectral-domain optical coherence tomography findings of myopic foveoschisis surgery using 25-gauge transconjunctival sutureless vitrectomy. Retina. 2012;32:486–92.

72. Ohno-Matsui K, Jonas JB, Spaide RF. Macular Bruch membrane holes in highly myopic patchy chorioretinal atrophy. Am J Ophthalmol. 2016;166:22–8.

73. Du R, Fang Y, Jonas JB, et al. Clinical features of patchy chorioretinal atrophy in pathologic myopia. Retina (Philadelphia, Pa). 2019;40:951.

74. Jonas JB, Ohno-Matsui K, Spaide RF, Holbach L, Panda-Jonas S. Macular Bruch's membrane defects and axial length: association with gamma zone and delta zone in peripapillary region. Invest Ophthalmol Vis Sci. 2013;54:1295–302.

75. Ohno-Matsui K, Akiba M, Moriyama M, Ishibashi T, Hirakata A, Tokoro T. Intrachoroidal cavitation in macular area of eyes with pathologic myopia. Am J Ophthalmol. 2012;154:382–93.

76. Asakuma T, Yasuda M, Ninomiya T, et al. Prevalence and risk factors for myopic retinopathy in a Japanese population: the Hisayama Study. Ophthalmology. 2012;10:10.

77. Ito-Ohara M, Seko Y, Morita H, Imagawa N, Tokoro T. Clinical course of newly developed or progressive patchy chorioretinal atrophy in pathological myopia. Ophthalmologica. 1998;212:23–9.

78. Baba T, Ohno-Matsui K, Futagami S, et al. Prevalence and characteristics of foveal retinal detachment without macular hole in high myopia. Am J Ophthalmol. 2003;135:338–42.

79. Fang X, Zheng X, Weng Y, et al. Anatomical and visual outcome after vitrectomy with triamcinolone acedonide-assisted epiretinal membrane removal in highly myopic eyes with retinal detachment due to macular hole. Eye. 2009;23:248–54.

80. Chen L, Wang K, Esmaili DD, Xu G. Rhegmatogenous retinal detachment due to paravascular linear retinal breaks over patchy chorioretinal atrophy in pathologic myopia. Arch Ophthalmol. 2010;128:1551–4.

81. Ohno-Matsui K, Yoshida T, Futagami S, et al. Patchy atrophy and lacquer cracks predispose to the development of choroidal neovascularisation in pathological myopia. Br J Ophthalmol. 2003;87:570–3.

82. Gaucher D, Erginay A, Lecleire-Collet A, et al. Dome-shaped macula in eyes with myopic posterior staphyloma. Am J Ophthalmol. 2008;145:909–14.

83. Imamura Y, Iida T, Maruko I, Zweifel SA, Spaide RF. Enhanced depth imaging optical coherence tomography of the sclera in dome-shaped macula. Am J Ophthalmol. 2011;151:297–302.

84. Caillaux V, Gaucher D, Gualino V, Massin P, Tadayoni R, Gaudric A. Morphologic characterization of dome-shaped macula in myopic eyes with serous macular detachment. Am J Ophthalmol. 2013;156:958–967.e1.

85. Ellabban AA, Tsujikawa A, Matsumoto A, et al. Three-dimensional tomographic features of dome-shaped macula by swept-source optical coherence tomography. Am J Ophthalmol. 2013;155:320–328 e2.

86. Liang IC, Shimada N, Tanaka Y, et al. Comparison of clinical features in highly myopic eyes with and without a dome-shaped macula. Ophthalmology. 2015;122:1591–600.

87. Zhao X, Ding X, Lyu C, et al. Observational study of clinical characteristics of dome-shaped macula in Chinese Han with high myopia at Zhongshan Ophthalmic Centre. BMJ Open. 2018;8:e021887.

88. Viola F, Dell'Arti L, Benatti E, et al. Choroidal findings in dome-shaped macula in highly myopic eyes: a longitudinal study. Am J Ophthalmol. 2015;159:44–52.

89. Ellabban AA, Tsujikawa A, Matsumoto A, et al. Three-dimensional tomographic features of dome-shaped macula by swept-source optical coherence tomography. Am J Ophthalmol. 2012;3:00578.

90. Xu X, Fang Y, Jonas JB, et al. Ridge-shaped macula in young myopic patients and its differentiation from typical dome-shaped macula in elderly myopic patients. Retina (Philadelphia, Pa). 2018;40:225.

91. Cohen SY, Quentel G, Guiberteau B, Delahaye-Mazza C, Gaudric A. Macular serous retinal detachment caused by subretinal leakage in tilted disc syndrome. Ophthalmology. 1998;105:1831–4.

92. Nakanishi H, Tsujikawa A, Gotoh N, et al. Macular complications on the border of an inferior staphyloma associated with tilted disc syndrome. Retina. 2008;28:1493–501.

93. Maruko I, Iida T, Sugano Y, Oyamada H, Sekiryu T. Morphologic choroidal and scleral changes at the macula in tilted disc syndrome with staphyloma using optical coherence tomography. Invest Ophthalmol Vis Sci. 2011;52:8763–8.

94. Chen H, Wen F, Li H, et al. The types and severity of high myopic maculopathy in Chinese patients. Ophthalmic Physiol Opt. 2012;32:60–7.

95. Choudhury F, Meuer SM, Klein R, et al. Prevalence and characteristics of myopic degeneration in an adult Chinese American population: the Chinese American Eye Study. Am J Ophthalmol. 2018;187:34–42.

96. Wong YL, Sabanayagam C, Ding Y, et al. Prevalence, risk factors, and impact of myopic macular degeneration on visual impairment

and functioning among adults in Singapore. Invest Ophthalmol Vis Sci. 2018;59:4603–13.

97. Ueda E, Yasuda M, Fujiwara K, et al. Trends in the prevalence of myopia and myopic maculopathy in a Japanese population: the Hisayama Study. Invest Ophthalmol Vis Sci. 2019;60:2781–6.

98. Li Z, Liu R, Jin G, et al. Prevalence and risk factors of myopic maculopathy in rural southern China: the Yangxi Eye Study. Br J Ophthalmol. 2019;103:1797.

99. Lin C, Li SM, Ohno-Matsui K, et al. Five-year incidence and progression of myopic maculopathy in a rural Chinese adult population: the Handan Eye Study. Ophthalmic Physiol Opt. 2018;38:337–45.

100. Li Z, Liu R, Xiao O, et al. Progression of myopic maculopathy in highly myopic Chinese eyes. Invest Ophthalmol Vis Sci. 2019;60:1096–104.

101. Gao LQ, Liu W, Liang YB, et al. Prevalence and characteristics of myopic retinopathy in a rural Chinese adult population: the Handan Eye Study. Arch Ophthalmol. 2011;129:1199–204.

102. Samarawickrama C, Mitchell P, Tong L, et al. Myopia-related optic disc and retinal changes in adolescent children from Singapore. Ophthalmology. 2011;118:2050–7.

103. Tong L, Saw SM, Chua WH, et al. Optic disk and retinal characteristics in myopic children. Am J Ophthalmol. 2004;138:160–2.

104. Steidl SM, Pruett RC. Macular complications associated with posterior staphyloma. Am J Ophthalmol. 1997;123:181–7.

105. Pruett RC. Complications associated with posterior staphyloma. Curr Opin Ophthalmol. 1998;9:16–22.

106. Lai TY, Fan DS, Lai WW, Lam DS. Peripheral and posterior pole retinal lesions in association with high myopia: a cross-sectional community-based study in Hong Kong. Eye. 2008;22:209–13.

107. Ohno-Matsui K, Akiba M, Modegi T, et al. Association between shape of sclera and myopic retinochoroidal lesions in patients with pathologic myopia. Invest Ophthalmol Vis Sci. 2012;9:9.

108. Shimada N, Ohno-Matsui K, Harino S, et al. Reduction of retinal blood flow in high myopia. Graefes Arch Clin Exp Ophthalmol. 2004;242:284–8.

109. Akyol N, Kukner AS, Ozdemir T, Esmerligil S. Choroidal and retinal blood flow changes in degenerative myopia. Can J Ophthalmol. 1996;31:113–9.

110. Benavente-Perez A, Hosking SL, Logan NS, Broadway DC. Ocular blood flow measurements in healthy human myopic eyes. Graefes Arch Clin Exp Ophthalmol. 2010;248:1587–94.

111. Li H, Mitchell P, Rochtchina E, Burlutsky G, Wong TY, Wang JJ. Retinal vessel caliber and myopic retinopathy: the Blue Mountains Eye Study. Ophthalmic Epidemiol. 2011;18:275–80.

112. Fujiwara T, Imamura Y, Margolis R, Slakter JS, Spaide RF. Enhanced depth imaging optical coherence tomography of the choroid in highly myopic eyes. Am J Ophthalmol. 2009;148:445–50.

113. Ikuno Y, Tano Y. Retinal and choroidal biometry in highly myopic eyes with spectral-domain optical coherence tomography. Invest Ophthalmol Vis Sci. 2009;50:3876–80.

114. Barteselli G, Chhablani J, El-Emam S, et al. Choroidal volume variations with age, axial length, and sex in healthy subjects: a three-dimensional analysis. Ophthalmology. 2012;119:2572–8.

115. Nishida Y, Fujiwara T, Imamura Y, Lima LH, Kurosaka D, Spaide RF. Choroidal thickness and visual acuity in highly myopic eyes. Retina (Philadelphia, Pa). 2012;32:1229–36.

116. Pang CE, Sarraf D, Freund KB. Extreme choroidal thinning in high myopia. Retina (Philadelphia, Pa). 2015;35:407-15.

117. Ogata N, Imaizumi M, Miyashiro M, et al. Low levels of pigment epithelium-derived factor in highly myopic eyes with chorioretinal atrophy. Am J Ophthalmol. 2005;140:937–9.

118. Shin YJ, Nam WH, Park SE, Kim JH, Kim HK. Aqueous humor concentrations of vascular endothelial growth factor and pigment epithelium-derived factor in high myopic patients. Mol Vis. 2012;18:2265–70.

Overview of OCT-Based Classification of Macular Lesions Due to Pathologic Myopia

18

Kyoko Ohno-Matsui and Yuxin Fang

18.1 Introduction

Over the past two decades, optical coherence tomography (OCT) has greatly enhanced our understanding of various retinal pathologies. Recent advanced technology in OCT, including enhanced depth imaging OCT and swept-source OCT, provided the high-resolution images and highly reliable measurements of choroid in highly myopic eyes. It has been well known that choroid in high myopia is markedly thin [1–20]. All of previous studies support the theory that choroidal abnormality may play a key role in the pathogenesis of myopic maculopathy. In addition, swept-source OCT showed that patchy atrophy and myopic macular neovascularization (MNV)-related macular atrophy were not simply an atrophy but were macular Bruch's membrane defect [21–25]. Recently, it showed that some of myopic MNV were continuous with scleral vessels mainly the short posterior ciliary arteries, so the term "myopic macular neovascularization" (Myopic MNV) is more appropriate. Moreover, OCT revealed new macular lesions which were not detected by fundus photographs, such as myopic traction maculopathy and dome-shaped macula. In 2015, an international panel of researchers in myopia reviewed previous published studies and classifications and proposed a simplified, uniform classification system for pathologic myopia called META-PM classification for use in future studies [26]. However, based on the reasons above, OCT-based classification of myopic maculopathy is needed.

In this chapter, based on OCT features of each lesion of myopic maculopathy, OCT-based classification is presented. This objective classification is useful for clinical management of pathologic myopia.

18.2 META-PM Classification of Myopic Maculopathy (Table 18.1) [26]

18.2.1 The Details of META-PM and Several Supplements for Myopic Maculopathy

META-PM classification is based on funduscopic appearance of myopic maculopathy. In this classification, myopic maculopathy lesions are categorized into five categories from "no myopic retinal lesions" (category 0), "tessellated fundus only" (category 1), "diffuse chorioretinal atrophy" (category 2), "patchy chorioretinal atrophy" (category 3), to "macular atrophy" (category 4). Three additional features were added to these categories and were included as "plus signs": (1) lacquer cracks, (2) myopic MNV, and (3) Fuchs spot. Representative fundus photographs of each lesion of myopic maculopathy are shown in Fig. 18.1. Diffuse choroidal atrophy as assessed upon ophthalmoscopy is an ill-defined yellowish lesion in the posterior fundus; patchy atrophy is a grayish-white, well-defined atrophy; and lacquer cracks were fine, irregular, yellowish lines often crisscross over the underlying choroidal vessels.

Macular atrophy can be sub-classified into MNV-related macular atrophy developing centered on the fovea and into patchy atrophy-related macular atrophy first developing outside of the foveal area and enlarging, or coalescing with other patchy atrophies, into the foveal center. The differentiation of these macular atrophies is based on a history of myopic MNV) or based on its funduscopic features. Myopic MNV includes three stages: the active stage with proliferation of a fibrovascular membrane including MNV, exudation, and hemorrhage; the scar stage exemplified by a Fuchs spot; and the atrophic stage represented by a MNV-related macular atrophy. Because Fuchs spots are one aspect of myopic MNV, Fuchs spots were not analyzed as independent lesions.

K. Ohno-Matsui (✉) · Y. Fang
Department of Ophthalmology and Visual Science, Tokyo Medical and Dental University, Bunkyo-Ku, Tokyo, Japan
e-mail: k.ohno.oph@tmd.ac.jp

© Springer Nature Switzerland AG 2021
R. F. Spaide et al. (eds.), *Pathologic Myopia*, https://doi.org/10.1007/978-3-030-74334-5_18

18.2.2 Why the OCT-Based Classification Is Needed?

Although META-PM classification is very useful, the diagnosis of diffuse atrophy relies solely on its yellowish appearance on ophthalmoscopy. However, the fundus color may look different according to the degree of fundus pigmentation among races, which could affect an accurate diagnosis of atrophic lesions. Earlier studies showed that diffuse atrophy was represented by marked choroidal thinning by OCT [3, 17, 20, 27]. Thus, integrating choroidal thickness into the classification system would offer the objective information which should be accurate and reproducible. Besides, other myopic

macular lesions such as myopic traction maculopathy and dome-shaped macula were not included in the META-PM classification because only fundus photographs were used.

18.3 OCT Features of Each Lesion of Myopic Maculopathy

18.3.1 Choroidal Thinning

It has been well known that the choroid in high myopia is markedly thin compared to the normal eyes [1–20]. OCT shows an extreme thinning of choroid with presence of sporadically large choroidal vessels in the area of diffuse choroidal atrophy [20, 27]. The extent of the diffuse atrophy varies from a restricted area around the optic disc and a part of the macula to the entire posterior pole. Thus, diffuse choroidal atrophy can be additionally sub-classified as peripapillary diffuse choroidal atrophy (PDCA) and macular diffuse choroidal atrophy (MDCA) [28] (Fig. 18.2).

A retrospective case series study conducted in the high myopia clinic at Tokyo Medical and Dental University (TMDU) included children and adolescents aged 15 years or

Table 18.1 META-PM classification of myopic maculopathy

	Myopic maculopathy	"Plus" lesions
Category 0	No macular lesions	+ Lacquer cracks (Lc)
Category 1	Tessellated fundus	Macular neovascularization (MNV)
Category 2	Diffuse chorioretinal atrophy	Fuchs spots
Category 3	Patchy chorioretinal atrophy	
Category 4	Macular atrophy	

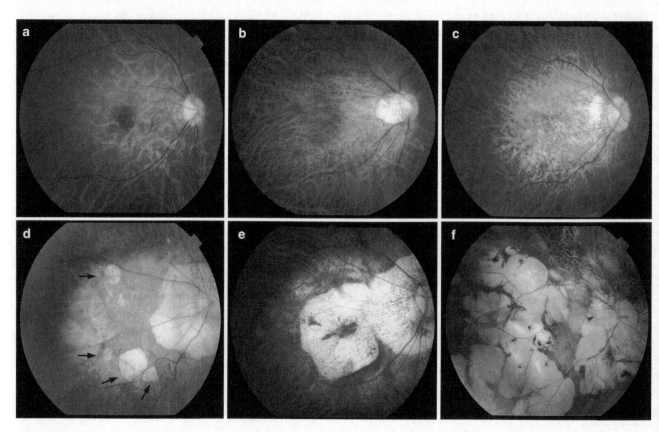

Fig. 18.1 Representative fundus photographs of each lesion of myopic maculopathy. (**a**) Tessellated fundus in a 52-year-old man with axial length of 28.15 mm. (**b**) Peripapillary diffuse choroidal atrophy in a 53-year-old man with axial length of 28.39 mm. (**c**) Macular diffuse choroidal atrophy in a 58-year-old man with axial length of 33.40 mm.

(**d**) Patchy atrophy (arrows) in a 73-year-old woman with axial length of 32.63 mm. (**e**) Myopic macular neovascularization-related macular atrophy in a 73-year-old woman with axial length of 29.24 mm. (**f**) Patchy atrophy-related macular atrophy in a 74-year-old woman. Reproduced by *Ophthalmology*

younger who had been followed up for over 20 years [29]. At the last visit, 35 eyes (63%) showed features of pathologic myopia in adulthood, of which 29 eyes (83%) showed pre-existing PDCA during childhood or adolescence. This suggests that the presence of PDCA in children with high axial myopia may be an indicator for the eventual development of advanced myopic maculopathy in later life. In addition, PDCA is significantly associated with thinner choroidal thickness in the parapapillary region [30].

18.3.2 Bruch's Membrane Holes

The defects of Bruch's membrane in the macular region were reported in a histological study of highly myopic eyes [31]. These macular Bruch's membrane defects were accompanied by a complete loss of RPE and choriocapillaris and an almost complete loss of the outer and middle retinal layers and of the middle-sized choroidal vascular layer. Later, by using swept-source OCT, Bruch's membrane defect was found in association with two different macular lesions spe-

cific to pathologic myopia, i.e., with MNV-related macular atrophy and with patchy atrophy [21–23] (Fig. 18.3). These studies showed that patchy atrophy and MNV-related macular atrophy which had previously been considered to be chorioretinal atrophies were not simply atrophy but were a hole of Bruch's membrane.

Lacquer cracks are yellowish linear lesions in and around the macula. It is difficult to detect lacquer cracks by OCT because the lesions are usually too narrow. In some cases, lacquer cracks are observed as discontinuities of the RPE and increased hyper-transmission into the deeper tissue beyond the RPE [32, 33] (Fig. 18.3).

18.3.3 Other Myopic Lesions (Myopic Traction Maculopathy and Dome-Shaped Macula)

Myopic traction maculopathy [34, 35] and dome-shaped macula [36] are two important and common complications that closely related with highly myopia. OCT is an indis-

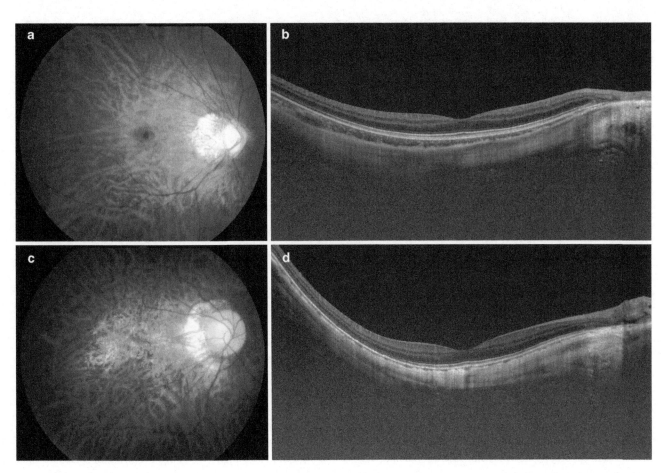

Fig. 18.2 Representative fundus photographs and swept-source optical coherence tomographic image for peripapillary diffuse chorioretinal atrophy and macular diffuse chorioretinal atrophy. (**a** and **b**) Peripapillary diffuse chorioretinal atrophy in a 30-year-old woman with axial length of 30.92 mm. The subfoveal CT was 95 μm, temporal CT was 146 μm, and nasal CT was 47 μm. (**c** and **d**) Macular diffuse chorioretinal atrophy in a 44-year-old woman with axial length of 30.91 mm. The subfoveal CT was 52 μm, temporal CT was 36 μm, and nasal CT was 27 μm. Reproduced by Ophthalmology

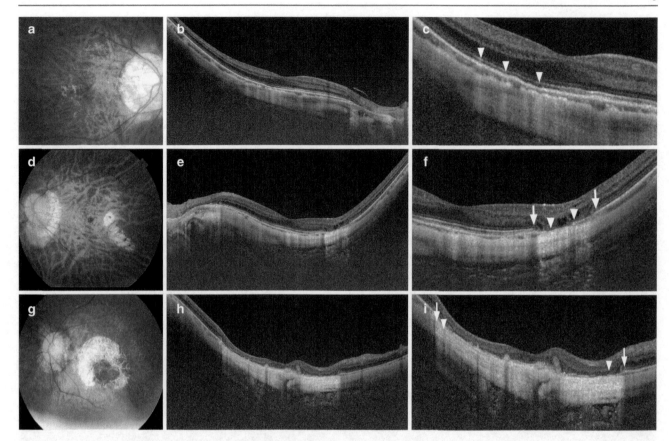

Fig. 18.3 Representative fundus photographs and swept-source optical coherence tomographic image for lacquer cracks, patchy atrophy, and MNV-related macular atrophy. (**a**–**c**) Lacquer cracks in a 35-year-old male with axial length of 30.98 mm. The lacquer cracks are seen as yellowish linear lesion in the macular area. The subfoveal CT was 39 μm and the temporal CT was 123 μm. There was no choroid on the nasal side. OCT image across the lacquer cracks shows the slight discontinuities of RPE and an increase in the light penetrance into the deeper tissues. (**d**–**f**) Patchy atrophy in a 49-year-old woman with axial length of 30.48 mm. The subfoveal CT was 53 μm and the temporal CT was 63 μm. There was no choroid on the nasal side. OCT image across the area of patchy atrophy shows the end of the retinal pigment epithe-

lium (RPE, white arrows). Bruch's membrane shows discontinuities and stops within the margin of the RPE defect (white arrowheads). In the area of the defective Bruch's membrane, almost the entire choroid is lacking, and the inner retina is in direct contact with the sclera. (**g**–**i**) MNV-related macular atrophy in a 59-year-old woman with axial length of 28.94 mm. The black arrow indicates the direction of the OCT scans. The subfoveal CT was 25 μm, temporal CT was 96 μm, and nasal CT was 38 μm. OCT images of the area of macular atrophy show the end of RPE (arrows). Bruch's membrane in the defective area of RPE is fragmented. The end of the Bruch's membrane is shown in arrowheads

pensable tool to diagnose both entities although the presence can be suspected ophthalmoscopically in a few cases. Myopic traction maculopathy is generally defined by OCT examinations including schisis-like inner retinal fluid, schisis-like outer retina fluid, foveal detachment, lamellar or full-thickness macular hole, and/or macular detachment [37]. Dome-shaped macula is first described using OCT as inward bulge in the macular area inside the staphyloma which may be responsible for visual disturbance in myopic patients [36]. According to the following expanded definition, it can be diagnosed quantitatively as macular bulge height of >50 μm in the most convex scan in either vertical or horizontal scan [38].

18.4   Establishment of OCT-Based Classification

18.4.1 Choroidal Thickness Profile in Each Lesion

18.4.1.1   Profile in Myopic Maculopathy Is Different from Normal Fundus

The topography of the choroidal thickness in highly myopic eyes with normal fundus is different from that in eyes with myopic maculopathy, i.e., being equal or more severe than tessellated fundus. In highly myopic eyes with normal fundus, the subfoveal choroidal thickness is the thickest in the horizontal sections, that is, in same pattern with non-highly myopic eyes [39], whereas in eyes with myopic maculopathy, the temporal choroidal thickness is the thickest (Fig. 18.4a). In the vertical sections, the inferior choroidal thickness is the thinnest in normal fundus, whereas in eyes with myopic maculopathy, the subfoveal choroidal thickness is the thinnest (Fig. 18.4b). The observation is also confirmed in vertical scan by another study comparing choroidal thickness in eyes with tessellated and normal fundus [40]. Actually, the distribution pattern of choroidal thickness in eyes with tessellation is similar to the eyes with other lesions of myopic maculopathy, e.g., PDCA, MDCA, and patchy atrophy. This suggested that the tessellation might be the first sign for myopic eyes to become pathologic.

18.4.1.2 Progressive Thinning from Tessellated to PDCA and to MDCA, but Not Thereafter

Earlier literatures showed that the choroidal thickness was negatively correlated with severity of myopic maculopathy based on META-PM classification [11, 17, 20]. From a clinic-based cross-sectional study on 1487 eyes of 884 high myopic patients (241 men and 643 women) who were examined by swept-source OCT, Fang et al. showed that the mean subfoveal choroidal thickness in eyes with a normal fundus (category 0) was 274.5 μm, tessellated fundus is 129.1 μm, PDCA was 84.6 μm, MDCA was 50.2 μm, patchy atrophy was 48.6 μm, MNV-related macular atrophy was 27.3 μm,

and patchy-related macular atrophy was 3.5 μm (Fig. 18.5) [20]. In our series, choroidal thickness in all locations decreased from normal fundus to tessellated fundus, to PDCA, and to MDCA, as the severity of the myopic maculopathy increased. But there was no significant difference in choroidal thickness between eyes with MDCA and patchy atrophy in all locations except for those at nasally.

The subfoveal choroidal thickness of eyes with macular atrophy (both MNV-related macular atrophy and patchy-related macular atrophy or either of them) was significantly thinner than that in any other groups. The subfoveal choroidal thickness in eyes with patchy-related macular atrophy was even thinner than choroidal thickness in MNV-related macular atrophy. It is noted that there was no difference among MNV-related macular atrophy, MDCA) and patchy atrophy in choroidal thickness at temporal, nasal, superior, and inferior locations.

Another high myopia clinic-based study from Zhongshan Ophthalmic Center [17] also investigated the choroidal thickness in a large population of highly myopic eyes with different categories of myopic maculopathy according to META-PM classification. In this study, the median subfoveal choroidal thickness was 165 μm in normal fundus (C0), 80 μm in tessellated fundus (C1), 49 μm in diffuse atrophy (C2), 35 in patchy atrophy(C3), and 6.5 μm in macular atrophy(C4). It showed that the subfoveal choroidal thickness became significantly thinner with the increasing severity of maculopathy in C0 to C4, but the eyes with C3 to C4

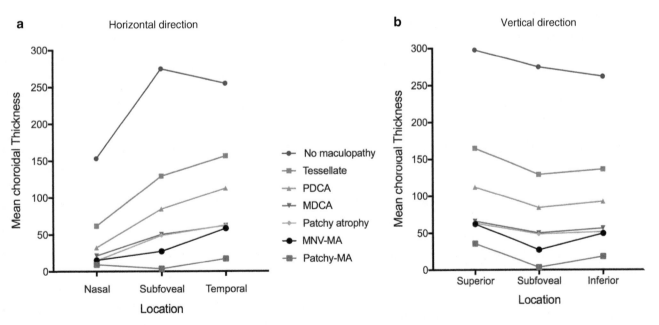

Fig. 18.4 Graph showing the topography of choroidal thickness (CT) for each type of myopic maculopathy in the horizontal direction (**a**) and in the vertical direction (**b**). The CT was measured at the subfoveal region and at 3 mm nasal, temporal, superior, and inferior to the fovea. The pattern of the CT in highly myopic eyes with normal fundus (=no maculopathy) was different from that in eyes with myopic maculopathy, i.e., ≥tessellated fundus. In eyes with myopic maculopathy (≥tessellated fundus), the temporal CT was thicker than the subfoveal CT or nasal CT (A). In the vertical scan, the subfoveal CT was thinner than the superior CT or inferior CT (Fig. 18.1b)

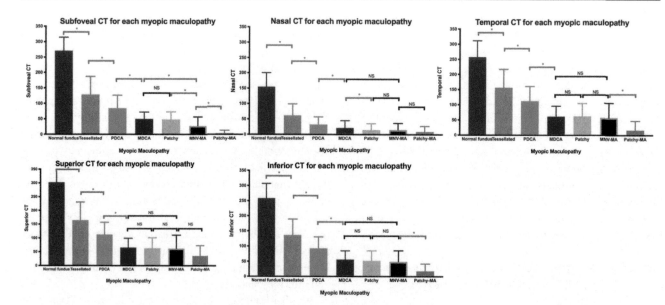

Fig. 18.5 The choroidal thickness (CT) (mean with standard deviation) at each location in each myopic maculopathy is shown. Choroidal thickness decreased significantly from normal fundus to tessellated fundus, to PDCA, and to MDCA in all locations. There is no significant difference in CT between eyes with MDCA and patchy atrophy in all locations except for nasal CT. It is noted that only subfoveal CT in MNV-related macula atrophy is significantly thinner than CT in MDCA and patchy atrophy, but there is no difference in CT with other locations. *P < 0.05; NS, not significant. PDCA, peripapillary diffuse choroidal atrophy, MDCA, macular diffuse choroidal atrophy

shared similar parafoveal choroidal thickness, leading to the conclusion that C4 was not the result of progression from C3 which was consistent with long-term follow-up study by Fang et al. [28].

18.4.2 Cut-Off Value of Choroidal Thickness for Identifying PDCA and MDCA

The diagnosis of peripapillary diffuse choroidal atrophy (PDCA) and macular diffuse choroidal atrophy (MDCA) now is solely based on fundus examination, which is somewhat subjective. Since there was a significant difference in choroidal thickness between tessellation and PDCA, as well as PDCA and MDCA, it is interesting to see if choroidal thickness can be used as a diagnostic tool for both entities.

The use of receiver operating characteristic (ROC) curve and Youden's index allowed us to determine the optimal cut-off CT value for the diagnosis of PDCA and MDCA (Fig. 18.6) [20]. In predicting the eyes with PDCA from the tessellation group, the cut-off value for the nasal choroidal thickness (3000 μm from fovea) was 56.5 μm with a high sensitivity of 90% and a good specificity of 88% in the age <20 group which is consistent with previous findings [30]. The area under curve (AUC) of choroidal thickness in each location became lower in the older age group. For the 60–79 years group, only the subfoveal choroidal thickness can be used for diagnosis.

To differentiate eyes with MDCA from PDCA, the nasal choroidal thickness cannot be used. Instead, the choroidal thickness cut-off value of 62 μm at subfovea (sensitivity, 71%; specificity, 72%), 73 μm at temporal (sensitivity, 67%; specificity, 90%), 83 μm at superior (sensitivity, 67%; specificity, 80%), and 84.5 μm at inferior (sensitivity, 81%; specificity, 65%) can be used to define the eyes with MDCA [20]. Although the area under curve (AUC) of subfoveal choroidal thickness is not the largest among all the locations, the cut-off value differentiating MDCA from PDCA is still based on the subfoveal choroidal thickness since the detection of the fovea is easier and more accurate than the parafoveal points.

18.5 Summary of OCT-Based Classification of Myopic Maculopathy (Table 18.2)

Combining all the hallmarks of myopic maculopathy in pathologic myopia, we propose a new classification based on OCT findings. In this new system, diffuse choroidal atrophy, for PDCA to MDCA, is suggested to be named as "peripapillary choroidal thinning" and "macular choroidal thinning." Learn from our results; the cut-off value of choroidal thickness as diagnostic tool for diffuse atrophy is added into this system. That is, peripapillary choroidal thinning is defined as choroidal thickness <56.5 mm at 3000 mm nasal from the fovea, and macular choroidal thinning is defined as choroidal thickness <62 mm at subfovea. Patchy atrophy and MNV-related macular atrophy are not simply due to atrophy but the holes in

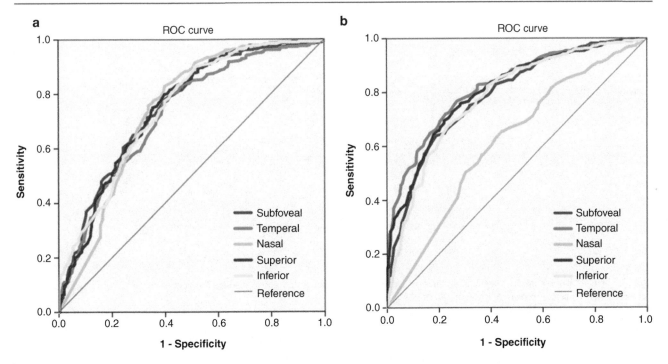

Fig. 18.6 Graphs showing the receiver operating curve (ROC) of optimal choroidal thickness for each location to predict PDCA (**a**) and MDCA (**b**). PDCA peripapillary diffuse choroidal atrophy, MDCA macular diffuse choroidal atrophy

Table 18.2 OCT-based classification of myopic maculopathy

New terminology	Details	Old terminology
Peripapillary choroidal thinning	CT < 56.5 μm at 3000 μm nasal from the fovea	PDCA
Macular choroidal thinning	CT < 62 μm at subfovea	MDCA
Linear BM defects	Yellowish linear lesions. Discontinuities of the RPE and increased hyper-transmission into deeper tissues beyond the RPE in OCT image	Lacquer cracks
Extrafoveal BM defects	Well-defined, grayish white, round lesion(s) in the macular, extrafoveal area. The BM defect is usually surrounded by a slightly wider RPE defect, the size and shape of which determines the ophthalmoscopical size and shape of the lesion. In the region of the BM defect, the outer retinal layer, the RPE, the choriocapillaris, and most of the medium-sized choroidal vessel layer are absent, and a medium-sized or large choroidal vessel may occasionally be present. The middle and inner retinal layers, more or less thinned, are in direct contact with the inner scleral surface	Patchy atrophy
Myopic MNV	MNV occurring in eyes with at least peripapillary or macular choroidal thinning	MNV
Foveal BM defect		Macular atrophy
MNV-related	Well-defined, round lesion centered on the fovea and expanding centrifugally around the fovea. The edges of the macular BM defect are often upturned. In the center, remnants of BM can be present, folded up in the process of the RPE-associated scar formation	MNV-MA
Patchy-related	Develops outside of the foveal area and enlarges in direction to the fovea or coalesces with other extrafoveal BM defects in direction to the fovea	Patchy-MA
Macular traction maculopathy	Schisis-like inner retinal fluid, schisis-like outer retina fluid, foveal detachment, lamellar or full-thickness macular hole, and/or macular detachment	
Dome-shaped macula	Inward bulge of the RPE line of >50 μm above a base line connecting the RPE lines on either the vertical or horizontal scans	

OCT optical coherence tomography, *PDCA* peripapillary diffuse choroidal atrophy, *MDCA* macular diffuse choroidal atrophy, *CT* choroidal thickness, *MNV* myopic macular neovascularization, *MNV* macular neovascularization, *MNV-MA* macular neovascularization-related macular atrophy, *patchy-MA* patchy atrophy-related macular atrophy, *BM* Bruch membrane, *RPE* retinal pigment epithelium

Bruch's membrane. Patchy atrophy is seen as a well-defined, grayish white lesion by fundus photograph seldomly involving the central fovea which is appropriately called as "extrafoveal planar Bruch membrane defects" by OCT definition. On the other hand, "macular Bruch membrane defects" is named for macular atrophy, i.e., category 4 in META-PM classification, for both MNV-related and patchy-related. In addition, myopic traction maculopathy and dome-shaped macula both as poten-

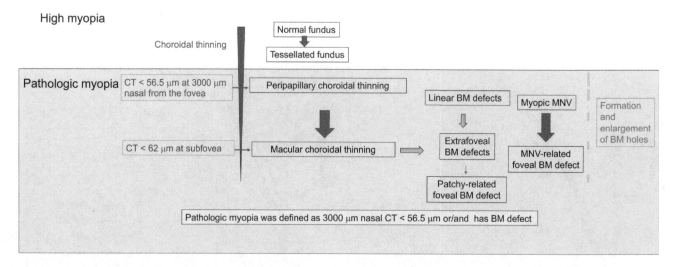

Fig. 18.7 Diagram showing the progression patterns of myopic maculopathy and corresponding characteristic of OCT finding. BM Bruch's membrane, MNV macular neovascularization, CT choroidal thickness

tial vision-threatening macular complications that only can be detected by OCT are also included in OCT-based classification of myopic maculopathy.

18.6 A Scheme Depicting the Progression Patterns of Myopic Maculopathy Combining with OCT Finding
(Fig. 18.7)

First, the progression from category 0 (no myopic maculopathy) to category 1 (fundus tessellation) was not associated with a decline of visual acuity. Although tessellation is not considered as pathologic myopia, a remarkable thinning of the choroid begins with the appearance of tessellation, which is the first sign of the progression of myopic maculopathy. Second, diffuse atrophy (category 2) primarily occurs in the peripapillary region (PDCA) and eventually extends into the macula (MDCA). Third, the eyes with patchy atrophy have a hole in the macular Bruch's membrane that either forms by an enlargement of lacquer cracks or develops in regions of advanced diffuse atrophy with a more vulnerable Bruch's membrane. Fourth, both patchy atrophy and macular atrophy (MNV-related and patchy-related) tend to enlarge with time. Fifth, macular atrophy is almost always MNV-related, although patchy-related MA can occasionally occur.

18.7 Future Perspective

Frist of all, further studies are needed to validate if the cut-off values of choroidal thickness in our series can work well in clinical practice. More studies should be done for investigating the role of choroid in high myopia not only by mea-

suring the thickness but also using other parameters such as choroidal blood flow and morphologic and vascular features of choroid. Longitudinal studies on choroidal change will help us to depict a real picture for choroidal changes in high myopic patients.

It is undoubtful that artificial intelligence (AI) is one of the greatest revolutions in many fields especially in the image analysis in ophthalmology. Researchers are now developing AI -based systems to better detect and evaluate ophthalmic conditions such as diabetic retinopathy. The automated grading of myopic maculopathy is expected. It would be helpful for using new OCT-based classification into artificial intelligence for better diagnose of the myopic maculopathy.

References

1. Fujiwara T, Imamura Y, Margolis R, Slakter JS, Spaide RF. Enhanced depth imaging optical coherence tomography of the choroid in highly myopic eyes. Am J Ophthalmol. 2009;148:445–50.
2. Ikuno Y, Tano Y. Retinal and choroidal biometry in highly myopic eyes with spectral-domain optical coherence tomography. Invest Ophthalmol Vis Sci. 2009;50:3876–80.
3. Wang NK, Lai CC, Chu HY, et al. Classification of early dry-type myopic maculopathy with macular choroidal thickness. Am J Ophthalmol. 2012;153:669–77, 677 e1–2.
4. Nishida Y, Fujiwara T, Imamura Y, Lima LH, Kurosaka D, Spaide RF. Choroidal thickness and visual acuity in highly myopic eyes. Retina. 2012;32:1229–36.
5. Takahashi A, Ito Y, Iguchi Y, Yasuma TR, Ishikawa K, Terasaki H. Axial length increases and related changes in highly myopic normal eyes with myopic complications in fellow eyes. Retina. 2012;32:127–33.
6. Flores-Moreno I, Lugo F, Duker JS, Ruiz-Moreno JM. The relationship between axial length and choroidal thickness in eyes with high myopia. Am J Ophthalmol. 2013;155:314–9. e1
7. Ho M, Liu DT, Chan VC, Lam DS. Choroidal thickness measurement in myopic eyes by enhanced depth optical coherence tomography. Ophthalmology. 2013;120:1909–14.

8. Flores-Moreno I, Ruiz-Medrano J, Duker JS, Ruiz-Moreno JM. The relationship between retinal and choroidal thickness and visual acuity in highly myopic eyes. Br J Ophthalmol. 2013;97:1010–3.

9. Gupta P, Saw SM, Cheung CY, et al. Choroidal thickness and high myopia: a case-control study of young Chinese men in Singapore. Acta Ophthalmol. 2015;93:e585–92.

10. Pang CE, Sarraf D, Freund KB. Extreme choroidal thinning in high myopia. Retina. 2015;35:407–15.

11. Wong CW, Phua V, Lee SY, Wong TY, Cheung CM. Is choroidal or scleral thickness related to myopic macular degeneration? Invest Ophthalmol Vis Sci. 2017;58:907–13.

12. Zhou LX, Shao L, Xu L, Wei WB, Wang YX, You QS. The relationship between scleral staphyloma and choroidal thinning in highly myopic eyes: the Beijing Eye Study. Sci Rep. 2017;7:9825.

13. Abdolrahimzadeh S, Parisi F, Plateroti AM, et al. Visual acuity, and macular and peripapillary thickness in high myopia. Curr Eye Res. 2017;42:1468–73.

14. Lee JH, Lee SC, Kim SH, et al. Choroidal thickness and chorioretinal atrophy in myopic choroidal neovascularization with anti-vascular endothelial growth factor therapy. Retina. 2017;37:1516–22.

15. Xiong S, He X, Deng J, et al. Choroidal thickness in 3001 Chinese children aged 6 to 19 years using swept-source OCT. Sci Rep. 2017;7:45059.

16. Liu B, Wang Y, Li T, et al. Correlation of subfoveal choroidal thickness with axial length, refractive error, and age in adult highly myopic eyes. BMC Ophthalmol. 2018;18:127.

17. Zhao X, Ding X, Lyu C, et al. Morphological characteristics and visual acuity of highly myopic eyes with different severities of myopic maculopathy. Retina. 2018;40(3):461–7.

18. Fledelius HC, Jacobsen N, Li XQ, Goldschmidt E. Choroidal thickness at age 66 years in the Danish high myopia study cohort 1948 compared with follow-up data on visual acuity over 40 years: a clinical update adding spectral domain optical coherence tomography. Acta Ophthalmol. 2018;96:46–50.

19. Chalam KV, Sambhav K. Choroidal thickness measured with swept source optical coherence tomography in posterior staphyloma strongly correlates with axial length and visual acuity. Int J Retina Vitreous. 2019;5:14.

20. Fang Y, Du R, Nagaoka N, et al. OCT-based diagnostic criteria for different stages of myopic maculopathy. Ophthalmology. 2019;126:1018–32.

21. Ohno-Matsui K, Jonas JB, Spaide RF. Macular Bruch membrane holes in choroidal neovascularization-related myopic macular atrophy by swept-source optical coherence tomography. Am J Ophthalmol. 2016;162:133–9. e1

22. Ohno-Matsui K, Jonas JB, Spaide RF. Macular Bruch membrane holes in highly myopic patchy chorioretinal atrophy. Am J Ophthalmol. 2016;166:22–8.

23. Du R, Fang Y, Jonas JB, et al. Clinical features of patchy chorioretinal atrophy in pathologic myopia. Retina. 2019;40(5):951–9.

24. Ishida T, Watanabe T, Yokoi T, Shinohara K, Ohno-Matsui K. Possible connection of short posterior ciliary arteries to choroidal neovascularisations in eyes with pathologic myopia. Br J Ophthalmol. 2019;103(4):457–62.

25. Xie S, Fang Y, Du R, Onishi Y, Yokoi T, Moriyama M, Watanabe T, Ohno-Matsui K. Role of dilated subfoveal choroidal veins in eyes with myopic macular neovascularization. Retina. 2021;41(5):1063–70.

26. Ohno-Matsui K, Kawasaki R, Jonas JB, et al. International photographic classification and grading system for myopic maculopathy. Am J Ophthalmol. 2015;159:877–83. e7

27. Marchese A, Carnevali A, Sacconi R, et al. Retinal pigment epithelium humps in high myopia. Am J Ophthalmol. 2017;182:56–61.

28. Fang Y, Yokoi T, Nagaoka N, et al. Progression of myopic maculopathy during 18-year follow-up. Ophthalmology. 2018;125:863–77.

29. Yokoi T, Jonas JB, Shimada N, et al. Peripapillary diffuse chorioretinal atrophy in children as a sign of eventual pathologic myopia in adults. Ophthalmology. 2016;123:1783–7.

30. Yokoi T, Zhu D, Bi HS, et al. Parapapillary diffuse choroidal atrophy in children is associated with extreme thinning of parapapillary choroid. Invest Ophthalmol Vis Sci. 2017;58:901–6.

31. Jonas JB, Ohno-Matsui K, Spaide RF, Holbach L, Panda-Jonas S. Macular Bruch's membrane defects and axial length: association with gamma zone and delta zone in peripapillary region. Invest Ophthalmol Vis Sci. 2013;54:1295–302.

32. Liu CF, Liu L, Lai CC, et al. Multimodal imaging including spectral-domain optical coherence tomography and confocal near-infrared reflectance for characterization of lacquer cracks in highly myopic eyes. Eye (Lond). 2014;28:1437–45.

33. Xu X, Fang Y, Uramoto K, et al. Clinical features of lacquer cracks in eyes with pathologic myopia. Retina. 2019;39:1265–77.

34. Panozzo G, Mercanti A. Optical coherence tomography findings in myopic traction maculopathy. Arch Ophthalmol. 2004;122:1455–60.

35. Baba T, Ohno-Matsui K, Futagami S, et al. Prevalence and characteristics of foveal retinal detachment without macular hole in high myopia. Am J Ophthalmol. 2003;135:338–42.

36. Gaucher D, Erginay A, Lecleire-Collet A, et al. Dome-shaped macula in eyes with myopic posterior staphyloma. Am J Ophthalmol. 2008;145:909–14.

37. Johnson MW. Myopic traction maculopathy: pathogenic mechanisms and surgical treatment. Retina. 2012;32(Suppl 2):S205–10.

38. Ellabban AA, Tsujikawa A, Matsumoto A, et al. Three-dimensional tomographic features of dome-shaped macula by swept-source optical coherence tomography. Am J Ophthalmol. 2013;155:320–8. e2

39. Margolis R, Spaide RF. A pilot study of enhanced depth imaging optical coherence tomography of the choroid in normal eyes. Am J Ophthalmol. 2009;147:811–5.

40. Zhou Y, Song M, Zhou M, Liu Y, Wang F, Sun X. Choroidal and retinal thickness of highly myopic eyes with early stage of myopic chorioretinopathy: tessellation. J Ophthalmol. 2018;2018:2181602.

Choroidal Neovascularization

19

Richard F. Spaide

The realization that highly myopic eyes were prone to develop choroidal neovascularization (CNV) occurred relatively recently. Fuchs spots [1], also known as Forster-Fuchs spots, were described as pigmentary changes in the posterior pole of myopes. These spots, sometimes associated with hemorrhage, were first described by Forster in 1862 and Fuchs in 1901. The reason for the hemorrhage was not known at the time. In 1953 Lloyd [2] wrote that Fuchs spots were often preceded by a cystic appearance of the macula and attributed the Fuchs spot to stretching of the choriocapillaris. In 1973, Focosi and coworkers [3] described a group of myopic eyes that developed serous and serosanguineous detachments of the macula. The authors found these patients had fluorescein angiographic evidence of leakage, sometimes from multiple lesions. Close inspection of the published angiograms shows the eyes had findings suggestive of multifocal choroiditis and panuveitis (MCP, a condition described much later) complicated by neovascularization. The authors thought the patients had serous pigment epithelial detachments with no neovascularization, and the blood present originated from the constituent vessels of the choroid. In 1977 fluorescein angiographic evidence was presented to show Fuchs spots were actually caused by choroidal neovascularization [4]. In this paper, Levy and coauthors hypothesized laser photocoagulation may prove to be a useful treatment. Since then the importance of CNV as a major cause of vision loss in highly myopic eyes has been more fully appreciated, and several successive treatment modalities have been developed.

19.1 Background

Myopic choroidal neovascularization mCNV is classified as a subtype of myopic maculopathy in which neovascularization originating from the choroid typically is type 2. It is the most significant cause of severe vision loss in more advanced forms of myopia. Pathologic myopia is generally taken to mean a myopic refractive error of at least −6 diopters. The proportion of people in Western countries with this level of myopia ranges from 1% to 5%, and in Asia the proportion can be up to 40%. A World Health Organization estimate places the proportion of myopes with a refractive error greater than −5 diopters to be approximately 4% of the world's population in 2020, and that number is expected to increase to 10% by 2050 [5]. Given the United Nations Department of Economic and Social Affairs projects world population in 2050 will be approximately 9.8 billion people [6], that means nearly a billion will have at least high myopia. This is in context of an estimated 52% having some degree of myopia.

The proportion of eyes developing mCNV with pathologic myopia is estimated [7] to be between 5.2% and 11.3% with up to 30% developing bilateral disease. Neovascularization can be a devastating development in eyes with pathologic myopia, as it occurs in extant regions of retina, often adjacent to areas affected by lacquer cracks, atrophy, or staphyloma. Neovascularization is a significant cause of severe visual loss in work-age adults worldwide, but particularly in Asia [8–13]. Without treatment, more than 90% of affected eyes progress to legal blindness in 10 years [14–16].

19.2 Clinical Characteristics

The principle symptoms from CNV in myopia are loss of acuity, scotomata, and distortion of vision. Some patients with advanced myopic degeneration have prior impairments to their vision from lacquer cracks, atrophy, or staphyloma such that the addition of CNV may not cause enough incremental change in their vision for them to notice any early irregularity. The presenting abnormalities of myopic CNV differ by degrees from that seen in AMD. The CNV in myopic eyes is less likely to have sub- or intraretinal fluid or lipid and seems to be associated with less proliferation in the

R. F. Spaide (✉)
Vitreous, Retina, Macula Consultants of New York, New York, NY, USA

© Springer Nature Switzerland AG 2021
R. F. Spaide et al. (eds.), *Pathologic Myopia*, https://doi.org/10.1007/978-3-030-74334-5_19

subretinal space than CNV in AMD. Myopic CNV almost never has associated serous pigment epithelial detachments. CNV in myopia is generally fairly small in contrast to that seen in AMD. The size of the CNV seems to vary inversely with the amount of myopia.

Growth of neovascularization occurs in eyes showing other signs of abnormalities related to high myopia. Mechanical dehiscence of Bruch's membrane occurs in eyes with high myopia to produce thin branching lines in the posterior pole called lacquer cracks. These ruptures affect the full thickness of Bruch's membrane and as a consequence involve the choriocapillaris as well. Thus it is common to see subretinal hemorrhage in eyes with high myopia that are overlying lacquer cracks or clear to show new lacquer cracks (Fig. 19.1) [17–20]. The defect caused by the break in Bruch's membrane appears to be repopulated by retinal pigment epithelium (RPE) producing a granular pigmentation. Over time the cracks can widen, presumably from tensile traction in Bruch's membrane. This can lead to broad cracks, addition of neighboring cracks, or development of patchy atrophy.

Eyes with high myopia have concurrent reduction in the thickness of the choroid [21–24], and with advanced amounts of myopia, particularly in older patients, the choroid may shrink to have nearly no thickness. These eyes appear to develop areas of full-thickness loss of the choroid and overlying retinal pigment epithelium. Both lacquer cracks and atrophy appear to be risk factors for development of CNV [17, 20, 25, 26]. While pre-existing lacquer cracks provide an easy avenue for the ingrowth of new vessels, neovascularization can erode directly through intact Bruch's membrane [27]. In most cases lacquer cracks appear to be the most significant risk factor, however [28]. Once the neovascular process begins, the vessel ingrowth can be partially or completely engulfed by proliferating pigment cells, producing a Fuchs spot. In the past, prior to the availability of treatment for myopic CNV, the visualization of pigmentation around the neovascularization was seen to be a favorable sign suggestive of stabilization of the process. If the neovascularization is not enveloped with RPE cells, it appears a grayish-white thickening under the retina. There may be associated small hemorrhages and sometimes subtle flecks of lipid. The con-

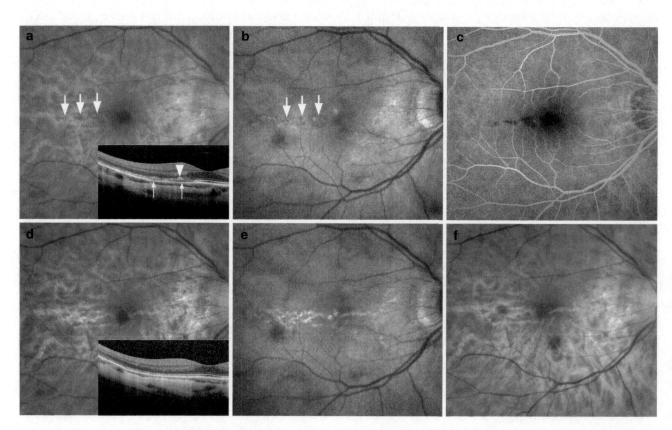

Fig. 19.1 Progression of lacquer cracks. (**a**) This highly myopic patient presented with a complaint of distortion of vision. There is a linear array of hemorrhages and a faintly visible crack (arrows). The inset shows the RPE is not elevated (arrows). The retina is elevated by collections of blood (arrowhead). (**b**) A near infrared scanning laser ophthalmoscopic image shows the lacquer crack in higher contrast (arrows). (**c**) A fluorescein angiogram shows no evidence of neovascu-

larization. (**d**) Two years later, after several instances of subretinal hemorrhage associated with the formation of new lacquer cracks, the patient had no hemorrhage. Inset shows no elevation of the RPE indicative of neovascularization. (**e**) The larger number of interconnected lacquer cracks is apparent. (**f**) Three months later the patient presented with subretinal hemorrhage, but no evidence of neovascularization

verse, big hemorrhages or large amounts of lipid exudation, are almost never seen.

Fluorescein angiography demonstrates the vascular ingrowth as early hyperfluorescence with variable amounts of leakage later in the angiographic sequence (Figs. 19.2, 19.3, and 19.4). Some eyes show nearly no leakage of fluorescein. Thus, the neovascularization seen in highly myopic eyes can show some, but not necessarily all, of the features required to classify the neovascularization as being "classic." The proportion of cases classified as predominantly classic were approximately 80% in the Verteporfin in Photodynamic Therapy-Pathologic Myopia (VIP-PM) study [28, 29], although some authors consider most [26] or all [30] neovascularization in high myopia to be classic.

Optical coherence tomography (OCT) can show signs of exudation such as intra- or subretinal fluid and hyperreflective subretinal material in eyes with myopic CNV. Small hemorrhages are usually not easy to visualize with OCT. The infiltration causes a low, flat alteration in the contour of the RPE monolayer. The exudation and infiltration related to the neovascularization cause the boundary between the lesion and outer retina to become less well-defined or "fuzzy." Loss of exudative manifestations, through history or natural course, is associated with the boundary becoming more well-defined [31]. OCT angiography demonstrates the neovascularization in both the B-scan with flow overlay and the en face sections (Fig. 19.5). It is common for highly myopic eyes to be segmented incorrectly, and consequently the en

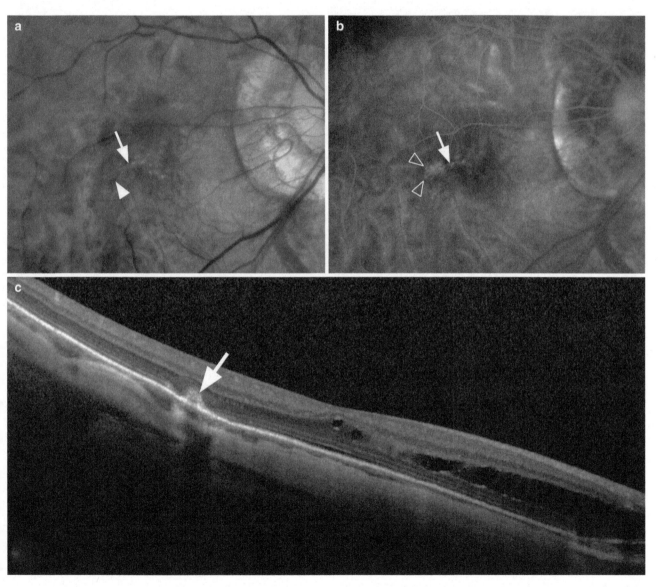

Fig. 19.2 (**a**) This −16 diopter myope developed a small scotoma near the center of the visual field. There were lacquer cracks, one of which was highlighted by the arrow. There were some associated pigmentary changes (arrowhead). (**b**) Fluorescein angiography showed a hyperfluo-rescent lesion consistent with choroidal neovascularization. (**c**) The optical coherence tomography scan shows a small elevated lesion (arrow) and also non-associated macular schisis

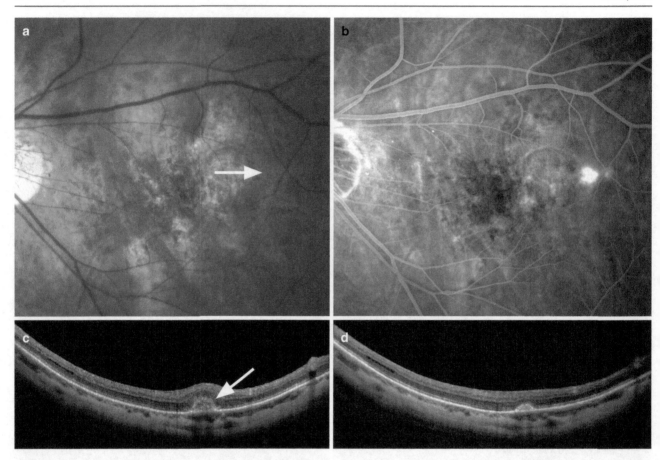

Fig. 19.3 Myopic choroidal neovascularization at the edge of a staphyloma. (**a**) The patient had distortion of her vision. There was a subtle gray-white thickening (arrow). (**b**) The fluorescein angiogram shows a hyperfluorescent lesion seen early with pronounced leakage consistent with type 2 neovascularization. (**c**) An OCT obtained by using a vertical scan to avoid the effects of the staphyloma showed a lesion in the deep retina. The borders of the lesion are not well defined. The outer nuclear layer over the lesion shows increased reflectivity as compared to the outer nuclear layer away from the lesion. The patient was given an intravitreal injection of an anti-VEGF agent. (**d**) The same lesion seen 1 month later shows the lesion has decreased in size and the outer border of the lesion is more sharply defined

face images may be difficult to evaluate. The value of the B-scan images with flow overlay is that they are not affected by segmentation issues, although image folding can be problematical in larger scans. Use of a 3 mm × 3 mm scan overcomes many current problems with segmentation and image folding. Commercial instruments with a deeper scan range and better segmentation, particularly employing artificial intelligence, may help overcome prevailing limitations of OCT angiography.

The subtlety of findings, along with the relatively small neovascular lesions, can make diagnosis of CNV difficult in some cases. The differential diagnosis for myopic CNV includes macular hole, small focal areas of chorioretinal atrophy or scarring, and inflammatory conditions such as MCP [20]. Because of the relative depigmentation of the fundus in a high myope, macular holes may not be that obvious. These holes are often associated with decreased acuity and can have associated subretinal fluid. The diagnosis is readily apparent using OCT. High myopes frequently have

small areas of altered pigmentation in the posterior pole. Small hyperpigmented spots are usually flat and do not have a surrounding area of atrophy. True CNV causes an elevation at the level of the RPE. Fluorescein angiography shows hyperfluorescence later in the angiographic sequence if new vessels are present. True Fuchs spots are usually surrounded by varying amounts of depigmentation or frank atrophy. MCP causes grayish-white inflammatory lesions at the level of the RPE that can have associated subretinal fluid during the acute, active phase. OCT shows the inflammatory lesions to be conical elevations of the RPE. During fluorescein angiography, these lesions can show early fluorescence with late staining. Clues that the eye harbors MCP are recurrent accumulations of new lesions, multiple lesions in the fundus, clinically evident inflammatory cells, and the characteristic OCT appearance of the inflammatory mounds that start as sub-RPE accumulations and then make break through the RPE monolayer. These same eyes may develop CNV, which is heralded by an increase in exudation and scarring, often

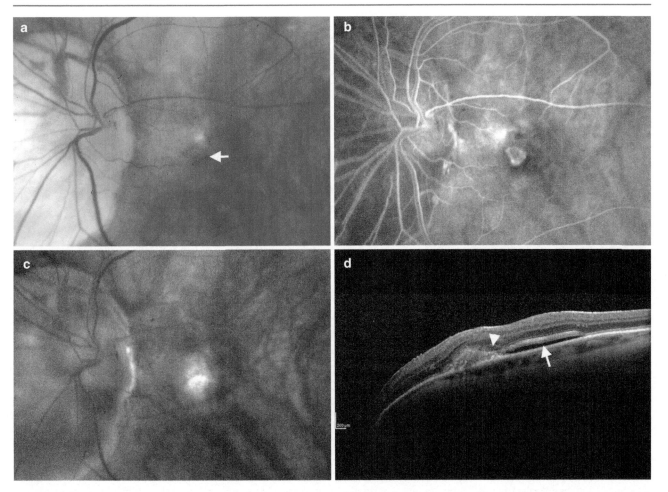

Fig. 19.4 Presentation of choroidal neovascularization in a high myope. (**a**) There is a small area of focal hypopigmentation with an adjacent, but not contiguous area of altered pigmentation and barely visible hemorrhage (arrow). (**b**) The early phase of the fluorescein angiogram shows early visualization of the vascular network. Note the separation between the vessels and the hypopigmented area. (**c**) In the later phases of the angiogram, there is leakage from the vessels, which is another angiographic characteristic required to make the diagnosis of classic choroidal neovascularization. (**d**) Optical coherence tomography shows a triangular elevation of the retina with poor delineation between the lesion and the retina. There is granular material in the space above the lesion (arrowhead) and subretinal fluid (arrow)

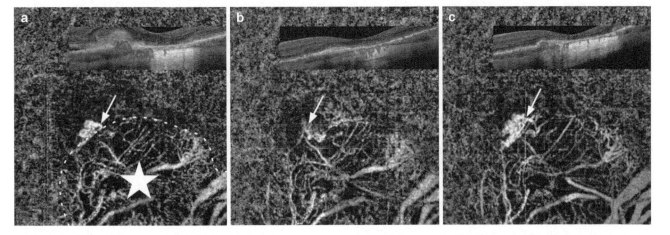

Fig. 19.5 Optical coherence tomography of myopic neovascularization. (**a**) The neovascularization appeared in a subfoveal location (arrow) at the border of an area of patchy atrophy (star, area outlined by a dashed line). The segmentation slab extended into the inner choroid intentionally to show the larger choroidal vessels effaced in the area of atrophy. The inset is a B-scan with flow overlay showing the ingress of the neovascularization. The patient was given an anti-VEGF injection. (**b**) One month later the lesion showed regression (arrow). The inset shows the lesion is much smaller, with no evident intralesional flow. (**c**) Two years later the patient had a recurrence of neovascularization (arrow). The inset shows the reappearance of flow signal in the lesion

with minimal hemorrhage. These eyes may have reactive changes in the RPE, which are hypofluorescent in fluorescein angiography and hyperautofluorescent with autofluorescence imaging [32, 33].

The incidence of CNV in high myopia probably is related to a number of factors, which may in turn influence estimates. These factors include age, refractive status, gender, and potentially involvement of the fellow eye [34–42]. Curtin and Karlin reported Fuchs spots were present in 5.2% of eyes with an axial length of 26.5 mm [34]. Grossniklaus and Green [43] found a similar proportion in what were reported to be myopic eyes coming to histopathologic evaluation, although no axial length or refractive error data for those eyes was presented. There appears to be a female predominance in myopic CNV.

19.3   Potential Pathologic Mechanisms

The actual pathogenic sequence of the early phases of any form of CNV is unclear, and myopic CNV is no exception. A variety of contributing factors have been proposed to explain why CNV occurs, but all of these seem to have shortcomings. What we do know is eyes with myopia have axial lengthening and apparent stretching of the structures in the posterior pole. The choroidal thickness decreases in high myopia [21, 22, 24], but the thickness of the overlying RPE cells and the packing density of the photoreceptors decrease in a manner than initially may be proportionate. With the passage of time, the choroid becomes even thinner, at which point decompensation secondary to outer retina ischemia seems possible. Coincident with, or perhaps in part related to, the choroidal thinning are alterations of Bruch's membrane manifested as lacquer cracks. Eyes with lacquer cracks have RPE alterations in the same general area. Lacquer cracks may offer avenues for the ingrowth of vessels or may indicate a general degeneration of Bruch's membrane such that CNV may be more likely to occur. Other conditions leading to the ingrowth of neovascularization in the context of breaks in Bruch's membrane include choroidal ruptures due to trauma, angioid streaks in pseudoxanthoma elasticum [44], and microbreaks in AMD [45]; however each of these has other factors at play that may encourage the growth of CNV. Most eyes with high myopia have lacquer cracks [17, 18, 25, 26], but only a minority develops CNV, so other factors may be involved in myopic CNV as well. Grossniklaus and Green proposed the growth of new vessels from the choroid may be a compensatory mechanism for the loss of choroidal blood flow through a degenerating choriocapillaris in AMD [46]. This same pathophysiologic mechanism may be operative in high myopia and offers a tantalizing explanation for CNV growth. However, observation of the growth characteristics of myopic CNV argues against simple ischemia.

The choroidal thickness decreases with increasing myopia, but neither the size nor the number of CNV lesions increases with increasing myopia. If CNV were a compensatory response, it is difficult to understand why the RPE would envelope and seemingly limit the growth of vessels. Ischemia would continue or increase with time, so one would expect ever increasing incidence of CNV in highly myopic eyes and multiple new lesions over time if ischemia was the sole cause.

19.4   Disease Characteristics

In 1981 several papers were published that showed many of the salient characteristics of myopic CNV. Hotchkiss and Fine published a case series in which nearly half of the eyes followed deteriorated to legal blindness [36]. The location of the CNV was found to be an important determinant of the final visual acuity. A significant proportion of eyes did not have neovascularization under the fovea, and these eyes appeared to have a lower risk of poor visual outcome. Some of the eyes in the series had laser photocoagulation, which was thought to potentially stabilize the visual acuity. The authors recommended a large prospective study to evaluate laser photocoagulation as a treatment. In the same year, Rabb and coauthors reported the clinical findings of a large series of patients with CNV secondary to high myopia [35]. They described choroidal atrophy, the need to recognize lacquer cracks as a potential precursor for choroidal neovascularization, eyes with CNV develop scars, atrophy, and even macular holes and mentioned laser photocoagulation of CNV could preserve visual acuity. The authors thought the development of atrophy to be the most common reason for eyes to have poor visual acuity. Also in 1981 Fried and coauthors described a series of eyes with Fuchs spots [37]. These generally occurred with increasing age of the patient but were seen in some as young as 14 years old. These authors described the use of laser photocoagulation. In 1983 Hampton and coworkers published a retrospective study of patients with visual loss secondary to myopic CNV [47]. They reported the visual acuity was related to the size and location of the neovascularization, the age of the patient, and duration of follow-up. At last follow-up 60% of the eyes in their study were 20/200 or worse. The visual acuity was lost in the eyes in a rapid early phase of disease and more slowly later, with development of atrophy, was a common endstage outcome. Avila and coworkers [36] reported a series of patients with CNV associated with degenerative myopia in 1984 and concluded CNV was a self-limited disorder. There is an old medical school joke that hemorrhage is a self-limited disorder; however the implication was the pathologic process caused a loss of function early after the development of the neovascularization and did not smolder on. They reported results of laser photocoagulation in 19 eyes, and the mean acuity of treated eyes did not improve. As a consequence of these "disappointing" results, the authors stated they stopped performing laser photocoagulation [48], which is curious given a theme this paper had with other contemporaneous publications was the poor natural history of the disease.

In 1999 Tabandeh and coworkers investigated patients aged 50 years or more in relation to the findings of CNV in high myopia [49]. As is typical for myopic CNV, the lesions were small, but a greater proportion of patients, as compared with historical controls, had a visual acuity of 20/200 or worse. Bottoni and Tilanus [50] showed that for a mean follow-up of 3 years, eyes with non-subfoveal CNV were more likely to retain good acuity as compared with eyes with subfoveal involvement. Yoshida and coauthors [14] reported 10-year follow-up of a retrospective series of 25 highly myopic eyes with CNV, and nearly all of them had a visual acuity less than 20/200 [14]. In examining the 5-year outcomes, Hayashi and coworkers found patients with a good prognosis for visual acuity preservation in the absence of treatment were more likely to be younger, with smaller areas of CNV, better initial acuity, and the lesions were more likely to be nonsubfoveal [51]. Secretan and coauthors [15] reported a group of 50 eyes with nonsubfoveal disease that were not treated. Over time all of the eyes developed subfoveal extension of neovascularization. Yoshida and coauthors reported, in agreement with previous reports, that older eyes were more likely to have decreased vision from myopic CNV [28]. The untreated group of the VIP-PM group showed a rapid initial loss of acuity, expansion of the CNV, and enlargement of macular scarring over time [28]. The initial phases of neovascularization appear to be the more significant in causing vision loss, but the process continues with a smoldering expansion of neovascularization in many and the late development of atrophy affecting the central macula.

19.5 Treatment of Myopic Choroidal Neovascularization

Successive forms of treatment have been developed for choroidal neovascularization (CNV) secondary to age-related macular degeneration (AMD). Most of the major developments were the product of extensive pre-clinical work, progression to small pilot studies, and then multicentered randomized clinical trials. Fortunately, the main multicentered clinical trials were large and well-designed, giving treating physicians enough information to formulate both a reasonable expected outcome and an appropriately narrow confidence interval of the treatment effect. Advances in the treatment of CNV secondary to pathologic myopia have trended those from AMD in both the proposed theoretical basis and practice.

The early myopia studies uniformly examined smaller numbers of patients and had various design defects. Consequently estimates of treatment effect, and the corresponding confidence intervals, had the potential to be less precise for any given study, but in aggregate they were surprisingly predictive of future results of larger studies. For each therapeutic modality, the development and multicentered trial results for AMD will be presented. Then the adaptation of the treatment to myopic CNV will be shown through review of applicable studies along with a discussion of their general strengths and weaknesses. The treatment response as it relates to the special characteristics of highly myopic eyes and the complication profiles will be presented. Several of these treatments seem to share a similar late-stage outcome, namely, the development of atrophy, and a set of possible mechanisms for the development of atrophy will be proposed.

19.6 Thermal Laser Photocoagulation

In the 1960s the idea that neovascularization was an important component of exudative AMD was derived from information gleaned from the then newly developed testing modality, fluorescein angiography [52]. The new blood vessels were seen to proliferate into regions not ordinarily containing vessels, and concurrently the eyes were seen to develop signs of exudation and bleeding. The contemporaneous development of laser technology provided a method to deliver high-density photothermal energy to selected areas in the eye [53, 54]. Many small series of laser photocoagulation for AMD-related CNV were published and helped define the clinical response that could be expected [55–57]. The results from these reports formed a base of knowledge to design a randomized clinical trial.

The efficacy of thermal laser photocoagulation was investigated in the late 1970s and early 1980s in the Macular Photocoagulation Study, a series of related multicentered clinical trials. The strategy employed was to photocoagulate neovascular lesions, along with a border of seemingly normal retina, in order to preserve surrounding areas of macula [58]. Refinement of the ideas about the fluorescein angiographic imaging of CNV occurred during this time, and the importance of differentiating classic from occult neovascularization became apparent. CNV located 200–2500 μm (extrafoveal lesions) and 1–199 μm (juxtafoveal lesions) from the geometric center of the fovea was evaluated in two related studies [58–61]. Thermal laser photocoagulation was found to reduce the incidence of severe visual loss, which was defined as a loss of six or more lines of visual acuity using a standardized measurement protocol [62], in both the extrafoveal and juxtafoveal studies. Recurrence of the CNV was a frequent occurrence after photocoagulation. The reappearance of new vessels was much more common on the foveal side of the photocoagulation scar and typically was associated with subfoveal extension of disease [61]. Eyes with no recurrence had much better acuity than eyes with recurrence. The problem with laser photocoagulation for CNV secondary to AMD is that a remarkably small proportion of the eyes do not have subfoveal involvement at presentation [63]. Later studies showed photocoagulation of lesions that were not classic neovascularization did not result in a treatment benefit and that choice of wavelength was not an important consideration in terms of treatment outcome [64].

19.7 Laser Photocoagulation for Myopic Choroidal Neovascularization

There are several potential reasons that thermal laser photocoagulation of CNV secondary to high myopia would be easier than for AMD. The neovascularization seen in high myopia is usually not masked by blood or lipid to the extent seen in eyes with AMD and as a consequence is readily visualized. They typically are small classic lesions that are frequently non-subfoveal. The enveloping pigmented cells are an attribute in terms of absorbing laser energy. Early reports of laser therapy for CNV demonstrated what was to be a recurrent theme: treated patients could have stabilization, and even improvement in some cases, but many eyes developed areas of atrophy that expanded over time [35, 36, 48, 65–68]. Some authors of the early papers questioned the value of laser, even though contemporaneous reports of the natural course of myopic CNV to be dismal in the long term [48]. A later study by Pece and coauthors with a larger patient sample showed laser photocoagulation resulted in a mean stabilization of acuity, even with longer-term follow-up [66]. A randomized trial of 70 eyes showed in the early phase after treatment, eyes receiving photocoagulation had a much better mean acuity than did non-treated eyes [67]. The difference at 5 years was no longer significant, the result of expansion of the area of atrophy in the treated eyes. A retrospective study from the same group showed laser-treated patients had less decline in acuity during the first 2 years as compared with historical controls, but the effect was not seen at 5 years [15].

Two main problems complicate thermal laser photocoagulation for myopic CNV. The first is recurrence of the neovascularization, much the same as in AMD. The majority of treated patients have recurrences, and most of these recurrences are at the foveal edge of the laser photocoagulation. The second problem is that an overwhelming majority of eyes develop enlargement of the area of atrophy that eventually involves the fovea with loss of acuity as the result. Mechanical stretching of the posterior pole of the eye appears to influence the expansion characteristics of the atrophic area [69]. The expansion of atrophy is more problematical in treating CNV in myopic eyes as compared with those having AMD. Laser photocoagulation has been studied only in eyes with nonsubfoveal lesions, which are the minority of cases of myopic CNV. Laser photocoagulation of subfoveal CNV would result in loss of central vision. Consequently, laser photocoagulation does not appear to be a good treatment for myopic CNV.

19.8 Surgical Treatment

The surgical treatment for age-related macular degeneration involves three main strategies used independently or in combination: direct surgical removal of neovascularization, removal of hemorrhage, or translocation of the macula to a more favorable location. Early reports of removal of neovascularization, hemorrhage, or both suggested most eyes had visual stabilization in AMD, with some patients showing substantial improvement [70–73]. Patients with neovascularization that was idiopathic or secondary to inflammatory conditions such as presumed ocular histoplasmosis syndrome were purported to have a better outcome [72]. The Subretinal Surgery Trials were organized, and this group of multicentered randomized trials examined the role of surgery in visual performance of affected patients [73–76]. In a study of 454 patients with CNV secondary to AMD, surgical removal did not show any benefit as compared with observation alone [74]. The median visual acuity decreased from 20/100 to 20/400 in both arms at 24 months. Cataracts and retinal detachments were more common in the surgical arm. In a group of 336 patients with subretinal hemorrhage secondary to CNV associated with AMD, drainage of the hemorrhage did not increase the chance of stable or improved visual acuity [75]. The surgical arm had a high proportion (16%) of patients going on to have rhegmatogenous retinal detachment. In a group of 225 patients with CNV lesions that were either idiopathic or associated with presumed ocular histoplasmosis, no treatment benefit was demonstrated for surgical removal as compared with observation [76]. Later the Visual Preference Value Scale findings from these patients showed no quality of life improvements among patients having surgery as compared with observation [77]. Following these reports and coincident with the availability of agents directed against vascular endothelial growth factor, there did not appear to be any compelling reason to undertake surgical extraction approaches to CNV lesions that were idiopathic or associated with AMD or inflammatory disorders.

Macular translocation is an attempt to move the macular region to an area not affected by neovascularization. This modality can be combined with removal of neovascularization and offers the possibility of placing the fovea on a relatively healthy RPE bed. The rotation of the retina causes a correspondingly large alteration of visual perception and can cause severe diplopia. Therefore in practice it was reserved to treat the second eye of a patient with bilateral disease [78–83]. In a series of 61 AMD patients who underwent 360 degree macular translocation, the median improvement of visual acuity was 7 letters [80]. There was a significant corresponding improvement in vision-related quality of life scores [81]. One randomized trial of 50 eyes in which translocation was compared with photodynamic therapy (PDT) for predominantly classic subfoveal membranes secondary to AMD found after 2 years of follow-up the translocation group had a mean change of +0.3 letters while the PDT group lost a mean of 12.6 letters [82]. Quality of life testing showed improved performance in the translocation group in several subsets [83]. The surgery required for macular translocation is difficult and time-consuming and has a high proportion of eyes eventually experiencing complications. A long-term follow-up study showed the development of atrophy was a common occurrence limiting visual potential [84].

Surgical removal of neovascularization in high myopia does not appear to cause visual acuity improvement. Uemura and Thomas reported the visual acuity results of 23 patients with myopic CNV followed for a mean of 24 months and 9 eyes had an improvement of 2 or more lines of Snellen acuity, 6 remained stable, and 8 had decreased acuity [85]. Recurrences were seen in 57% of the eyes. In a series of 22 eyes with a mean follow-up of nearly 30 months reported by Ruiz-Moreno and de la Vega, no substantive improvement of visual acuity was seen in eyes having surgical removal of CNV, but recurrences were seen in 4 eyes, cataract in 3, and retinal detachment in 1, and two patients required intraocular pressure-lowering agents [86]. In a series of 17 eyes with subfoveal CNV associated with high myopia, Hera and associates reported 4 had visual acuity improvement, 10 had no change, and 3 had a decrease in acuity [87]. Given the small sample size, lack of standardization of acuity measurement, absence of a control group, and no long-term follow-up information, it is difficult to gauge the magnitude of a benefit with this surgery, if any.

Macular translocation for subfoveal CNV in high myopia has been reported in case series and in one comparative trial. Hamelin and coauthors reported a retrospective study of 32 eyes treated by either limited macular translocation in 14 eyes or surgical extraction in 18 eyes [88]. The mean follow-up in the extraction group was 14 months, and the mean change in acuity was loss of 0.7 lines. The mean follow-up in the translocation group was 11 months, and the mean change in acuity was 3.8 lines. Recurrences were seen in 39% of the surgical removal and 14% of the translocation eyes. Retinal detachment occurred as a complication in two eyes of each group. The small sample size, lack of a control group, and any long-term information make analysis of translocation surgery for high myopia difficult.

19.9 Photodynamic Therapy

Photodynamic therapy for subfoveal CNV in AMD using verteporfin was investigated in the Treatment of Age-Related Macular Degeneration with Photodynamic Therapy (TAP) Study. Verteporfin was injected at a dose of 6 mg/m^2 of body surface area, and the neovascular lesion then was irradiated with a non-thermal laser spot (50 J/cm^2) 1000 μm larger than the greatest linear dimension of the lesion. Patients were retreated every 3 months if they showed leakage by fluorescein angiography [89]. Patients were given 3.4 treatments in the first year and 2.2 treatments in the second year. Patients with predominantly classic CNV had treatment benefit that extended to the second year of the study [90]. Patients with occult with no classic CNV did not have a statistically significant benefit at 1 year, but at 2 years there was a statistically significant treatment benefit [29]. Retrospective analysis of pooled data showed that lesion size was significantly related to the response to PDT with small lesions appearing to show response regardless of lesion composition, while larger lesions only showed treatment benefit if the lesion was predominantly classic [91]. Patients with predominantly classic CNV had a 39% chance of experiencing a three line or more visual acuity loss [89], and the expectation for treated patients was a slower decline in visual acuity than what would occur without treatment. Analysis of cases by the reading center suggested there was a slight undertreatment among patients in the registration trials. An open-label expanded access trial was performed with 4435 patients, and in a clinic setting, the number of treatments per year was lower than that seen in the registration trials [92]. There are many possible explanations for this finding, but one was in a real-world deployment of an as needed as opposed to a mandated strategy which may result in undertreatment.

Eyes with myopic CNV were evaluated in the Verteporfin in Photodynamic Therapy (VIP) Study. In contrast to studies done on AMD, the primary outcome was the proportion of eyes experiencing fewer than 8 letters, which is about 1.5 lines, of visual acuity loss. At 1 year fewer patients treated with photodynamic therapy lost 8 letters as compared with the untreated controls [28]. Contrast sensitivity was better in the treated eyes as well. The mean number of treatments was 3.4 in the treatment arm versus 3.2 in the sham group. The treatment effect began to wane so that by 2 years the advantage in the treated group was no longer significant [93]. (See Fig. 19.6.) In the second year, the mean number of treatments was 1.7 in the treatment group and 1.4 in the control group. The 3-year results showed stability from the 2-year results [94]. Several studies examining treated patient series reported longer-term follow-up, but it is difficult to put these studies into perspective because all of them lacked a control

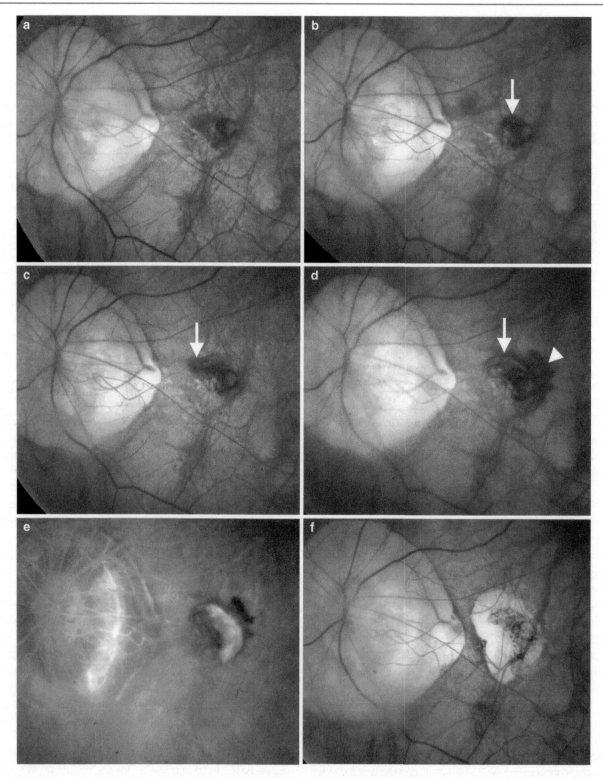

Fig. 19.6 Expansion of choroidal neovascularization with photodynamic therapy and subsequent treatment with bevacizumab. (**a**) This patient was treated with photodynamic therapy for myopic choroidal neovascularization. Note the rings of pigment centrally. Since the patient had leakage, he was treated with photodynamic therapy. (**b**) The patient had expansion of the lesion. Note the pigment (arrow). He was treated with photodynamic therapy again which was associated with expansion of the lesion, arrow in (**c**), and with further expansion (arrow in **d**) with hemorrhage. His visual acuity was 20/80. (**e**) The fluorescein angiographic image shows the extent of the neovascularization. The patient was given an injection of intravitreal bevacizumab 1.25 mg. (**f**) Over time the patient was given two additional injections. In this picture 6 years after first being treated with bevacizumab, the patient has some residual hyperpigmentation, but also a wide area of pigmentary loss. When last examined nearly 7 years after injection, his visual acuity was 20/60

group [95–112]. Krebs and coauthors [102] reported 3-year results of 20 treated eyes and found the distance acuity and central field threshold sensitivity showed stabilization, but reading acuity declined from year 1 to year 3. Pece and coworkers followed 62 eyes of 62 patients for a mean of 31 months and found 13% improved by one or more lines of Snellen acuity, 32% deteriorated, and 55% remained stable [103]. The authors thought younger eyes (≤55 years) did better than older eyes. Lam and colleagues [95] reported a 2-year study of pathologic myopia in Chinese patients comparing PDT to the results of the VIP-PM study. The authors stated the visual results were similar in the two studies, but Chinese patients seemed to require fewer treatments as compared with the VIP-PM study group. However the eyes had juxtafoveal CNV exclusively, which may have impacted the treatment frequency. Younger (<55 years) patients had a better final acuity than older patients. Hayashi and coworkers [110] reported the visual results of 48 eyes of 46 patients with subfoveal and nonsubfoveal CNV in Japanese patients with pathologic myopia. The visual acuity did not change in a significant way after PDT. A minority of eyes had follow-up for 4 years or more, but 70% of these developed chorioretinal atrophy, particularly if the neovascularization was initially subfoveal. Coutinho and coauthors reported the 5-year follow-up of 43 consecutive eyes of 36 patients [111]. There results were amazingly good, as 32.6% of the eyes had a visual acuity improvement of three or more lines and the mean acuity of the group was better at 5 years than at baseline.

Common to all studies was the need for treatment at closer intervals early after the treatment began with fewer needed later. In the controlled study, VIP-PM, the sham group showed visual stability while "requiring" fewer treatments in the second year. This is consistent with the known natural history of the disease; the lesions show fewer signs of disease activity over time, and the decline in vision is not as rapid as in the earlier phases. That is not to say the natural history is good; it appears PDT offers little help in changing the outcome over after the initial phases of neovascularization. Analysis of many of these cases showed a propensity to develop atrophy.

19.10 Agents Directed Against Vascular Endothelial Growth Factor

A requirement for tumor growth to recruit blood vessels for metabolite supply started a multiyear effort that ultimately resulted in the identification and modalities to block the effects of vascular endothelial growth factor (VEGF) [113–115]. The potential of anti-VEGF agents in use against CNV offered a second use for these agents. In parallel development tracks, bevacizumab, a full-length antibody, was devel-

oped for use in cancer therapy, and ranibizumab, an antibody fragment, was created for use in the eye. Bevacizumab was found to be effective in the treatment of colon cancer when used in combination with standard chemotherapy and was approved by the Federal Food and Drug Administration in 2004 [116]. Ranibizumab was shown to have remarkable efficacy in the treatment of CNV secondary to AMD in multicentered, randomized phase III trials [117, 118]. In open-label extension investigation, the rate of treatments in clinic settings was much lower than that seen under the registration trials [119]. The visual acuity concurrently decreased, suggesting that real-world implementation of an as needed strategy may have resulted in undertreatment.

The results of the trials were available well before ranibizumab was made available, due to the FDA approval process. In an attempt to get the same clinical efficacy, bevacizumab was given intravitreally and appeared to have beneficial effect [120–123]. Early studies being published show bevacizumab had effects mirroring those of ranibizumab. Investigators from around the world examined the potential safety and efficacy of bevacizumab in human and animal studies [113]. No significant ocular toxicity was found. Medicare reimbursement of bevacizumab enabled patients with AMD to have cost coverage early after it began to be used despite the lack of any randomized trial showing efficacy. The cost difference between ranibizumab and bevacizumab is astounding. A dose of ranibizumab is approximately $2000, while bevacizumab is about 1/50th the cost. The chief competitor for ranibizumab became bevacizumab, although each was made by the same company. In 2007 the company had a press release stating they would stop the sale of bevacizumab to compounding pharmacies [124]. Senator Herb Kohl sent a letter to Kerry Weems, the Acting Administrator of the Centers for Medicare and Medicaid Services, expressing concerns about the costs of the proposed ban [125]. In a compromise negotiated by the American Academy of Ophthalmology and the American Society of Retinal Surgeons, the ban was lifted.

Over time studies of bevacizumab for the treatment of CNV secondary to AMD became more refined and sophisticated, ultimately resulting in the Comparison of AMD Treatment Trials or CATT [126, 127]. This multicentered randomized trial had four arms, ranibizumab monthly, bevacizumab monthly, ranibizumab given on an as needed basis, and bevacizumab given as needed. The monthly dosing of ranibizumab was used in the trials used for FDA approval, and the other treatment arms were compared to that in a noninferiority design. At the end of 1 year, the four arms were rerandomized to more to examine how alterations in treatment frequency would affect visual acuity outcomes. At 1 year the visual acuity outcomes showed roughly similar outcomes for all arms, although that is not the exact primary goal of a noninferiority design [126]. The bevacizumab given as needed did not meet the non-inferiority endpoints as compared with ranibizumab given monthly or bevacizumab given monthly. The authors of the paper stated these results were inconclusive given the 1-year follow-up and the small mean difference in visual acuity seen. The report of the second year results condensed the multiple arms the patients were separated into to determine as needed approaches consistently resulted in lower visual acuity than did monthly dosing [127]. Of interest is the switch from monthly dosing to an as needed strategy which was met with a statistically significant loss of visual acuity even if the patients received 12 previous injections on a monthly interval.

Aflibercept is a recombinant fusion protein consisting of VEGF-binding portions from the extracellular domains of human VEGF receptors 1 and 2, which were fused to the Fc portion of the human IgG1 immunoglobulin. The medication was marketed, after successful registration trials, for ocular use as Eylea and for cancer treatment as Zaltrap. The initial ocular registration trials for ocular use were the VIEW 1 and VIEW 2 trials [128], for which the primary endpoint was noninferiority to ranibizumab in the proportion of patients maintaining vision (losing <15 letters on Early Treatment Diabetic Retinopathy Study chart) at week 52. The outcomes for aflibercept all were withing 0.5 letters of the reference ranibizumab, even for an every 8-week dosing.

Studies for myopic CNV started in a similar manner to that seen for AMD, except the sample sizes were much smaller [129–169]. Early studies showed rapid resolution of exudation along with improvement in mean visual acuity in patients treated with intravitreal bevacizumab independent of if they had previous PDT or not. Later studies reported longer duration of follow-up from the initial studies with only a few months to 1 year and later multiyear follow-up. The sample sizes increased in later studies as well. The visual acuity outcomes from these studies seemed robust, as far as can be discerned, and were associated with cessation of exudation and improvement of acuity. The reported studies for myopic CNV did not show comparable improvement in design or sophistication to the degree that the preceding AMD studies did.

The many early patient series involving ranibizumab for mCNV showed favorable results [135, 145, 155, 158, 159, 164, 166, 170–173]. These led to the design of the RADIANCE study, which was a phase III study comparing two different dosing regimens of ranibizumab to verteporfin photodynamic therapy [174]. The dosing was one mandated injection followed by as needed injections based on two different sets of criteria. The shorthand designation for one mandated dose followed by as needed dosing is 1 + PRN. For the visual acuity group, two monthly doses were given. If the visual acuity was stable, the patient did not get an injection.

If the visual acuity decreased, the patient was given monthly injections until the acuity was stable for three consecutive monthly assessments. For the disease activity group, one injection was given and thereafter only if the patient had visual impairment attributable to intra- or subretinal fluid or active leakage secondary to myopic neovascularization. As could be deduced from the treatment strategies, the visual acuity group had a larger mean number of injections, 4.6 versus 3.5 for the disease activity group. The visual acuity response was a gain of 10.5 and 10.6 ETDRS letters in the visual acuity and disease activity groups, respectively, at 3 months as contrasted with a 2.2 letter gain in the verteporfin PDT arm. By 1 year the visual acuities were +11.7 and +11.9 ETDRS letters in the visual acuity and disease activity arms, respectively. The verteporfin PDT arm could receive injections of ranibizumab after the third month and showed a +9.3 letter gain with a mean 2.4 injections.

A post-RADIANCE observation period was evaluated in patients who completed the RADIANCE study and had at least one subsequent follow-up visit [175]. Of the 267 patients who completed the RADIANCE trial, 41 were included in a long-term post-RADIANCE observational study. These were split into two groups; group A was stated to need additional treatments over the follow-up period, while group B did not. No information, other than it was up to the physicians' discretion, was given about how needed versus no needed was determined. Patients who needed additional treatment received a mean of five ranibizumab injections over a mean of 29.4 months of follow-up. Overall, the patients showed a +16.3 ± 18.7 letter change from baseline by 48 months; however this was based on only 16 patients.

The MYRROR study [176] examined the efficacy of intravitreal aflibercept in a phase III trial of patients with mCNV randomized in a 3:1 ratio to intravitreal aflibercept 2 mg or a sham control. The study had a 1 + PRN design. In the sham group, patients received a sham injection through week 20 and from week 24 on received a mandatory intravitreal aflibercept injection followed by PRN aflibercept or sham injection every 4 weeks. Patients in the treatment arm gained a mean of 12.1 ETDRS letters, while the sham group lost 2 letters. Patients in the aflibercept arm received a median of two injections (mean 2) in weeks 0–8 and a median of 0 injections (mean 2.2) thereafter until the study end at week 48 and gained 13.5 letters. The sham/aflibercept arm eventually received a median of three injections (mean 4.2) by week 48 but only had a 3.9 letter gain [176]. Thus, both arms received the same number of mean injections, but prompt treatment resulted in better visual acuity gains.

Hu and colleagues [177] performed a systematic review of three randomized controlled clinical trials examining bevacizumab as compared with ranibizumab. At 1 year, both treatments caused a significant improvement in visual acuity, but there was no significant difference between the two drugs in terms of outcome. Sayanagi et al. [178] conducted a retrospective review of 30 eyes of 28 patients who received either ranibizumab or aflibercept for mCNV. There was a significant improvement in visual acuity with both drugs, intravitreal aflibercept was associated with greater thinning of the choroid, but no difference was detected in visual acuity response. Chen and coworkers [179] performed a retrospective review of 64 eyes of 59 patients with mCNV treated with either conbercept or ranibizumab. Both drugs were associated with a significant improvement in visual acuity, but there was no significant difference in logMAR best-corrected visual acuity or central macular thickness change between the two groups. Wang and colleagues [180] retrospectively compared a series of 42 eyes treated with a 1 + PRN strategy with bevacizumab with a later series of 36 eyes treated with a 1 + PRN strategy using aflibercept. Both arms showed a significant improvement in acuity, but there was no significant difference in the change in best-corrected visual acuity or central foveal thickness between the two groups. The mean number of bevacizumab injections required in the first year was 3.23, which was greater than that required in the aflibercept group (2.11, $P = 0.01$). Korol et al. [181] conducted a randomized trial in which 97 eyes of 96 patients were randomized to either ranibizumab or aflibercept with a 1 + PRN strategy. In the first 12 months, there was a mean number of 2.5 injections in the ranibizumab group versus 2.6 in the aflibercept group. In the second year, the means were 0.4 and 0.2 injections, respectively. At the end of 24 months, there was no difference in visual acuity response which was noted between the two groups, and both arms showed a significant improvement in visual acuity. Howaidy and Eldaly randomized 48 eyes of 48 patients with mCNV to either aflibercept or ranibizumab for three consecutive monthly injections. At the third month of follow-up, the change in best-corrected visual acuity and central macular thickness was significantly improved in both groups, but there was no difference between the two groups. In comparing two roughly similar treatment arms using a PRN strategy with a consistent threshold for treatment, the likelihood is no difference will be detected [182]. If one drug is less effective than another, it would meet the treatment threshold more often and therefore be given more frequently, obviating the difference in underlying efficacy.

No published study administered a gold standard monthly dosing schedule such as that used in AMD. Therefore, the upper limit of expected visual acuity performance in myopic CNV is not known, but given the large gains and relatively stable visual acuity results with a low treatment frequency, a PRN strategy is likely to approach the theoretical maximum.

19.11 Recommended Treatment of Eyes with Myopic Choroidal Neovascularization

The first step in management of myopic CNV is to be absolutely sure the patient does not have MCP. Eyes with MCP have CNV as a frequent complication, and most eyes with MCP are myopic. It is common to see patients with MCP being considered to have myopic CNV as a consequence. Treating the CNV alone without treating the underlying inflammatory condition puts patients at risk for vision loss in both eyes because of scarring or atrophy. If the eye is thought to have myopic CNV that is active, the treatment with the highest probability of visual gain appears to be injection of an anti-VEGF agent. Choice of anti-VEGF medication appears to involve regulatory and funding issues and not efficacy of one drug over another. Patients are given a dose of medication at baseline (Figs. 19.7 and 19.8). A regimen of using one injection as compared with three initial doses has been evaluated in small studies [163, 183, 184]. There may be slightly less need for injections during the first year with a 3 + PRN approach, at the obvious expense of giving three loading injections instead of one.

The key unresolved problem with treatment of myopic CNV is treatment frequency. The neovascularization seems sensitive to anti-VEGF agents. A 1 + PRN strategy produces results that are "good" as compared with the natural course, but for myopic CNV we do not know what the outcome is with more frequent mandated doses. As needed strategies are based on a particular abnormality being detected; for fluorescein angiography leakage would be a threshold indicator, while for OCT the indications may be intra- or subretinal accumulation of fluid. The two main problems are that these tests may not be particularly sensitive in high myopes, and we do not have sufficient evidence that one or the other is better modality to follow patients. As a consequence, some retinal physicians treat myopes based on objective tests such as fluorescein angiography or OCT but also according to the subjective complaints of the patient. It is common to have patients complain about vision changes before any testing modality shows an abnormality and also for these same patients to return stating their vision improved after the injection.

There are numerous potential signs of recurrent disease. Patients may have a sudden decrease in acuity not explainable by the expansion of atrophy, which is generally slow. Patients have complaints of increased distortion, but measurements obtained with an Amsler grid are not quantifiable and therefore difficult to compare from one examination to the next. Recurrent activity of the lesion can produce the ophthalmoscopic signs of blurring of the margin of the neovascular lesion, visible hemorrhage, and rarely lipid.

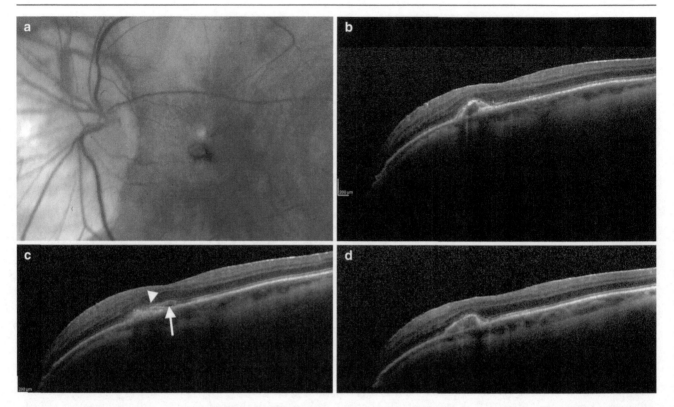

Fig. 19.7 Anti-VEGF treatment effect. (**a**) Two months after treatment of the lesion shown in Fig. 19.2 with ranibizumab, the lesion developed a ring of hyperpigmentation. (**b**) The optical coherence tomography image shows a smaller lesion with a well-defined outer surface interface with the overlying retina. (**c**) Several months later the patient developed signs of recurrent disease activity. The lesion had a change in internal reflectivity, the boundary between the lesion and the retina was blurred (arrowhead), and there was a small amount of subretinal fluid (arrow). (**d**) Following treatment the lesion regained signs of inactivity with decreased internal reflectivity, a sharp boundary between the lesion and retina, and no subretinal fluid. Over the following 2 years of follow-up, the patient needed repeat injections on a periodic basis, but the appearance of the lesion and his visual acuity, 20/25, remained stable

Fluorescein angiography can show modest amounts of increased leakage and faint increases in the size of staining. There are numerous potential indications using OCT imaging. When a treated lesion shows cessation of activity, the lesion becomes more compact, the internal reflectivity is often less than the surface, the boundary between the lesion and retina is sharp, and there is no associated intra- or subretinal fluid. When the lesion becomes active, any of these parameters may change. The lesion becomes larger, the reflectivity in the lesion can increase, the boundary between the lesion and retina becomes less distinct, and there can be subretinal fluid and less commonly intraretinal fluid.

Patients starting with good acuity, small lesions, or non-subfoveal location have better acuity over time, but none of these attributes are selectable by either the patient or physician. There have been studies using a combination of an anti-VEGF agent with photodynamic therapy, but much like in AMD, evidence is lacking showing any improvement in visual acuity performance as compared with the use of anti-VEGF agents alone [185, 186]. Patients with MCP are generally treated with a short course of corticosteroids, and long-term immunosuppression is commonly started simulta-

neously. Any concurrent CNV is treated with anti-VEGF agents. These eyes may have a rapid loss of visual acuity secondary to inflammatory disease exacerbation, to activity of the CNV or both. Evidence of inflammatory activity includes seeing an increase in cells in the vitreous, infiltration in the subretinal space, sub-RPE accumulation of material, fluid within or under the retina, and areas where the outer retinal architecture, particularly the ellipsoid band, shows widespread disruption. These changes are generally rapidly responsive to corticosteroids. Signs of active CNV include an increase in intra- or subretinal blood, thickening or expansion of the CNV lesion, or hemorrhage. Treatment of the CNV is done with anti-VEGF agents, although some patients may show some response to corticosteroids.

19.12 Retinal Pigment Epithelial Loss and Atrophy

High myopes have a number of anatomic disturbances prior to the development of CNV: they have RPE disturbances, lacquer cracks, and usually very thin choroids. There may be

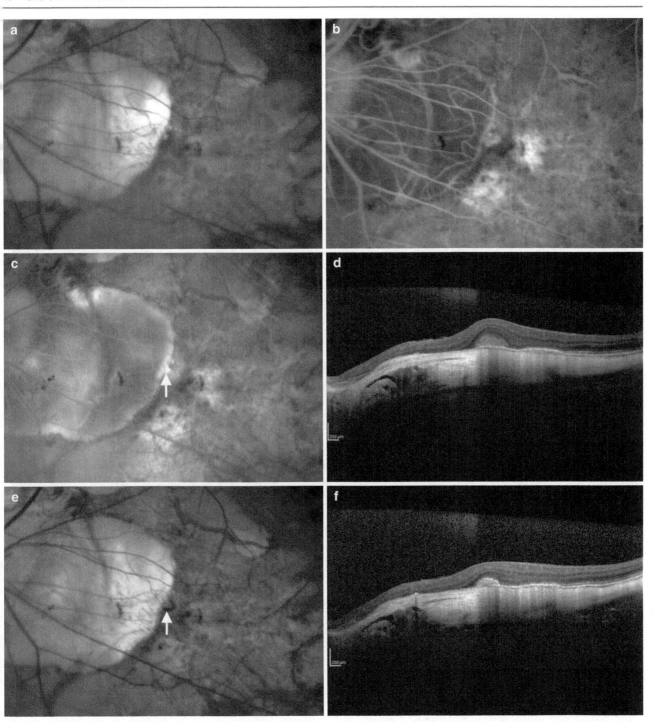

Fig. 19.8 This patient thought there may have been distortion in her vision, but was not quite certain. (**a**) The color fundus photograph shows a large area of peripapillary atrophy, but little in the way of an explanation of a cause of the symptoms. (**b**) The early phase fluorescein angiogram shows multiple transmission defects. (**c**) Later in the angiographic sequence, there is an increase in the fluorescence of one spot (arrow). (**d**) In one section of the optical coherence tomographic examination, there was an elevation of reflective material under the retina, in the region corresponding to the increased brightness in the angiogram.

(**e**) Two months after presentation, and following two intravitreal injections of an agent directed against vascular endothelial growth factor, a rim of pigment around the neovascularization could be seen. (**f**) The optical coherence tomographic section shows a smaller lesion with a sharp boundary between the lesion and the outer retina. Note the lack of any intra- or subretinal fluid in either (**d**) or (**f**). This case illustrates the use of an anti-VEGF injection not only as a therapeutic agent but also as a potential diagnostic one as well

concurrent focal areas of chorioretinal atrophy. With no treatment the CNV follows a stereotypical life cycle in which the vessels proliferate and cause exudation and bleeding and then in many cases there is enveloping of the neovascularization with proliferating pigment cells. The CNV complex shrinks, and there can be a centripetal retraction of the lesion from the surrounding RPE monolayer, causing a halo of absent RPE around the CNV. This absent RPE is not really atrophy, in that the word atrophy implies a withering of the normally present cells.

Laser photocoagulation uses thermal energy to destroy the newly growing vessels, but there is significant collateral dam-

age to the underlying RPE, Bruch's membrane, and choroid (Fig. 19.9). This induces a region of cell loss that is commonly called atrophy even though the RPE and choriocapillaris were actively killed by the treatment. Atrophy implies the cells withered and became less active, while laser photocoagulation increases the temperature of the cells to the point where they are destroyed. The choriocapillaris is a confluent layer of vascular channels with the spaces between vessels nearly vanishing in the posterior pole because of the packing density of the vessels. The blood flow is functionally lobular, but regionally blood from any one section has the potential to flow to adjacent areas based on instantaneous pressure differ-

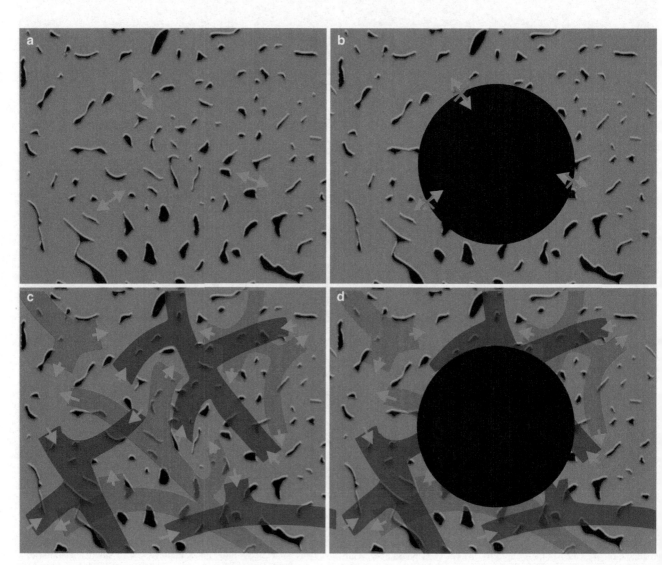

Fig. 19.9 Hypothesis of atrophy generation post-treatment for myopic choroidal neovascularization. (**a**) The choriocapillaris is a densely packed interconnected set of specialized capillaries. There are no anatomical lobules per se, but local flow is a function of regional pressure differences as illustrated by the green arrows. (**b**) Laser photocoagulation has the potential to destroy the choriocapillaris. Clearly the area treated will be harmed, but the regional flow coming from this area will also be absent. (**c**) Under the choriocapillaris are larger vessels of

Haller's and Sattler's layers drawn in a stylized way with green arrows showing the flow in the respective arterioles (red) or venules (blue). Laser photocoagulation has the propensity of altering this flow as well, thus affecting local choriocapillaris areas by more than one mechanism. The choroid in highly myopic eyes is thin and with each passing year gets thinner. By affecting the flow in the choroid, localized laser could hasten this process. The same argument could be made for the effects of photodynamic therapy

ences. The area destroyed by laser photocoagulation cannot participate in this shared flow across the choriocapillaris network, so one would expect the regional flow immediately around the laser photocoagulation to be somewhat less than in comparable people without CNV or laser photocoagulation. Under the choroid are layers of larger vessels, Haller's and Sattler's layers that feed into the choriocapillaris in the superjacent or adjacent choriocapillaris. Laser destruction of these layers also affects regional choriocapillaris flow. High myopes have thinning of the choroid that often progresses to areas of complete absence of the choroid and overlying RPE. Since there is an absence of pigmented tissue (only a thin remnant of retina remains), the sclera is directly visible, so consequently these lesions appear as ovoid or round areas that are white. Decreases in regional blood supply could be expected to advance the process and may explain why the "atrophic" area of tissue absence related to laser photocoagulation increases with size over time.

PDT also causes collateral damage to the choroid. Early on in the investigation of treatment of CNV secondary to AMD, indocyanine green angiography showed patients treated with PDT could develop choroidal hypoperfusion abnormalities. The first paper looking at the choroidal thickness of myopes as measured by enhanced depth imaging OCT noted that patients who had a history of PDT for CNV had thinner subfoveal choroidal thicknesses [21]. It is conceivable that PDT damages an already infirm choroidal vas-

cular system, which may encourage or hasten the atrophic, degenerative processes seen in high myopia. Eyes with high myopia are on a path to develop increasing manifestations of atrophy over time, and the occurrence of CNV, along with any trauma its attendant treatment may induce, may well hasten this fated process.

Some eyes treated with anti-VEGF agents may also develop atrophy or loss of the RPE, and if it occurs, it is usually located around the outer border. Some of these eyes show further outward expansion of the outer border of the area of absent RPE, and the inner, formerly hyperpigmented, central region can gradually become increasingly hypopigmented. It is possible that pharmacologically induced scarring and shrinkage of the CNV lesion could lead to circumferential rips of the RPE. Some eyes develop areas of atrophy, but not necessarily where the CNV is located. Figure 19.10 shows an eye that developed an area of CNV, was treated with an anti-VEGF agent, and a year later developed another region of CNV. This second lesion was treated with an anti-VEGF agent as well. After 3 years of follow-up, the patient had areas of profound atrophy, but not exactly where the CNV was located. The patient presented with choroidal atrophy, which progressed to chorioretinal atrophy over time. The invasion of neovascularization into the subretinal space necessitates a penetration of Bruch's membrane. The defects in Bruch's membrane appear to expand over time [187].

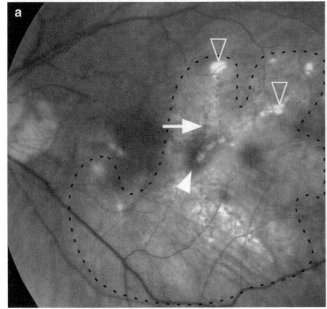 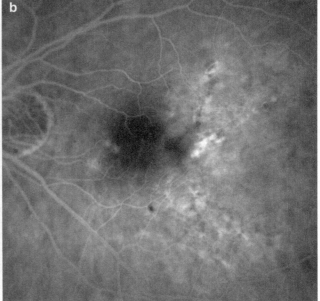

Fig. 19.10 (**a**) This 61-year-old high myopic patient presented with a dot of hemorrhage in the temporal macula (arrow) and an area of increased pigmentation (arrowhead) straddling a lacquer crack. There was an area of choroidal thinning (contained in the dashed line) with small regions of more profound tissue loss (open arrowheads). (**b**) Early and late (**c**) fluorescein angiogram shows expanding hyperfluorescence caused by leakage from an area of choroidal neovascularization. The patient was treated with injections of an agent directed against vascular

endothelial growth factor, and the neovascularization became quiescent. (**d**) Nearly a year later, the patient presented with new symptoms caused by a second area of neovascularization located under the fovea. This showed leakage in the later phases of the angiogram (**e**). The patient was treated with additional injections. (**f**) Three years later the patient showed multiple regions of profound atrophy, located within the area of choroidal thinning identified in (**a**). Note that the areas of neovascularization themselves did not show atrophy

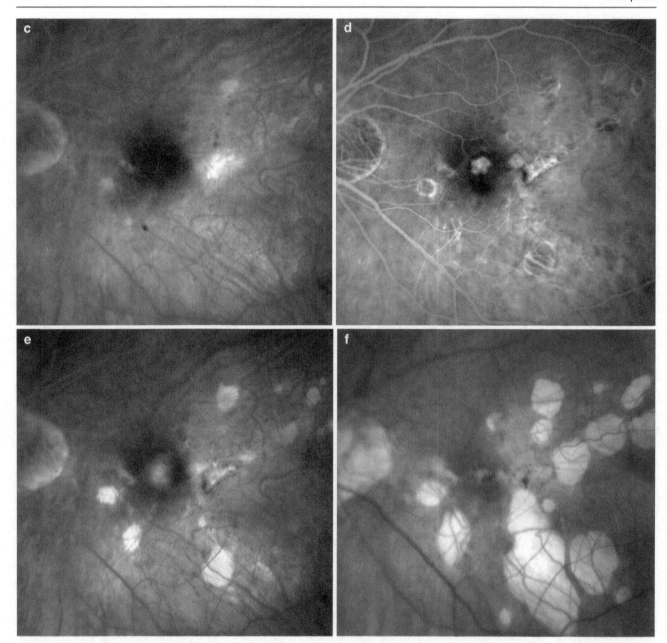

Fig. 19.10 (continued)

References

1. Fuchs E. Der centrale schwarze Fleck bei Myopie. Z Augenheilkunde. 1901;5:171–8.
2. Lloyd RI. Clinical studies of the myopic macula. Trans Am Ophthalmol Soc. 1953;51:273–84.
3. Focosi M, Brancato R, Frosini R. Serous maculopathy of myopes. Fluorescein retinography and possibilities for treatment. Doc Ophthalmol. 1973;34:157–64.
4. Levy JH, Pollock HM, Curtin BJ. The Fuchs' spot: an ophthalmoscopic and fluorescein angiographic study. Ann Ophthalmol. 1977;9:1433–43.
5. Vision Institute Institute. The impact of myopia and high myopia: report of the Joint World Health Organization–Brien Holden Vision Institute Global Scientific Meeting on Myopia. University of New South Wales, Sydney, Australia, 16–18 March 2015. Geneva World Health Organization. 2017.
6. United Nations Department of Economic and Social Affairs. World population prospects 2019 highlights. New York: United Nations; 2019.
7. Wong TY, Ferreira A, Hughes R, et al. Epidemiology and disease burden of pathologic myopia and myopic choroidal neovascularization: an evidence-based systematic review. Am J Ophthalmol. 2014;157(1):9–25.e12.
8. Buch H, Vinding T, La Cour M, et al. Prevalence and causes of visual impairment and blindness among 9980 Scandinavian adults: the Copenhagen City Eye Study. Ophthalmology. 2004;111(1):53–61.
9. Cedrone C, Culasso F, Cesareo M, et al. Incidence of blindness and low vision in a sample population: the Priverno Eye Study, Italy. Ophthalmology. 2003;110(3):584–8.

10. Krumpaszky HG, Lüdtke R, Mickler A, Klauss V, Selbmann HK. Blindness incidence in Germany. A population-based study from Württemberg-Hohenzollern. Ophthalmologica. 1999;213(3):176–82.

11. Xu L, Wang Y, Li Y, et al. Causes of blindness and visual impairment in urban and rural areas in Beijing: the Beijing Eye Study. Ophthalmology. 2006;113(7):1134.e1–11.

12. Hsu WM, Cheng CY, Liu JH, et al. Prevalence and causes of visual impairment in an elderly Chinese population in Taiwan: the Shihpai Eye Study. Ophthalmology. 2004;111(1):62–9.

13. Iwase A, Araie M, Tomidokoro A, et al. Prevalence and causes of low vision and blindness in a Japanese adult population: the Tajimi Study. Ophthalmology. 2006;113(8):1354–62.

14. Yoshida T, Ohno-Matsui K, Yasuzumi K, et al. Myopic choroidal neovascularization: a 10-year follow-up. Ophthalmology. 2003;110:1297–305.

15. Secretan M, Kuhn D, Soubrane G, Coscas G. Long-term visual outcome of choroidal neovascularization in pathologic myopia: natural history and laser treatment. Eur J Ophthalmol. 1997;7:307–16.

16. Yoshida T, Ohno-Matsui K, Ohtake Y, et al. Long-term visual prognosis of choroidal neovascularization in high myopia: a comparison between age groups. Ophthalmology. 2002;109:712–9.

17. Klein RM, Curtin BJ. Lacquer crack lesions in pathologic myopia. Am J Ophthalmol. 1975;79:386–92.

18. Klein RM, Green S. The development of lacquer cracks in pathologic myopia. Am J Ophthalmol. 1988;106:282–5.

19. Hayasaka S, Uchida M, Setogawa T. Subretinal hemorrhages with or without choroidal neovascularization in the maculas of patients with pathologic myopia. Graefes Arch Clin Exp Ophthalmol. 1990;228:277–80.

20. Curtin BJ. The myopias. Basic science and clinical management. Philadelphia: Harper & Row; 1985.

21. Fujiwara T, Imamura Y, Margolis R, Slakter JS, Spaide RF. Enhanced depth imaging optical coherence tomography of the choroid in highly myopic eyes. Am J Ophthalmol. 2009;148:445–50.

22. Ikuno Y, Tano Y. Retinal and choroidal biometry in highly myopic eyes with spectral-domain optical coherence tomography. Invest Ophthalmol Vis Sci. 2009;50:3876–80.

23. Ikuno Y, Maruko I, Yasuno Y, et al. Reproducibility of retinal and choroidal thickness measurements in enhanced depth imaging and high-penetration optical coherence tomography. Invest Ophthalmol Vis Sci. 2011;52:5536–40.

24. Nishida Y, Fujiwara T, Imamura Y, Lima LH, Kurosaka D, Spaide RF. Choroidal thickness and visual acuity in highly myopic eyes. Retina. 2012;32:1229–36.

25. Ohno-Matsui K, Yoshida T, Futagami S, et al. Patchy atrophy and lacquer cracks predispose to the development of choroidal neovascularisation in pathological myopia. Br J Ophthalmol. 2003;87:570–3.

26. Ikuno Y, Sayanagi K, Soga K, et al. Lacquer crack formation and choroidal neovascularization in pathologic myopia. Retina. 2008;28:1124–31.

27. Heriot WJ, Henkind P, Bellhorn RW, Burns MS. Choroidal neovascularization can digest Bruch's membrane. A prior break is not essential. Ophthalmology. 1984;91:1603–8.

28. Verteporfin in Photodynamic Therapy Study Group. Photodynamic therapy of subfoveal choroidal neovascularization in pathologic myopia with verteporfin. 1-year results of a randomized clinical trial – VIP report no. 1. Ophthalmology. 2001;108:841–52.

29. Verteporfin in Photodynamic Therapy Study Group. Verteporfin therapy of subfoveal choroidal neovascularization in age-related macular degeneration: two-year results of a randomized clinical trial including lesions with occult with no classic choroidal neovascularization—verteporfin in photodynamic therapy report 2. Am J Ophthalmol. 2001;131:541–60.

30. Hayashi K, Shimada N, Moriyama M, Hayashi W, Tokoro T, Ohno-Matsui K. Two-year outcomes of intravitreal bevacizumab for choroidal neovascularization in Japanese patients with pathologic myopia. Retina. 2012;32:687–95.

31. Lee DH, Kang HG, Lee SC, Kim M. Features of optical coherence tomography predictive of choroidal neovascularisation treatment response in pathological myopia in association with fluorescein angiography. Br J Ophthalmol. 2018;102(2):238–42.

32. Vance SK, Khan S, Klancnik JM, Freund KB. Characteristic spectral-domain optical coherence tomography findings of multifocal choroiditis. Retina. 2011;31:717–23.

33. Haen SP, Spaide RF. Fundus autofluorescence in multifocal choroiditis and panuveitis. Am J Ophthalmol. 2008;145:847–53.

34. Curtin BJ, Karlin DB. Axial length measurements and fundus changes of the myopic eye. Am J Ophthalmol. 1971;71:42–53.

35. Rabb MF, Garoon I, LaFranco FP. Myopic macular degeneration. Int Ophthalmol Clin. 1981;21:51–69.

36. Hotchkiss ML, Fine SL. Pathologic myopia and choroidal neovascularization. Am J Ophthalmol. 1981;91:177–83.

37. Fried M, Siebert A, Meyer-Schwickerath G. A natural history of Fuchs' spot: a long-term follow-up study. Doc Ophthalmol. 1981;28:215–21.

38. Cohen SY, Laroche A, Leguen Y, Soubrane G, Coscas GJ. Etiology of choroidal neovascularization in young patients. Ophthalmology. 1996;103:1241–4.

39. Steidl SM, Pruett RC. Macular complications associated with posterior staphyloma. Am J Ophthalmol. 1997;123:181–7.

40. Shih YF, Ho TC, Hsiao CK, Lin LL. Visual outcomes for high myopic patients with or without myopic maculopathy: a 10 year follow up study. Br J Ophthalmol. 2006;90:546–50.

41. Vongphanit J, Mitchell P, Wang JJ. Prevalence and progression of myopic retinopathy in an older population. Ophthalmology. 2002;109:704–11.

42. Gao LQ, Liu W, Liang YB, et al. Prevalence and characteristics of myopic retinopathy in a rural Chinese adult population: the Handan Eye Study. Arch Ophthalmol. 2011;129:1199–204.

43. Grossniklaus HE, Green WR. Pathologic findings in pathologic myopia. Retina. 1992;12:127–33.

44. Wright RE, Freudenthal W. Angioid streaks with pseudoxanthoma elasticum (Gronblad-Strandberg Syndrome). Proc R Soc Med. 1943;36:290–1.

45. Spraul CW, Lang GE, Grossniklaus HE, Lang GK. Histologic and morphometric analysis of the choroid, Bruch's membrane, and retinal pigment epithelium in postmortem eyes with age-related macular degeneration and histologic examination of surgically excised choroidal neovascular membranes. Surv Ophthalmol. 1999;44(Suppl 1):S10–32.

46. Grossniklaus HE, Green WR. Choroidal neovascularization. Am J Ophthalmol. 2004;137:496–503.

47. Hampton GR, Kohen D, Bird AC. Visual prognosis of disciform degeneration in myopia. Ophthalmology. 1983;90:923–6.

48. Avila MP, Weiter JJ, Jalkh AE, Trempe CL, Pruett RC, Schepens CL. Natural history of choroidal neovascularization in degenerative myopia. Ophthalmology. 1984;91:1573–81.

49. Tabandeh H, Flynn HW Jr, Scott IU, et al. Visual acuity outcomes of patients 50 years of age and older with high myopia and untreated choroidal neovascularization. Ophthalmology. 1999;106:2063–7.

50. Bottoni F, Tilanus M. The natural history of juxtafoveal and subfoveal choroidal neovascularization in high myopia. Int Ophthalmol. 2001;24:249–55.

51. Hayashi K, Ohno-Matsui K, Yoshida T, et al. Characteristics of patients with a favorable natural course of myopic choroi-

dal neovascularization. Graefes Arch Clin Exp Ophthalmol. 2005;243:13–9.

52. Gass JD. Pathogenesis of disciform detachment of the neuroepithelium. Am J Ophthalmol. 1967;63(Suppl):1–139.

53. L'Esperance FA Jr. The treatment of ophthalmic vascular disease by argon laser photocoagulation. Trans Am Acad Ophthalmol Otolaryngol. 1969;73:1077–96.

54. L'Esperance FA Jr. Clinical photocoagulation with the krypton laser. Arch Ophthalmol. 1972;87:693–700.

55. Little HL, Zweng HC, Peabody RR. Argon laser slit-lamp retinal photocoagulation. Trans Am Acad Ophthalmol Otolaryngol. 1970;74:85–97.

56. Patz A, Maumenee AJ, Ryan SJ. Argon laser photocoagulation in macular diseases. Trans Am Ophthalmol Soc. 1971;69:71–83.

57. Gass JD. Photocoagulation of macular lesions. Trans Am Acad Ophthalmol Otolaryngol. 1971;75:580–608.

58. Macular Photocoagulation Study Group. Argon laser photocoagulation for senile macular degeneration. Results of a randomized clinical trial. Arch Ophthalmol. 1982;100:912–8.

59. Macular Photocoagulation Study Group. Argon laser photocoagulation for neovascular maculopathy. Three-year results from randomized clinical trials. Arch Ophthalmol. 1986;104:694–701.

60. Macular Photocoagulation Study Group. Laser photocoagulation for juxtafoveal choroidal neovascularization. Five-year results from randomized clinical trials. Arch Ophthalmol. 1994;112:500–9.

61. Zimmer-Galler IE, Bressler NM, Bressler SB. Treatment of choroidal neovascularization: updated information from recent macular photocoagulation study group reports. Int Ophthalmol Clin. 1995;35:37–57.

62. Blackhurst DW, Maguire MG. Reproducibility of refraction and visual acuity measurement under a standard protocol. The Macular Photocoagulation Study Group. Retina. 1989;9:163–9.

63. Berkow JW. Subretinal neovascularization in senile macular degeneration. Am J Ophthalmol. 1984;97:143–7.

64. Willan AR, Cruess AF, Ballantyne M. Argon green vs. krypton red laser photocoagulation for extrafoveal choroidal neovascularization secondary to age-related macular degeneration: 3-year results of a multicentre randomized trial. Canadian Ophthalmology Study Group. Can J Ophthalmol. 1996;31:11–7.

65. Jalkh AE, Weiter JJ, Trempe CL, Pruett RC, Schepens CL. Choroidal neovascularization in degenerative myopia: role of laser photocoagulation. Ophthalmic Surg. 1987;18:721–5.

66. Pece A, Brancato R, Avanza P, Camesasca F, Galli L. Laser photocoagulation of choroidal neovascularization in pathologic myopia: long-term results. Int Ophthalmol. 1994;18:339–44.

67. Fardeau C, Soubrane G, Coscas G. Photocoagulation des néovaisseaux sous-rétiniens compliquant la dégénérescence myopique. Bull Soc Ophtalmol Fr. 1992;92:239–42.

68. Ruiz-Moreno JM, Montero JA. Long-term visual acuity after argon green laser photocoagulation of juxtafoveal choroidal neovascularization in highly myopic eyes. Eur J Ophthalmol. 2002;12:117–22.

69. Brancato R, Pece A, Avanza P, Radrizzani E. Photocoagulation scar expansion after laser therapy for choroidal neovascularization in degenerative myopia. Retina. 1990;10:239–43.

70. de Juan E Jr, Machemer R. Vitreous surgery for hemorrhagic and fibrous complications of age-related macular degeneration. Am J Ophthalmol. 1988;105:25–9.

71. Berger AS, Kaplan HJ. Clinical experience with the surgical removal of subfoveal neovascular membranes. Short-term postoperative results. Ophthalmology. 1992;99:969–75.

72. Thomas MA, Grand MG, Williams DF, Lee CM, Pesin SR, Lowe MA. Surgical management of subfoveal choroidal neovascularization. Ophthalmology. 1992;99:952–68.

73. Bressler NM, Bressler SB, Hawkins BS, et al. Submacular surgery trials randomized pilot trial of laser photocoagulation versus surgery for recurrent choroidal neovascularization secondary to age-related macular degeneration: I. Ophthalmic outcomes submacular surgery trials pilot study report number 1. Am J Ophthalmol. 2000;130:387–407.

74. Hawkins BS, Bressler NM, Miskala PH, et al. Surgery for subfoveal choroidal neovascularization in age-related macular degeneration: ophthalmic findings: SST report no. 11. Ophthalmology. 2004;111:1967–80.

75. Bressler NM, Bressler SB, Childs AL, et al. Surgery for hemorrhagic choroidal neovascular lesions of age-related macular degeneration: ophthalmic findings: SST report no. 13. Ophthalmology. 2004;111:1993–2006.

76. Hawkins BS, Bressler NM, Bressler SB, et al. Surgical removal vs observation for subfoveal choroidal neovascularization, either associated with the ocular histoplasmosis syndrome or idiopathic: I. Ophthalmic findings from a randomized clinical trial: Submacular Surgery Trials (SST) Group H Trial: SST report no. 9. Arch Ophthalmol. 2004;122:1597–611.

77. Bass EB, Gilson MM, Mangione CM, et al. Surgical removal vs observation for idiopathic or ocular histoplasmosis syndrome-associated subfoveal choroidal neovascularization: vision preference value scale findings from the randomized SST Group H Trial: SST report no. 17. Arch Ophthalmol. 2008;126:1626–32.

78. Fujii GY, de Juan E, Thomas MA, Pieramici DJ, Humayun MS, Au Eong KG. Limited macular translocation for the management of subfoveal retinal pigment epithelial loss after submacular surgery. Am J Ophthalmol. 2001;131:272–5.

79. Ohji M, Fujikado T, Kusaka S, et al. Comparison of three techniques of foveal translocation in patients with subfoveal choroidal neovascularization resulting from age-related macular degeneration. Am J Ophthalmol. 2001;132:888–96.

80. Mruthyunjaya P, Stinnett SS, Toth CA. Change in visual function after macular translocation with 360 degrees retinectomy for neovascular age-related macular degeneration. Ophthalmology. 2004;111:1715–24.

81. Cahill MT, Stinnett SS, Banks AD, Freedman SF, Toth CA. Quality of life after macular translocation with 360 degrees peripheral retinectomy for age-related macular degeneration. Ophthalmology. 2005;112:144–51.

82. Lüke M, Ziemssen F, Völker M, et al. Full macular translocation (FMT) versus photodynamic therapy (PDT) with verteporfin in the treatment of neovascular age-related macular degeneration: 2-year results of a prospective, controlled, randomised pilot trial (FMT-PDT). Graefes Arch Clin Exp Ophthalmol. 2009;247:745–54.

83. Lüke M, Ziemssen F, Bartz-Schmidt KU, Gelisken F. Quality of life in a prospective, randomised pilot-trial of photodynamic therapy versus full macular translocation in treatment of neovascular age-related macular degeneration--a report of 1 year results. Graefes Arch Clin Exp Ophthalmol. 2007;245:1831–6.

84. Yamada Y, Miyamura N, Suzuma K, Kitaoka T. Long-term follow-up of full macular translocation for choroidal neovascularization. Am J Ophthalmol. 2010;149:453–7.e1.

85. Uemura A, Thomas MA. Subretinal surgery for choroidal neovascularization in patients with high myopia. Arch Ophthalmol. 2000;118(3):344–50.

86. Ruiz-Moreno JM, de la Vega C. Surgical removal of subfoveal choroidal neovascularisation in highly myopic patients. Br J Ophthalmol. 2001;85:1041–3.

87. Hera R, Mouillon M, Gonzalvez B, Millet JY, Romanet JP. Surgery for choroidal subfoveal neovascularization in patients with severe myopia. Retrospective analysis of 17 patients. J Fr Ophtalmol. 2001;24:716–23.

88. Hamelin N, Glacet-Bernard A, Brindeau C, Mimoun G, Coscas G, Soubrane G. Surgical treatment of subfoveal neovascularization in myopia: macular translocation vs surgical removal. Am J Ophthalmol. 2002;133:530–6.

89. Treatment of age-related macular degeneration with photodynamic therapy (TAP) Study Group. Photodynamic therapy of subfoveal choroidal neovascularization in age-related macular degeneration with verteporfin: one-year results of 2 randomized clinical trials--TAP report. Arch Ophthalmol. 1999;117:1329–45.

90. Bressler NM, Treatment of Age-Related Macular Degeneration with Photodynamic Therapy (TAP) Study Group. Photodynamic therapy of subfoveal choroidal neovascularization in age-related macular degeneration with verteporfin: two-year results of 2 randomized clinical trials-TAP report 2. Arch Ophthalmol. 2001;119:198–207.

91. Blinder KJ, Bradley S, Bressler NM, et al. Effect of lesion size, visual acuity, and lesion composition on visual acuity change with and without verteporfin therapy for choroidal neovascularization secondary to age-related macular degeneration: TAP and VIP report no. 1. Am J Ophthalmol. 2003;136:407–18.

92. Bressler NM, VAM Study Writing Committee. Verteporfin therapy in age-related macular degeneration (VAM): an open-label multicenter photodynamic therapy study of 4,435 patients. Retina. 2004;24:512–20.

93. Blinder KJ, Blumenkranz MS, Bressler NM, Verteporfin in Photodynamic Therapy Study Group, et al. Verteporfin therapy of subfoveal choroidal neovascularisation in pathologic myopia: 2-year results of a randomized clinical trial – VIP report no. 3. Ophthalmology. 2003;110:667–72.

94. Bandello F, Blinder K, Bressler NM, et al. Verteporfin in photodynamic therapy: report no. 5. Ophthalmology. 2004;111:2144.

95. Lam DS, Chan WM, Liu DT, Fan DS, Lai WW, Chong KK. Photodynamic therapy with verteporfin for subfoveal choroidal neovascularisation of pathologic myopia in Chinese eyes: a prospective series of 1 and 2 year follow up. Br J Ophthalmol. 2004;88:1315–9.

96. Gelisken F, Inhoffen W, Hermann A, Grisanti S, Bartz-Schmidt KU. Verteporfin photodynamic therapy for extrafoveal choroidal neovascularisation in pathologic myopia. Graefes Arch Clin Exp Ophthalmol. 2004;242:926–30.

97. Axer-Siegel R, Ehrlich R, Weinberger D, et al. Photodynamic therapy of subfoveal choroidal neovascularization in high myopia in a clinical setting: visual outcome in relation to age at treatment. Am J Ophthalmol. 2004;138:602–7.

98. Ergun E, Heinzl H, Stur M. Prognostic factors influencing visual outcome of photodynamic therapy for subfoveal choroidal neovascularization in pathologic myopia. Am J Ophthalmol. 2004;138:434–8.

99. Gibson J. Photodynamic therapy with verteporfin for juxtafoveal choroidal neovascularisation secondary to pathological myopia. Eye (Lond). 2005;19:829–30.

100. Lam DS, Liu DT, Fan DS, Lai WW, So SF, Chan WM. Photodynamic therapy with verteporfin for juxtafoveal choroidal neovascularization secondary to pathologic myopia-1-year results of a prospective series. Eye (Lond). 2005;19:834–40.

101. Schnurrbusch UE, Jochmann C, Wiedemann P, Wolf S. Quantitative assessment of the long-term effect of photodynamic therapy in patients with pathologic myopia. Graefes Arch Clin Exp Ophthalmol. 2005;243:829–33.

102. Krebs I, Binder S, Stolba U, Glittenberg C, Brannath W, Goll A. Choroidal neovascularization in pathologic myopia: three-year results after photodynamic therapy. Am J Ophthalmol. 2005;140:416–25.

103. Pece A, Isola V, Vadala M, Matranga D. Photodynamic therapy with verteporfin for subfoveal choroidal neovasculariza-tion secondary to pathologic myopia: long-term study. Retina. 2006;26:746–51.

104. Ohno-Matsui K, Moriyama M, Hayashi K, Mochizuki M. Choroidal vein and artery occlusion following photodynamic therapy in eyes with pathologic myopia. Graefes Arch Clin Exp Ophthalmol. 2006;244:1363–6.

105. Chen YS, Lin JY, Tseng SY, Yow SG, Hsu WJ, Tsai SC. Photodynamic therapy for Taiwanese patients with pathologic myopia: a 2-year follow-up. Retina. 2007;27:839–45.

106. Virgili G, Varano M, Giacomelli G, et al. Photodynamic therapy for nonsubfoveal choroidal neovascularization in 100 eyes with pathologic myopia. Am J Ophthalmol. 2007;143:77–82.

107. Pece A, Vadala M, Isola V, Matranga D. Photodynamic therapy with verteporfin for juxtafoveal choroidal neovascularization in pathologic myopia: a long-term follow-up study. Am J Ophthalmol. 2007;143:449–54.

108. Ruiz-Moreno JM, Montero JA, Gomez-Ulla F. Photodynamic therapy may worsen the prognosis of highly myopic choroidal neovascularisation treated by intravitreal bevacizumab. Br J Ophthalmol. 2009;93:1693–4.

109. Ruiz-Moreno JM, Amat P, Montero JA, Lugo F. Photodynamic therapy to treat choroidal neovascularisation in highly myopic patients: 4 years' outcome. Br J Ophthalmol. 2008;92:792–4.

110. Hayashi K, Ohno-Matsui K, Shimada N, et al. Long-term results of photodynamic therapy for choroidal neovascularization in Japanese patients with pathologic myopia. Am J Ophthalmol. 2011;151:137–147.e1.

111. Coutinho AM, Silva RM, Nunes SG, Cachulo ML, Figueira JP, Murta JN. Photodynamic therapy in highly myopic eyes with choroidal neovascularization: 5 years of follow-up. Retina. 2011;31:1089–94.

112. Giansanti F, Virgili G, Donati MC, et al. Long-term results of photodynamic therapy for subfoveal choroidal neovascularization with pathologic myopia. Retina. 2012;32(8):1547–52.

113. Folkman J. Tumor angiogenesis: therapeutic implications. N Engl J Med. 1971;285:1182–6.

114. Ferrara N, Gerber HP, LeCouter J. The biology of VEGF and its receptors. Nat Med. 2003;9:669–76.

115. Ferrara N, Hillan KJ, Novotny W. Bevacizumab (Avastin), a humanized anti-VEGF monoclonal antibody for cancer therapy. Biochem Biophys Res Commun. 2005;333:328–35.

116. Hurwitz H, Fehrenbacher L, Novotny W, et al. Bevacizumab plus irinotecan, fluorouracil, and leucovorin for metastatic colorectal cancer. N Engl J Med. 2004;350:2335–42.

117. Brown DM, Kaiser PK, Michels M, et al. Ranibizumab versus verteporfin for neovascular age-related macular degeneration. N Engl J Med. 2006;355:1432–44.

118. Rosenfeld PJ, Brown DM, Heier JS, et al. Ranibizumab for neovascular age-related macular degeneration. N Engl J Med. 2006;355:1419–31.

119. Singer MA, Awh CC, Sadda S, et al. HORIZON: an open-label extension trial of ranibizumab for choroidal neovascularization secondary to age-related macular degeneration. Ophthalmology. 2012;119:1175–83.

120. Rosenfeld PJ, Moshfeghi AA, Puliafito CA. Optical coherence tomography findings after an intravitreal injection of bevaci-zumab (Avastin) for neovascular age-related macular degeneration. Ophthalmic Surg Lasers Imaging. 2005;36:331–5.

121. Avery RL, Pieramici DJ, Rabena MD, Castellarin AA, Nasir MA, Giust MJ. Intravitreal bevacizumab (Avastin) for neovascular age-related macular degeneration. Ophthalmology. 2006;113:363–372.e5.

122. Spaide RF, Laud K, Fine HF, et al. Intravitreal bevacizumab treatment of choroidal neovascularization secondary to age-related macular degeneration. Retina. 2006;26:383–90.

123. El-Mollayess GM, Noureddine BN, Bashshur ZF. Bevacizumab and neovascular age related macular degeneration: pathogenesis and treatment. Semin Ophthalmol. 2011;26:69–76.

124. http://online.wsj.com/article/SB119213222981256309.html?mod=home_health_right

125. http://aging.senate.gov/letters/genentechcmsltr.pdf

126. CATT Research Group, Martin DF, Maguire MG, Ying GS, et al. Ranibizumab and bevacizumab for neovascular age-related macular degeneration. N Engl J Med. 2011;364:1897–908.

127. Comparison of Age-related Macular Degeneration Treatments Trials (CATT) Research Group, Martin DF, Maguire MG, Fine SL, Ying GS, et al. Ranibizumab and bevacizumab for treatment of neovascular age-related macular degeneration: two-year results. Ophthalmology. 2012;119:1388–98.

128. Heier JS, Brown DM, Chong V, et al. Intravitreal aflibercept (VEGF trap-eye) in wet age-related macular degeneration. Ophthalmology. 2012;119(12):2537–48.

129. Laud K, Spaide RF, Freund KB, Slakter J, Klancnik JM Jr. Treatment of choroidal neovascularization in pathologic myopia with intravitreal bevacizumab. Retina. 2006;26:960–3.

130. Yamamoto I, Rogers AH, Reichel E, Yates PA, Duker JS. Intravitreal bevacizumab (Avastin) as treatment for subfoveal choroidal neovascularisation secondary to pathological myopia. Br J Ophthalmol. 2007;91:157–60.

131. Sakaguchi H, Ikuno Y, Gomi F, et al. Intravitreal injection of bevacizumab for choroidal neovascularisation associated with pathological myopia. Br J Ophthalmol. 2007;91:161–5.

132. Hernández-Rojas ML, Quiroz-Mercado H, Dalma-Weiszhausz J, et al. Short-term effects of intravitreal bevacizumab for subfoveal choroidal neovascularization in pathologic myopia. Retina. 2007;27:707–12.

133. Chan WM, Lai TY, Liu DT, Lam DS. Intravitreal bevacizumab (Avastin) for myopic choroidal neovascularization: six-month results of a prospective pilot study. Ophthalmology. 2007;114:2190–6.

134. Rensch F, Spandau UH, Schlichtenbrede F, et al. Intravitreal bevacizumab for myopic choroidal neovascularization. Ophthalmic Surg Lasers Imaging. 2008;39:182–5.

135. Silva RM, Ruiz-Moreno JM, Nascimento J, et al. Short-term efficacy and safety of intravitreal ranibizumab for myopic choroidal neovascularization. Retina. 2008;28:1117–23.

136. Arias L, Planas N, Prades S, et al. Intravitreal bevacizumab (Avastin) for choroidal neovascularisation secondary to pathological myopia: 6-month results. Br J Ophthalmol. 2008;92:1035–9.

137. Chang LK, Spaide RF, Brue C, Freund KB, Klancnik JM Jr, Slakter JS. Bevacizumab treatment for subfoveal choroidal neovascularization from causes other than age-related macular degeneration. Arch Ophthalmol. 2008;126:941–5.

138. Rheaume MA, Sebag M. Intravitreal bevacizumab for the treatment of choroidal neovascularization associated with pathological myopia. Can J Ophthalmol. 2008;43:576–80.

139. Wong D, Li KK. Avastin in myopic choroidal neovascularisation: is age the limit? Br J Ophthalmol. 2008;92:1011–2.

140. Ruiz-Moreno JM, Montero JA, Gomez-Ulla F, Ares S. Intravitreal bevacizumab to treat subfoveal choroidal neovascularisation in highly myopic eyes: 1-year outcome. Br J Ophthalmol. 2009;93:448–51.

141. Hayashi K, Ohno-Matsui K, Teramukai S, et al. Comparison of visual outcome and regression pattern of myopic choroidal neovascularization after intravitreal bevacizumab or after photodynamic therapy. Am J Ophthalmol. 2009;148:396–408.

142. Yodoi Y, Tsujikawa A, Nakanishi H, et al. Central retinal sensitivity after intravitreal injection of bevacizumab for myopic choroidal neovascularization. Am J Ophthalmol. 2009;147:816–24. 24.e1.

143. Ikuno Y, Soga K, Wakabayashi T, Gomi F. Angiographic changes after bevacizumab. Ophthalmology. 2009;116:2263.e1.

144. Hayashi K, Ohno-Matsui K, Shimada N, et al. Intravitreal bevacizumab on myopic choroidal neovascularization that was refractory to or had recurred after photodynamic therapy. Graefes Arch Clin Exp Ophthalmol. 2009;247:609–18.

145. Konstantinidis L, Mantel I, Pournaras JA, Zografos L, Ambresin A. Intravitreal ranibizumab (Lucentis) for the treatment of myopic choroidal neovascularization. Graefes Arch Clin Exp Ophthalmol. 2009;247:311–8.

146. Dithmar S, Schaal KB, Hoh AE, Schmidt S, Schutt F. Intravitreal bevacizumab for choroidal neovascularization due to pathological myopia. Ophthalmologe. 2009;106:527–30.

147. Chan WM, Lai TY, Liu DT, Lam DS. Intravitreal bevacizumab (Avastin) for myopic choroidal neovascularisation: 1-year results of a prospective pilot study. Br J Ophthalmol. 2009;93:150–4.

148. Ruiz-Moreno JM, Gomez-Ulla F, Montero JA, et al. Intravitreous bevacizumab to treat subfoveal choroidal neovascularization in highly myopic eyes: short-term results. Eye (Lond). 2009;23:334–8.

149. Ikuno Y, Sayanagi K, Soga K, et al. Intravitreal bevacizumab for choroidal neovascularization attributable to pathological myopia: one-year results. Am J Ophthalmol. 2009;147:94–100.e1.

150. Sayanagi K, Ikuno Y, Soga K, Wakabayashi T, Tano Y. Marginal crack after intravitreal bevacizumab for myopic choroidal neovascularization. Acta Ophthalmol. 2009;87:460–3.

151. Cohen SY. Anti-VEGF drugs as the 2009 first-line therapy for choroidal neovascularization in pathologic myopia. Retina. 2009;29:1062–6.

152. Monés JM, Amselem L, Serrano A, Garcia M, Hijano M. Intravitreal ranibizumab for choroidal neovascularization secondary to pathologic myopia: 12-month results. Eye (Lond). 2009;23:1275–80.

153. Gharbiya M, Allievi F, Mazzeo L, Gabrieli CB. Intravitreal bevacizumab treatment for choroidal neovascularization in pathologic myopia: 12-month results. Am J Ophthalmol. 2009;147:84–93.e1.

154. Wu PC, Chen YJ. Intravitreal injection of bevacizumab for myopic choroidal neovascularization: 1-year follow-up. Eye (Lond). 2009;23:2042–5.

155. Lai TY, Chan WM, Liu DT, Lam DS. Intravitreal ranibizumab for the primary treatment of choroidal neovascularization secondary to pathologic myopia. Retina. 2009;29:750–6.

156. Ruiz-Moreno JM, Montero JA. Intravitreal bevacizumab to treat myopic choroidal neovascularization: 2-year outcome. Graefes Arch Clin Exp Ophthalmol. 2010;248:937–41.

157. Voykov B, Gelisken F, Inhoffen W, Voelker M, Bartz-Schmidt KU, Ziemssen F. Bevacizumab for choroidal neovascularization secondary to pathologic myopia: is there a decline of the treatment efficacy after 2 years? Graefes Arch Clin Exp Ophthalmol. 2010;248:543–50.

158. Lalloum F, Souied EH, Bastuji-Garin S, et al. Intravitreal ranibizumab for choroidal neovascularization complicating pathologic myopia. Retina. 2010;30:399–406.

159. Silva RM, Ruiz-Moreno JM, Rosa P, et al. Intravitreal ranibizumab for myopic choroidal neovascularization: 12-month results. Retina. 2010;30:407–12.

160. Vadala M, Pece A, Cipolla S, et al. Is ranibizumab effective in stopping the loss of vision for choroidal neovascularisation in pathologic myopia? A long-term follow-up study. Br J Ophthalmol. 2010;95:657–61.

161. Scupola A, Tiberti AC, Sasso P, et al. Macular functional changes evaluated with MP-1 microperimetry after intravitreal bevacizumab for subfoveal myopic choroidal neovascularization: one-year results. Retina. 2010;30:739–47.

162. Gharbiya M, Allievi F, Conflitti S, et al. Intravitreal bevacizumab for treatment of myopic choroidal neovascularization: the second year of a prospective study. Clin Ter. 2010;161:e87–93.

163. Wakabayashi T, Ikuno Y, Gomi F. Different dosing of intravitreal bevacizumab for choroidal neovascularization because of pathologic myopia. Retina. 2011;31:880–6.

164. Calvo-Gonzalez C, Reche-Frutos J, Donate J, Fernandez-Perez C, Garcia-Feijoo J. Intravitreal ranibizumab for myopic choroidal neovascularization: factors predictive of visual outcome and need for retreatment. Am J Ophthalmol. 2011;151:529–34.

165. Nakanishi H, Tsujikawa A, Yodoi Y, et al. Prognostic factors for visual outcomes 2-years after intravitreal bevacizumab for myopic choroidal neovascularization. Eye (Lond). 2011;25:375–81.

166. Franqueira N, Cachulo ML, Pires I, et al. Long-term follow-up of myopic choroidal neovascularization treated with ranibizumab. Ophthalmologica. 2012;227:39–44.

167. Peiretti E, Vinci M, Fossarello M. Intravitreal bevacizumab as a treatment for choroidal neovascularisation secondary to myopia: 4-year study results. Can J Ophthalmol. 2012;47:28–33.

168. Gharbiya M, Cruciani F, Parisi F, Cuozzo G, Altimari S, Abdolrahimzadeh S. Long-term results of intravitreal bevacizumab for choroidal neovascularisation in pathological myopia. Br J Ophthalmol. 2012;96(8):1068–72.

169. Ruiz-Moreno JM, Montero JA, Arias L, et al. Twelve-month outcome after one intravitreal injection of bevacizumab to treat myopic choroidal neovascularization. Retina. 2010;30:1609–15.

170. Gharbiya M, Giustolisi R, Allievi F, et al. Choroidal neovascularization in pathologic myopia: intravitreal ranibizumab versus bevacizumab – a randomized controlled trial. Am J Ophthalmol. 2010;149:458–64.

171. Nor-Masniwati S, Shatriah I, Zunaina E. Single intravitreal ranibizumab for myopic choroidal neovascularization. Clin Ophthalmol. 2011;5:1079–82.

172. Wu TT, Kung YH. The 12-month outcome of three consecutive monthly intravitreal injections of ranibizumab for myopic choroidal neovascularization. J Ocul Pharmacol Ther. 2012;28(2):129–33.

173. Tufail A, Narendran N, Patel PJ, et al. Ranibizumab in myopic choroidal neovascularization: the 12-month results from the REPAIR study. Ophthalmology. 2013;120(9):1944–5.e1.

174. Wolf S, Balciuniene VJ, Laganovska G, et al. RADIANCE: a randomized controlled study of ranibizumab in patients with choroidal neovascularization secondary to pathologic myopia. Ophthalmology. 2014;121(3):682–92.e2.

175. Tan NW, Ohno-Matsui K, Koh HJ, et al. Long-term outcomes of ranibizumab treatment of myopic choroidal neovascularization in east-Asian patients from the RADIANCE study. Retina. 2018;38(11):2228–38.

176. Ikuno Y, Ohno-Matsui K, Wong TY, et al. Intravitreal aflibercept injection in patients with myopic choroidal neovascularization: the MYRROR study. Ophthalmology. 2015;122(6):1220–7.

177. Hu Q, Li H, Du Y, et al. Comparison of intravitreal bevacizumab and ranibizumab used for myopic choroidal neovascularization: a PRISMA-compliant systematic review and meta-analysis of randomized controlled trials. Medicine (Baltimore). 2019;98(12):e14905.

178. Sayanagi K, Uematsu S, Hara C, et al. Effect of intravitreal injection of aflibercept or ranibizumab on chorioretinal atrophy in myopic choroidal neovascularization. Graefes Arch Clin Exp Ophthalmol. 2019;257(4):749–57.

179. Chen C, Yan M, Huang Z, et al. The evaluation of a two-year outcome of intravitreal conbercept versus ranibizumab for pathological myopic choroidal neovascularization. Curr Eye Res. 2020;45(11):1415–21.

180. Wang JK, Huang TL, Chang PY, et al. Intravitreal aflibercept versus bevacizumab for treatment of myopic choroidal neovascularization. Sci Rep. 2018;8(1):14389.

181. Korol A, Kustryn T, Zadorozhnyy O, et al. Comparison of efficacy of intravitreal ranibizumab and aflibercept in eyes with myopic choroidal neovascularization: 24-month follow-up. J Ocul Pharmacol Ther. 2020;36(2):122–5.

182. Spaide RF. The as-needed treatment strategy for choroidal neovascularization: a feedback-based treatment system. Am J Ophthalmol. 2009;148(1):1–3.

183. Niwa Y, Sawada O, Miyake T, et al. Comparison between one injection and three monthly injections of intravitreal bevacizumab for myopic choroidal neovascularization. Ophthalmic Res. 2012;47:135–40.

184. Ruiz-Moreno JM, Montero JA, Amat-Peral P. Myopic choroidal neovascularization treated by intravitreal bevacizumab: comparison of two different initial doses. Graefes Arch Clin Exp Ophthalmol. 2011;249:595–9.

185. Yoon JU, Byun YJ, Koh HJ. Intravitreal anti-VEGF versus photodynamic therapy with verteporfin for treatment of myopic choroidal neovascularization. Retina. 2010;30:418–24.

186. Kaiser PK, Boyer DS, Cruess AF, et al. Verteporfin plus ranibizumab for choroidal neovascularization in age-related macular degeneration: twelve-month results of the DENALI study. Ophthalmology. 2012;119:1001–10.

187. Ohno-Matsui K, Jonas JB, Spaide RF. Macular Bruch membrane holes in choroidal neovascularization-related myopic macular atrophy by swept-source optical coherence tomography. Am J Ophthalmol. 2016;162:133–139.e1.

Myopic Macular Retinoschisis

20

Kyoko Ohno-Matsui

20.1 Myopic Macular Retinoschisis and Associated Lesions

In 1997, Takano and Kishi first identified and reported that the foveal retinal detachment and myopic macular retinoschisis (MRS) were observed in highly myopic eyes before developing macular hole retinal detachment by using OCT [1]. This finding provided a clue why macular holes in highly myopic eyes tend to develop retinal detachment unlike idiopathic macular holes in non-myopic eyes. The schisis was found to occur in the outer retinal layer unlike congenital macular retinoschisis; however, the morphological details of the separated retina were unclear at this point mainly due to a limited resolution of OCT [1–3]. With the advent of OCT, MRS has been increasingly recognized as important causes of vision decrease in eyes with pathologic myopia. MRS is found in 9–34% of highly myopic eyes with posterior staphyloma [1, 2, 4].

Despite numerous publications on this condition, no clear definition of MRS has been found in the literature. The hallmark of MRS is the appearance of schisis of the retinal layers, most commonly in the outer plexiform layer (outer retinoschisis) (Fig. 20.1) [5–7]. In some cases, the appearance of schisis may also occur within more internal retinal layers (inner retinoschisis) with detachment of the internal limiting membrane (ILM) (Fig. 20.1) [7, 8]. Although the terminology "myopic macular retinoschisis" still prevails, it is now believed (due in part to improved imaging with recent OCT) that eyes with myopic retinoschisis have traction, resulting in elongation of Henle's nerve fiber rather than a splitting of the retina. Thus, MRS is a totally different condition from congenital macular retinoschisis, which is a splitting of the retinal nerve fiber layer from the rest of the sensory retina disrupting a synaptic transfer between bipolar cells and ganglion cells. A lack of central scotoma in eyes with MRS supports this concept.

Pannozzo and Mercanti [4] proposed to unify all of the pathologic features generated by traction in the myopic environment under the name of myopic traction maculopathy.

20.2 Clinical Features of MRS

Most of the patients with MRS may be relatively asymptomatic especially while the eyes do not develop more serious complications like full-thickness MH or foveal RD [2], and MRS may persist for many years before affecting vision significantly. Vision loss attributed to MRS has been associated with the development of foveal RD and/or macular holes in most cases. The best-corrected visual acuity (BCVA) of the patients with MRS ranged widely from 20/40 to 20/200 [2, 9]. Some patients complain of metamorphopsia or distorted vision before the visual acuity is decreased. However, what makes difficult for clinicians to suspect the MRS is that some of the patients with MRS do not notice the change in vision [2], due to co-existing myopic retinochoroidal lesions like myopic CNV, myopic chorioretinal atrophy, or myopic optic neuropathy. Thus, a periodic examination using OCT is recommended for highly myopic eyes with posterior staphyloma even when they do not recognize the change of visual symptoms.

The mean age of diagnosis of MRS in highly myopic patients was in 60s [2, 9], and it is uncommon to detect MRS in the patients under the age 40, although MRS in the patients with age 28 was reported [9]. Baba et al. [2] reported that the mean refractive error of the eyes with MRS was −18.4 D (range, −13.0 to −27.0) and the mean axial length was 29.8 mm (range, 28.6 to 32.2 mm). Similarly, Fujimoto et al. [5] reported that the axial lengths ranged from 26.8 to 34.2 mm (mean, 29.7 ± 2.0 mm).

MRS was initially reported to exclusively develop in severely myopic eyes with posterior staphyloma and does not develop in eyes without staphyloma [2, 5]. Although

K. Ohno-Matsui (✉)
Department of Ophthalmology and Visual Science, Tokyo Medical and Dental University, Bunkyo-Ku, Tokyo, Japan
e-mail: k.ohno.oph@tmd.ac.jp

R. F. Spaide et al. (eds.), *Pathologic Myopia*, https://doi.org/10.1007/978-3-030-74334-5_20

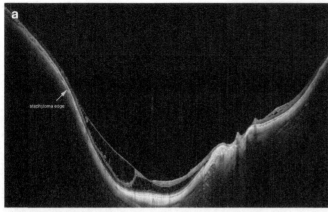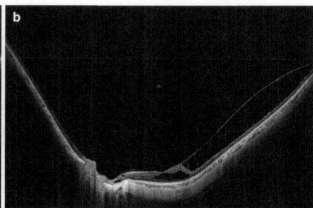

Fig. 20.1 Wide-field OCT image of myopic macular retinoschisis. The tissue splitting of outer retina is observed, and many columnar structures are seen within the outer retinoschisis in the macular area. The columnar structures are almost perpendicular to the line of retinal pigmented epithelium at the fovea and tend to be slightly inclined away from the fovea. The inner retinoschisis is seen temporal to the fovea, and in this area, the inner limiting membrane (ILM) is detached from the rest of the retinal tissue. (**a**) The area of inner and outer retinoschisis is restricted within the staphylomatous area and does not go beyond the staphyloma edge (arrow). (**b**) OCT features suggesting staphyloma edges (changes of choroidal thickness as well as scleral inward protrusion according to Shinohara et al. [10]) are not evident. Although outer retinoschisis is seen in macular area, the inner retinoschisis is widely observed beyond the scan range

there were no good technologies to objectively identify the presence of staphylomas, Shinohara et al. [10] used ultra-wide field OCT prototype and succeeded in identifying the staphyloma edges objectively (see Chap. XX for details). The recent study using ultra-wide field OCT showed that 14% of the eyes with MRS did not have an evident staphyloma (Fig. 20.1b), suggesting that staphyloma was not a mandatory requirement for development of MRS [11].

20.3 Diagnosis of MRS

OCT is an indispensable tool to diagnose MRS and associated lesions, although the presence of MRS can be suspected opthalmoscopically in some cases. In some cases, the MRS can be observed as a shallow retinal elevation by the stereoscopic fundus examinations using magnified lens (e.g., +90D lens). Such retinal elevations are more easily detected along and within the patchy chorioretinal atrophy, along the retinal vascular arcade, and along the temporal margin of myopic conus.

By using SD-OCT, MRS is observed as the splitting of the inner retina from the outer retinal layers with multiple columnar structures connecting the split retinal layers (Fig. 20.1) [3, 5, 9]. Different from retinal detachment, the remnants of outer retina are observed on the RPE layer. On enhanced SD-OCT images, Fujimoto et al. [5] reported that the splitting of the outer retina appeared to be present between the outer plexiform layer and the outer nuclear layer. Columnar structures are almost perpendicular to the RPE at the fovea and tend to become inclined away from the fovea, which corresponds to the course of Henle's nerve fiber layer in the macula [12]. Thus, columnar structures are con-

sidered to represent a retention of Henle's fiber layer. In addition to the retinoschisis in the outer retina, retinoschisis was also found at the level of the inner plexiform layer or an ILM detachment (Fig. 20.1) [7, 8]. Foveal RD often co-exists with MRS. An outer lamellar MH is reported to predispose to the MRS to a foveal RD [13]. Mostly, an outer lamellar MH is observed in eyes with foveal RD if we analyze multiple OCT sections. MRS tends to be present in and around the macular atrophy around the regressed CNV due to pathologic myopia [2]. MRS in the eyes with atrophic stage of myopic CNV appeared markedly less column-like than the MRS seen in highly myopic eyes without CNV [14], and it was difficult to differentiate a foveal RD from MRS in the eyes with atrophic stage of myopic CNV.

Other methods than OCT might help in the diagnosis of MRS or visualization of the full extent of MRS in the posterior fundus. Retromode of the F10 (Nidek, Aichi, Japan) scanning laser confocal ophthalmoscope (SLO) uses an infrared laser and an aperture with a modified central stop. This optical arrangement allows for pseudo-three-dimensional image, which can detect abnormalities in the deeper retinal layers. By using retromode imaging by F10, Tanaka et al. [15] showed a characteristic fingerprint pattern at the corresponding area of the MRS (Fig. 20.2). The fingerprint pattern consisted of radiating retinal striae centered on the fovea and many light dots and lines that ran in parallel to the striae or formed a whorled pattern surrounding the radiating striae. Also, the area of MRS showed various retinal vascular abnormalities (capillary telangiectasia, microaneurysm formation, and dye leakage) by fluorescein angiography [16]. Sayanagi and associates [17] reported the different patterns of fundus autofluorescence (FAF) between macular hole retinal detachment and MRS.

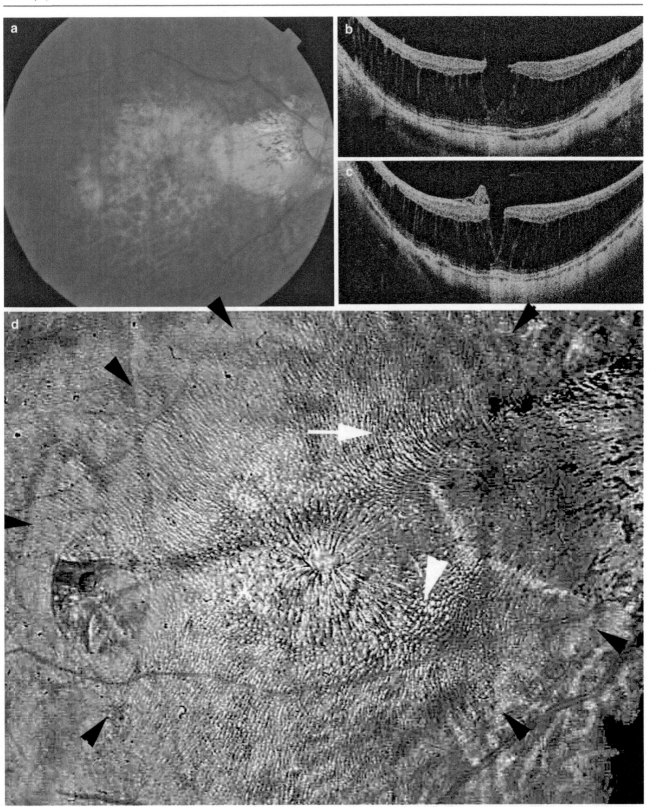

Fig. 20.2 Representative retromode images of an eye with an outer macular retinoschisis. (**a**) Fundus photograph of the right eye of a 77-year-old woman showing diffuse chorioretinal atrophy in the posterior fundus. (**b, c**) Horizontal and vertical scans across the central fovea by optical coherence tomography (OCT) showing the macular retinoschisis with inner lamellar hole in the central fovea. (**d**) Retromode image by F10 showing a fingerprint pattern (black arrowheads) consisting of central radiating retinal striae and surrounding multiple dots (arrowhead) and lines (arrow). Many lines appear in parallel or in a whorled pattern. The inner lamellar hole is observed as a circular defect at the central fovea

Various macular lesions co-exist in eyes with MRS, such as lamellar macular hole (lamellar MH), full-thickness macular hole (FTMH), and foveal retinal detachment (RD) (Fig. 20.3).

20.4   Pathological Findings of MRS

Tang and associates [6] examined both eyes of a 73-year-old woman with high myopia and showed that the degenerative retinoschisis with interbridging strands in the outer plexiform layer of the macular region was found (Fig. 20.4). Interestingly, there were multiple cystic degenerations in the outer plexiform layer, and there appeared to be folding of the inner layers of the retina, which were novel findings not observed previously with OCT.

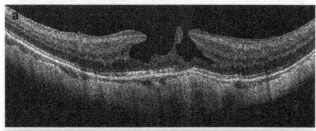
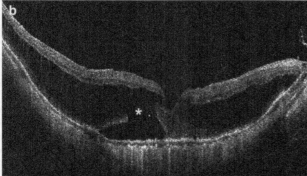
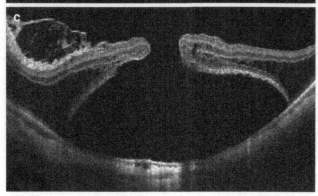

Fig. 20.3 Macular lesions associated with myopic macular retinoschisis. (**a**) Inner lamellar macular hole. (**b**). Outer lamellar macular hole (asterisk). (**c**) Full-thickness macular hole and foveal retinal detachment

20.5   Factors Related to MRS Development

MRS is considered to be caused by various factors. Wu and associates [18] reported that three factors were independently associated with MRS and foveal RD without MH in high myopia in the multivariate analysis: axial length, macular chorioretinal atrophy, and vitreoretinal interface factors. MRS tends to develop in highly myopic eyes with advanced chorioretinal atrophy [2]. Johnson [19, 20] suggested four major traction mechanisms: vitreomacular traction (from perifoveal PVD), remnant cortical vitreous layer (after PVD), epiretinal membrane, and intrinsic noncompliance of the ILM. Using electron microscopy, Bando et al. [21] reported that collagen fiber and cell debris were identified on the inner surface of ILM in 70% of the eyes with MRS, whereas none in ILM from control subjects (idiopathic MH). More fibrous glial cells were found on the inner surface of ILM from the eyes with myopic MRS [21], and they concluded that the cell migration and consequent collagen synthesis on the ILM can be another contributor for developing MRS. Chen et al. [22] histologically examined the ILM specimens peeled from eye MRS and those with idiopathic MHs. The vitreal side stiffness of the MRS ILMs was markedly higher than that of idiopathic MH ILMs, and astrocytes were frequently observed in MRS ILMS, whereas none of idiopathic MH ILM did not have astrocytes. Based on these results, they suggested that MRS ILMs appeared to be associated with Muller cell and astrocyte reactive gliosis.

Johnson [19] also suggested retinal arteriolar stiffness as minor mechanism contributing to the MRS development. The OCT examinations of serious sections along the entire posterior vascular arcade showed that the paravascular abnormalities such as paravascular lamellar holes [23], vascular microfolds [23–26], and paravascular retinal cysts [23] are frequently found in eyes with MRS (Figs. 20.5). Following to the formation of paravascular lamellar holes, the glial cells like astrocytes which exist abundantly around the retinal vessels can migrate and proliferate through the paravascular lamellar holes. These cells can produce collagen and facilitate the proliferative and contractile response of ILM. In some OCT sections, we directly can see images suggestive of cell migration toward the vitreous through paravascular lamellar holes (Fig. 20.5a).

MRS tends to develop in eyes with severe myopic fundus changes (patchy chorioretinal atrophy or bare sclera) more than those with mild myopic fundus changes [2]. Although the reason for this association is not fully clear, the scleral shape alterations are considered to affect the MRS development [27–38]. The slope and shape of posterior staphyloma in highly myopic eyes have long been analyzed by using OCT [30–38]. Smiddy et al. [39] hypothesized that progressive staphyloma formation generated a posteriorly applied

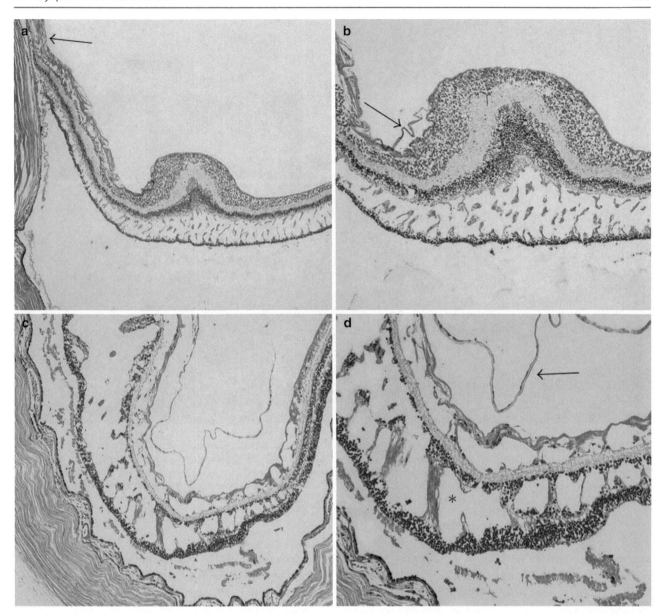

Fig. 20.4 Photomicrograph of the right eye demonstrating areas of macular retinoschisis (MRS). (**a**) Lower magnification showing the tissue splitting in the outer retina. A region containing the staphyloma is also seen (black arrow). (**b**) Higher magnification of MRS seen in multiple layers of the retina including the outer plexiform layer, inner plexiform layer, nerve fiber layer, and the outer plexiform layer in the perifoveal region. A thin fibrous preretinal membrane is seen (black

arrow). (Hematoxylin and eosin, original magnification, (**a**) ×50; (**b**) ×100). (**c**) Photomicrograph of the left eye demonstrating MRS in the outer plexiform layer, ganglion cell layer, and nerve fiber layer. (**d**) Higher magnification demonstrating neuronal bridges between both nuclear layers (asterisk). A fibrous preretinal membrane is seen (black arrow). (hematoxylin and eosin, original magnification, (**c**) ×50; (**d**) ×100)

force that gives the appearance that there is primary (anterior or tangentially directed) preretinal traction.

Recent studies using swept-source OCT support the association between scleral curvature alterations and MRS [27–29]. Intrachoroidal cavitation (ICC) is yellowish-orange lesion located inferior to the optic disc (see "Choroid" chapter) [40–43]. Ohno-Matsui et al. [28] recently found that ICC was located in the macular area on and around the patchy chorioretinal atrophy. As seen in peripapillary ICC, the sclera in the area of macular ICC was bowed posteriorly (Fig. 20.6).

The eyes with macular ICC had retinoschisis around the patchy atrophy significantly more frequently than the eyes without cavitation. Swept-source OCT also showed that the curvature of inner scleral surface of highly myopic eyes could be divided into those whose curvature sloped toward the optic nerve, was symmetrical and centered on the fovea, was asymmetrical, and was irregular [29]. Patients with irregular curvature were significantly older with significantly longer axial lengths than the eyes with other curvatures. MRS was present significantly more frequently in the eyes

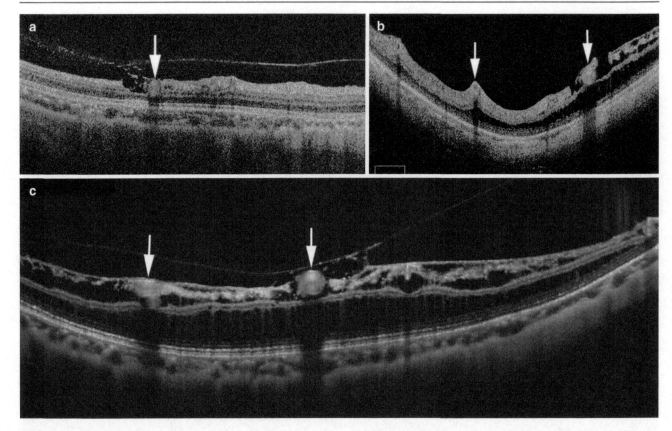

Fig. 20.5 Paravascular abnormalities seen in eyes with myopic macular retinoschisis (MRS). In (**a–c**), arrows indicate the retinal vessels. (**a**) The upper roof of paravascular retinal cyst is avulsed by the detached posterior hyaloid and is observed as paravascular lamellar hole. Through the paravascular lamellar hole, it seems that the cells migrate toward the vitreous, shown as many granular hyper-reflective dots. (**b**) Paravascular lamellar holes are observed along both sides of the retinal vessel (shown by a right arrow). Retinal vessels seem to protrude toward the vitreous and are observed as retinal vascular microfolds. (**c**) Paravascular retinal cysts are observed along the retinal vessels. A wide MRS is also noted in the inner as well as outer retina

with irregular curvature [29]. These descriptions suggested that a scleral contour might affect the development of MRS. In contrary, some other kinds of scleral contour might act preferably against the MRS development. Dome-shaped macula (DSM) was first described by Gaucher and associates [31] as an unexpected finding in myopic staphyloma and was characterized as an inward convexity of the macula (see "Sclera" chapter). By using EDI-OCT, Imamura and Spaide [33] reported that the DSM is the result of a localized variation in thickness of the sclera in the macular area. Ellabban and associates [44] recently found that among nine eyes with extrafoveal retinal schisis, only one eye had foveal schisis without either foveal RD or MH formation. They suggested that the bulge in eyes with a DSM may act as a macular buckle-like mechanism and thus may prevent or alleviate tractional forces over the fovea, thereby preventing schisis or detachment.

Progression of MRS into foveal RD after IVB against myopic CNV has been reported [45]. In the eyes with a myopic CNV, the neural retina is pushed vitreally by the protrusion of the CNV. In addition, there is a tractional force of the ILM on the retina in the eyes with a retinoschisis. IVB causes

a rapid shrinkage of the CNV accompanied by an absorption of the subretinal hemorrhage and exudated fluid. Under these conditions, the continuous inward tractional force by the ILM enhanced by the rapid contraction of the CNV leads to further splitting of the retina and finally to a RD.

20.6 Natural Course

Earlier studies have reported the progression of a MRS into more serious complications such as foveal RD or full-thickness MH during its natural course [9, 13, 39, 46–49]. Benhamou et al. [9] reported that 1 of the 21 highly myopic eyes (4.8%) with MRS without MH evolved into a full-thickness MH, and this eye had a vitreous traction on the fovea. Fujimoto and associates [5] reported that a foveal RD developed in 6 of 21 eyes (28.6%) with myopic MRS and FTMH developed in 2 of the 21 eyes (9.5%) with MRS during a follow-up. Gaucher and associates [48] reported that 6 of 18 eyes (33.3%) with MRS that did not undergo surgical intervention developed full-thickness MH during a mean follow-up of 34.7 months (range, 12–60 months). Shimada

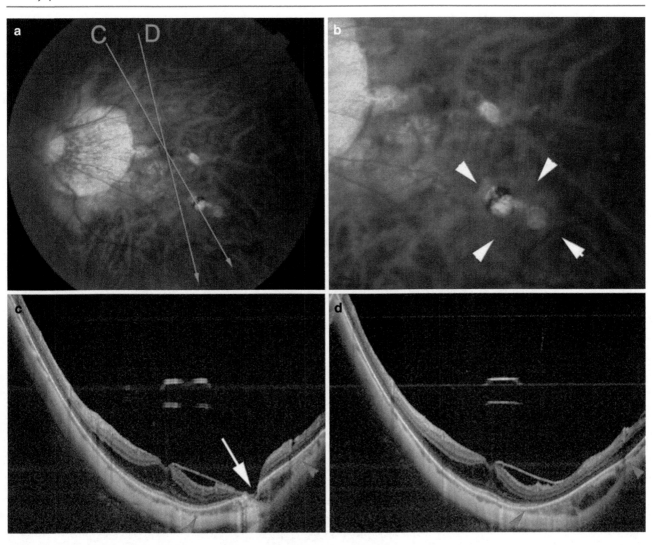

Fig. 20.6 Macular retinoschisis (MRS) seen in the area of macular intrachoroidal cavitation (macular ICC). (**a**) Photograph of the left fundus of a 60-year-old woman showing 3 areas of patchy chorioretinal atrophy temporal to and inferotemporal to the fovea. (**b**) Magnified image of top left image shows 3 areas of patchy chorioretinal atrophy. The area around the patchy atrophy is orange (arrowheads). (**c**) B-scan swept-source optical coherence tomographic (OCT) image of line C in Fig. A shows that the sclera is bowed posteriorly (between arrowheads) compared to neighboring sclera beyond the retinal pigment epithelium (RPE) defects. The choroid seems to be thickened in the area, and the retina is caved into the intrachoroidal cavitation (arrow). Inner retinoschisis is observed around the intrachoroidal cavitation. (**d**) In the section shown by line B in top left image, a bowing of the sclera is observed (between arrowheads). The hyporeflective space suggests the presence of fluid in the space of the intrachoroidal cavitation

et al. [47] also reported that four of eight eyes (50.0%) with MRS progressed to foveal RD or full-thickness MH in a follow-up period of more than 2 years. Sun et al. [49] reported five eyes of five patients with myopic MRS who developed full-thickness MH. The natural evolution from MRS to full-thickness MH was classified into two patterns by OCT findings. In full-thickness MH formation pattern 1, a focal area of the external retinal layer was elevated and followed by the development of a small outer lamellar MH and retinal detachment (RD). The outer lamellar MH and RD were then enlarged horizontally and elevated vertically until the outer lamellar MH was attached to the overlying retinal layer. A full-thickness MH finally developed when the roof of RD opened. In full-thickness MH formation pattern 2, the opening of the roof of MRS or cystoid space caused an inner lamellar MH. The MRS was then gradually resolved except the residual MRS beneath the inner lamellar MH; the inner lamellar MH would finally proceed into a full-thickness MH. As a mechanism of progression from MRS to foveal RD, Shimada et al. [13] investigated five eyes of five consecutive patients with myopic MRS who developed an RD during the follow-up period. The results showed that the progression from MRS to foveal RD passed through four stages: (1) a focal irregularity of the thickness of external retina, (2) an outer lamellar MH development within the thickened area and subsequent development of small RD, (3) horizontal separation of the column-like structures overlying the outer lamellar hole and vertical enlargement of outer lamellar hole, and (4) the elevation of the upper edge of the external retina and the attachment to the upper part of retinoschisis layer accompanied with further enlargement of RD. The interval from stage 1 to 3 was relatively short (mean, 4.5 months) indicating that we should be very cautious about the progression to RD when the findings in stage 1 are observed in OCT images. Once the outer lamellar hole develops, an RD will develop in a short time. Sayanagi and Ikuno [50] reported a case which showed a spontaneous resolution of MRS and a consequent development of foveal RD.

Shimada et al. [51] recently analyzed the natural course in as many as 207 eyes with MRS with a follow-up ≥ 24 months. Shimada et al. have classified MRS according to its extent and location from S_0 through S_4 (Fig. 20.7a, b): no MRS (S_0),

Fig. 20.7 (**a**) Schematic illustration of classification of myopic macular retinoschisis (MRS) according to the area. S_0, no MRS; S_1, extrafoveal; S_2, foveal; S_3, include both fovea and extrafovea but do not involve the entire macula; S_4, entire macula. (**b**) Modified classification of outer retinoschises according to their location and size by using ultra-wide field OCT. (Cited with permission from the Ref. [11]). S0, no outer retinoschisis; S1, extrafoveal outer retinoschisis; S2, foveal outer retinoschisis; S3, foveal but not entire macular outer retinoschisis; S4, entire macular outer retinoschisis; S4(D), dome-shaped macula and entire macular outer retinoschisis except for the foveal region; and S5d, outer retinoschisis beyond the range of the scan length

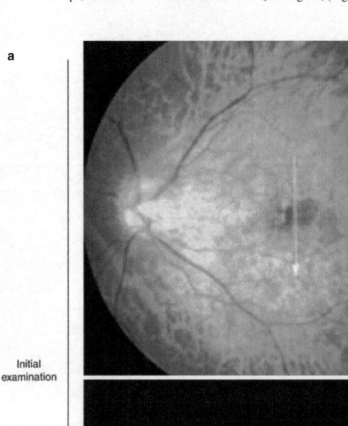

Initial examination

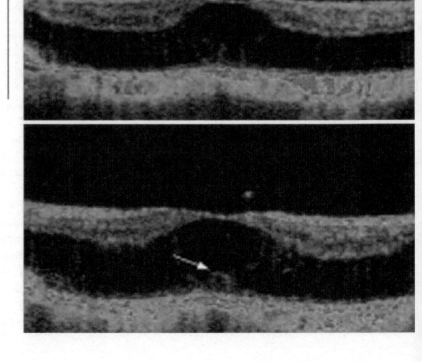

Stage 1

Fig. 20.7 (continued)

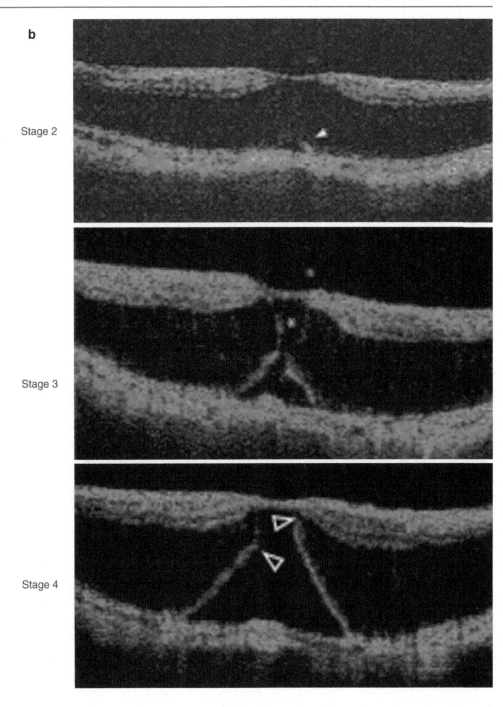

Stage 2

Stage 3

Stage 4

extra-foveal MRS (S_1), foveal only MRS (S_2), foveal but not entire macular area MRS (S_3), and entire macular area MRS (S_4). The progression of MRS was defined as (1) an increase of the extent or height of MRS (an increase of the height means the change >100 μm) and (2) new development of lamellar MH, foveal RD, or FTMH. The results showed that the progression was found in 26 of 207 eyes (12.6%) (Fig. 20.8). According to the extent of MRS at the initial examination, the progression was found in 6.2% of the eyes with S_0, in 3.6% of the eyes with S_1, in 8.9% of the eyes with S_2, in 13.0% of the eyes with S_3, and in 42.9% of the eyes with S_4. The eyes with S_4 MRS significantly more frequently showed a progression of MRS than the eyes with S_0 to S_3. In the eyes with S_0 and S_1, a development or increase of MRS was found. In the eyes with S_2, a development of full-thickness MH was a main progression pattern. In the eyes with S_4, a development of foveal RD was a main progression pattern. Figure 20.9a shows the representative cases with progression. By using ultra-wide field OCT, the MRS area can be observed in a wide area{Shinohara, 2018 #2200} In addition, a spatial relationship between MRS and other lesions (staphylomas and dome-shaped macula) is clearly visible. Based on the results with ultra-wide field OCT, the MRS classification has been updated (Fig. 20.10). The

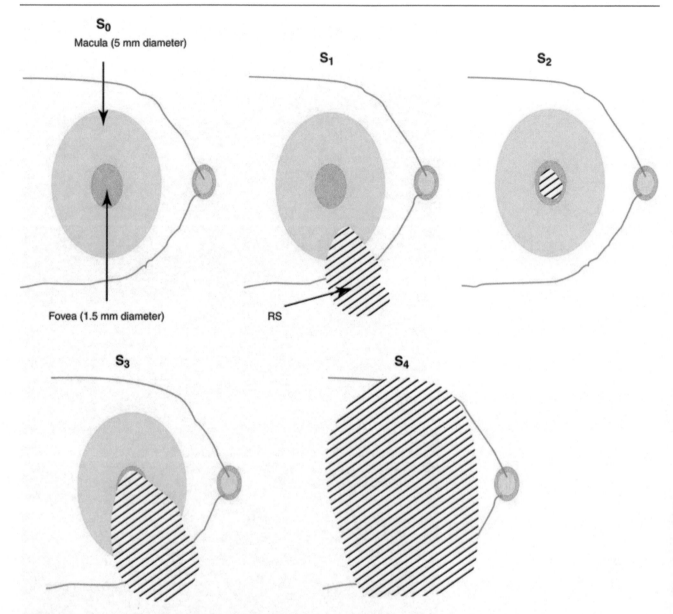

Fig. 20.8 Different stages in the progression from myopic macular retinoschisis to early retinal detachment. Top row: posterior fundus photographs at the initial examination. Second to fifth rows: optical coherence tomographic (OCT) images at the initial examination and at stages 1, 2, 3, and 4. At the initial examination, the OCT images show macular retinoschisis without a retinal detachment. The outer retinal layer appears to be normal. At stage 1, the OCT images show a focal thickening of the outer retinal layers (arrow), and at stage 2, a lamellar hole (arrowhead) is present beneath the thickened area. At stage 3, the retinoschisis layer overlying the outer lamellar hole is separated horizontally (asterisks), and the outer lamellar hole appears enlarged. At stage 4, the upper edge of the external retina (open arrowhead) is attached to the upper part of retinoschisis layer. The RD is larger and is accompanied by the resolution of the retinoschisis

updated classification is more useful for making surgical strategies for MRS.

For the natural course of the lesions associated with MRS, Tanaka et al. [52] reported that a lamellar MH might be a relatively stable condition in highly myopic eyes, as we observe for lamellar MH in non-myopic eyes. Twenty-three of 24 eyes (95.8%) with a lamellar MH did not show any changes in the OCT images during a mean follow-up of 19.2 ± 10.2 months, although the remaining eye progressed to a full-thickness MH.

Spontaneous resolution of MRS has also been reported. Polito et al. [53] reported a case whose foveal RD as well as MRS spontaneously disappeared in the follow-up by developing spontaneous posterior vitreous detachment (PVD). Using the MRS classification into S_0 to S_4, Shimada et al. [51] also analyzed the spontaneous resolution of MRS. The improvement of MRS was defined as a decrease of the extent or height of MRS without developing new lamellar MH, RD, or full-thickness MH. Interestingly, 8 among a total of 175 eyes showed a resolution of MRS: a decrease of MRS in 2

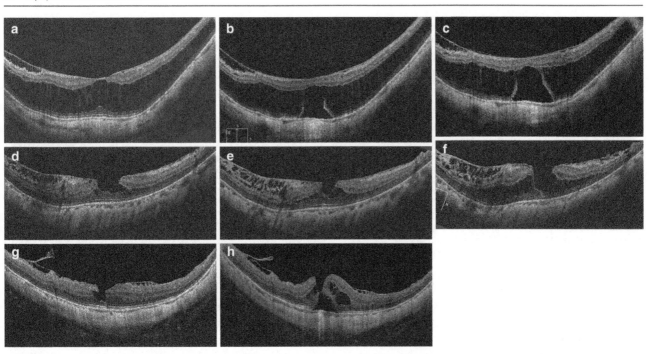

Fig. 20.9 Cases which show progression of myopic traction macu-lopathy (MTM.). (**a–c**) Progression from macular retinoschisis (MRS) to foveal retinal detachment (RD). Left eye of a 69-year-old man with an axial length of 30.9 mm. (**a**) Vertical OCT scan across the fovea shows a wide MRS in the macular area. (**b**) Fifteen months later, a foveal RD has developed. An outer lamellar macular hole is also formed. (**c**) At 20 months after the initial examination, the foveal RD is seen. (**d–f**) An increased extent of MRS. The right eye of a 52-year-old man with an axial length of 30.1 mm. (**d**) Vertical OCT section across

the fovea shows a limited MRS on the fovea. Inner lamellar macular hole is also seen. ILM detachment is seen inferior to the fovea. (**e**) Nine months later, the MRS area has slightly enlarged. (**f**) Two more months later, the MRS area has further enlarged. (**g, h**) Development of full-thickness macular hole in the left eye of a 62-year-old man with an axial length of 31.9 mm. (**g**) Vertical OCT section across the fovea shows an inner lamellar macular hole. ILM detachment is observed around the fovea. (**h**) Eight months later, a full-thickness macular hole has developed

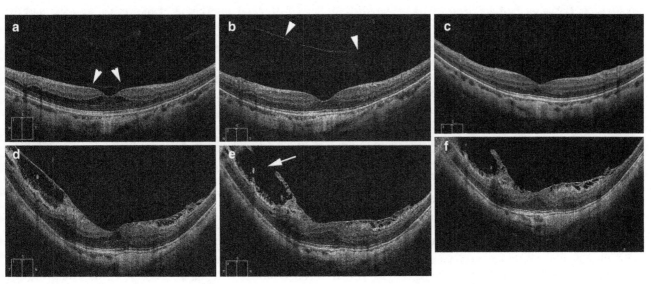

Fig. 20.10 Cases which show a resolution of myopic traction macu-lopathy (MTM). (**a–c**) Complete resolution of macular retinoschisis (MRS) subsequent to a development of posterior vitreous detachment (PVD). Left eye of a 46-year-old woman with a refractive error (spheri-cal equivalent) of −16.0 D and an axial length of 29.3 mm. (**a**) Vertical OCT scan across the fovea at the initial examination shows a shallow MRS on and around the fovea. Partial PVD is seen (arrowheads). (**b**) One month later, a complete PVD has occurred (arrowheads) and MRS has almost disappeared. (**c**) Fifteen months after the initial visit. MRS

has been completely resolved. (**d–f**) Resolution of macular retinoschisis (MRS) secondary to spontaneous disruption of internal limiting mem-brane (ILM). Right eye of a 52-year-old man with an axial length of 30.9 mm. (**d**) Vertical OCT scan across the fovea at the initial examina-tion shows a shallow MRS on and upper to the fovea. ILM detachment is also noted. (**e**) Fourteen months later, a spontaneous disruption of ILM has occurred upper to the fovea (arrow). MRS appears to decrease. (**f**) Twenty-four months after the initial visit, MRS has been completely resolved

eyes and complete resolution of MRS in 6 eyes (Fig. 20.10). Resolution of MRS was seen in three eyes with each of S_3 and S_4 and in one eye of each S_1 and S_2. Six of the eight eyes with improvement of MRS showed a release of retinal traction before resolution of MRS. PVD developed in four eyes, and spontaneous disruption of ILM was developed in two eyes before resolution of MRS. Figure 20.10 shows the representative cases with spontaneous resolution. Although the number of the patients is limited, it suggests that a spontaneous disruption of ILM occurs, and it causes a subsequent resolution of MRS.

20.7 Treatment for MRS

The literature on treatment options for MRS and its complications is limited by a lack of prospective data and small numbers in treated series. However, the usefulness of pars plana vitrectomy (PPV) in resolving the foveal RD and MRS has been reported in many studies [54–60]. The functional and anatomical outcome of vitrectomy in earlier studies is summarized in Table 20.1.

The indication of PPV for MRS without full-thickness MH has not been consistent. It is generally considered that we should perform vitrectomy for the eyes which developed foveal RD in addition to MRS. However, we are not certain what the indications are and when the optimal time is for surgery especially for myopic MRS without RD. The majority of eyes with MRS without foveal RD retain relatively good vision. Based on the four distinct stages from MRS to foveal RD, Shimada et al. [13] recommend that we had better consider surgical treatment between stages 3 (development of outer lamellar MH and small RD around it) and 4 (the upper edge of outer retina is attached to the upper part of the retinoschisis layer), because the vitrectomy at stage 4 has an increased risk of developing full-thickness MH postoperatively.

ILM peeling was first reported by Kuhn [61] to treat macular retinal detachment without macular hole in a highly myopic patient, although OCT was not performed in this report. The need for ILM peeling during vitrectomy remains a controversy; however, it is necessary when apparent ILM traction is recognized on preoperative OCT images. The cases with myopic MRS and foveal RD which were successfully treated with vitrectomy without ILM peeling were reported [60]; however, Futagami and Hirakata [62] reported a case whose MRS recurred 3 years after the vitrectomy without ILM peeling and was successfully treated by the second surgery involving the ILM peeling.

Besides the dispute whether we should perform ILM peeling or not to treat MRS, another option would be to remove ILM completely in the macular area or outside the foveal area only. The development of a full-thickness MH is a serious complication in highly myopic eyes with a foveal

RD during and after vitrectomy [58]. This is important because a full-thickness MH is associated not only with reduced vision but also with a risk of developing a MH retinal detachment in highly myopic eyes [63–66]. It is difficult to obtain a closure of full-thickness MH in highly myopic eyes [67, 68].

The mechanisms of why and how full-thickness MHs develop postoperatively in eyes with foveal RD have not been fully determined; however, it is hypothesized that ILM peeling itself will increase the risk of developing a full-thickness MH. The mechanical traction on such a thinned central fovea by peeling the ILM off of the fovea could induce a break of the central foveal tissue. Another possibility is that when the retina moves backward to match the contour of the staphyloma after vitrectomy, the removal of ILM may reduce the structural strength of the fovea. Based on these concerns, Ho et al. [69] and Shimada et al. [70] reported the "foveola nonpeeling technique" or "fovea-sparing ILM peeling", respectively. For fovea-sparing ILM peeling, the ILM was grasped with an ILM forceps and peeled off in a circular fashion (Fig. 20.11), but the ILM was not completely removed and was left attached to the fovea. After the ILM was peeled from the entire macula area except the foveal area (in a circular area with a diameter approximately that of the vertical extent of the optic disc), the peeled ILM was trimmed with a vitreous cutter. Shimada et al. [70] reported that at around 3 months after fovea-sparing ILM peeling, a contraction of the remaining ILM at the fovea was observed as an irregular thickening of the retinal surface, and the outer lamellar hole became smaller or indistinct (Fig. 20.12). No further contraction of the remaining ILM was obvious after 3 months. None of the eyes with the fovea-sparing ILM peeling developed full-thickness MH [69, 70]. Although the longer follow-up in a large number of the patients as well as appropriate controls is necessary, these results are promising for the prevention of postoperative full-thickness MH formation. The combined release of macular traction and less surgical trauma to the central fovea led to a centripetal contraction of the remaining ILM, which is most likely why full-thickness MH did not develop.

The usefulness of scleral buckling with macular prombe for eyes with MRS and foveal RD without MH has also been reported [71–74]. However, complications including chorioretinal atrophy development and pre-existing fibrovascular proliferation were found [72], probably due to mechanical pressure and stretching of the retina-choroid by the protrusion of macular plombe. In addition, the posterior scleral reinforcement surgery [75, 76], an intraocular expansible gas, and prone posturing [77, 78] have been reported to treat MRS.

Recently, it has been reported that an intravitreal injection of the vitreolytic agent ocriplasmin resolved vitreomacular

Table 20.1 Summary of earlier studies reporting the functional and anatomical outcome of vitreous surgery against myopic traction maculopathy

Year	Author(s)	No. of eyes (patients)	Age (years) (mean) (range)	Axial length (mm) (mean) (range)	Preoperative OCT findings			Vitreous surgery		Postoperative OCT findings			Complications	Mean BCVA		Mean follow-up period (months)
					MRS	Foveal RD	FTMH	ILM peeling	Gas tamponade	Complete resolution of RD and MRS	Partial resolution of RD and MRS	Unchanged		Before surgery	After surgery	
2003	Kobayashi and Kishi	9 (7)	54.7 (36–74)	27.5 (26.5–28.5)	9/9 eyes	9/9 eyes	–	+	+	8/9 eyes	1/9 eyes	–	FTMH in 1 eye	0.17 (0.02–0.4)	0.48 (0.4–0.6)[a]	20.4
2003	Kanda	2 (2)	52 and 84	N/A	2/2 eyes	1/2 eyes	–	+	1/2 eyes	1/2 eyes	1/2 eyes	–	–	N/A	N/A	8 and 12
2004	Ikuno	6 (5)	59.5 (51–63)	29.2 (27.9–29.9)	6/6 eyes	6/6 eyes	–	+	+	5/6 eyes	1/6 eyes	–	–	N/A	N/A	14
2005	Spaide	6 (5)	61	N/A	4/6 eyes?	4/6 eyes?	–	–	+	6/6 eyes	–	–	–	20/100	20/60	19.1
2005	Kwok	9 (8)	52.7 (40–65)	29.0 (26.3–32.1)	9/9 eyes	9/9 eyes	–	+	+	7/9 eyes	2/9 eyes	–	–	20/80	20/50	17.2
2006	Hirakata	16 (14)	64.9 (53–77)	28.0 (24.9–30.2)	16/16 eyes	11/16 eyes	2/16 eyes	6/16 eyes	12/16 eyes	16/16 eyes	–	–	FTMH in 5 eyes	N/A	N/A	25.6
2006	Scott	3 (3)	53, 31, 69	32.6 mm in 1 case	3/3 eyes	2/3 eyes	–	2/3 eyes	3/3 eyes	3/3 eyes	–	–	–	N/A	N/A	8, 7, 1
2007	Pannozzo	24	58 (32–79)	N/A	24/24 eyes	5/24 eyes	–	24/24 eyes	–	23/24 eyes	–	1/24 eyes	FTMH in 5 eyes	logMAR 0.6 (1.1–0.2)	logMAR 0.43 (1.1 to –0.1)	29.6
2007	Gaucher	11	55 (43–70)	N/A	11/11 eyes	5/11 eyes	–	1/11 eyes	6/11 eyes	4/11 eyes	4/11 eyes	–	FTMH in 3 eyes	logMAR 0.97	logMAR 0.63	26.9
2008	Yeh	3 (3)	61, 62, 52	30.1, 28.8, 31.1	3/3 eyes	3/3 eyes	–	–	+	1/2 eyes	2/2 eyes	–	RRD and retinal breaks in one eye each	N/A	N/A	12
2008	Ikuno	44 (42)	63.3 (43–79)	29.1 (24.4–34.6)	16/44 eyes	17/44 eyes	11/44 eyes	+	+	44/44 eyes	–	–	FTMH in 2 eyes	N/A	N/A	12
2009	Fang	6 (6)	53.1	29	6/6 eyes	6/6 eyes	–	–	+	4/6 eyes	2/6 eyes	–	–	20/400	20/160	9.8
2010	Kumagai	39 (39)	66.3±8.3 (44–80)	28.6±2.3 (24.2–34.7)	39/39 eyes	27/39 eyes	–	+	34/39 eyes	39/39 eyes	–	–	–	logMAR 0.79±0.60	logMAR 0.54±0.60	6
2011	Zhang	18 (17)	51.3±13.7 (25–78)	29.7±2.1 (26.8–34.1)	18/18 eyes	12/18 eyes	–	+	11/18 eyes	18/18 eyes	–	–	–	logMAR 0.94 (2–0.15)	logMAR 0.49 (1.3–0.15)	17.5
2012	Kim	17 (17)	61.9 (44–78)	29.75 (27.80–32.95)	17/17 eyes	9/17 eyes	–	+	9/17 eyes	12/17 eyes	2/17 eyes	3/17 eyes	FTMH in 2 eyes	logMAR 0.81–0.83	logMAR 0.56	13 or 15.3
2012	Shin	38 (36)	63.5±9.5 (32–84)	29.16±1.92 (26.61–36.17)	38/38 eyes	7/38 eyes	2/38 eyes	+	+	34/38 eyes	3/38 eyes	–	FTMH in 1 eye	logMAR 0.841±0.534	logMAR 0.532±0.536	6

OCT optical coherence tomography, MRS macular retinoschisis, RD retinal detachment, FTMH full-thickness macular hole, ILM inner limiting membrane, BCVA best-corrected visual acuity, logMAR logarithm of minimum angle of resolution, N/A not applicable, RRD rhegmatogenous retinal detachment

[a]In the eight eyes without developing FTMH during surgery

Fig. 20.11 Schematic drawings of fovea-sparing internal limiting membrane (ILM) peeling. (**1**) Start ILM peeling away from the central fovea. (**2**) Proceed with the ILM peeling. (**3**) When the peeled ILM flap comes close to the central fovea, stop and start ILM peeling from a new site. (**4**) Proceed with ILM peeling from the new site with special attention not to peel the ILM around the central fovea. (**5**) Start the ILM peeling from several new sites, and proceed to peel ILM from the entire macular area away from the central fovea. (**6**) Trim the ILM that remains on and around the fovea with a vitreous cutter. (**7**) Completed fovea-sparing ILM peeling

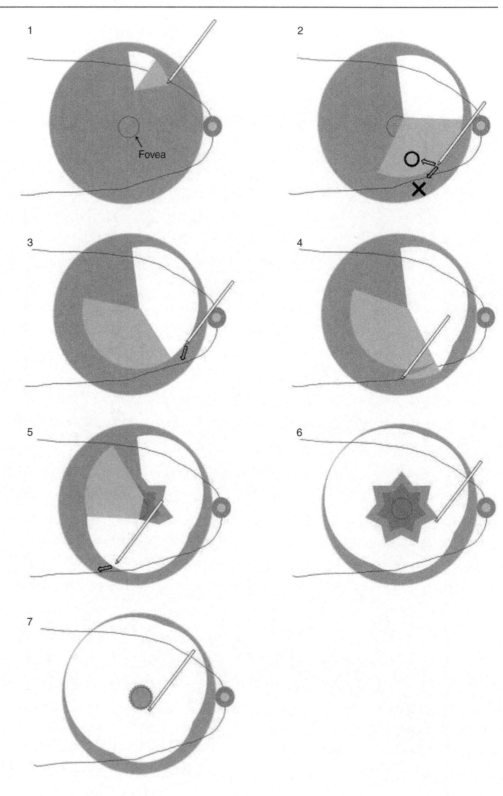

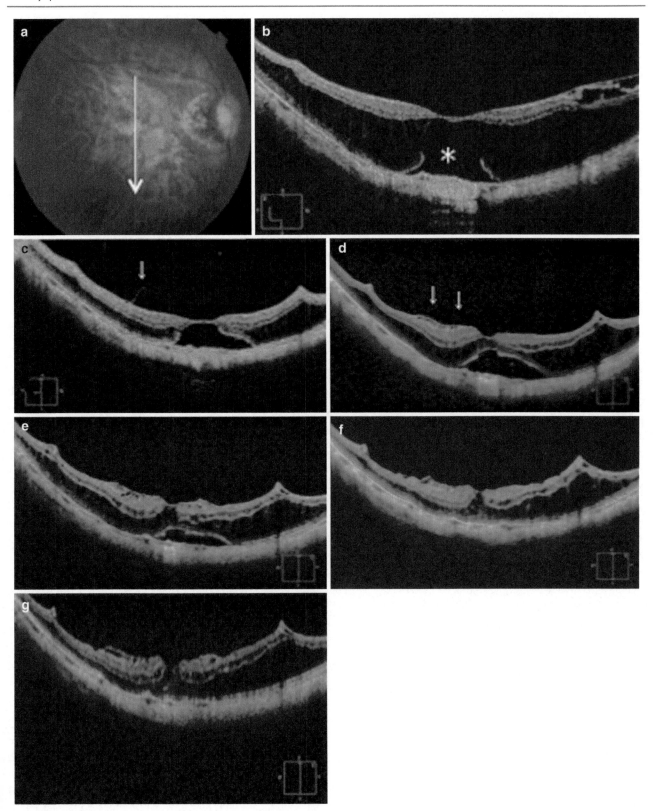

Fig. 20.12 Changes in optical coherence tomographic (OCT) findings after vitrectomy with fovea-sparing internal limiting membrane peeling and gas tamponade to treat myopic foveal retinal detachment (RD). (**a**) Preoperative fundus photograph. An arrow indicates the OCT scan line. (**b**) Preoperative OCT image of the same eye. Foveal RD with large outer lamellar macular hole (asterisk) and macular retinoschisis can be seen. (**c**) At 1 month after fovea-sparing ILM peeling, the retinoschisis is decreased along with the intraocular gas absorption. The foveal RD is still present although reduced. The rolled edges of the ILM (arrow) can be seen. (**d**) At

3 months after surgery, the residual ILM (between arrowheads) appears to have contracted and thickened. The retinoschisis is slightly increased and foveal RD is still present. However, the outer lamellar hole has become small (asterisk). (**e**) At 6 months after surgery, the retinoschisis and foveal RD are still present but decreased. (**f**) At 12 months after surgery, the foveal RD is completely resolved, and the retinoschisis is also decreased except at the lower macular area around the retinal artery which is observed as a retinal vascular microfold (arrow). (**g**) At 18 months (left) and 24 months (right) after surgery, the retinoschisis has been absorbed

traction and closed macular holes [79]. The usefulness of ocriplasmin fora MRS should be investigated in the future.

Also, a new approach involves suprachoroidal buckling using a catheter to deliver long-acting hyaluronic acid into the suprachoroidal space, which creates a choroidal indentation, thereby supporting the macula in the area of the posterior staphyloma. In a study of highly myopic eyes (five with MRS and seven with MHRD) treated with this technique, all patients with MRS achieved anatomical improvement, and four out of five improved vision by at least one line [80]. Among the eyes with MHRD, 57% showed improvement in visual acuity with no recurrence of RD at 1 year. The long-term outcomes of this approach are currently unknown. The scleral shortening in addition to vitrectomy might also be useful for difficult cases.

20.8 Other Types of Macular Retinal Detachments in Pathologic Myopia

20.8.1 Macular Hole Retinal Detachment (MHRD)

RD resulting from full-thickness MH occurs most commonly in highly myopic eyes [63, 66, 81]. Ripandelli et al. [46] reviewed OCT findings of 214 eyes with pathologic myopia (axial length >30 mm and posterior staphyloma) and found full-thickness MH in 18 eyes (8.4%). FTMH in highly myopic eyes is sometimes asymptomatic. Coppe et al. [82] examined 373 highly myopic patients with no visual disturbance and found FTMH in 24 eyes (6.26%). The absence of symptoms could be related to the localization of the hole in a juxtafoveal area. Akiba et al. [66] retrospectively analyzed 52 consecutive eyes with MH and severe myopia and found that an extensive RD was observed in 37 eyes (71%). Morita et al. [64] found the incidence of MHRD was 97.6% in myopia over −8.25 D, 67.7% in myopia between −8.0 and 3.25 D, and 1.1% in eyes under −3.0 D; 100% in widespread chorioretinal atrophy, 90.6% in spotty or linear chorioretinal atrophy, 64.3% in myopic tigroid fundus, and 0% in eyes without myopic tigroid or atrophy; and 96.0% in eyes with posterior staphyloma and 8.2% in eyes without staphyloma. Oie and Ikuno [83] reported that among various types of staphyloma by Curtin, the rate of type II staphyloma was significantly higher in the Japanese patients with MHRD. The fellow eyes of MHRD are reportedly at high risk of MHRD [84–86]. Oie and Emi [85] analyzed the fellow eyes of MHRD and found that the incidence of MHRD among the highly myopic fellow eyes was 12.8%.

Despite the surgical interventions, MHRD is still one of the most difficult types of RD to treat, with poor visual prognosis [87]. Nonclosure or reopening of the MH and RD may still develop, and in some patients, anatomical success may require multiple procedures.

MHRD in highly myopic eyes has been reported to develop following to some medical interventions like hypotony after trabeculectomy [88], after YAG laser capsulotomy [89], after cataract surgery [90], after clear lens extraction [91], and after LASIK [92, 93]. Shimada et al. [14] reported that a macular hole was detected by OCT in 14% of the eyes with CNV and large chorioretinal atrophy (>1 disc area). The hole always existed at the border between an old CNV and the surrounding chorioretinal atrophy. RD developed in 89% of eyes with complete PVD; thus it is suggested that posterior staphyloma rather than antero-posterior vitreomacular traction may contribute to the development of RD associated with MH in severely myopic eyes.

Surgical treatments for MHRD have been reported in many studies. The most common procedures appear to include the vitrectomy, removal of adherent vitreous cortex, removal of ERM, fluid-gas exchange, and intraocular gas (or silicone oil, if necessary) tamponade [81, 90, 94–101], although some studies reported the successful reattachment of MHRD without removal of ILM. Nakanishi et al. [102] analyzed prognostic factors in PPV for initial reattachment of MHRD and found that an axial length was the only significant prognostic factor for initial reattachment after PPV with gas tamponade for MHRD in high myopia. Jo et al. [34] reported that the presence of MRS negatively impacts the visual and anatomical prognosis of vitrectomy for full-thickness MH in highly myopic patients. The effectiveness of macular buckling has also been reported [103]. The inverted ILM flap technique was originally reported for idiopathic macular hole by Michalewska et al. [104]. In this technique, the ILM was not removed completely from the retina during vitrectomy but was left attached to the edge of the MH. The ILM was them massaged gently over the MH so that the MH was covered with the inverted ILM flap. Recently, Kuriyama et al. [105] reported that it was effective for a closure of myopic macular hole. Further studies are expected to confirm the effectiveness of this new technique.

20.8.2 Macular RD Associated with Peripapillary Intrachoroidal Cavitation (ICC)

ICC is a yellowish-orange lesion inferior to the optic disc seen in 4.9% of highly myopic eyes [40–43]. Spaide et al. [43] demonstrated the posterior deformation of the sclera in the area of ICC (see "Choroid" chapter). Shimada et al. [106] reported a case with high myopia in which a macular RD is accompanied with peripapillary ICC. In their patient, OCT examination revealed that the vitreous cavity was connected to the ICC space through a full-thickness tissue defect in the retina overlying the ICC and the ICC was continuous with the RD through the subretinal path at the conus area (Fig. 20.13). This suggested that the eyes with peripapillary ICC might be

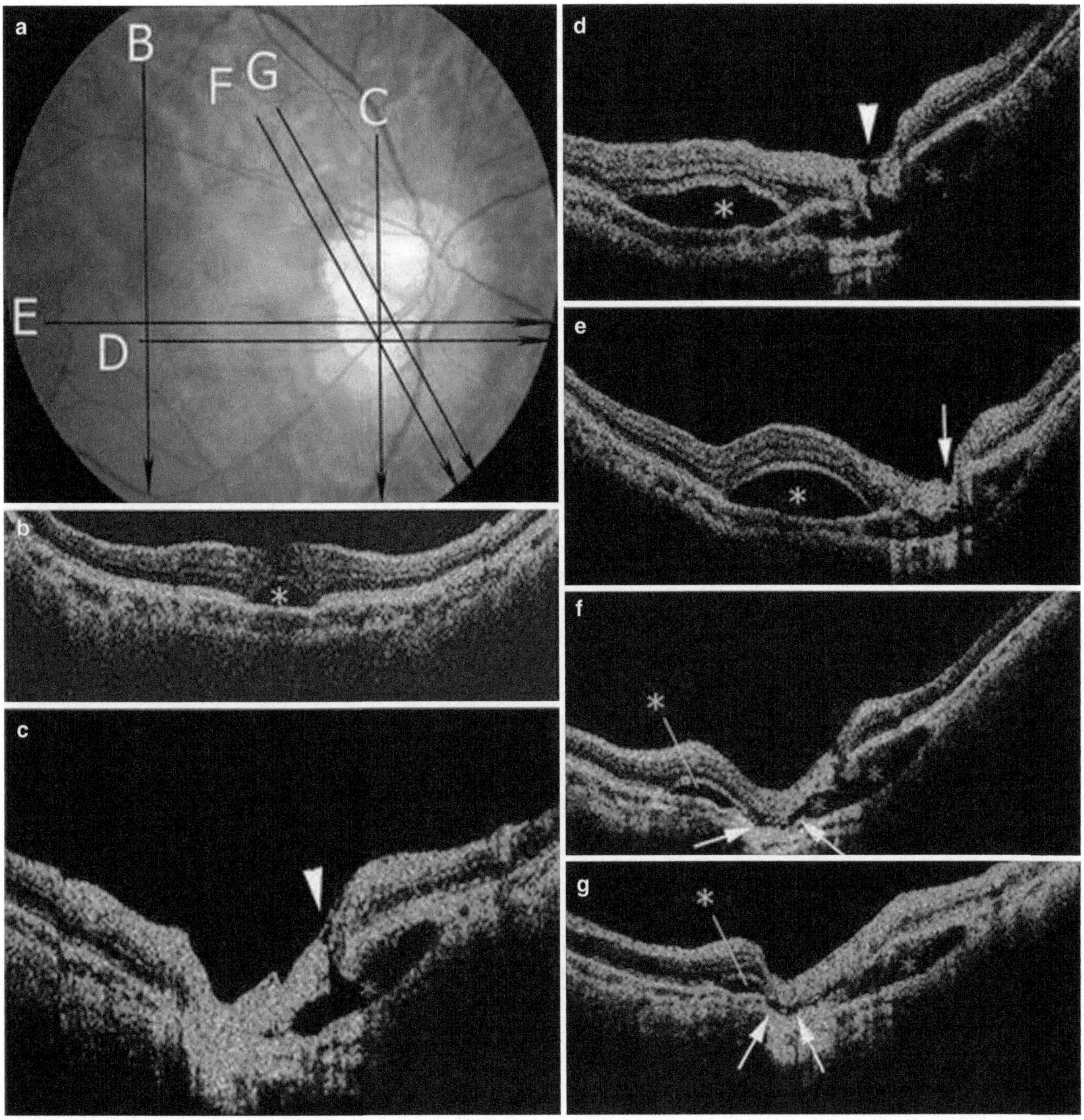

Fig. 20.13 Optical coherence tomographic images of the macular retinal detachment and intrachoroidal cavitation (ICC). (**a**) Each line shows an optical coherence tomography (OCT) scan for the images shown in (**b**–**f**) (scan length, 10 mm). (**b**)Vertical OCT section across the central fovea showing a retinal detachment (*asterisk*). (**c**) Vertical OCT section through the hole-like lesion within the area of chorioretinal atrophy showing a full-thickness defect at the hole-like lesion (*arrowhead*). The vitreous cavity is connected to the intrachoroidal cavity through this defect, suggestive of ICC (*red asterisk*). (**d**) Horizontal OCT section through the hole-like lesion within the area of chorioretinal atrophy shows an empty space at this lesion (*arrowhead*). The vitreous cavity is connected to the intrachoroidal cavity through this defect, suggestive of ICC (*red asterisks*). Retinal detachment is also detected (*yellow aster-*

isk) and is separated from ICC by the retinal pigment epithelial (RPE) layer. (**e**) Horizontal OCT section across the hole-like lesion at the border between myopic conus and chorioretinal atrophy shows a small hollow of the retina at the site (*arrow*). A full-thickness retinal defect is not observed in any adjacent sections. Intrachoroidal cavity suggestive of ICC (*red asterisks*) and retinal detachment (*yellow asterisk*) can also be seen. (**f**) Oblique OCT section through the hole-like lesion within the chorioretinal atrophy shows that the ICC (*red asterisks*) seems continuous with the retinal detachment (*yellow asterisk*) through the outer retinal schisis-like path at the conus area (*arrows*). (**g**) In the adjacent section of (**f**), the continuity of ICC with macular RD through the outer retinal schisis-like path is clearly observed

at risk of developing macular RD. Akimoto et al. [107] reported a similar case with macular RD and peripapillary ICC and without high myopia. Recently, Yeh and colleagues [108] analyzed 122 eyes with peripapillary ICC and found that 26.2% of the eyes with ICC were not highly myopic (< −6 D). These suggest that peripapillary ICC was not exclusive to highly myopic eyes, and peripapillary structural alterations like disc tilting might relate to the ICC development and subsequent formation of ICC-related macular RD.

20.8.3 RD Caused by a Retinal Break in and Along the Macular Atrophy or Patchy Atrophy

In addition to the MH, a retinal break reportedly develops within or along the margin of macular atrophy [109, 110]. Macular atrophy develops around the regressed CNV in the atrophic stage of myopic CNV [111, 112]; thus, these suggest that myopic CNV acts on the development of MRS and RD in various manners and in various stages of CNV. Chen et al. [110] reported cases which developed RD caused by paravascular linear retinal breaks over areas of patchy atrophy. Considering that patchy chorioretinal atrophy contributes on the development of MRS by forming macular ICC, patchy atrophy also acts on the development of MRS and RD in various manners, as seen in macular atrophy.

20.9   Closing Remarks

MRS is the macular lesion which was most recently identified by new imaging modalities in highly myopic eyes. However, after its discovery, the pathologies, the pathogenesis, and treatment options have been greatly investigated due to the advance of OCT technologies as well as the surgical techniques. It is certain that there will be a great improvement for understanding this pathology and preventing a vision loss due to MRS in the near future.

References

1. Takano M, Kishi S. Foveal retinoschisis and retinal detachment in severely myopic eyes with posterior staphyloma. Am J Ophthalmol. 1999;128(4):472–6.
2. Baba T, Ohno-Matsui K, Futagami S, et al. Prevalence and characteristics of foveal retinal detachment without macular hole in high myopia. Am J Ophthalmol. 2003;135(3):338–42.
3. Menchini U, Brancato R, Virgili G, Pierro L. Unilateral macular retinoschisis with stellate foveal appearance in two females with myopia. Ophthalmic Surg Lasers. 2000;31(3):229–32.
4. Panozzo G, Mercanti A. Optical coherence tomography findings in myopic traction maculopathy. Arch Ophthalmol. 2004;122(10):1455–60.
5. Fujimoto M, Hangai M, Suda K, Yoshimura N. Features associated with foveal retinal detachment in myopic macular retinoschisis. Am J Ophthalmol. 2010;150(6):863–70.
6. Tang J, Rivers MB, Moshfeghi AA, et al. Pathology of macular foveoschisis associated with degenerative myopia. J Ophthalmol. 2010;2010
7. Jiang C, Wang W, Xu G, Wang L. Retinoschisis at macular area in highly myopic eye by optic coherence tomography. Yan Ke Xue Bao. 2006;22(3):190–4.
8. Sayanagi K, Ikuno Y, Tano Y. Tractional internal limiting membrane detachment in highly myopic eyes. Am J Ophthalmol. 2006;142(5):850–2.
9. Benhamou N, Massin P, Haouchine B, et al. Macular retinoschisis in highly myopic eyes. Am J Ophthalmol. 2002;133(6):794–800.
10. Shinohara K, Shimada N, Moriyama M, et al. Posterior staphylomas in pathologic myopia imaged by widefield optical coherence tomography. Invest Ophthalmol Vis Sci. 2017;58(9):3750–8.
11. Shinohara K, Tanaka N, Jonas JB, et al. Ultra-widefield optical coherence tomography to investigate relationships between myopic macular retinoschisis and posterior staphyloma. Ophthalmology. 2018;125(10):1575–86.
12. Curcio CA, Allen KA. Topography of ganglion cells in human retina. J Comp Neurol. 1990;300(1):5–25.
13. Shimada N, Ohno-Matsui K, Yoshida T, et al. Progression from macular retinoschisis to retinal detachment in highly myopic eyes is associated with outer lamellar hole formation. Br J Ophthalmol. 2008;92(6):762–4.
14. Shimada N, Ohno-Matsui K, Yoshida T, et al. Development of macular hole and macular retinoschisis in eyes with myopic choroidal neovascularization. Am J Ophthalmol. 2008;145(1):155–61.
15. Tanaka Y, Shimada N, Ohno-Matsui K, et al. Retromode retinal imaging of macular retinoschisis in highly myopic eyes. Am J Ophthalmol. 2010;149(4):635–40 e1.
16. Hayashi W, Shimada N, Hayashi K, et al. Retinal vessels and high myopia. Ophthalmology. 2011;118(4):791–e2.
17. Sayanagi K, Ikuno Y, Tano Y. Different fundus autofluorescence patterns of retinoschisis and macular hole retinal detachment in high myopia. Am J Ophthalmol. 2007;144(2):299–301.
18. Wu PC, Chen YJ, Chen YH, et al. Factors associated with foveoschisis and foveal detachment without macular hole in high myopia. Eye. 2009;23(2):356–61.
19. Johnson MW. Myopic traction maculopathy: pathogenic mechanisms and surgical treatment. Retina. 2012;32(2).
20. Johnson MW. Perifoveal vitreous detachment and its macular complications. Trans Am Ophthalmol Soc. 2005;103:537–67.
21. Bando H, Ikuno Y, Choi JS, et al. Ultrastructure of internal limiting membrane in myopic foveoschisis. Am J Ophthalmol. 2005;139(1):197–9.
22. Chen L, Wei Y, Zhou X, et al. Morphologic, biomechanical, and compositional features of the internal limiting membrane in pathologic myopic foveoschisis. Invest Ophthalmol Vis Sci. 2018;59(13):5569–78.
23. Shimada N, Ohno-Matsui K, Nishimuta A, et al. Detection of paravascular lamellar holes and other paravascular abnormalities by optical coherence tomography in eyes with high myopia. Ophthalmology. 2008;115(4):708–17.
24. Shimada N, Ohno-Matsui K, Nishimuta A, et al. Peripapillary changes detected by optical coherence tomography in eyes with high myopia. Ophthalmology. 2007;114(11):2070–6.

25. Ikuno Y, Gomi F, Tano Y. Potent retinal arteriolar traction as a possible cause of myopic foveoschisis. Am J Ophthalmol. 2005;139(3):462–7.
26. Sayanagi K, Ikuno Y, Gomi F, Tano Y. Retinal vascular microfolds in highly myopic eyes. Am J Ophthalmol. 2005;139(4):658–63.
27. Ohno-Matsui K, Akiba M, Moriyama M. Macular pits and scleral dehiscence in highly myopic eyes with macular chorioretinal atrophy. Retinal Cases & Brief Reports. 2013; 7(4):334–7.
28. Ohno-Matsui K, Akiba M, Moriyama M, et al. Intrachoroidal cavitation in macular area of eyes with pathologic myopia. Am J Ophthalmol. 2012;154(2):382–93.
29. Ohno-Matsui K, Akiba M, Modegi T, et al. Association between shape of sclera and myopic retinochoroidal lesions in patients with pathologic myopia. Invest Ophthalmol Vis Sci. 2012;53(10):6046–61.
30. Chae JB, Moon BG, Yang SJ, et al. Macular gradient measurement in myopic posterior staphyloma using optical coherence tomography. Korean J Ophthalmol. 2011;25(4):243–7.
31. Gaucher D, Erginay A, Lecleire-Collet A, et al. Dome-shaped macula in eyes with myopic posterior staphyloma. Am J Ophthalmol. 2008;145(5):909–14.
32. Ikuno Y, Jo Y, Hamasaki T, Tano Y. Ocular risk factors for choroidal neovascularization in pathologic myopia. Invest Ophthalmol Vis Sci. 2010;51(7):3721–5.
33. Imamura Y, Iida T, Maruko I, et al. Enhanced depth imaging optical coherence tomography of the sclera in dome-shaped macula. Am J Ophthalmol. 2011;151(2):297–302.
34. Jo Y, Ikuno Y, Nishida K. Retinoschisis: a predictive factor in vitrectomy for macular holes without retinal detachment in highly myopic eyes. Br J Ophthalmol. 2012;96(2):197–200.
35. Maruko I, Iida T, Sugano Y, et al. Morphologic choroidal and scleral changes at the macula in tilted disc syndrome with staphyloma using optical coherence tomography. Invest Ophthalmol Vis Sci. 2011;52(12):8763–8.
36. Maruko I, Iida T, Sugano Y, et al. Morphologic analysis in pathologic myopia using high-penetration optical coherence tomography. Invest Ophthalmol Vis Sci. 2012;15:15.
37. Hayashi M, Ito Y, Takahashi A, et al. Scleral thickness in highly myopic eyes measured by enhanced depth imaging optical coherence tomography. Eye. 2013;27(3):410–7.
38. Alkabes M, Padilla L, Salinas C, et al. Assessment of OCT measurements as prognostic factors in myopic macular hole surgery without foveoschisis. Graefes Arch Clin Exp Ophthalmol. 2013;22:22.
39. Smiddy WE, Kim SS, Lujan BJ, Gregori G. Myopic traction maculopathy: spectral domain optical coherence tomographic imaging and a hypothesized mechanism. Ophthalmic Surg Lasers Imaging. 2009;40(2):169–73.
40. Freund KB, Ciardella AP, Yannuzzi LA, et al. Peripapillary detachment in pathologic myopia. Arch Ophthalmol. 2003;121(2):197–204.
41. Shimada N, Ohno-Matsui K, Yoshida T, et al. Characteristics of peripapillary detachment in pathologic myopia. Arch Ophthalmol. 2006;124(1):46–52.
42. Toranzo J, Cohen SY, Erginay A, Gaudric A. Peripapillary intrachoroidal cavitation in myopia. Am J Ophthalmol. 2005;140(4):731–2.
43. Spaide RF, Akiba M, Ohno-Matsui K. Evaluation of peripapillary intrachoroidal cavitation with swept source and enhanced depth imaging optical coherence tomography. Retina. 2012;32(6):1037–44.
44. Ellabban AA, Tsujikawa A, Matsumoto A, et al. Three-dimensional tomographic features of dome-shaped macula by swept-source optical coherence tomography. Am J Ophthalmol. 2012;3(12):578.
45. Shimada N, Ohno-Matsui K, Hayashi K, et al. Macular detachment after successful intravitreal bevacizumab for myopic choroidal neovascularization. Jpn J Ophthalmol. 2011;55(4):378–82.
46. Ripandelli G, Rossi T, Scarinci F, et al. Macular vitreoretinal interface abnormalities in highly myopic eyes with posterior staphyloma: 5-year follow-up. Retina. 2012;32(8):1531–8.
47. Shimada N, Ohno-Matsui K, Baba T, et al. Natural course of macular retinoschisis in highly myopic eyes without macular hole or retinal detachment. Am J Ophthalmol. 2006;142(3):497–500.
48. Gaucher D, Haouchine B, Tadayoni R, et al. Long-term follow-up of high myopic foveoschisis: natural course and surgical outcome. Am J Ophthalmol. 2007;143(3):455–62.
49. Sun CB, Liu Z, Xue AQ, Yao K. Natural evolution from macular retinoschisis to full-thickness macular hole in highly myopic eyes. Eye (Lond). 2010;24(12):1787–91.
50. Sayanagi K, Ikuno Y, Tano Y. Spontaneous resolution of retinoschisis and consequent development of retinal detachment in highly myopic eyes. Br J Ophthalmol. 2006;90(5):652–3.
51. Shimada N, Tanaka Y, Tokoro T, Ohno-Matsui K. Natural course of myopic traction maculopathy and factors associated with progression or resolution. Am J Ophthalmol. 2013;156(5):948–957.e1.
52. Tanaka Y, Shimada N, Moriyama M, et al. Natural history of lamellar macular holes in highly myopic eyes. Am J Ophthalmol. 2011;152(1):96–9.
53. Polito A, Lanzetta P, Del Borrello M, Bandello F. Spontaneous resolution of a shallow detachment of the macula in a highly myopic eye. Am J Ophthalmol. 2003;135(4):546–7.
54. Kanda S, Uemura A, Sakamoto Y, Kita H. Vitrectomy with internal limiting membrane peeling for macular retinoschisis and retinal detachment without macular hole in highly myopic eyes. Am J Ophthalmol. 2003;136(1):177–80.
55. Kobayashi H, Kishi S. Vitreous surgery for highly myopic eyes with foveal detachment and retinoschisis. Ophthalmology. 2003;110(9):1702–7.
56. Ikuno Y, Sayanagi K, Ohji M, et al. Vitrectomy and internal limiting membrane peeling for myopic foveoschisis. Am J Ophthalmol. 2004;137(4):719–24.
57. Kwok AK, Lai TY, Yip WW. Vitrectomy and gas tamponade without internal limiting membrane peeling for myopic foveoschisis. Br J Ophthalmol. 2005;89(9):1180–3.
58. Hirakata A, Hida T. Vitrectomy for myopic posterior retinoschisis or foveal detachment. Jpn J Ophthalmol. 2006;50(1):53–61.
59. Scott IU, Moshfeghi AA, Flynn HW Jr. Surgical management of macular retinoschisis associated with high myopia. Arch Ophthalmol. 2006;124(8):1197–9.
60. Yeh SI, Chang WC, Chen LJ. Vitrectomy without internal limiting membrane peeling for macular retinoschisis and foveal detachment in highly myopic eyes. Acta Ophthalmol. 2008;86(2):219–24.
61. Kuhn F. Internal limiting membrane removal for macular detachment in highly myopic eyes. Am J Ophthalmol. 2003;135(4):547–9.
62. Futagami S, Inoue M, Hirakata A. Removal of internal limiting membrane for recurrent myopic traction maculopathy. Clin Experiment Ophthalmol. 2008;36(8):782–5.
63. Siam A. Macular hole with central retinal detachment in high myopia with posterior staphyloma. Br J Ophthalmol. 1969;53(1):62–3.
64. Morita H, Ideta H, Ito K, et al. Causative factors of retinal detachment in macular holes. Retina. 1991;11(3):281–4.
65. Stirpe M, Michels RG. Retinal detachment in highly myopic eyes due to macular holes and epiretinal traction. Retina. 1990;10(2):113–4.
66. Akiba J, Konno S, Yoshida A. Retinal detachment associated with a macular hole in severely myopic eyes. Am J Ophthalmol. 1999;128(5):654–5.

67. Wu TT, Kung YH. Comparison of anatomical and visual outcomes of macular hole surgery in patients with high myopia vs. non-high myopia: a case-control study using optical coherence tomography. Graefes Arch Clin Exp Ophthalmol. 2012;250(3):327–31.

68. Patel SC, Loo RH, Thompson JT, Sjaarda RN. Macular hole surgery in high myopia. Ophthalmology. 2001;108(2):377–80.

69. Ho TC, Chen MS, Huang JS, et al. Foveola nonpeeling technique in internal limiting membrane peeling of myopic foveoschisis surgery. Retina. 2012;32(3):631–4.

70. Shimada N, Sugamoto Y, Ogawa M, et al. Fovea-Sparing Internal Limiting Membrane Peeling for Myopic Traction Maculopathy. Am J Ophthalmol. 2012;154(4):693–701.

71. Ripandelli G, Coppe AM, Fedeli R, et al. Evaluation of primary surgical procedures for retinal detachment with macular hole in highly myopic eyes: a comparison [corrected] of vitrectomy versus posterior episcleral buckling surgery. Ophthalmology. 2001;108(12):2258–64.

72. Baba T, Tanaka S, Maesawa A, et al. Scleral buckling with macular plombe for eyes with myopic macular retinoschisis and retinal detachment without macular hole. Am J Ophthalmol. 2006;142(3):483–7.

73. Mateo C, Bures-Jelstrup A, Navarro R, Corcostegui B. Macular buckling for eyes with myopic foveoschisis secondary to posterior staphyloma. Retina. 2012;32(6):1121–8.

74. Theodossiadis GP, Theodossiadis PG. The macular buckling procedure in the treatment of retinal detachment in highly myopic eyes with macular hole and posterior staphyloma: mean follow-up of 15 years. Retina. 2005;25(3):285–9.

75. Zhu Z, Ji X, Zhang J, Ke G. Posterior scleral reinforcement in the treatment of macular retinoschisis in highly myopic patients. Clin Experiment Ophthalmol. 2009;37(7):660–3.

76. Ward B, Tarutta EP, Mayer MJ. The efficacy and safety of posterior pole buckles in the control of progressive high myopia. Eye. 2009;23(12):2169–74.

77. Gili P, Yanguela J, Martin JC. Intraocular gas treatment for myopic foveoschisis. Eur J Ophthalmol. 2010;20(2):473–5.

78. Wu TY, Yang CH, Yang CM. Gas tamponade for myopic foveoschisis with foveal detachment. Graefes Arch Clin Exp Ophthalmol. 2012;10:10.

79. Stalmans P, Benz MS, Gandorfer A, et al. Enzymatic vitreolysis with ocriplasmin for vitreomacular traction and macular holes. N Engl J Med. 2012;367(7):606–15.

80. El Rayes EN. Supra choroidal buckling in managing myopic vitreoretinal interface disorders: 1-Year Data. Retina. 2013;23:23.

81. Ortisi E, Avitabile T, Bonfiglio V. Surgical management of retinal detachment because of macular hole in highly myopic eyes. Retina. 2012;32(9):1704–18.

82. Coppe AM, Ripandelli G, Parisi V, et al. Prevalence of asymptomatic macular holes in highly myopic eyes. Ophthalmology. 2005;112(12):2103–9.

83. Oie Y, Ikuno Y, Fujikado T, Tano Y. Relation of posterior staphyloma in highly myopic eyes with macular hole and retinal detachment. Jpn J Ophthalmol. 2005;49(6):530–2.

84. Tsujikawa A, Kikuchi M, Ishida K, et al. Fellow eye of patients with retinal detachment associated with macular hole and bilateral high myopia. Clin Experiment Ophthalmol. 2006;34(5):430–3.

85. Oie Y, Emi K. Incidence of fellow eye retinal detachment resulting from macular hole. Am J Ophthalmol. 2007;143(2):203–5.

86. Ripandelli G, Coppe AM, Parisi V, Stirpe M. Fellow eye findings of highly myopic subjects operated for retinal detachment associated with a macular hole. Ophthalmology. 2008;115(9):1489–93.

87. Kuriyama S, Matsumura M, Harada T, et al. Surgical techniques and reattachment rates in retinal detachment due to macular hole. Arch Ophthalmol. 1990;108(11):1559–61.

88. Higashide T, Nishimura A, Torisaki M, Sugiyama K. Retinal redetachment involving a macular hole resulting from hypotony after trabeculectomy in a highly myopic eye. Ophthalmic Surg Lasers Imaging. 2007;38(5):406–9.

89. Sakimoto S, Saito Y. Acute macular hole and retinal detachment in highly myopic eyes after neodymium:YAG laser capsulotomy. J Cataract Refract Surg. 2008;34(9):1592–4.

90. Zheng Q, Yang S, Zhang Y, et al. Vitreous surgery for macular hole-related retinal detachment after phacoemulsification cataract extraction: 10-year retrospective review. Eye. 2012;26(8):1058–64.

91. Ripandelli G, Billi B, Fedeli R, Stirpe M. Retinal detachment after clear lens extraction in 41 eyes with high axial myopia. Retina. 1996;16(1):3–6.

92. Arevalo JF, Rodriguez FJ, Rosales-Meneses JL, et al. Vitreoretinal surgery for macular hole after laser assisted in situ keratomileusis for the correction of myopia. Br J Ophthalmol. 2005;89(11):1423–6.

93. Arevalo JF, Mendoza AJ, Velez-Vazquez W, et al. Full-thickness macular hole after LASIK for the correction of myopia. Ophthalmology. 2005;112(7):1207–12.

94. Xie A, Lei J. Pars plana vitrectomy and silicone oil tamponade as a primary treatment for retinal detachment caused by macular holes in highly myopic eyes: a risk-factor analysis. Curr Eye Res. 2013;38(1):108–13.

95. Feng LG, Jin XH, Li JK, et al. Surgical management of retinal detachment resulting from macular hole in a setting of high myopia. Yan Ke Xue Bao. 2012;27(2):69–75.

96. Nadal J, Verdaguer P, Canut MI. Treatment of retinal detachment secondary to macular hole in high myopia: vitrectomy with dissection of the inner limiting membrane to the edge of the staphyloma and long-term tamponade. Retina. 2012;32(8):1525–30.

97. Kumar A, Tinwala S, Gogia V, Sinha S. Clinical presentation and surgical outcomes in primary myopic macular hole retinal detachment. Eur J Ophthalmol. 2012;22(3):450–5.

98. Nishimura A, Kimura M, Saito Y, Sugiyama K. Efficacy of primary silicone oil tamponade for the treatment of retinal detachment caused by macular hole in high myopia. Am J Ophthalmol. 2011;151(1):148–55.

99. Avitabile T, Bonfiglio V, Buccoliero D, et al. Heavy versus standard silicone oil in the management of retinal detachment with macular hole in myopic eyes. Retina. 2011;31(3):540–6.

100. Mete M, Parolini B, Maggio E, Pertile G. 1000 cSt silicone oil vs heavy silicone oil as intraocular tamponade in retinal detachment associated to myopic macular hole. Graefes Arch Clin Exp Ophthalmol. 2011;249(6):821–6.

101. Li KK, Tang EW, Li PS, Wong D. Double peel using triamcinolone acetonide and trypan blue in the management of myopic macular hole with retinal detachment: a case-control study. Clin Experiment Ophthalmol. 2010;38(7):664–8.

102. Nakanishi H, Kuriyama S, Saito I, et al. Prognostic factor analysis in pars plana vitrectomy for retinal detachment attributable to macular hole in high myopia: a multicenter study. Am J Ophthalmol. 2008;146(2):198–204.

103. Siam AL, El Maamoun TA, Ali MH. Macular buckling for myopic macular hole retinal detachment: a new approach. Retina. 2012;32(4):748–53.

104. Michalewska Z, Michalewski J, Adelman RA, Nawrocki J. Inverted internal limiting membrane flap technique for large macular holes. Ophthalmology. 2010;117(10):2018–25.

105. Kuriyama S, Hayashi H, Jingami Y, et al. Efficacy of inverted internal limiting membrane flap technique for the treatment of macular hole in high myopia. Am J Ophthalmol. 2013;24(13):00141–4.

106. Shimada N, Ohno-Matsui K, Iwanaga Y, et al. Macular retinal detachment associated with peripapillary detachment in pathologic myopia. Int Ophthalmol. 2009;29(2):99–102.

107. Akimoto M, Akagi T, Okazaki K, Chihara E. Recurrent macular detachment and retinoschisis associated with intrachoroidal cavitation in a normal eye. Case Report Ophthalmol. 2012;3(2):169–74.

108. Yeh SI, Chang WC, Wu CH, et al. Characteristics of peripapillary choroidal cavitation detected by optical coherence tomography. Ophthalmology. 2012;1(12):00812–3.

109. Baba T, Moriyama M, Nishimuta A, Mochizuki M. Retinal detachment due to a retinal break in the macular atrophy of a myopic choroidal neovascularization. Ophthalmic Surg Lasers Imaging. 2007;38(3):242–4.

110. Chen L, Wang K, Esmaili DD, Xu G. Rhegmatogenous retinal detachment due to paravascular linear retinal breaks over patchy chorioretinal atrophy in pathologic myopia. Arch Ophthalmol. 2010;128(12):1551–4.

111. Hayashi K, Ohno-Matsui K, Shimada N, et al. Long-term pattern of progression of myopic maculopathy: a natural history study. Ophthalmology. 2010;117(8):1595–611.

112. Yoshida T, Ohno-Matsui K, Yasuzumi K, et al. Myopic choroidal neovascularization: a 10-year follow-up. Ophthalmology. 2003;110(7):1297–305.

Surgical Approaches for Complications of PM

21

Ramin Tadayoni, Hiroko Terasaki, and Jun Takeuchi

21.1 Indication for Surgery

21.1.1 Introduction and Definitions

Recent improvements in surgical techniques, including visualization methods and specialized surgical instruments, have greatly expanded the options to improve visual function in patients with myopia. In particular, surgery has become more common for highly myopic eyes with complicated pathological conditions resulting from an extension of the axial length and expansion of the eyewall. Phillips first reported on retinal detachment without a full-thickness macular hole (FTMH) in eyes with high myopia in 1958, long before the development of optical coherence tomography (OCT) [1]. After the development of OCT, Takano and Kishi detected retinoschisis-like structures and tractional retinal detachment in eyes with high myopia and posterior staphylomas in 1999 [2]. These lesions are now considered to represent the prodromal stages of retinal detachment with a macular hole (MHRD) [3].

Use of the term "myopic traction maculopathy" (MTM) to describe all pathologic macular features generated by traction and associated with high myopia was proposed in 2004 by Panozzo and Mercanti [4]. MTM includes retinal thickening, macular retinoschisis-like structures, lamellar macular holes (lamellar MH), and foveal retinal detachment (FRD) (Fig. 21.1). These pathological features are thought to develop from the complex of traction forces from the adherent vitreous cortex, epiretinal membrane (ERM), internal limiting membrane (ILM), retinal vessel, and posterior staphyloma.

The incidence of MTM in highly myopic eyes has been reported to be from 9% to 34% [4, 5]. Gaucher et al. [6] reported that 6 of 18 eyes (33.3%) in patients with MTM who did not undergo surgery developed FTMH over a 3-year follow-up period. Shimada et al. [7] also reported on the natural course of 207 eyes of MTM over a minimum follow-up period of 24 months. According to their report, 26 of 207 eyes (12.6%) showed a progression of MTM. The authors also developed a new classification system where the eyes were divided into five groups based on the area of macular retinoschisis: no macular retinoschisis (stage 0); extra-foveal macular retinoschisis (stage 1); fovea-only macular retinoschisis (stage 2); foveal but not entire macular area macular retinoschisis (stage 3); and entire macular area macular retinoschisis (stage 4). Thirteen of twenty-eight eyes (42.9%) with stage 4 retinoschisis showed MTM progression, while 10.7% of these eyes improved without surgical treatment.

Therefore, surgical treatment such as pars plana vitrectomy (PPV) combined with internal limiting membrane (ILM) peeling at an appropriate time is recommended in order to release traction generated by the adherent vitreous cortex and ILM and prevent the development of FTMH and MHRD. However, because of the possibility of post-surgical complications that can reduce visual acuity, it is important to determine the best timing for surgical treatment.

21.1.2 Indications for Surgery

There are three conditions of surgical indications in pathologic myopia: MTM, FTMH, and MHRD. In FTMH and MHRD, surgery is indicated in most cases to prevent a significant loss of visual function. However, the value of surgery for MTM is much more controversial and requires careful consideration as to whether, and if so when, the surgery should be performed.

R. Tadayoni (✉)
Department of Ophthalmology, Université de Paris, AP-HP, Hôpital Lariboisière, Hôpital Fondation Adolphe de Rothschild, Paris, France
e-mail: ramin.tadayoni@aphp.fr

H. Terasaki · J. Takeuchi
Department of Ophthalmology, Nagoya University Hospital, Nagoya, Aichi, Japan
e-mail: terasaki@med.nagoya-u.ac.jp; takeuchi.jun@med.nagoya-u.ac.jp

© Springer Nature Switzerland AG 2021
R. F. Spaide et al. (eds.), *Pathologic Myopia*, https://doi.org/10.1007/978-3-030-74334-5_21

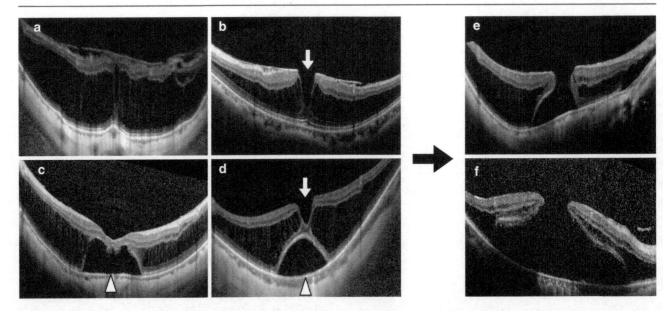

Fig. 21.1 Representative fovea in myopic traction maculopathy (MTM). (**a**) Retinoschisis. (**b**) Lamellar macular hole (lamellar MH). (**c**) Foveal retinal detachment (FRD). (**d**) FRD with lamellar MH. (**e**) Full-thickness macular hole (FTMH). (**f**) Macular hole retinal detachment (MHRD). Arrows indicate an intraretinal split and arrowheads indicate FRD

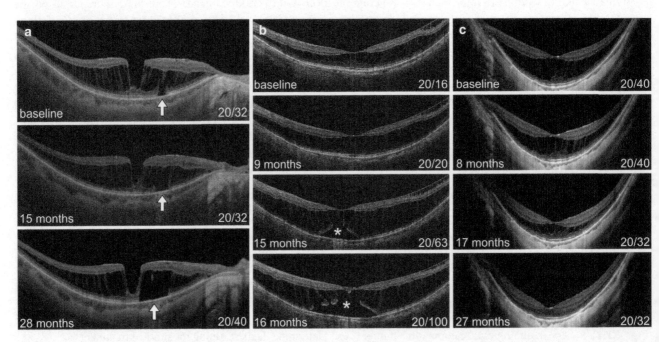

Fig. 21.2 Typical myopic traction maculopathy progression process. (**a**) 74 years old, female. The axial length is 27.43 mm. A pseudo-hole with a schisis-like structure is shown. Due to the progression of the defective ellipsoid zone and loss of intraretinal structure (white arrows), the risk of progression to the full-thickness macular hole was high, and surgery was performed. (**b**) 56 years old, male. The axial length is 29.37 mm. Macular schisis was observed from baseline. Gradually, the height of the macular schisis increased, and there was an accelerated expansion of the foveal retinal detachment (asterisks) and a decrease in visual acuity. Surgery was performed at this point. (**c**) 68 years old, male. The axial length is 29.00 mm. The macular schisis observed from baseline decreased gradually over the natural course and was completely resolved at 27 months. Visual acuity was maintained or increased during the follow-up period

21.1.2.1 Myopic Traction Maculopathy

In MTM, myopic retinoschisis is thought to progress to lamellar MH and/or FRD (Fig. 21.2a, b); some cases will also develop FTMH and/or MHRD. The onset of FTMH or MHRD irreversibly leads to a significant loss of visual function. Therefore, the important issue is at what point we should intervene.

Previous studies have reported that postoperative best-corrected visual acuity (BCVA) is correlated with preoperative BCVA [8, 9]. Additionally, a correlation between visual improvement resulting from surgical treatment for MTM and symptom duration has been reported [9]. Over a 24-month natural history, stage 4 macular retinoschisis will progress to foveal detachment or FTMH in about 43% eyes, whereas about 10% of the eyes will have a regression of the retinoschisis (Fig. 21.2c). Accordingly, eyes that have advanced past stage 4 may be at the earliest surgical indication of MTM.

To further evaluate indications for MTM surgery, we analyzed the relationships between pre-surgical OCT findings and surgical outcomes in a large case series of patients who underwent PPV for MTM [10]. Eyes with MTM were categorized into four types: retinoschisis-like structure without FRD (retinoschisis type), lamellar MH without FRD (lamellar MH type), FRD without lamellar MH (FRD type), and FRD with lamellar MH without FTMH (FRD + lamellar MH type) (Fig. 21.1). All except the lamellar MH type showed significantly increased BCVA after surgery, and all four types had moderately strong to strong positive correlations with pre- and postoperative BCVA. Eyes with FRD (FRD type and FRD + lamellar MH type) had significantly worse BCVA both pre- and postoperatively than did eyes without FRD (retinoschisis type and lamellar MH type). These results suggest that preoperative BCVA and the presence of FRD are important indicators for MTM surgery. Surgical intervention may also be recommended in stages without FRD but with good BCVA.

However, it should also be considered that there is potential for surgical complications. The most worrisome complication of MTM surgery is the formation of FTMH or MHRD. Postoperative FTMH and MHRD significantly reduce visual acuity and are often refractory, even with secondary surgery. In our data, postoperative FTMH or MHRD developed in 4 of 79 eyes (5.1%; FTMH in 3 eyes, MHRD in 1 eye) covering all MTM types except for macular schisis, and it should be noted that all of the complications occurred within 1 month of surgery. Similarly, Hwang et al. [11] reported that postoperative FTMH or MHRD developed in 1 of 28 eyes (3.6%) after PPV with ILM peeling, while Ikuno et al. [8] reported the same for 2 of 33 eyes (6.1%). However, in a more recent report, Gao et al. [12] reported a higher postoperative complication rate, with FTMH or MHRD developing in 8 of 42 eyes (19.0%) after PPV with ILM peeling. Reasons for these different results are not clear. However, the Gao et al. report was from a smaller case series (42 eyes). Further, they chose SF_6 for all intraocular tamponades, while we changed the tamponade material (air, SF_6, C_3F_8, silicone oil, or fluid) according to the preoperative stage of MTM. The authors also mentioned that the presence of an inner segment/outer segment junction defect, including FRD, was a risk factor for postoperative FTMH or MHRD. In our data [10], the risk of postoperative FTMH or MHRD in eyes of retinoschisis type without FRD and lamellar MH was lower

when compared with the other types. High-quality images and precise OCT evaluations are essential for the accurate assessment of risk factors for postoperative complications. Regardless, the incidence of FTMH or MHRD after PPV for MTM is not low, so the risk of surgical complications must be considered when assessing surgical indications. Conversely, it may be excessive to perform surgery in eyes that have gone without change for a long time. Therefore, a close monitoring of precise OCT, at a minimum of a monthly basis, is recommended.

As an additional factor in determining surgical indications, a new technique for MTM surgery called "foveal sparing" is becoming popular [13–15]. More details on this method will be described in a later chapter, but if the technique reduces the incidence of postoperative FTMH, surgical indications for MTM may become apparent at an earlier stage [16, 17].

In summary, patients with advanced MTM who have developed FRD with decreased visual acuity are indicated for surgery. Foregoing intervention may result in a further loss of visual acuity, and the macular retinoschisis may progress to FTMH in a natural course. However, indications are more controversial for MTM without FRD and with good visual acuity. In these cases, surgery at the early stage may suppress the progression of MTM and maintain visual acuity. Nevertheless, it is necessary to consider the risk of complications such as glaucoma. Therefore, we emphasize the importance of thorough preoperative anatomical examinations such as spectral-domain OCT or swept-source OCT to determine the exact changes in the outer retinal layer.

21.1.2.2 Full-Thickness Macular Hole

The goal of FTMH surgery is to close the MH and prevent progression to MHRD. In cases of chronic FTMH without a schisis-like structure or with non-progressive schisis and severe chorioretinal atrophy, follow-up without surgery is an option, although surgery is indicated in most cases.

The gold standard treatment for idiopathic FTMH is PPV with total ILM peeling, with reported anatomical closure rates greater than 90% [18–20]. In highly myopic MH, however, achieving anatomic and functional success in initial surgeries remains challenging [21]. Several techniques, such as the inverted ILM flap technique, have been proposed and put into practice to increase the closure rate of MH [22–25].

21.1.2.3 Retinal Detachment with a Macular Hole

The goal of surgery for MHRD is retinal reattachment and MH closure. Left untreated, regional retinal detachment with MH can progress to total retinal detachment so that surgical intervention is nearly always indicated.

Vitrectomy for MHRD was first reported in 1982 [26]. The procedure is approximately the same as for FTMH, but the reported MH closure rates of 35–60% are much lower than the rates of successful retinal reattachment [27–29]. However, as with FTMH, new techniques such as the ILM flap and autologous transplant have increased the rates of successful MH closure, further expanding indications for surgery [23, 29, 30].

21.2 Surgical Procedures

Complications of pathological myopia described before are treated when indicated by vitrectomy or scleral buckling. Scleral buckling is covered in another chapter. The term vitrectomy is used by extension for all intraocular surgeries that include vitrectomy but often other intraocular procedures too. Intraocular procedures for treating complications of pathological myopia include techniques used in other conditions too, as peeling of posterior hyaloid, but often with specific difficulties. Other techniques are mainly used for these pathological myopia-related complications as fovea sparing ILM peeling.

21.2.1 Vitrectomy

Vitrectomy is a common procedure for vitreoretinal surgery. However, in pathological myopia it has specificities at each stage. Sclera in these myopic eyes seems less elastic and fragile and then tends to release the cannulas and leak at the end of the surgery. Incision needs then higher attention than usual. They should be made with a blade inclined at 30–45° from the surface of the sclera. If the blade is not round shape but flattened, the flat face should be parallel to the surface of the sclera. During surgery one should be careful not to tension the edges of the incisions as they tend to easily enlarge and release the cannula or leak.

The volume of myopic eyes and the vitrectomy may need more time than usual. However, in many cases, the vitreous is liquefied with fibers concentrated in some areas of the vitreous cavity, mostly in the anterior part. Then vitreous seems as detached with a vitrectomy that seems quick and easy. In these cases, it should be suspected than other parts of the vitreous are remaining in the posterior part with the hyaloid still attached. When the visualization of the vitreous is difficult, a visualization agent can be used [31]. The most used agent is triamcinolone for which approved formulations are available in many countries. The trick here is to dilute the suspension far more than usual (e.g., 4–5 times more). This makes the vitreous conveniently visible without need to washout the excess. A good visualization is particularly critical for properly detaching the posterior hyaloid.

21.2.2 Posterior Hyaloid Detachment

Posterior vitreous attachment in pathological myopic eyes is abnormal [32]. In most of the eyes operated for macular complications of pathological myopia, the posterior vitreous is attached [32]. However, in some case condensations of vitreous fibers associated with large lacunas in the vitreous create the illusion of a posterior detachment. It will seem to the surgeon that he peels two layers of posteriori hyaloid which is sometimes referred to as posterior vitreoschisis [33]. If the hyaloid is not detached, it may preclude proper treatment of the complication indicating the vitrectomy. To avoid that, the surgeon must always consider the possibility of posterior hyaloid attachment and properly check it. Triamcinolone as described above can be used to reveal residual hyaloid. In some situation blue dyes can be used instead of triamcinolone to reveal the hyaloid if it is planned to use them for retinal staining [34]. Once the hyaloid is spotted, it should be peeled with caution. In highly myopic eyes, the vitreous base can be attached more posteriorly than usual. In some eyes abnormal attachments of the hyaloid around posterior vessels may induce a retinal break if peeled without caution. It still happens then that the dissection of the hyaloid has to be stopped more posteriorly than expected due to the high risk of a creating a break.

21.2.3 Epiretinal Membrane Peeling

When an epiretinal membrane is present, it is usually peeled. The basic principles remain unchanged compared to other eyes. A few particularities must be considered. Myopic eyes are longer than usual, and in some eyes it may be difficult to access the macula at the bottom of a deep staphyloma. Before injecting anything, one should check if he can aspirate it afterward. Longer instruments are proposed by several manufacturers and may be necessary in eyes with highest axial length. A trick that can help to increase the attainable depth by a too short instrument is to pull out the cannula, which remove a few millimeters of thickness at entry side, and enter the eye directly through sclerotomy. Staining of the epiretinal membrane is often needed in a low-contrast fundus. In some myopic eyes, the epiretinal membrane is in fact an epiretinal proliferation as described for lamellar macular holes [35]. In this case the proliferation is often yellowish and often attached to the center of the fovea. The attach may be firm, and one should take care not to open the center of the macula by pulling too hard on it. If needed, it can be just shortened close to the surface of the macula and left.

21.2.4 Internal Limiting Membrane Peeling

The basic techniques of internal limiting membrane (ILM) peeling are similar to other eyes. Here, due to low contrast, even more than in emmetropic eyes, staining is needed to allow a safe and controlled peeling. In myopic eyes, specific patterns of ILM peeling have been proposed. Fovea-sparing ILM peeling has been proposed to avoid fragilizing the center of the fovea and by doing this to reduce the risk of induced macular hole [15–17]. ILM flap techniques have been described in different varieties with the same goal of covering a hole by the ILM to increase its chances of closure [22, 23, 30]. One of the easiest and reproducible techniques is to leave piece of ILM attached to the temporal side the hole and to invert it to cover the hole. As often last drops of intraocular fluid are aspirated close to the optic nerve head, the liquid flow will help to pull the flap over the hole and increase chance of the flap sticking over the hole.

21.2.5 Other Procedures

Macular indentation, which is also proposed for treating macular complications of pathological myopia, is described in another chapter. Other procedures can be needed or useful to treat retinal conditions related to pathological myopia. They differ little or no from the techniques in the other eyes. These can include all classical techniques as laser, gas, or silicone injections. Indications of techniques to treat complications of pathological myopia are specified with the description of diseases in this chapter and in other chapters.

21.3 Intraoperative and Postoperative Complications

21.3.1 Intraoperative Complications

Some complications of intraocular surgery occur more frequently in the eyes with pathological myopia. Vitreous in pathological myopia can be firmly attached to the posterior part of the retina in particular around large retinal vessels. Posterior vitreous detachment can then cause a posterior break that can lead to a retinal detachment later. The risk is of particular significance if the tear is in a staphyloma and/or the vitreous can't be detached further and may apply traction on the edge of the break postoperatively. This complication can be prevented by cautious peeling of the posterior detachment and can be treated by applying laser around the break.

Peeling of the internal limiting membrane in particular when the macula is detached and very thin can induce a macular hole. The diagnosis of such a hole may not be easy and can be facilitated by an intraoperative OCT [36]. This complication can be prevented by cautious dissection of any structure close to the center of the fovea and by fovea sparing dissection when possible. If a macular hole appears during the surgery, the following steps of the surgery must be adapted to treat it as a myopic macular hole. For holes that are so small that intraoperative OCT can reveal them, they may not be yet proof that treating them is mandatory, but the rate of postoperative macular hole after macular surgery was high enough to be in favor of not ignoring a hole as small as it is [15, 36].

Highly myopic eyes are at high risk of presenting intraoperative suprachoroidal hemorrhage that can be massive and severe. Prevention of this complication is done by avoiding low intraocular pressure and any trauma to the choroid during surgery. If a hemorrhage appears and tends to increase, the intraocular pressure should be raised as much as possible for at least 2 minutes. If the hemorrhage does not stop, in some case it would be safer to stop the surgery and close the eye to avoid an expulsive hemorrhage.

As the sclera is thin and less elastic in pathological myopia, sclerotomies tend more to leak at the end of the surgery. This can be prevented by reducing as much as possible any force applied by instruments at their level. If a leakage is noticed, it should be treated by appropriate suturing to avoid any postoperative hypotonia that can lead to a dramatic suprachoroidal hemorrhage.

21.3.2 Postoperative Complications

Several postoperative complications echo intraoperative complications exposed in the previous section: a macular hole can appear even with best intraoperative precautions; if a posterior break is induced and not treated, it will lead to a posterior retinal detachment, and if the eyes remain hypotonic, a postoperative suprachoroidal hemorrhage can appear postoperatively. Even in the eyes perfectly handled, such a hemorrhage can appear in particular after general anesthesia followed by violent coughing fits, which should be avoided by the anesthesia team. All these impose a close postoperative surveillance by a team trained for such surgeries. Myopic eyes can also present all the main usual complications of vitrectomies (endophthalmitis, cataract, and retinal detachment) with sometimes higher rates. One is of particular interest and should be discussed even before the surgery: cataract. Pathological myopic eyes tend to present cataract at earlier ages, and vitrectomy that accelerate cataract formation, in particular when tamponade is also used, will be often followed by a cataract that can decrease again the visual acuity. This complication here is more problematic than in emmetropes as cataract surgery is often a chance for these patients to reduce their high myopia. However, if the other eye doesn't present any cataract and only the eye that had vitrectomy need cataract extraction, reducing myopia will lead to anisometropia. If contact lens is used, this may not be a problem as contacts eliminate the anisometropia, but when patients can only wear eyeglasses, the anisometropia can be a complicated condition to handle.

21.4   Usefulness of Intraoperative OCT

In macular disease surgery, pre- and postoperative morphological evaluations are mainly performed using optical coherence tomography (OCT). However, intraoperative OCT (iOCT) remains uncommon, even in macular surgery. In surgery for myopic macular retinoschisis with or without a foveal-sparing technique, enhanced three-dimensional visualization of the retinal morphology is important to find intraoperative complications, such as a macular hole (MH), and to

prevent a second surgery for postoperative MH or macular hole retinal detachment (MHRD) [36, 37]. Correct positioning of the internal limiting membrane (ILM) flap in the inverted ILM flap technique for highly myopic MH and MHRD requires visualization of the ILM [38–41]. Dyes such as indocyanine green (ICG) and brilliant blue G (BBG) can enable visualization of the ILM in en face mode, but there is a potential for toxicity by illumination. The thickness of the retinal tissue and the depth of the MH when staffing the ILM are very important for ILM management. In this section, we introduce some examples of iOCT use in the management of complications associated with high myopia surgery.

The first application is foveal-sparing ILM peeling in surgery for myopic retinoschisis. Here, a three-dimensional assessment with iOCT will inform the surgeon's judgment of how close the ILM should be peeled toward the foveal center (Fig. 21.3).

Second, iOCT can be used to find MH development during surgery and to decide on additional procedures,

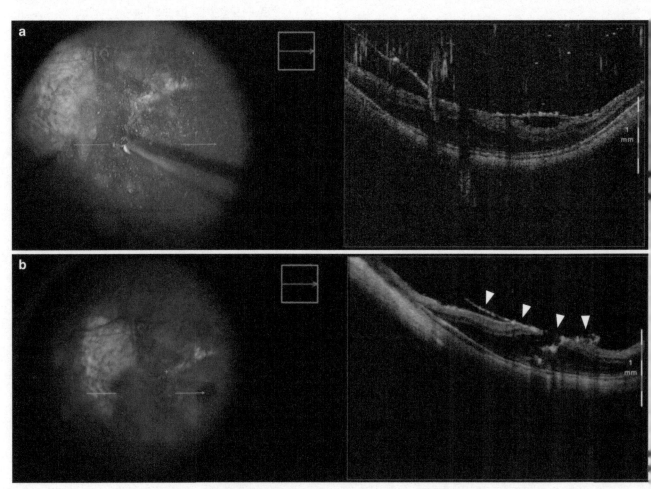

Fig. 21.3 A case of foveal-sparing ILM peeling for myopic traction maculopathy. A 55-year-old female presented macular schisis-like structure with an epiretinal membrane (ERM). The axial length was 29.16 mm. Intraoperative OCT (iOCT) revealed ERM peeling enhanced by triamcinolone acetonide particles (**a**) and foveal-sparing ILM peeling using BBG as staining. Finally, a partially preserved ILM can be seen at the fovea (**b**, arrowheads)

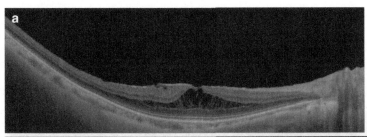

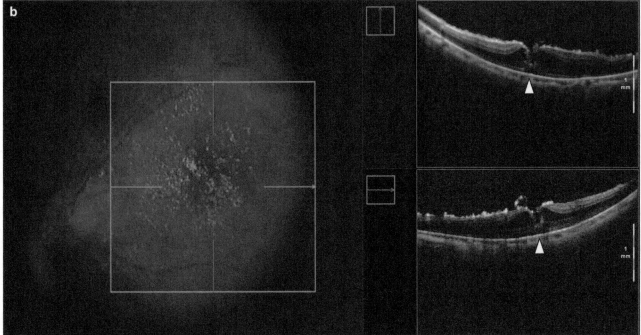

Fig. 21.4 A case of myopic traction maculopathy in which micro MH developed intraoperatively. A 65-year-old woman with myopic schisis-like structure in the preoperative OCT (**a**). The axial length was 26.84 mm. Initially, foveal sparing peeling was attempted, but the ILM was totally peeled unintentionally. Precise examination of the fovea by iOCT revealed a micro MH with an ellipsoid zone defect (**b**, arrowheads). Therefore, C_3F_8 was used for intraocular tamponade, followed by a postoperative face-down position to close the MH. As a result, the MH closed, and the defect of the ellipsoid zone disappeared

such as the selection of tamponade to prevent postoperative MH opening and subsequent MHRD development (Fig. 21.4).

Third, iOCT allows surgeons to check the positioning of the ILM flap during the stuffing of the ILM in the MH and after the fluid-air exchange before the end of the procedure, ensuring the success of the inverted ILM flap technique for large MHs (Fig. 21.5)..

Another extraordinary indication for the complication of myopic eye surgery is autologous neurosensory retinal flap transplantation (ART) for refractory highly myopic MH [42, 43]. In this surgery, the MH is closed by implanting an autologous retinal flap harvested from the peripheral retina. To ensure closure of the refractory MH, the retinal flap must be implanted in an appropriate location. Here, iOCT can indicate the correct position of the retinal graft (Fig. 21.6)..

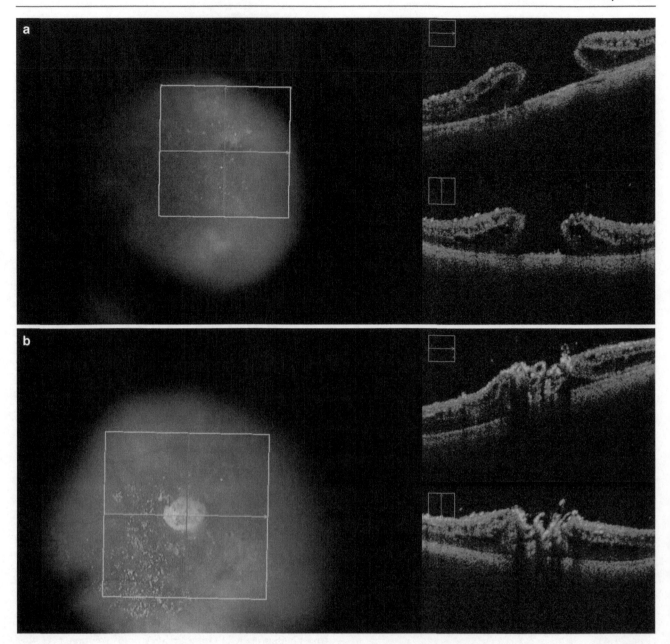

Fig. 21.5 A case of an inverted ILM flap technique for a MH developed after previous surgery. A 69-year-old female. The axial length was 27.75 mm. The MH developed after the first pars plana vitrectomy for the epiretinal membrane in the myopic eye, so a second surgery was performed. iOCT showed MH with remaining ILM during surgery (**a**).

Therefore, an inverted ILM flap was inserted into the MH with iOCT guidance (**b**). Immediately before the end of surgery after fluid-air exchange, it was confirmed that the ILM flap remained in an appropriate position

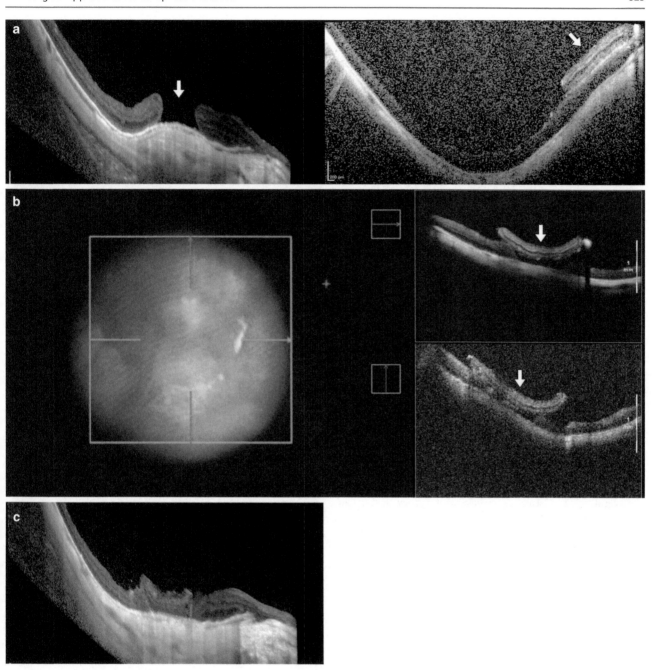

Fig. 21.6 A case in which the retinal flap was dislocated after the autologous retinal transplant (ART) and repositioned. An 80-year-old male with refractory MH after pars plana vitrectomy with ILM peeling and macular buckling. The axial length is 28.78 mm. ART was performed to close the refractory MH, but the retinal flap dislocated 4 days after surgery. Therefore, retinal flap repositioning was performed. Preoperative OCT images showing the dislocated retinal flap and recurrent MH (**a**, arrows). Retinal flap repositioning was performed, and the anatomical closure of the MH was confirmed by iOCT during surgery (**b**, arrows) and postoperative OCT (**c**)

References

1. Phillips CI. Retinal detachment at the posterior pole. Br J Ophthalmol. 1958;42(12):749–53.
2. Takano M, Kishi S. Foveal retinoschisis and retinal detachment in severely myopic eyes with posterior staphyloma. Am J Ophthalmol. 1999;128(4):472–6.
3. Kobayashi H, Kishi S. Vitreous surgery for highly myopic eyes with foveal detachment and retinoschisis. Ophthalmology. 2003;110(9):1702–7.
4. Panozzo G, Mercanti A. Optical coherence tomography findings in myopic traction maculopathy. Arch Ophthalmol. 2004;122(10):1455–60.
5. Baba T, Ohno-Matsui K, Futagami S, Yoshida T, Yasuzumi K, Kojima A, et al. Prevalence and characteristics of foveal reti-

nal detachment without macular hole in high myopia. Am J Ophthalmol. 2003;135(3):338–42.

6. Gaucher D, Haouchine B, Tadayoni R, Massin P, Erginay A, Benhamou N, et al. Long-term follow-up of high myopic foveoschisis: natural course and surgical outcome. Am J Ophthalmol. 2007;143(3):455–62.

7. Shimada N, Tanaka Y, Tokoro T, Ohno-Matsui K. Natural course of myopic traction maculopathy and factors associated with progression or resolution. Am J Ophthalmol. 2013;156(5):948–57.e1.

8. Ikuno Y, Sayanagi K, Soga K, Oshima Y, Ohji M, Tano Y. Foveal anatomical status and surgical results in vitrectomy for myopic foveoschisis. Jpn J Ophthalmol. 2008;52(4):269–76.

9. Kumagai K, Furukawa M, Ogino N, Larson E. Factors correlated with postoperative visual acuity after vitrectomy and internal limiting membrane peeling for myopic foveoschisis. Retina. 2010;30(6):874–80.

10. Hattori K, Kataoka K, Takeuchi J, Ito Y, Terasaki H. Predictive factors of surgical outcomes in vitrectomy for myopic traction maculopathy. Retina. 2018;38(1):S23–30.

11. Hwang JU, Joe SG, Lee JY, Kim JG, Yoon YH. Microincision vitrectomy surgery for myopic foveoschisis. Br J Ophthalmol. 2013;97(7):879–84.

12. Gao X, Ikuno Y, Fujimoto S, Nishida K. Risk factors for development of full-thickness macular holes after pars plana vitrectomy for myopic foveoschisis. Am J Ophthalmol. 2013;155(6):1021–7.e1.

13. Ho TC, Chen MS, Huang JS, Shih YF, Ho H, Huang YH. Foveola nonpeeling technique in internal limiting membrane peeling of myopic foveoschisis surgery. Retina. 2012;32(3):631–4.

14. Ho TC, Yang CM, Huang JS, Yang CH, Yeh PT, Chen TC, et al. Long-term outcome of foveolar internal limiting membrane nonpeeling for myopic traction maculopathy. Retina. 2014;34(9):1833–40.

15. Shimada N, Sugamoto Y, Ogawa M, Takase H, Ohno-Matsui K. Fovea-sparing internal limiting membrane peeling for myopic traction maculopathy. Am J Ophthalmol. 2012;154(4):693–701.

16. Iwasaki M, Miyamoto H, Okushiba U, Imaizumi H. Fovea-sparing internal limiting membrane peeling versus complete internal limiting membrane peeling for myopic traction maculopathy. Jpn J Ophthalmol. 2020;64(1):13–21.

17. Shiraki N, Wakabayashi T, Ikuno Y, Matsumura N, Sato S, Sakaguchi H, et al. Fovea-sparing versus standard internal limiting membrane peeling for myopic traction maculopathy: a study of 102 consecutive cases. Ophthalmol Retina. 2020;4(12):1170–80. https://doi.org/10.1016/j.oret.2020.05.016.

18. Lois N, Burr J, Norrie J, Vale L, Cook J, McDonald A, et al. Internal limiting membrane peeling versus no peeling for idiopathic full-thickness macular hole: a pragmatic randomized controlled trial. Invest Ophthalmol Vis Sci. 2011;52(3):1586–92.

19. Spiteri Cornish K, Lois N, Scott NW, Burr J, Cook J, Boachie C, et al. Vitrectomy with internal limiting membrane peeling versus no peeling for idiopathic full-thickness macular hole. Ophthalmology. 2014;121(3):649–55.

20. Ando F, Sasano K, Ohba N, Hirose H, Yasui O. Anatomic and visual outcomes after indocyanine green-assisted peeling of the retinal internal limiting membrane in idiopathic macular hole surgery. Am J Ophthalmol. 2004;137(4):609–14.

21. Wu TT, Kung YH. Comparison of anatomical and visual outcomes of macular hole surgery in patients with high myopia vs. non-high myopia: a case-control study using optical coherence tomography. Graefes Arch Clin Exp Ophthalmol. 2012;250(3):327–31.

22. Michalewska Z, Michalewski J, Adelman RA, Nawrocki J. Inverted internal limiting membrane flap technique for large macular holes. Ophthalmology. 2010;117(10):2018–25.

23. Kuriyama S, Hayashi H, Jingami Y, Kuramoto N, Akita J, Matsumoto M. Efficacy of inverted internal limiting membrane flap technique for the treatment of macular hole in high myopia. Am J Ophthalmol. 2013;156(1):125–31.

24. Hayashi H, Kuriyama S. Foveal microstructure in macular holes surgically closed by inverted internal limiting membrane flap technique. Retina. 2014;34(12):2444–50.

25. Michalewska Z, Michalewski J, Dulczewska-Cichecka K, Nawrocki J. Inverted internal limiting membrane flap technique for surgical repair of myopic macular holes. Retina. 2014;34(4):664–9.

26. Gonvers M, Machemer R. A new approach to treating retinal detachment with macular hole. Am J Ophthalmol. 1982;94(4):468–72.

27. Arias L, Caminal JM, Rubio MJ, Cobos E, Garcia-Bru P, Filloy A, et al. Autofluorescence and axial length as prognostic factors for outcomes of macular hole retinal detachment surgery in high myopia. Retina. 2015;35(3):423–8.

28. Nishimura A, Kimura M, Saito Y, Sugiyama K. Efficacy of primary silicone oil tamponade for the treatment of retinal detachment caused by macular hole in high myopia. Am J Ophthalmol. 2011;151(1):148–55.

29. Chen SN, Yang CM. Inverted internal limiting membrane insertion for macular hole–associated retinal detachment in high myopia. Am J Ophthalmol. 2016;162:99–106.e1.

30. Kinoshita T, Onoda Y, Maeno T. Long-term surgical outcomes of the inverted internal limiting membrane flap technique in highly myopic macular hole retinal detachment. Graefes Arch Clin Exp Ophthalmol. 2017;255(6):1101–6.

31. Sakamoto T, Ishibashi T. Visualizing vitreous in vitrectomy by triamcinolone. Graefes Arch Clin Exp Ophthalmol. 2009;247(9):1153–63.

32. Philippakis E, Couturier A, Gaucher D, Gualino V, Massin P, Gaudric A, et al. Posterior vitreous detachment in highly myopic eyes undergoing vitrectomy. Retina. 2016;36(6):1070–5.

33. Liu HY, Zou HD, Liu K, Song ZY, Xu X, Sun XD. Posterior vitreous cortex contributes to macular hole in highly myopic eyes with retinal detachment. Chin Med J. 2011;124(16):2474–9.

34. Vote BJ, Russell MK, Joondeph BC. Trypan blue-assisted vitrectomy. Retina. 2004;24(5):736–8.

35. Hubschman JP, Govetto A, Spaide RF, Schumann R, Steel D, Figueroa MS, et al. Optical coherence tomography-based consensus definition for lamellar macular hole. Br J Ophthalmol. 2020;104(12):1741–7.

36. Bruyère E, Philippakis E, Dupas B, Nguyen-Kim P, Tadayoni R, Couturier A. Benefit of intraoperative optical coherence tomography for vitreomacular surgery in highly myopic eyes. Retina. 2018;38(10):2035–44.

37. Itoh Y, Inoue M, Kato Y, Koto T, Hirakata A. Alterations of foveal architecture during vitrectomy for myopic retinoschisis identified by intraoperative optical coherence tomography. Ophthalmologica. 2019;242(2):87–97.

38. Jenkins TL, Adam MK, Hsu J. Intraoperative optical coherence tomography of internal limiting membrane flap. Ophthalmology. 2017;124(10):1456.

39. Lytvynchuk LM, Falkner-Radler CI, Krepler K, Glittenberg CG, Ahmed D, Petrovski G, et al. Dynamic intraoperative optical coherence tomography for inverted internal limiting membrane flap technique in large macular hole surgery. Graefes Arch Clin Exp Ophthalmol. 2019;257(8):1649–59.

40. Borrelli E, Palmieri M, Aharrh-Gnama A, Ciciarelli V, Mastropasqua R, Carpineto P. Intraoperative optical coherence tomography in the full-thickness macular hole surgery with internal limiting membrane inverted flap placement. Int Ophthalmol. 2019;39(4):929–34.

41. Lorusso M, Micelli Ferrari L, Cicinelli MV, Nikolopoulou E, Zito R, Bandello F, et al. Feasibility and safety of intraoperative optical coherence tomography-guided short-term posturing prescription after macular hole surgery. Ophthalmic Res. 2020;63(1):18–24.

42. Grewal DS, Mahmoud TH. Autologous neurosensory retinal free flap for closure of refractory myopic macular holes. JAMA Ophthalmol. 2016;134(2):229–30.

43. Grewal DS, Charles S, Parolini B, Kadonosono K, Mahmoud TH. Autologous retinal transplant for refractory macular holes: Multicenter International Collaborative Study Group. Ophthalmology. 2019;126(10):1399–408.

Peripheral Retinal Abnormalities

Peripheral Retinal Abnormalities

22

22

Sarah Mrejen, Gerardo Ledesma-Gil,
and Michael Engelbert

22.1 Introduction

The major peripheral vitreoretinal and/or chorioretinal changes associated with pathologic myopia are lattice degeneration, white-without-pressure, pigmentary degeneration, paving stone degeneration, retinal holes, retinal tears, and retinal detachment. Each of these entities has a distinct morphology and prevalence varying with age and axial length. They are all prone to progression, although the number and extent of the lattice lesions tend to not progress after the teens. The dynamic interaction between the vitreous and the retina plays an important role in the development, appearance, and progression of these peripheral retinal changes. The combination of abnormal vitreoretinal adhesion, traction by posterior vitreous detachment, and liquefied vitreous gel that can enter the subretinal space through retinal breaks is necessary to produce a rhegmatogenous retinal detachment. High myopes have an increased liquid component of the vitreous gel, associated with reduced viscosity and stability [1] and abnormal vitreoretinal adhesion, whether visible, such as lattice degeneration, or invisible, possibly leading to retinal breaks. They also tend to experience vitreous detachment at a younger age compared to emmetropic subjects [2]. Therefore, high myopes have an increased frequency of rhegmatogenous retinal detachments, often at a younger age.

The recognition of the peripheral retinal changes associated with high myopia through careful ophthalmoscopic examination and possibly additional wide-field retinal imaging is critical because lattice degeneration is frequently associated with retinal breaks and rhegmatogenous retinal detachments while white-without-pressure, paving stone, and pigmentary degeneration are usually benign. Some important peripheral findings are seen in syndromic myopia such as Stickler syndrome.

22.2 Lattice Degeneration

Lattice degeneration is acknowledged to be the most important clinically recognizable vitreoretinal abnormality in pathologic myopia [3]. In 1904, Gonin was the first to describe the histologic appearance of an equatorial lesion consistent with lattice degeneration in an enucleated globe from a patient with retinal detachment [4]. Lattice is known to be closely associated with retinal breaks and therefore to be a potential precursor of rhegmatogenous retinal detachment. Even though this entity has been widely described both clinically and histologically, some aspects of the condition remain controversial especially with regard to its management.

22.2.1 Historical Background

A wide variety of names has been given to lattice degeneration. Gonin gave the first description of lattice degeneration in 1920 and introduced the terms *snail-track degeneration (Schneckenspuren)*, *palissades*, and *état-givre* [3]. In 1930, Vogt provided the first complete clinical description of the disease and demonstrated that the white lines represented blood vessels and were not essential to the diagnosis. His mistaken hypothesis was that the entity corresponded to peripheral *cystoid degeneration* of the retina. These dissimilar designations for lattice degeneration may be confusing but reflect the variety of its clinical appearances.

22.2.2 Clinical Features

The shape, location, and orientation of lattice degeneration are characteristic: they typically appear as sharply demarcated

S. Mrejen
15-20 Ophthalmologic National Hospital, Paris, France

G. Ledesma-Gil · M. Engelbert (✉)
Vitreous Retina Macula Consultants of New York,
New York, NY, USA

© Springer Nature Switzerland AG 2021
R. F. Spaide et al. (eds.), *Pathologic Myopia*, https://doi.org/10.1007/978-3-030-74334-5_22

oval, round, or linear areas oriented circumferentially and parallel to the ora serrata at or anterior to the equator. Many features can be observed separately or in combination. One or many of the following features can predominate in an individual lesion, explaining the striking differences between one lesion and another [3]. These features are localized round, oval, or linear areas of retinal thinning; pigmentation; glistening whitish-yellow surface flecks; round, oval, or linear white patches; round, oval, or linear red craters; small atrophic round holes in approximately 25%; branching white lines corresponding to retinal vessels with thickened or hyalinized walls; yellow atrophic spots; and sometimes tractional retinal tears at the posterior margins of lesions in the context of vitreous separation (Fig. 22.1). The presence of white lines is not a defining feature [3]. A variable amount of pigment may be seen with these lesions, probably due to retinal pigment epithelial proliferation into the retina, but it is not essential to the diagnosis (Fig. 22.1) [3]. Lattice degeneration is associated with liquefaction of the overlying vitreous gel and firm vitreoretinal adhesion along the edges of the lesion. Vitreous traction on these areas during posterior vitreous detachment is often responsible for retinal tears. The size of the lattice degeneration can vary from a small solitary lesion to extensive lesions covering almost the complete circumference of the peripheral retina [3]. Areas of lattice degeneration are usually multiple, with the average number ranging from a low of two at 60 years and above to a high of 4.5 lesions at ages 20–29 [5]. Given that these lesions do not disappear over time, these variations are probably related to sampling variation.

22.2.3 Prevalence

The prevalence of lattice degeneration has been found to vary from 7.1 [5] to 8% [6] in clinical surveys and was 10.7% [7] in a histologic survey in the general population. No statistically significant difference in prevalence between men and women or between left and right eyes has been reported in the literature. Lattice degeneration is not known to show any racial preference either. Cambiaggi [8] reported palissade degeneration in 4.5% of normal eyes and in 19% of myopic eyes with increased prevalence in those over −8.00 diopter (D). The disease appears to reach its maximum prevalence prior to the age of 10 years [5], but this is subject to small sample size and sampling variation. Bansal and Hubbard [9] evaluated 54 eyes of 30 highly myopic children under the age of 10 years and identified peripheral retinal changes in 33% of eyes, the most common being lattice degeneration in 20% of eyes. Karlin and Curtin showed an increased prevalence of lattice degeneration with increased axial length in adult myopia with an overall prevalence of 6.1% in a series of 1437 myopic eyes [10]. Celorio and Pruett found a prevalence of lattice degeneration of 33% among 218 highly myopic patients (436 eyes) and an inverse relationship between axial length and the prevalence of lattice degeneration [11]. More recently, Lai et al. reported that 13.6% of 337 highly myopic adults in China with a mean axial length of 26.84 mm had lattice degeneration [12]. The discrepancies between these different studies in the prevalence of lattice degeneration may be due to the differences in axial length, refractive error, and age of the evaluated populations.

It is often the bilateral (34 [5], 40 [10], 50 [13], 63% [14]) and the temporal quadrants [10, 13, 15, 16] and the vertical axis are predominantly involved [5, 6].

22.2.4 Clinical Variants

22.2.4.1 Snail-Track Degeneration

Linear nonpigmented lesions that have a glistening, frostlike appearance have been termed *snail-tracks* (Fig. 22.1). They usually have borders that are less discrete than typical lattice degeneration, and the interstitial spaces between the dots have a translucent appearance. The presence of tiny glistening whitish-yellow flecks at their surface is essential to the diagnosis (Fig. 22.1). The lesion reported by Gärtner as *Milky Way-like* or *galaxy-like degeneration* falls within the group of snail-track lesions [3]. These lesions lack both the white lines and pigmentation and are not commonly seen with lattice degeneration [17]. They seem to pose a greater risk of retinal detachment [18]. Therefore, there is controversy as to whether they represent a variant of lattice degeneration or a separate entity. However, *snail-track* degeneration is usually clinically classified as lattice degeneration because they closely resemble the characteristic shape and orientation of lattice lesions [3]. They are located very anteriorly, typically behind the ora serrata. Moreover, the white flecks of the snail-track appearance occur to varying degrees in 80% of lattice lesions [5], and the *snail-track* appearance is frequently combined with other classic features of lattice lesions such as round atrophic holes, horseshoe tears, or a reddish base [3]. Overall, a snail-track appearance may actually represent a variant or an early stage of lattice degeneration [19].

22.2.5 Associations with Hereditary Disorders

Lattice degeneration has been observed in various hereditary disorders such as Ehlers-Danlos syndrome [20], Wagner's hereditary vitreoretinal degeneration [21–24], and Turner's syndrome [25].

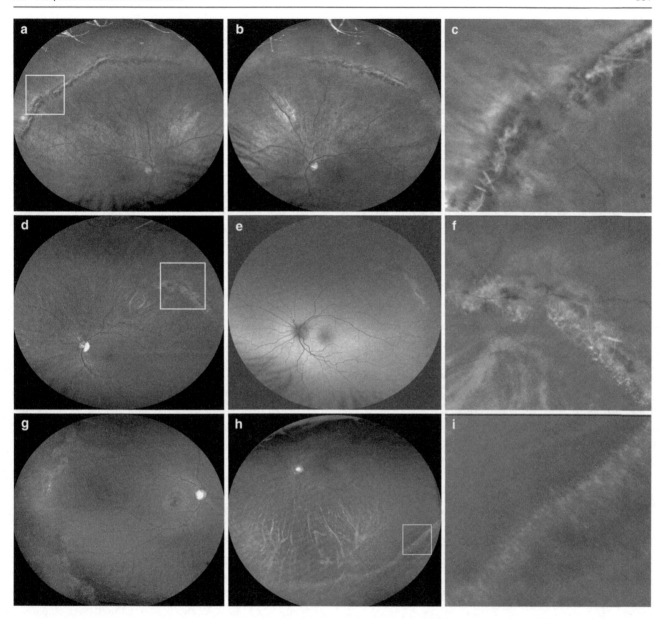

Fig. 22.1 Various clinical appearances of lattice degeneration, all located at the level of or anterior to the equator and oriented circumferentially parallel to the ora serrata, in four highly myopic patients, a 65-year-old male (**a–c**), a 29-year-old female (**d–f**), a 34-year-old female (**g**), and a 31-year-old female (**h, i**), using ultrawide-field imaging. (**a–c**) Bilateral lattice degeneration superotemporal with magnification of the area in the *white rectangle* (**c**) showing linear areas of retinal thinning, pigmentation, branching *white lines* corresponding to hyalinized walls of retinal vessels, and areas of whitish atrophy, glistening whitish-yellow surface flecks, and sheathing of the overlying retinal vessels. (**d–f**) The lattice degeneration appears hyperautofluorescent on fundus autofluorescence imaging (**e**). Note on magnification of the area in the *white rectangle* (**f**) the glistening whitish-yellow surface flecks, round white patches, moderate pigmentation, and sheathing of the overlying retinal vessels. (**g**) Multiple lattice lesions with white patches, glistening white flecks, and no pigmentation. (**h, i**) Lattice degeneration showing a pure snail-track feature with magnification of the area in the white rectangle in (**i**) showing discrete yellow-white glistening flecks on the surface and abrupt borders

22.2.6 Histologic Features

Straatsma et al. [7] evaluated a series of 86 autopsy cases with lattice degeneration. Three constant features were found in all the 286 lesions evaluated: retinal thinning, vitreous liquefaction, and vitreous condensation with exaggerated vit-

reoretinal adherence at the edges of the lesion. The autopsy reports also mention accumulation of glial proliferation within the lesion. The authors evaluated lattice degeneration with electron microscopy as well, demonstrating retinal thinning, fibrosis of blood vessels, loss of retinal neurons, accumulation of extracellular glial material, and pigment abnormalities. The retinal thinning and degeneration were more advanced toward the center of the lesions [7]. Electron microscopic analysis revealed focal thinning and intermittent absence of the inner limiting membrane in the center of the lattice degeneration [7]. There was no age-related trend in regard to the size, location, or orientation of lesions, but there was an age-related increase in degree of vitreoretinal attachment, prevalence of pigmentation, white lines, retinal holes, posterior vitreous detachment, and retinal tears. Of interest, it has also been observed histologically that the earliest and most severe degenerative changes occur at the level of the inner retinal layers [7] and that the choroid was most often not involved in lattice lesions [26].

22.2.7 Pathogenesis

The etiology of lattice degeneration is still uncertain. Their bilateral occurrence in patients with unilateral pathologic myopia [27] suggests a hereditary etiology. It is likely that both genetic and environmental factors play important roles in its development. Michaelson had postulated that the primary event in lattice degeneration was at the level of the choroid, leading to a focal loss of perfusion to the outer retina from the choriocapillaris [28], but this hypothesis has not been reinforced by histologic observations which have shown that the choroid was most often not involved in lattice lesions and that the earliest changes were actually at the level of the inner retina. Tolentino et al. hypothesized that lattice degeneration was primarily a vitreous disease with secondary retinal degeneration [29]. A primary retinal vascular etiology leading to retinal ischemia has also been proposed [7].

The pathogenesis may also be due to a developmental abnormality involving primarily the Müller cells resulting in an aplasia or focal defect of the internal limiting membrane [30].

22.2.8 Evolution and Management

Lattice degeneration may not only contain round holes within the confines of the lesion but is also predisposed to developing retinal tears at the posterior margin and ends of the lesion (Fig. 22.2). In one large study, the majority of eyes demonstrating retinal breaks (55%) showed lattice degeneration [31]. These breaks frequently lead to detachment of the retina. Approximately 6–8% of patients in the general population have lattice degeneration [32, 33], and up to 35% of these will have atrophic holes in the lattice [33]. Some of the atrophic holes are associated with subretinal fluid. Any collection of fluid greater than 1 disc diameter is generally considered to be a retinal detachment, although collections of about 1 disc diameter are sometimes called subclinical

detachments. Tillery et al. found that 2.8% of all retinal detachments were due to atrophic retinal holes in lattice degeneration [34]. It is therefore not surprising that approximately 20–30% of patients with retinal detachments have lattice degeneration [33]. In a series of 553 consecutive retinal detachments, 29% were due to lattice degeneration. Forty-five percent of these were due to atrophic holes in the lattice degeneration, and 55% were due to tears caused by traction posterior to or at the end of a patch of lattice [32].

Retinal detachment secondary to retinal holes is more commonly seen in young myopes, whereas detachments due to tears tend to occur in older, less myopic patients [32]. The detachments secondary to atrophic holes in lattice degeneration show a more insidious course than those due to traction breaks, which generally occur in the context of a symptomatic posterior vitreous detachment. The formation of demarcation lines is not uncommon in chronic round hole detachments. The risk of detachment in lattice degeneration with round holes was estimated at about 1 in 90 [35], but this risk has to be tempered by the refractive error. Lattice degeneration increases the risk by a factor of 6–7 [36]. Detachment of the retina can therefore be readily appreciated as a frequent sequel to lattice degeneration.

Whether to treat lattice degeneration in adult eyes has previously been a source of controversy. A high proportion of eyes with retinal detachment were found to have lattice lesions: 20 [28], 29 [32], 30 [13, 16], or 38.5% [14], and even 65% [37]. Therefore, treatment of such lesions was generally favored in the 1970s and 1980s. However, eyes with lattice degeneration may experience retinal detachment from tears which are not in an area of lattice in 40% [33]. In a long-term natural history study, Byer showed that in 276 adults (423 eyes) with lattice degeneration followed for an average of 10.8 years, retinal detachment occurred in only 1.08% of patients (0.7% of eyes) [33]. Byer concluded that prophylactic treatment of lattice lesions with or without holes in phakic eyes should be discontinued if the fellow eye had no history of rhegmatogenous retinal detachment [33]. Prophylactic treatment of lattice in fellow eyes of patients with rhegmatogenous retinal detachment has been shown by Folk et al. to reduce the risk of retinal detachment from 5.1 to 1.8% [38]. In a consensus between a panel of vitreoretinal experts based on a review of the literature regarding the prevention of retinal detachment in adults in 2000, there was not sufficient data to support prophylactic treatment of lesions other than symptomatic flap tears [39]. In the same consensus, there was substantial evidence to recommend to "sometimes treat" lattice lesions with or without retinal holes in fellow eyes of patients with a history of retinal detachment in the first eye, to "rarely treat" asymptomatic lattice lesions in aphakic eyes, and not to treat asymptomatic lattice lesions in phakic and myopic eyes [39]. However, treatment of fellow eyes of patients with a history of retinal detachment with

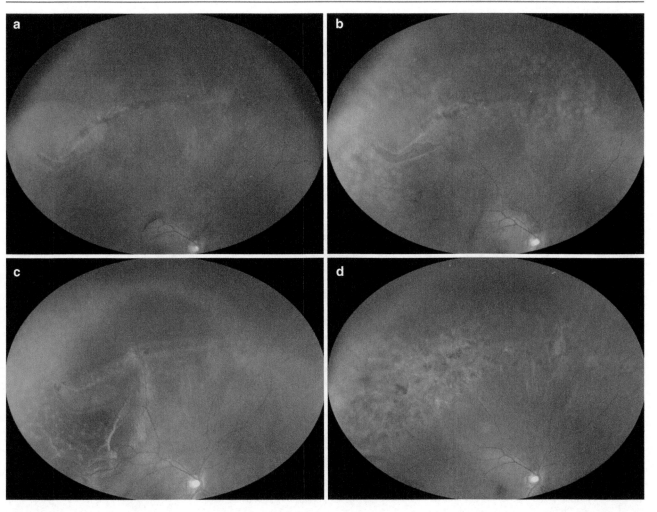

Fig. 22.2 This 42-year-old high myope developed a horseshoe tear at the lateral and posterior edge of a patch of pigmented lattice after vitreous separation (**a**). This tear and the associated lattice were surrounded with retinopexy (**b**), but the subretinal fluid progressed through the laser barrier and involved the macula (**c**). Vitrectomy with removal of subretinal fluid through the preexisting tear and endolaser were performed to reattach the retina (**d**)

lattice degeneration seems to be more beneficial if the eye has less than 6 diopters of myopia, if the lesion is present in less than 6 clock hours, and especially if there is no posterior vitreous separation [38].

22.3 White-Without-Pressure

22.3.1 Clinical Features

Since the first clinical description by Schepens in 1952 [40], the terms white-without-pressure and white-with-pressure refer to opacification of the retina noticed either spontaneously or upon scleral depression. This white to gray opacification partially obscures the normal choroidal vascular color and pattern as if it was visualized through a "semi-translucent veil" [41]. This phenomenon tends to run cir-

cumferentially in wide swatches affecting the retina immediately posterior to the ora serrata (Fig. 22.3). The lesions may extend more posteriorly and reach the equator and sometimes even the vascular arcades of the posterior pole [10, 41]. Karlin and Curtin found that the white-without-pressure areas can assume various shapes and locations [10]. White-without-pressure can be diffused with ill-defined margins or may have a very distinct edge with an abrupt transition to a zone of normal choroidal coloration (Fig. 22.3) [41]. It can be flat or have a slightly elevated appearance. They often cover diffusely almost the entire retinal periphery but can also appear as smaller focal patches, with a predilection for the temporal quadrants, particularly the inferior [10]. Similar to lattice degeneration [5], retinoschisis [42], or snowflake degeneration [43], white-without-pressure can also be covered by glistening yellow-white dots and fine lines (Fig. 22.3).

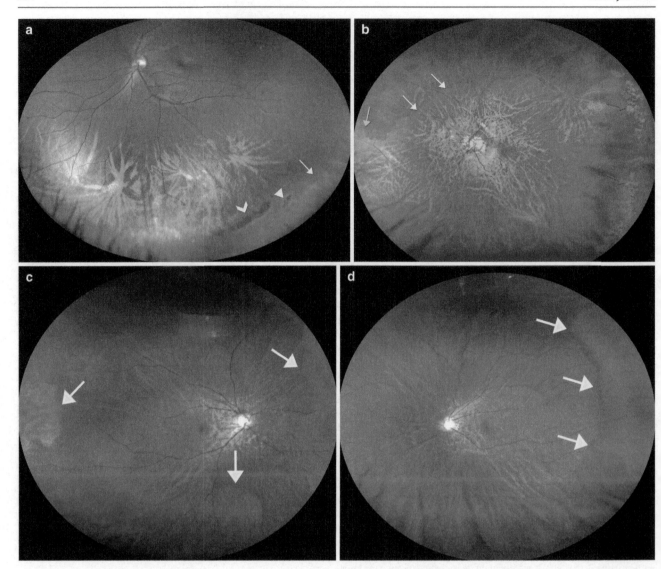

Fig. 22.3 Various shapes and locations of white-without-pressure in three highly myopic males, a 27-year-old (**a**), a 52-year-old (**b**), and a 37-year-old (**c, d**), using ultrawide-field multicolor fundus photographs. (**a**) White-without-pressure appears as a focal patch oriented circumferentially, located immediately posterior to the ora serrata in the temporal inferior quadrant (*white arrow*). The lesion is covered by glistening *yellow-white dots* and has relatively ill-defined margins. Note the presence of pigmented lattice degeneration (*arrowhead*) as well as atrophic retinal holes (*white triangles*). (**b**) White-without-pressure appears as a wide area immediately posterior to the ora serrata in the nasal quadrant (*yellow arrow*) and extends more posteriorly to the equator (*white arrows*) with a very distinct edge and an abrupt transition to a zone of normal choroidal coloration. Note the presence of paving stone degeneration in the temporal periphery as well (*red arrows*). (**c, d**) Bilateral multiple areas of white-without-pressure appearing as wide swatches oriented circumferentially temporal, inferior, and nasal in the right eye (**c**, *white arrows*) and temporal in the left eye (**d**, *white arrows*)

22.3.2 Prevalence

White-without-pressure has been demonstrated to be significantly more prevalent in young patients [10, 44]. Its prevalence in patients under the age of 20 years is 36% and decreases considerably to 9.5% in patients over the age of 40 [10]. White-without-pressure is also easier to visualize in pigmented individuals [45].

Karlin and Curtin found a tendency for white-without-pressure to affect eyes of individuals 19 years of age or younger and more myopic, with a prevalence reaching 100% in this age group when the axial length was 33 mm or more [10]. Pierro et al. evaluated 513 patients (513 eyes) with an axial length superior to 24 mm and a mean age of 48 years and found a prevalence of white-without-pressure of 22.8%, the second most common peripheral retinal change after paving stone degeneration (27.1%) [44]. They also found that white-without-pressure was significantly more common in younger patients [44]. Bansal and Hubbard evaluated 54 eyes of 30 highly myopic children under the age of 10 years and identified white-without-pressure in 11% of eyes, the second most common change after lattice degeneration (20%) [9]. Lai et al. found a prevalence of white-without-pressure of 21.1% among 337 highly myopic Chinese subjects with a mean age of 36 years and a mean axial length of 26.84 mm [12]. The most prevalent peripheral retinal change in this population was pigmentary retinal degeneration (37.7%) [12]. Lam et al. evaluated 213 highly myopic Chinese patients (213 eyes) with a mean age of 33.5 years and a mean axial length of 26.69 mm and found a prevalence of white-without-pressure of 31%. The most frequent peripheral retinal change in this population was pigmentary degeneration (51.2%) [46]. This higher prevalence of white-without-pressure in young patients could be explained if the lesion is viewed as an earlier stage of another lesion type [10] or if the lesion can change or fade in time [47].

22.3.3 Pathogenesis and Histology

Since its first description by Schepens in 1952 [40], there have not been many reports about white-without-pressure pathogenesis in the literature. Karlin and Curtin postulated that white-without-pressure may represent advanced retinal cystoid degeneration, flat retinal detachment, or flat retinoschisis [10]. Nagpal and coworkers reported that all their patients had posterior vitreous detachment except in the areas of white-without-pressure, suggesting that white-without-pressure may be due to areas of vitreoretinal traction [47]. White-without-pressure is considered by many to be an advanced form of white-with-pressure. White-with-pressure is commonly found in elderly fundi, almost invariably in areas of lattice degeneration and around small retinal breaks [41]. It is also frequently seen in the attached retina of eyes with partial retinal detachment or in the asymptomatic fellow eye of patients with unilateral rhegmatogenous retinal detachment [41]. However, Fawzi and coworkers demonstrated with multimodal imaging that the fundus color change in white- or dark-without-pressure corresponds to a change in the OCT reflectivity of the outer retina and were unable to demonstrate any associated vitreoretinal interface changes [48].

22.3.4 Evolution and Prognosis

Nagpal and coworkers described the peculiar phenomenon of migratory white-without-pressure areas in nine patients with various hemoglobinopathies [47]. In their series, follow-up examinations revealed a change in configuration of the lesions: some receded while others progressed [47]. The authors also claim that the migratory nature of white-without-pressure was not restricted to hemoglobinopathies.

In their series, the white-without-pressure areas were not associated with vascular occlusions or tortuosity or sea fans, nor did fluorescein angiography show any vascular abnormality. The fact that these lesions may change with time is also supported by the dramatic reduction in prevalence between age groups. White-without-pressure is essentially a benign lesion.

22.3.5 Associations and Variants

22.3.5.1 Associations
A number of retinal disorders can give rise to areas of peripheral retinal whitening quite similar to white-without-pressure. Condon and Serjeant in 1972 described peripheral whitening of the retina in 76 patients with sickle cell anemia [49], but this may have been because these patients were pigmented and the prevalence of white-without-pressure in pigmented patients with sickle cell anemia may not be greater than in pigmented patients without sickle cell anemia [48]. These patients had condensation of the overlying vitreous base. Most of the white areas were ill defined, but some were well demarcated and associated with vascular abnormalities. These lesions may have represented white-without-pressure. In 1966, Tasman and coworkers reported that the characteristic appearance of the premature fundus included white-without-pressure [50]. Pars planitis, snowflake degeneration [43], retinoschisis, and flat retinal detachment have also been associated with white-without-pressure.

White-without-pressure is mainly an incidental finding, and its chief importance is that it may be confused with a retinal detachment. Children may need an examination under anesthesia to distinguish between both entities [9, 51].

22.3.5.2 Dark-Without-Pressure
Nagpal and coworkers also described homogeneous, geographical, flat, brown areas surrounded by a halo of pale retina in the fundi of seven Black patients, of whom six had various hemoglobinopathies (Fig. 22.4). These lesions were called "dark-without-pressure fundus lesions" [52]. These lesions were associated with iridescent glistening spots and varied in size, shape, location, and orientation. They could be oriented either radially or circumferentially. Most of these lesions were transient. Fluorescein angiography in these areas did not reveal any vascular abnormality. The authors hypothesized that these dark areas may represent focal and relatively preserved retinal areas surrounded by more diffuse white-without-pressure areas. Like white-without-pressure, these dark lesions can vary in size, shape, and location and can also fade in time. Unlike white-without-pressure, these dark lesions occur usually near the posterior pole or in the midperiphery, and they seem to be unrelated to the status of the vitreous [52]. Indeed, Fawzi and colleagues demonstrated

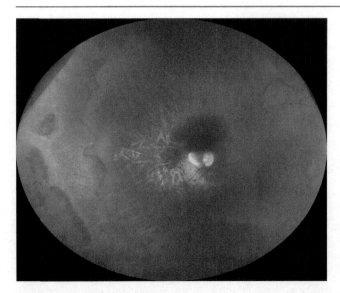

Fig. 22.4 Dark-without-pressure in the right eye of a 25-year-old black female with high myopia and pigmented lattice degeneration. The central dark opacity stems from a posterior subcapsular cataract

the fundus appearance to correlate with changes in outer retinal reflectivity, as in white-without-pressure [48].

22.4　Pigmentary Degeneration

22.4.1　Clinical Features

Pigmentary degeneration corresponds to a variable degree of pigmentation in the extreme periphery. This pigmentation may vary widely from a light dusting of fine particles to large discrete pigment clumps (Fig. 22.5). The temporal quadrants especially the superior are involved preferentially. The posterior margin can extend several disc diameters from the ora serrata and is typically indistinct. The border may be contiguous with a relatively depigmented zone of the fundus. This retinal lesion is typically bilateral.

22.4.2　Prevalence

Pigmentary degeneration affects an increasing proportion of eyes as the axial length and the age increase [10]. No sex preference has been reported in the literature. Karlin found them in only 6% of eyes in young patients and 41% of patients age 40 and above in a series of 1437 predominantly myopic eyes [10]. Two community-based studies reported pigmentary degeneration to be the most frequent peripheral retinal change in highly myopic Chinese patients [12, 46]. Lam et al. found pigmentary degeneration in 51.2% of 213 patients with a mean age of 33.5 years and a mean axial length of 26.69 mm [46], and Lai et al. found it in 37.7% of

337 patients with a mean age of 36 years and a mean axial length of 26.84 mm [12]. In a population of 30 children under the age of 10 years, there was no pigmentary degeneration [9].

22.4.3　Pathogenesis and Evolution

Despite its frequency, this retinal peripheral change is the least studied and therefore least understood. Vascular, inflammatory, and toxic agents may be involved in their development. This higher prevalence of pigmentary degeneration in older patients could be explained if the lesion is viewed as a later stage of another lesion type. For example, it is plausible that lattice degeneration may become increasingly pigmented over time and become indistinguishable from pigmentary degeneration. Pigmentary degeneration of the retina can be associated with both retinal holes and tears [10]. Everett evaluated fellow eyes of patients with retinal detachment and found that 32% of patients with pigmentary degeneration had retinal breaks [53]. Pigmentary degeneration appears to be essentially a benign lesion, and its morbidity however may be attributed to unidentified underlying areas of lattice degeneration prone to formation of retinal breaks.

22.4.4　Differential Diagnosis

Areas of pigmentary changes may appear in the periphery of myopic eyes after a spontaneously flattening retinal detachment. These regions can adopt a variety of appearances to include nummular, bone-spicule, or a densely packed granular hyperpigmentation. Bilateral and extensive areas of pigmentary degeneration in a myopic eye could be leading to an erroneous diagnosis of retinal dystrophy with bone-spicule formation, such as retinitis pigmentosa.

22.5　Paving Stone Degeneration (Cobblestone Degeneration)

22.5.1　Clinical Features

Paving stone degeneration is a distinctive and fairly common disease process found in the evaluation of the peripheral fundus. During the past century, a number of appellations have been applied to this lesion: some of them presume of an etiology such as chorioretinal atrophy [54] or equatorial chorioditis [55], and some are purely descriptive such as punched-out chorioretinal degeneration [53], paving stone degeneration, or cobblestone degeneration [37]. Paving stone degeneration can be used interchangeably with cobblestone degeneration. Paving stone degeneration is the preferred

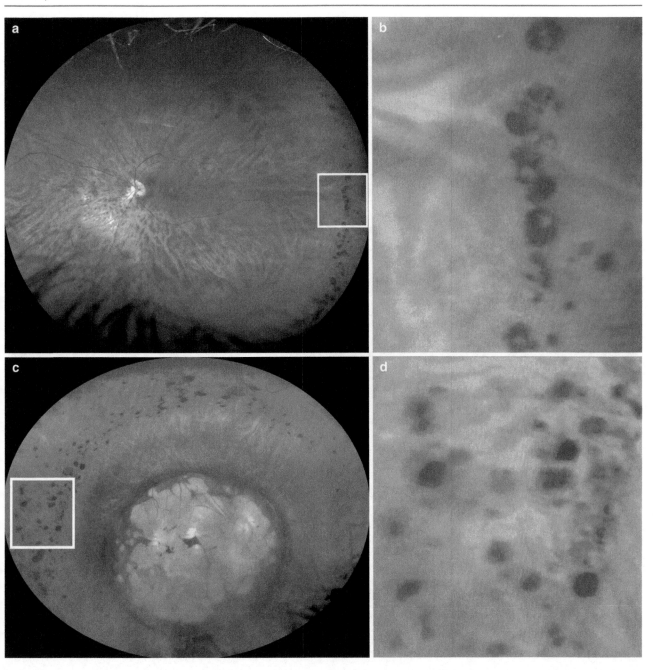

Fig. 22.5 Ultrawide-field fundus multicolor photographs of pigmentary degeneration in two highly myopic patients. (**a**) Pigmentary degeneration in the temporal periphery of a 52-year-old male, with magnification in (**b**) Note the presence of glistening *yellow-white dots* surrounding the pigmentary degeneration. (**c**) Pigmentary degeneration in 360° periphery of a 34 D myopic male, with magnification in (**d**). Note that the areas of pigmentary degeneration are surrounded by relatively depigmented zones of the fundus. (*Bottom image* courtesy of Jerome Sherman)

designation in the United States because cobblestone may suggest the connotation of elevation although these lesions are typically flat or depressed [37]. First described in 1855 by Donders [56], they usually appear as small, sharply demarcated, flat or slightly depressed, rounded, flat yellow to whitish areas of depigmentation and retinal thinning, with subsequent increased visualization of the relatively pre-

served underlying major choroidal vessels (Fig. 22.6). They often possess pigmented margins. They are usually located one or two disc diameters posterior to the ora serrata and are separated from the ora serrata by a band of intact retinal pigment epithelium. The basic unit can vary in size from 0.1 to 1.5 mm in diameter [55]. They can occur singly or in groups. When in group, they have a tendency to coalesce and form

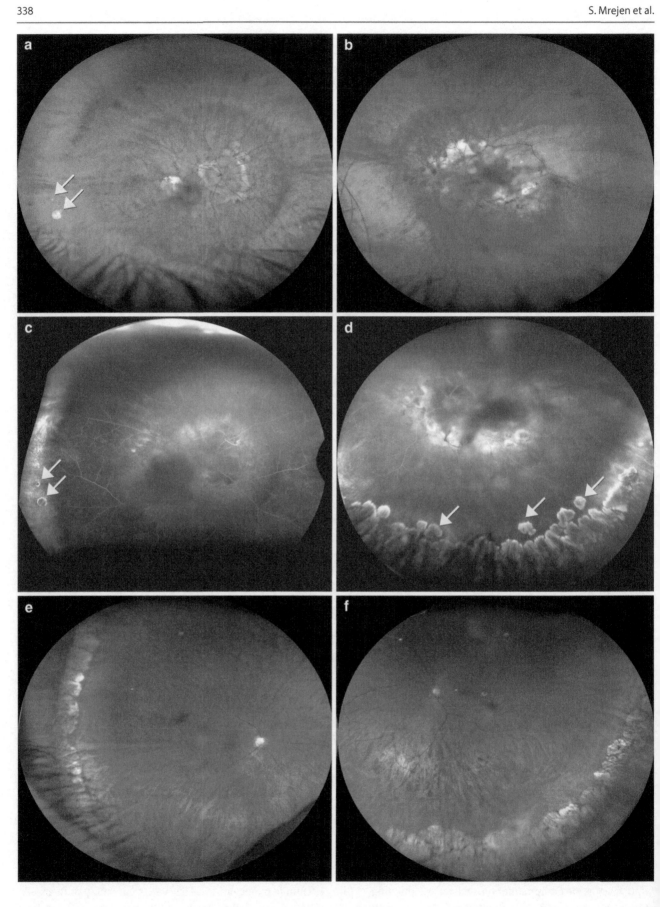

Fig. 22.6 Ultrawide-field fundus multicolor photographs and fluorescein angiography (late phase) of bilateral paving stone degeneration in a 63-year-old highly myopic female (**a–d**) and a 58-year-old highly myopic male (**e, f**). (**a, c**) In the right eye, the paving stone degeneration appears as two small, sharply demarcated, flat, rounded, whitish areas of depigmentation with subsequent increased visualization of the relatively preserved underlying major choroidal vessels (*white arrows*), located in the temporal periphery approximately two disc diameters posterior to the ora serrata. The lesions appear hyperfluorescent by window defect with increased visualization of the major choroidal vessels through a focal defect of the retinal pigment epithelium. (**b, d**) In the left eye, the paving stone degeneration appears as multiple coalescent lesions in the inferior periphery visualized as hyperfluorescent lesions in the fluorescein angiography by window defect as well (*white arrows*). (**e, f**) In both eyes, the paving stone degeneration appears as multiple coalescent lesions in the temporal (*right eye*) and inferior (*left eye*) periphery, at the level of and anterior to the equator

bands with scalloped borders (Fig. 22.6). The inferior and temporal retinal quadrants are affected most frequently [10, 55], and the lesion has been reported to be bilateral in 38 [57] to 57% [10].

22.5.2 Prevalence

The prevalence of paving stone degeneration has a clear significant association with increasing age and axial length [10]. In young subjects, Karlin and Curtin found a prevalence of less than 1%, whereas 40% of patients over the age of 40 years were affected [10]. Pierro et al. evaluated 513 patients (513 eyes) with an axial length superior to 24 mm and a mean age of 48 years and found that the most common peripheral degenerative change was paving stone degeneration with a frequency of 27.1% [44]. Lam et al. evaluated a younger population of 213 highly myopic Chinese patients (213 eyes) with a mean age of 33.5 years and a mean axial length of 26.69 mm and found a prevalence of cobblestone degeneration of only 5.2% [46]. Bansal and Hubbard evaluated 54 eyes of 30 highly myopic children under the age of 10 years and did not identify any cobblestone degeneration [9]. At autopsy, 27% of eyes over 20 years demonstrate these changes, and clinically, they are seen in 30% of the general population over the age of 60 years [55]. There does not appear to be a strong gender predilection for these lesions [55] although one report found males to be three times more likely to be affected [54].

22.5.3 Histologic Features and Pathogenesis

This entity is not fully understood. O'Malley et al. evaluated 1223 consecutive eyes obtained from 614 autopsies and found paving stone lesions in 186 eyes from 134 patients. The histologic features of all the lesions evaluated were remarkably similar showing a thinned retina closely applied to Bruch's membrane at an area devoid of RPE [55]. The RPE ended abruptly at the margins of the lesion and appeared normal in the surrounding areas. Hyperpigmented margins corresponded to proliferated RPE. The degree of retinal thinning was poorly correlated to the size of the lesions. The reti-

nal thinning was mainly due to the loss of the rods and cones and outer limiting membrane. The vitreous body was unchanged in the presence of the lesions, and when detached posteriorly, it showed no tendency to remain adherent to the retina at the site of the lesions. At the level of the choroid, the choriocapillaris was the only structure showing significant changes, with thinning, and even occasionally completely absent. The color of paving stone is generally very white due to the absence of underlying choriocapillaris. Brown and Shields showed that paving stone degeneration frequently developed peripheral to choroidal melanomas [58]. They theorized that the melanoma caused a steal syndrome and the paving stone developed secondary to decreased peripheral choroidal blood flow [58].

The pathogenesis of paving stone degeneration is unknown, but O'Malley postulated the likelihood of a vascular etiology due to the topography of the lesions limited to the portions of retina supplied by the choriocapillaris, the histologic appearance of the choriocapillaris altered beneath the lesions, and the absence of gliosis, fibrosis, or inflammatory infiltrate [55]. The anatomy of the choriocapillaris appears consistent with the size and shape of the basic lesion. The mechanical stretching of the highly myopic globe may generate vascular compromise and the development of choroidal ischemic atrophy of the RPE and overlying retina.

22.5.4 Evolution

Paving stone is not significantly associated with retinal breaks. Considering its prevalence and histologic features, a prophylactic treatment of this relatively benign process is not warranted. In fact, Meyer-Schwickerath suggested that treatment applied to these areas may even be detrimental, producing shrinkage of the retina and possibly a retinal break (quoted in [55]).

22.6 Retinal Breaks

What is called a full-thickness break in retinal continuity can be either a retinal hole or retinal tear. These two types of retinal breaks are labeled differently because they have different morphological characteristics, pathogenic mechanism, and distinct risks for retinal detachment. Retinal holes are related to chorioretinal degenerative changes. Retinal tears result from the traction of adherent vitreous on a weakened retinal area or from zonuloretinal tractions.

22.6.1 Prevalence

The prevalence of retinal breaks has varied among histopathological and clinical studies. These variations may be due to sampling variations since the prevalence of retinal breaks increases with age [59] and axial length [10, 46]. Histopathological studies have reported a prevalence of retinal breaks between 4.8% of cases (2.4% of eyes) [60] and 18.3% of cases (10.6% of eyes) [61]. Byer performed a clinical study on 1700 patients presenting for a complete eye examination and found that 5.8% of cases had one or more retinal breaks, in whom only two patients had symptoms: light flashes or floaters [31]. Lai et al. reported that 6.2% of 337 highly myopic Chinese adults (337 eyes) with a mean axial length of 26.84 mm and mean age of 36 years had retinal breaks [12]. Lam et al. evaluated 213 highly myopic Chinese patients (213 eyes) with a mean age of 33.5 years and a mean axial length of 26.69 mm and found a prevalence of retinal breaks of 7.5%. In this study, the prevalence of retinal breaks was 6.4% in eyes with an axial length inferior to 30 mm and increased to 30% in eyes with an axial length superior to 30 mm [46]. Pierro et al. evaluated 513 patients (513 eyes) with an axial length superior to 24 mm and a mean age of 48 years and found a prevalence of retinal breaks of 12.1% [44]. Bansal and Hubbard evaluated 54 eyes of 30 highly myopic children under the age of 10 years, with a mean age of 6 years and a mean refractive error of −13.88 D, and identified retinal holes in two eyes (3.7% of eyes) and a vitreoretinal tuft in one eye (1.9% of eyes) [9].

22.7 Tractional Retinal Tears

22.7.1 Clinical Features and Classification

Retinal tears can be flap (or arrowhead or horseshoe) tears (64% of all tears) [62] (Figs. 22.7 and 22.8) or operculated tears. They occur suddenly and can be symptomatic but are most commonly asymptomatic [31, 63]. The chief complaints are usually light flashes, floaters, or rarely blurred vision in the visual field corresponding to the quadrant of the retinal tear. The size can vary considerably from less than a quarter of a disc diameter to a giant tear if extending for one or more retinal quadrants. Byer found that 76% of

156 retinal breaks found in 1700 patients evaluated were less than a quarter of a disc diameter in size [31]. Retinal tears have been found to occur preferentially in the upper half and temporal half of the retina in both myopes and nonmyopes [64].

Foos proposed a classification of retinal tears in autopsy eyes based on their relationship to the vitreous base and pathogenic mechanism [62]. This anatomical classification helps to determine the clinical prognosis of retinal tears. The four categories are oral, at the level of the ora serrata; intrabasal, located within the vitreous base; juxtabasal, at the posterior border of the vitreous base; and extrabasal, in the equatorial zone of the peripheral retina posterior to the vitreous base. Retinal tears were postoral in 92% of eyes in Foos' analysis [62]. An oral tear is due to traction of the vitreous base primarily in the posterior direction and is usually associated with trauma and developmental abnormalities. Therefore, they are more common in younger subjects, with a peak of occurrence at the age of 20 years [65]. Oral tears do not have an anterior flap but rather rolling of the posterior flap and are traditionally called dialysis.

Intrabasal tears are due to zonuloretinal traction, resulting from the avulsion of a zonular traction tuft. These tears have been found to represent only 6.1% of all retinal tears in an autopsy study [66]. Most of them are operculated tears [62]. They carry a good prognosis and rarely lead to retinal detachment because the retina surrounding them is not under traction from the vitreous base.

Juxtabasal tears are typically flap tears. They result from an acute change in the vitreous body conformation, typically after a posterior vitreous detachment or a cataract surgery. The traction is exerted from the posterior border of the vitreous base on the anterior margins of the flap tear. The posterior edge of the tear is free of any traction. These tears carry the highest risk of retinal detachment among all postoral retinal tears, and this risk is highest acutely after a posterior vitreous detachment or a cataract surgery and then decreases [65]. Extrabasal tears are usually operculated and are considered relatively benign because they are free of traction at the margins of the tear.

Lattice lesion can lead to a tractional retinal tear at the time of posterior vitreous detachment depending on its precise location toward the vitreous base: intrabasal and extrabasal lesions are less likely than juxtabasal lesions to produce a flap tear [62, 66]. Foos found that 17% of eyes with flap tears had lattice degeneration in an autopsy series of 4812 eyes, but only 20% of these lattice lesions were actually adjacent to the flap tears, suggesting that in eyes with lattice degeneration, there are more widespread vitreoretinal traction and retinal weakness than just limited to the areas of visible lattice [66].

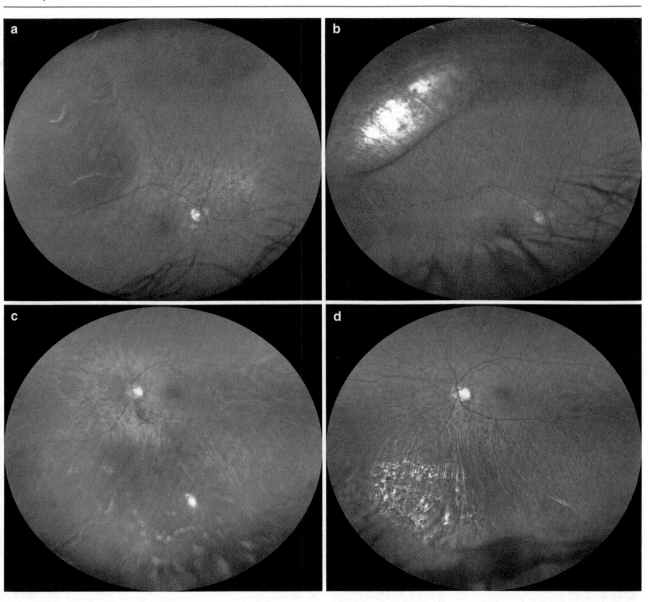

Fig. 22.7 Various clinical features of horseshoe tears in two highly myopic patients, a 58-year-old male (**a, b**) and a 41-year-old female (**c, d**), using ultrawide-field fundus multicolor photographs. (**a, b**) Two horseshoe tears with superotemporal retinal detachment. One month after a radial scleral buckle and cryotherapy, the retina is flat (**b**). (**c, d**) Three horseshoe tears inferonasal with retinal detachment despite prophylactic laser therapy (**c**). One month after vitrectomy, gas, and endolaser, the retina is flat (**d**)

22.7.2 Giant Tear

Giant retinal tears are tears of one or more retinal quadrant in the presence of a posterior vitreous detachment [67, 68]. It is a rare condition representing approximately 0.5% of all retinal detachments [69]. It is associated with a bad prognosis due to complicated retinal detachment, a high incidence of proliferative vitreoretinopathy, and therefore a high recurrence rate [70]. The identified predisposing factors are high myopia [70], trauma [71], hereditary vitreoretinopathies such as Stickler syndrome [72], and intraocular surgical procedures [73]. The fellow eyes of patients with giant retinal tears, especially nontraumatic, are at higher risk of developing a giant retinal tear (11.3%) and retinal detachment of any cause (up to 36%) [69, 74]. Therefore, it is recommended to perform 360° laser prophylactic therapy in the fellow eye, even though there is no prospective or case-control study demonstrating the benefit of this procedure [70].

22.7.3 Iatrogenic Retinal Tears

Iatrogenic retinal tears can be induced during pars plana vitrectomy and represent one of the most serious complications

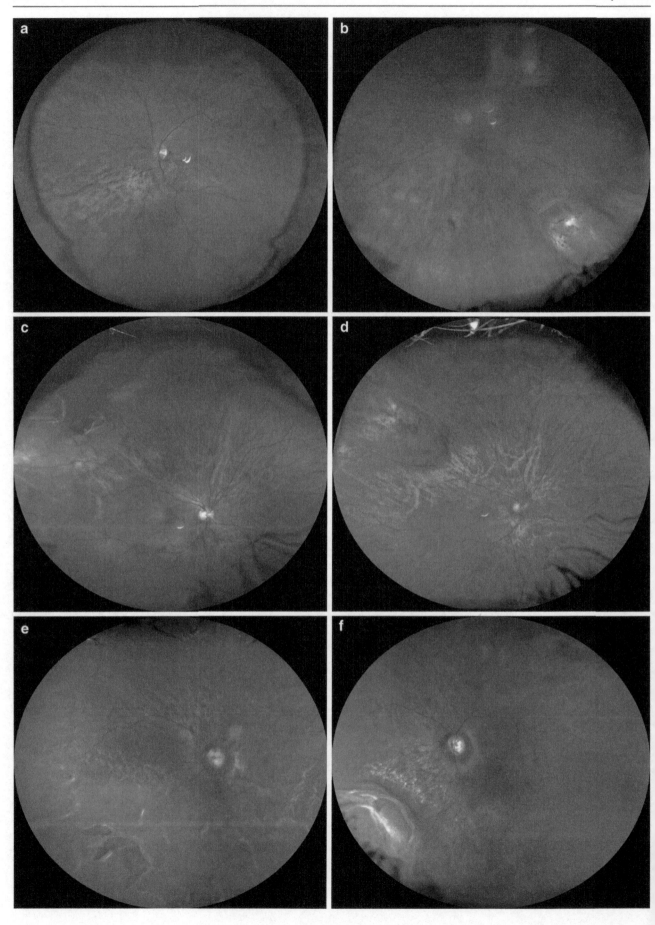

Fig. 22.8 Three examples of myopic patients with retinal detachment caused by horseshoes tears treated with radial scleral buckles, a 57-year-old male (**a**, **b**), a 55-year-old male (**c**, **d**), and a 63-year-old monocular male (**e**, **f**), illustrated with ultrawide-field fundus multicolor photographs. (**a**, **b**) Inferior retinal detachment caused by a single large horseshoe tear inferotemporal of approximately 2 disc diameters (**a**) and treated successfully with a radial scleral buckle and subsequent thermal laser the day after the surgical procedure, when the retina was reattached (**b**). The patient is pseudophakic and the edges of the implant are visualized in the color photograph (**a**). (**c**, **d**) Superonasal retinal detachment caused by two horseshoe tears radially aligned (**c**) and treated successfully with a radial scleral buckle and cryotherapy (**d**). (**e**, **f**) Inferior macula-off detachment caused by two large horseshoe tears at the level of the equator (**e**) and treated successfully with a large radial scleral buckle and cryotherapy (**f**) without drainage

of elective vitreoretinal surgery. These iatrogenic tears are more common when there is surgical induction of the posterior vitreous detachment [75] and in phakic eyes [76, 77]. There were significantly fewer entry-site breaks associated with transconjunctival 23-gauge vitrectomy compared with 20-gauge conventional vitrectomy [76, 78]. It is possible that the trocars' extension into the eye past the vitreous base enables instruments to pass repeatedly into the eye without engaging vitreous gel and leads to less vitreous traction and fewer iatrogenic breaks [76].

22.8 Atrophic Retinal Holes

Atrophic retinal holes are typically tiny and located near the ends of lattice lesions (Fig. 22.9). They usually occur early in life independent of a detaching posterior vitreous and do not produce symptoms [3]. Foos found that 75% of all round atrophic holes are within lattice lesions in 5600 autopsy eyes [79]. They are usually located at the level of or anterior to the equator. They typically favor the inferior retina but have been found to be more common superiorly in myopes [64].

These atrophic retinal holes may favor the equator due to the vascular anatomy of this region. The equator is a kind of watershed zone where the deep retinal capillary plexus disappears. The uveal circulation may be unable to compensate the blood flow in this region under certain circumstances such as age-related or myopia-related choroidal vascular atrophy [64]. The vascular hypothesis is reinforced by fluorescein angiographic observations that there was no perfusion of the choroid and retina in areas of retinal holes and the retina surrounding them [80]. Since 75% of round holes are in lattice lesions and lattice has been demonstrated to have genetic susceptibility [81], the vascular atrophic hypothesis may not be the only pathogenic mechanism involved though.

Retinal holes are more common than tractional retinal tears but lead to retinal detachment less frequently [3]. Tulloh evaluated 422 patients with primary retinal detachment and found 516 round retinal holes and 222 flap tears (ratio 2.3:1) [64]. Of interest, 65% of patients who develop new retinal holes are under 35 [6], and therefore, there is a decrease in retinal detachments due to round holes with increasing age [3]. Tillery and Lucier found that 2.8% of all primary retinal detachments were due to round holes of lattice lesions [34].

Retinal detachments caused by retinal holes occurred in younger and myopic patients (half under age 30, 75% exceeding −3.00 D) and were inferior, with slow progression and good prognosis [34].

22.9 Risk of Retinal Detachment and Prophylactic Therapy of Retinal Breaks

Identifying the retinal breaks at higher risk of progression to retinal detachment is essential because the prophylactic treatment of these is relatively safe and reduces this risk of retinal detachment significantly. Davis evaluated 213 patients (222 eyes) with one or more retinal breaks without clinical retinal detachment (defined as greater than two disc diameters) and found symptomatic breaks in 39 eyes and asymptomatic breaks in 183 eyes [63]. All the 39 symptomatic breaks were tears (33 flap tears and 6 operculated tears), and 101 out of 183 asymptomatic breaks were tears (71 flap tears and 30 operculated tears) [63]. Davis found that 9 out of 25 patients (36%) with fresh symptomatic flap tears developed a clinical retinal detachment within 6 weeks if left untreated [63]. Colyear and Pischel had found that 11 out of 20 patients (55%) with symptomatic flap tears developed a retinal detachment [82]. Symptomatic flap tears are at high risk of retinal detachment and are the only lesions with a strong evidence-based recommendation for systematic prophylactic therapy [39].

Fresh symptomatic operculated tears are very rare and have been shown to lead to retinal detachment only in one out of six cases in Davis' study [63]. They are usually considered relatively benign, but if the vitreous is adherent to the edge of the operculated tear, it can be considered an equivalent of a flap tear and should therefore be treated [83].

The progression to retinal detachment in phakic eyes with asymptomatic retinal breaks has been found to be very low in multiple studies, whether it is flap tears with less than 10% [63, 84, 85] or retinal holes with less than 5% [6, 63]. The consensus is usually not to treat asymptomatic breaks, except for dialysis or in aphakic, myopic, and fellow eyes of patients who had a retinal detachment [39]. The consensus is to always treat dialysis, whether they are symptomatic or not, with three rows of laser if feasible or cryotherapy [39].

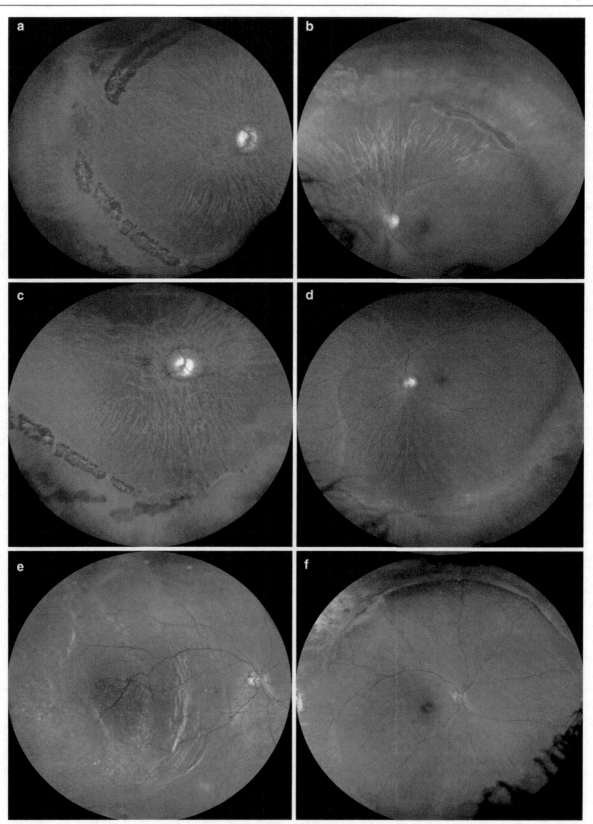

Fig. 22.9 Various clinical features of atrophic retinal holes in two myopic patients, a 39-year-old male (**a–d**) and a 29-year-old male (**e, f**), using ultrawide-field fundus multicolor photographs. (**a–d**) Bilateral multiple atrophic round holes in lattice lesions: most of them are tiny (**b–d**) and one is 1 disc diameter (**a**). There was a superior retinal detachment caused by an atrophic retinal hole in lattice degeneration in the left eye (not shown) treated with cryotherapy and encircling band because of the multiplicity of the peripheral atrophic holes in lattice degeneration (**b, d**). Note the white-without-pressure that may be confused with a retinal detachment in the temporal midperiphery of the left eye (**d**). (**e, f**) Bullous temporal retinal detachment caused by an atrophic round hole (**e**) treated successfully with cryotherapy and encircling band due to the multiplicity of peripheral breaks (not shown) (**f**)

22.9.1 Modulation of the Risk in Myopic, Aphakic, and Fellow Eyes

Börhinger reported that the lifetime risk of retinal detachment was 0.2% for emmetropes and hyperopes and myopes to −1.00 D, 4% for myopes −5 to −9 D, and reached 7% for high myopes greater than −9 D (quoted in [86]). The prevalence of retinal detachment after cataract extraction has been reported to be as high as 6.7% in 136 highly myopic eyes in 1975 in the era of intracapsular extractions and 0.28% according to the same authors in emmetropic eyes [87]. More recently, the risk for postoperative retinal detachment in high myopes has been reported to be 1.5–2.2% in 2356 eyes [88].

Breaks in aphakic eyes have been found to be more prone to progression [63]. Fellow eyes of patients who had a retinal detachment develop a retinal detachment in 5–10% of cases [89–91]. Aphakic fellow eyes have been found to develop retinal detachment in 26% of cases [92]. Therefore, the consensus is to sometimes treat asymptomatic flap tears in myopic eyes, aphakic eyes, and fellow eyes of patients who had a retinal detachment [39].

References

1. Holekamp NM, Harocopos GJ, Shui YB, Beebe DC. Myopia and axial length contribute to vitreous liquefaction and nuclear cataract. Arch Ophthalmol. 2008;126(5):744; author reply.
2. Akiba J. Prevalence of posterior vitreous detachment in high myopia. Ophthalmology. 1993;100(9):1384–8.
3. Byer NE. Lattice degeneration of the retina. Surv Ophthalmol. 1979;23(4):213–48.
4. Gonin J. La pathogénie du décollement spontané de la rétine. Ann d'Oculist (Paris). 1904;132:30–54.
5. Byer NE. Clinical study of lattice degeneration of the retina. Trans Am Acad Ophthalmol Otolaryngol. 1965;69(6):1065–81.
6. Byer NE. Changes in and prognosis of lattice degeneration of the retina. Trans Am Acad Ophthalmol Otolaryngol. 1974;78(2):OP114–25.
7. Straatsma BR, Zeegen PD, Foos RY, et al. Lattice degeneration of the retina. XXX Edward Jackson memorial lecture. Am J Ophthalmol. 1974;77(5):619–49.
8. Cambiaggi A. Research on the role of myopic chorioretinal changes in the pathogenesis of retinal detachment. Ophthalmologica. 1968;156(2):124–32.
9. Bansal AS. Hubbard 3rd GB. Peripheral retinal findings in highly myopic children < or =10 years of age. Retina. 2010;30(4 Suppl):S15–9.
10. Karlin DB, Curtin BJ. Peripheral chorioretinal lesions and axial length of the myopic eye. Am J Ophthalmol. 1976;81(5):625–35.
11. Celorio JM, Pruett RC. Prevalence of lattice degeneration and its relation to axial length in severe myopia. Am J Ophthalmol. 1991;111(1):20–3.
12. Lai TY, Fan DS, Lai WW, Lam DS. Peripheral and posterior pole retinal lesions in association with high myopia: a cross-sectional community-based study in Hong Kong. Eye (Lond). 2008;22(2):209–13.
13. Straatsma BR, Allen RA. Lattice degeneration of the retina. Trans Am Acad Ophthalmol Otolaryngol. 1962;66:600–13.
14. Morse PH. Lattice degeneration of the retina and retinal detachment. Am J Ophthalmol. 1974;78(6):930–4.
15. Arruga H. Ocular surgery. In: Hogan MJ, Chaparro LE, editors. . 4th ed. New York: Mc-Graw-Hill; 1956.
16. Dumas J, Schepens CL. Chorioretinal lesions predisposing to retinal breaks. Am J Ophthalmol. 1966;61(4):620–30.
17. Aaberg TM, Stevens TR. Snail track degeneration of the retina. Am J Ophthalmol. 1972;73(3):370–6.
18. Chignell AH, editor. Retinal detachment surgery. Berlin: Springer; 1980.
19. Shukla M, Ahuja OP. A possible relationship between lattice and snail track degenerations of the retina. Am J Ophthalmol. 1981;92(4):482–5.
20. Pemberton JW, Freeman HM, Schepens CL. Familial retinal detachment and the Ehlers-Danlos syndrome. Arch Ophthalmol. 1966;76(6):817–24.
21. Alexander RL, Shea M. Wagner's disease. Arch Ophthalmol. 1965;74:310–8.
22. Hagler WS, Crosswell HH Jr. Radial perivascular chorioretinal degeneration and retinal detachment. Trans Am Acad Ophthalmol Otolaryngol. 1968;72(2):203–16.
23. Hirose T, Lee KY, Schepens CL. Wagner's hereditary vitreoretinal degeneration and retinal detachment. Arch Ophthalmol. 1973;89(3):176–85.
24. Urrets-Zavalia A Jr. Lesions predisposing to retinal detachment. Annee Ther Clin Ophthalmol. 1969;20:11–34.
25. Jesberg DO. Vitreoretinal degeneration in Turner's syndrome. In: McPherson A, editor. New and controversial aspects of retinal detachment. New York: Harper Row; 1968. p. 127–34.
26. Pau H. Which retinal areas are disposed to idiopathic retinal detachment and may be considered for prophylactic operation? Klin Monbl Augenheilkd Augenarztl Fortbild. 1959;134:848–62.
27. Zauberman H, Merin S. Unilateral high myopia with bilateral degenerative fundus changes. Am J Ophthalmol. 1969;67(5):756–9.
28. Michaelson IC. Role of a distinctive choroido-retinal lesion in the pathogenesis of retinal hole; a clinical and pathological report. Br J Ophthalmol. 1956;40(9):527–35.
29. Tolentino FI, Schepens CL, Freeman HM. Vitreoretinal disorders, diagnosis and management. Philadelphia: Saunders; 1976.
30. Foos RY, Simons KB. Vitreous in lattice degeneration of retina. Ophthalmology. 1984;91(5):452–7.
31. Byer NE. Clinical study of retinal breaks. Trans Am Acad Ophthalmol Otolaryngol. 1967;71(3):461–73.
32. Benson WE, Morse PH. The prognosis of retinal detachment due to lattice degeneration. Ann Ophthalmol. 1978;10(9):1197–200.
33. Byer NE. Long-term natural history of lattice degeneration of the retina. Ophthalmology. 1989;96(9):1396–401. discussion 401–2
34. Tillery WV, Lucier AC. Round atrophic holes in lattice degeneration – an important cause of phakic retinal detachment. Trans Sect Ophthalmol Am Acad Ophthalmol Otolaryngol. 1976;81(3 Pt 1):509–18.
35. Murakami-Nagasako F, Ohba N. Phakic retinal detachment associated with atrophic hole of lattice degeneration of the retina. Graefe's archive for clinical and experimental ophthalmology. Albrecht von Graefes Archiv fur klinische und experimentelle Ophthalmologie. 1983;220(4):175–8.
36. Tielsch JM, Legro MW, Cassard SD, et al. Risk factors for retinal detachment after cataract surgery. A population-based case–control study. Ophthalmology. 1996;103(10):1537–45.
37. Meyer-Schwickerath G, editor. Light coagulation. St Louis: Mosby; 1960.
38. Folk JC, Arrindell EL, Klugman MR. The fellow eye of patients with phakic lattice retinal detachment. Ophthalmology. 1989;96(1):72–9.
39. Wilkinson CP. Evidence-based analysis of prophylactic treatment of asymptomatic retinal breaks and lattice degeneration. Ophthalmology. 2000;107(1):12–5. discussion 5–8
40. Schepens CL. Subclinical retinal detachments. AMA Arch Ophthalmol. 1952;47(5):593–606.

41. Watzke RC. The ophthalmoscopic sign "white with pressure". A clinicopathologic correlation. Arch Ophthalmol. 1961;66:812–23.

42. Shea M, Schepens CL, Von Pirquet SR. Retinoschisis. I. Senile type: a clinical report of one hundred seven cases. Arch Ophthalmol. 1960;63:1–9.

43. Hirose T, Lee KY, Schepens CL. Snowflake degeneration in hereditary vitreoretinal degeneration. Am J Ophthalmol. 1974;77(2):143–53.

44. Pierro L, Camesasca FI, Mischi M, Brancato R. Peripheral retinal changes and axial myopia. Retina. 1992;12(1):12–7.

45. Hunter JE. Retinal white without pressure: review and relative incidence. Am J Optom Physiol Optic. 1982;59(4):293–6.

46. Lam DS, Fan DS, Chan WM, et al. Prevalence and characteristics of peripheral retinal degeneration in Chinese adults with high myopia: a cross-sectional prevalence survey. Optom Vis Sci. 2005;82(4):235–8.

47. Nagpal KC, Huamonte F, Constantaras A, et al. Migratory white-without-pressure retinal lesions. Arch Ophthalmol. 1976;94(4):576–9.

48. Fawzi AA, Nielsen JS, Mateo-Montoya A, et al. Multimodal imaging of white and dark without pressure fundus lesions. Retina. 2014;34(12):2376–87.

49. Condon PI, Serjeant GR. Ocular findings in homozygous sickle cell anemia in Jamaica. Am J Ophthalmol. 1972;73(4):533–43.

50. Tassman W, Annesley W Jr. Retinal detachment in the retinopathy of prematurity. Arch Ophthalmol. 1966;75(5):608–14.

51. Chen DZ, Koh V, Tan M, et al. Peripheral retinal changes in highly myopic young Asian eyes. Acta Ophthalmol. 2018;96(7):e846–51.

52. Nagpal KC, Goldberg MF, Asdourian G, et al. Dark-without-pressure fundus lesions. Br J Ophthalmol. 1975;59(9):476–9.

53. Everett WG. The fellow-eye syndrome in retinal detachment. Am J Ophthalmol. 1963;56:739–48.

54. Rutnin U, Schepens CL. Fundus appearance in normal eyes. 3. Peripheral degenerations. Am J Ophthalmol. 1967;64(6):1040–62.

55. O'Malley P, Allen RA, Straatsma BR, O'Malley CC. Paving-stone degeneration of the retina. Arch Ophthalmol. 1965;73:169–82.

56. Donders FC. Beitrage zur Pathologischen Anatomie des Auges. Albrecht Von Graefes Arch Ophthalmol. 1855;1:106.

57. Allen RA. Cobblestone degeneration of the retina. In: Kimura SM, Caygill WB, editors. Pathology in retinal diseases. Philadelphia: Lea & Febiger; 1966.

58. Brown GC, Shields JA. Choroidal melanomas and paving stone degeneration. Ann Ophthalmol. 1983;15(8):705–8.

59. Hyams SW, Neumann E. Peripheral retina in myopia. With particular reference to retinal breaks. Br J Ophthalmol. 1969;53(5):300–6.

60. Okun E. Gross and microscopic pathology in autopsy eyes. III. Retinal breaks without detachment. Am J Ophthalmol. 1961;51:369–91.

61. Foos RY, Allen RA. Retinal tears and lesser lesions of the peripheral retina in autopsy eyes. Am J Ophthalmol. 1967;64(Suppl 3):643–55.

62. Foos RY. Tears of the peripheral retina; pathogenesis, incidence and classification in autopsy eyes. Mod Probl Ophthalmol. 1975;15:68–81.

63. Davis MD. Natural history of retinal breaks without detachment. Arch Ophthalmol. 1974;92(3):183–94.

64. Tulloh CG. Distribution of holes and tears in primary retinal detachment. Br J Ophthalmol. 1965;49(8):413–31.

65. Sigelman J. Vitreous base classification of retinal tears: clinical application. Surv Ophthalmol. 1980;25(2):59–70.

66. Foos RY. Postoral peripheral retinal tears. Ann Ophthalmol. 1974;6(7):679–87.

67. Schepens CL, Dobble JG, Mc MJ. Retinal detachments with giant breaks: preliminary report. Trans Am Acad Ophthalmol Otolaryngol. 1962;66:471–9.

68. Scott JD. Giant tear of the retina. Trans Ophthalmol Soc U K. 1975;95(1):142–4.

69. Freeman HM. Fellow eyes of giant retinal breaks. Trans Am Ophthalmol Soc. 1978;76:343–82.

70. Ang GS, Townend J, Lois N. Interventions for prevention of giant retinal tear in the fellow eye. Cochrane Database Syst Rev. 2012;(2):CD006909.

71. Aylward GW, Cooling RJ, Leaver PK. Trauma-induced retinal detachment associated with giant retinal tears. Retina. 1993;13(2):136–41.

72. Ang A, Poulson AV, Goodburn SF, et al. Retinal detachment and prophylaxis in type 1 Stickler syndrome. Ophthalmology. 2008;115(1):164–8.

73. Aaberg TM Jr, Rubsamen PE, Flynn HW Jr, et al. Giant retinal tear as a complication of attempted removal of intravitreal lens fragments during cataract surgery. Am J Ophthalmol. 1997;124(2):222–6.

74. Freeman HM. Fellow eyes of giant retinal breaks. Mod Probl Ophthalmol. 1979;20:267–74.

75. Muselier A, Dugas B, Burelle X, et al. Macular hole surgery and cataract extraction: combined vs consecutive surgery. Am J Ophthalmol. 2010;150(3):387–91.

76. Gosse E, Newsom R, Lochhead J. The incidence and distribution of iatrogenic retinal tears in 20-gauge and 23-gauge vitrectomy. Eye (Lond). 2012;26(1):140–3.

77. Sjaarda RN, Glaser BM, Thompson JT, et al. Distribution of iatrogenic retinal breaks in macular hole surgery. Ophthalmology. 1995;102(9):1387–92.

78. Nakano T, Uemura A, Sakamoto T. Incidence of iatrogenic peripheral retinal breaks in 23-gauge vitrectomy for macular diseases. Retina. 2011;31(10):1997–2001.

79. Foos RY. Retinal holes. Am J Ophthalmol. 1978;86(3):354–8.

80. Tolentino FI, Lapus JV, Novalis G, et al. Fluorescein angiography of degenerative lesions of the peripheral fundus and rhegmatogenous retinal detachment. Int Ophthalmol Clin. 1976;16(1):13–29.

81. Meguro A, Ideta H, Ota M, et al. Common variants in the COL4A4 gene confer susceptibility to lattice degeneration of the retina. PLoS One. 2012;7(6):e39300.

82. Colyear BH Jr, Pischel DK. Preventive treatment of retinal detachment by means of light coagulation. Trans Pac Coast Otoophthalmol Soc Annu Meet. 1960;41:193–217.

83. Kramer SG, Benson WE. Prophylactic therapy of retinal breaks. Surv Ophthalmol. 1977;22(1):41–7.

84. Byer NE. Prognosis of asymptomatic retinal breaks. Arch Ophthalmol. 1974;92(3):208–10.

85. Neumann E, Hyams S. Conservative management of retinal breaks. A follow-up study of subsequent retinal detachment. Br J Ophthalmol. 1972;56(6):482–6.

86. Burton TC. The influence of refractive error and lattice degeneration on the incidence of retinal detachment. Trans Am Ophthalmol Soc. 1989;87:143–55. discussion 55–7

87. Hyams SW, Bialik M, Neumann E. Myopia-aphakia. I. Prevalence of retinal detachment. Br J Ophthalmol. 1975;59(9):480–2.

88. Neuhann IM, Neuhann TF, Heimann H, et al. Retinal detachment after phacoemulsification in high myopia: analysis of 2356 cases. J Cataract Refract Surg. 2008;34(10):1644–57.

89. Merin S, Feiler V, Hyams S, et al. The fate of the fellow eye in retinal detachment. Am J Ophthalmol. 1971;71(2):477–81.

90. Mitry D, Singh J, Yorston D, et al. The fellow eye in retinal detachment: findings from the Scottish retinal detachment study. Br J Ophthalmol. 2012;96(1):110–3.

91. Tornquist R. Bilateral retinal detachment. Acta Ophthalmol. 1963;41:126–33.

92. Benson WE, Grand MG, Okun E. Aphakic retinal detachment. Management of the fellow eye. Arch Ophthalmol. 1975;93(4):245–9.

Retinal Detachment

C. P. Wilkinson

23.1 Introduction

The relationship between rhegmatogenous retinal detachment (RRD) and myopia has been recognized since soon after the introduction of the ophthalmoscope [1]. More than half of retinal detachments appear to occur in eyes with some degree of myopia [2], and the risk of retinal detachment is three to eight times greater in myopic eyes than in emmetropic and hyperopic cases [2, 3]. The relationship between risk of detachment and amount of myopia is linear, with 1–3 diopters (D) of myopia being associated with four times increased risk and greater than 3 D having a tenfold increased risk [2]. The relative risk appears to be higher in relatively youthful eyes than in patients over age 65 [2, 4], presumably due to an increased frequency of prior posterior vitreous detachment (PVD) in the older patients.

Retinal detachments remain an important cause of reduced vision, and their prevention has long been considered a worthy goal. However, efforts to accomplish this task have not been particularly successful except in eyes with acute symptomatic horseshoe tears [5]. And to date, there are no level I evidence-based guidelines regarding the prevention of retinal detachment [6]. Since RRDs always require the presence of retinal breaks and some degree of vitreous liquefaction and usually feature persistent vitreoretinal traction in the region of retinal breaks, changes in the vitreous gel are of critical importance in the pathogenesis of this form of retinal detachment. Still, most efforts to prevent retinal detachment have involved treatment of visible peripheral retinal lesions, including degenerative lesions such as lattice degeneration and retinal breaks of various types [5–7]. An additional strategy has involved the creation of a 360° peripheral zone of chorioretinal adhesive burns anterior to the equator. This will be described in more detail later, but to date it has not been demonstrated to be of proven value [7], and an effective means of preventing RRD remains an elusive goal.

The purpose of this review is to discuss the relatively unique vitreoretinal features of significantly myopic eyes that predispose them to RRD, to examine the results of specific efforts to prevent this problem, and to present a brief review of surgical reattachment methods. Vitreous changes and peripheral vitreoretinal degenerative lesions associated with myopia will be initially emphasized.

23.2 The Myopic Eye: Features Predisposing to Retinal Detachment

Vitreous gel changes and peripheral vitreoretinal degenerative disorders associated with anomalous vitreoretinal adhesions are responsible for most RRDs, and these factors are particularly common in myopic eyes.

23.2.1 Alterations in the Myopic Vitreous Gel

The usual sequence of vitreous changes that lead to clinical RRD begins with vitreous liquefaction leading to increased mobility and decreased stability of the vitreous gel [8]. This is followed by the critical event of posterior vitreous detachment (PVD), during which the posterior cortical surface of the vitreous separates from the inner surface of most of the retina (Fig. 23.1).

23.2.2 Vitreous Liquefaction and Myopia

There is an abundance of biochemical, experimental, histopathologic, and clinical evidence that the vitreous gel in myopic eyes has a substantially increased liquid component

C. P. Wilkinson (✉)
Department of Ophthalmology, Greater Baltimore Medical Center, Baltimore, MD, USA

Department of Ophthalmology, Johns Hopkins University, Baltimore, MD, USA

R. F. Spaide et al. (eds.), *Pathologic Myopia*, https://doi.org/10.1007/978-3-030-74334-5_23

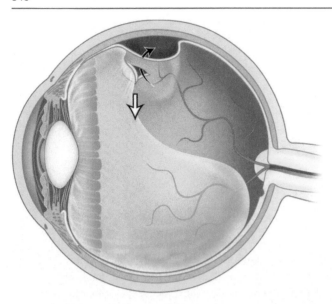

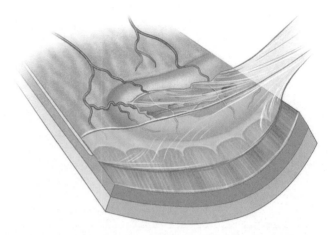

Fig. 23.2 Although holes in lattice lesions are considered to be "atrophic," nearby vitreoretinal traction upon the margins of the lattice lesions can facilitate passage of vitreous fluids into the subretinal space

Fig. 23.1 Retinal tears most commonly occur at sites of firm vitreoretinal adhesions following a posterior vitreous detachment. Traction (*white arrow*) from the detached cortical vitreous surface upon the retina creates the retinal break(s). Liquids in the vitreous cavity then can pass through the tear(s) into the subretinal space (*black arrow*)

compared to emmetropic and hyperopic control eyes [8]. This is associated with relative reductions in vitreous viscosity and vitreous stability.

23.2.3 Posterior Vitreous Detachment (PVD)

In the myopic eye, the relative increase in vitreous liquification combined with the relative elongation of the globe results in an increased frequency of PVD at relatively young ages [8–10]. In addition, there is increasing evidence that there appear to be increased vitreous stresses upon the myopic retina that promote relatively early PVD [11]. Until recently, PVD was believed to be a sudden rapidly progressive event, but modern studies with ultrasound and optical coherence tomography (OCT) have demonstrated that PVD usually evolves slowly in the posterior pole over months and years [12]. Still, ultimately, large areas of cortical vitreous separate rapidly from much of the retina, an event typically heralded by symptoms of "flashes and floaters." PVD does not cause retinal breaks in most eyes, because the cortical vitreous surface usually separates completely from the inner surface of the retina from the posterior pole to the posterior margin of the vitreous base. However, if vitreoretinal adhesions between vitreous and retinal surfaces are present, they are the sites of the majority of retinal tears that cause most RRDs (Fig. 23.1) [8, 13, 14]. Vitreoretinal adhesions, therefore, are of critical importance in the pathogenesis of retinal detachment.

23.2.4 Vitreoretinal Adhesions Associated with Peripheral Vitreoretinal Degenerative Disorders

In the most common forms of RRD, separation of the cortical vitreous from the retinal surface is not completed at sites of abnormal vitreoretinal adhesions, and flap ("horseshoe") tears develop at such locations (Fig. 23.1). Vitreous traction upon lattice lesions containing atrophic holes is another form of common retinal detachment (Fig. 23.2). Only in cases in which vitreoretinal traction is completely released from a retinal break, as when an operculum occurs at the site of the retinal tear, are subsequent clinical retinal detachments exceptionally rare. Once a localized retinal detachment is associated with a retinal tear and persistent vitreoretinal traction, a variety of forces promote an accumulation of subretinal fluid and an enlarging clinical detachment (Fig. 23.3). In some eyes especially in cases with high myopia, the initial PVD is not always complete, and retinal tears and detachments occur only after later progression of the PVD produces retinal tears at sites of vitreoretinal adhesions that were not previously included in the areas of vitreous separation [15, 16]. Vitreoretinal adhesions may be visible or invisible, and the latter lesions become apparent only after the development of a PVD and retinal tears. Although visible vitreoretinal adhesions have been most commonly discussed as preoperative risk factors for RRD, invisible adhesions appear to be very common, particularly in myopic eyes [16, 17].

23.2.5 Visible Vitreoretinal Adhesions

Lattice degeneration is the most common visible peripheral retinal vitreoretinal degenerative disorder associated with an

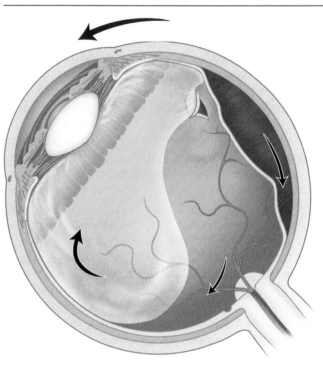

Fig. 23.3 Ocular saccades increase vitreoretinal traction forces. Rotation of the globe (*upper large arrow*) results in slightly delayed movement (*larger black arrow* in vitreous cavity) of the vitreous gel which in turn exerts more traction at sites of vitreoretinal adhesion. In addition, liquid currents within the vitreous cavity (*smaller intravitreal arrow*) promote increased vitreoretinal traction, whereas currents in the subretinal space (*arrow*) promote extension of subretinal fluid

Table 23.1 Vitreoretinal findings in highly myopic retinal detachment cases (*n* = 496)

Group	Mean age	Mean myopia (D)	Lattice breaks (%)	Tears (%)	Giant tears (%)
PVD complete	54	−15.5	45	40	15
PVD incomplete	59	−18.5	44	31	0
V liquefaction, no PVD	39	−19.5	0	0	71
V lacunae, no PVD	57	−24	N/A	N/A	0
Minimal PVD	23	−10.5	84	84	0

Adopted from Stirpe and Heimann [20]

increased risk of RRD. These lesions feature a variety of clinical appearances and have been described in a number of different ways, including "snail track degeneration," "peripheral retinal degeneration," and "pigmentary degeneration." Nevertheless, all have in common an exaggerated adhesion between the retina and cortical vitreous at the margins of the respective lesion. Lattice degeneration is more common in myopic eyes than in emmetropic and hyperopic cases, although there may not be a precise relationship between the degree of myopia and the prevalence of the lesion. Lattice lesions combined with myopia appear to increase the risk of later retinal detachment.

Additional sites of visible vitreoretinal adhesions that can be sites of retinal tears following PVD include cystic retinal tufts, chorioretinal scars, and foci of active or inactive retinitis [7].

23.2.6   Invisible Vitreoretinal Adhesions

Invisible vitreoretinal adhesions become evident only after at least some degree of PVD has taken place and/or a retinal tear develops [17]. Although these adhesions are responsible for many retinal tears and detachments, they cannot be

considered for direct prophylactic therapy because they occur in areas that appear "normal" prior to PVD. Irregularities in the contour of the margin of the posterior vitreous base as remodeling of this zone occurs with age may be responsible for a significant percentage of anterior horseshoe tears occurring in association with PVD [18]. Additional invisible sites of vitreoretinal adhesions typically occur along retinal blood vessels, and clinical retinal detachments due to such tears may be particularly common in highly myopic eyes [18, 19].

Sebag [8, 13, 14] has demonstrated that the strength of the attachment between the cortical vitreous and retina is stronger in relatively youthful eyes than in older cases. Thus, the combination of accelerated vitreous changes leading to PVD in relatively youthful eyes, combined with relatively strong invisible vitreoretinal attachments between a young vitreous cortex and the retina, appears to play a critical role in the production of retinal tears and detachments in relatively young myopic patients. In this context, a "normal" youthful adhesion between vitreous and cortex may become an "abnormal" vitreoretinal adhesion if relatively early "anomalous PVD" [13] occurs. This scenario is clearly most likely in highly myopic eyes. Vitreous changes typically occur slowly, and this may explain the relatively late appearance of retinal tears and detachments following procedures known to alter the vitreous gel.

Stirpe and Heimann [20] have added important descriptions of vitreous changes and associated vitreoretinal adhesions in highly myopic eyes with RRDs. They studied 496 such phakic eyes with myopia ranging from −18 to −30 D. These cases were subdivided into five classifications based on pre- and intraoperative observations of the vitreous gel, retina, and vitreoretinal adhesions. Vitreous liquefaction and vitreoretinal adhesions were demonstrated to be essential components of RRDs, and the amount of vitreous detachment correlated with the specific types of cases described. A selection of these findings in these highly myopic eyes is summarized in Table 23.1. Anomalous posterior vitreoretinal adhesions and subtotal PVDs appeared to be much more common in these highly myopic cases than in those associated with lower degrees of myopia.

In terms of the pathogenesis of relatively routine retinal tears and detachments, the following important observations in the report of Stirpe and Heimann [20] and others [18] appear to be most important:

- Complete, significant but incomplete, and limited PVDs are all observed in highly myopic eyes.
- Detachments due to routine retinal tears, including those associated with lattice degeneration, usually occur at areas of vitreoretinal adhesions that are surrounded by zones in which PVD had occurred.
- Retinal detachments due to atrophic holes in lattice degeneration usually occur in eyes with complete or partial PVD, in which PVD has occurred in the zones surrounding the lattice lesions.
- Detachments associated with extensive vitreous liquefaction or posterior lacunae but without significant PVD are usually due to giant retinal tears or unusual posterior breaks due to vitreoretinal traction in eyes with relatively high degrees of myopia.
- Detachments associated with extremely limited PVDs are not unusual, frequently occurring in relatively youthful eyes with relatively low degrees of high myopia and relatively common lesions, including atrophic holes in lattice lesions, retinal dialyses, and horseshoe tears.

These observations are important in supporting the classic concepts that (1) access of liquid vitreous to retinal breaks is essential for all RRDs, (2) vitreoretinal adhesions and traction upon retinal breaks are usually responsible for retinal detachments, and (3) PVD causes most RRDs by producing retinal tears or increased traction upon existing lattice lesions containing atrophic holes. Attempts to both prevent and repair retinal detachments should include the recognition of all of these realities.

23.3 Prevention of Rhegmatogenous Retinal Detachment in Myopia

As previously stated, the usual sequence of events leading to the production of retinal tears includes vitreous liquefaction leading to complete or large but incomplete PVD and the production of new retinal tears due to vitreoretinal traction at the sites of vitreoretinal adhesions including lattice lesions with atrophic holes (Figs. 23.1, 23.2, and 23.3). A not uncommon exception to this pattern is retinal detachment due to atrophic holes in lattice degeneration but unassociated with a major PVD. These cases are particularly likely to occur in youthful myopic eyes in which relatively early vitreous liquefaction has occurred [4], and vitreoretinal traction, in the absence of substantial PVD, exists in the region of the lattice lesions. The second common exceptions to the rule that

major PVD precedes retinal detachment are retinal detachment due to retinal dialyses or giant retinal tears, and these cases are usually discovered following ocular trauma or unequivocal symptoms, and prophylactic therapy to prevent small or huge retinal dialyses prior to their development is rarely considered except in fellow eyes of patients with nontraumatic giant tears.

In view of the pathogenesis of most RRDs in myopic eyes, theoretical means of preventing most retinal detachment in myopic eyes would include techniques to reduce the rates of (1) vitreous liquefaction, (2) PVD, (3) vitreoretinal traction, (4) retinal breaks at the sites of vitreoretinal adhesions, and (5) extension of subretinal fluid surrounding retinal breaks. No means are available to prevent vitreous liquefaction and/or PVD, although maintenance of an intact posterior lens capsule following cataract surgery may delay such changes. A reduction of vitreoretinal traction could be accomplished by vitrectomy or scleral buckling, but these are impractical maneuvers as widespread prophylactic procedures. Most contemporary preventative therapies have been proposed to reduce the frequency of retinal tears at sites of visible vitreoretinal adhesive lesions or to prevent the accumulation of subretinal fluid around retinal breaks [6, 7, 21]. Treatment has usually consisted of creation of chorioretinal adhesions, with lasers or cryotherapy, around visible focal degenerative lesions or retinal breaks. Others have proposed creating a peripheral ring of chorioretinal adhesions to prevent the development of tears at both visible and invisible vitreoretinal adhesions [7].

23.3.1 Treatment of Visible Vitreoretinal Adhesions in Myopia

The results of treating visible vitreoretinal adhesions such as lattice degeneration to prevent retinal detachment have been evaluated by expert panels that have employed contemporary methods of rating the quality of evidence contained in the multitude of articles that have been published on this topic, and the American Academy of Ophthalmology (AAO) has published a "Preferred Practice Pattern (PPP)" regarding prophylactic therapy [6].

In the AAO PPP, no prospective randomized trials regarding preventative therapy of any vitreoretinal lesions, including all types of retinal breaks, were identified. The best evidence indicated that treatment of focal retinal detachments associated with *symptomatic* horseshoe tears was effective. There was "substantial" evidence that treatment of lattice degeneration in all myopic eyes was of no benefit. In myopic eyes in which retinal detachment due to lattice had occurred in the first eye, there was "substantial" evidence that treating the lattice lesions in the fellow eye was of limited value [22]. However, the same evidence base demonstrated that such treatment was of no value if the degree of myopia exceeded −6 D or if there were more than 6 clock hours of lattice degeneration. Thus, prophylactic therapy is of less value in these higher-risk myopic eyes.

Table 23.2 provides a list of the AAO-PPP grading of recommendations for therapy of a variety of lesions in myopic eyes [6]. Most of these recommendations were graded as "level III (consensus of expert opinion)", the weakest level of evidence. Unfortunately, the apparent value of treating lesions other than symptomatic horseshoe tears is exceptionally limited.

23.3.2 Treatment of Invisible Vitreoretinal Adhesions in Myopia

The major limitation in treating visible vitreoretinal adhesions is that subsequent retinal tears and detachments occur in areas that appear normal prior to PVD (Fig. 23.4) [7, 17]. These tears that occur at sites of invisible vitreoretinal adhesions must be considered in any scheme for a genuinely effective preventative therapy. To accomplish a goal of treating invisible adhesions, some authors have recommended the placement of chorioretinal burns over a 360° zone of peripheral retina extending from near the anterior equator to anterior to the posterior margin of the vitreous base (Fig. 23.5)

[7, 23, 24]. Both laser and cryotherapy have been employed for this purpose. The majority of publications on this topic have appeared in the European literature, and they have been thoroughly summarized by Byer [9]. The evidence that this form of therapy is effective appears to be lacking, but there are data demonstrating that some risk may be associated with this form of treatment. It is possible that the pathophysiolog-

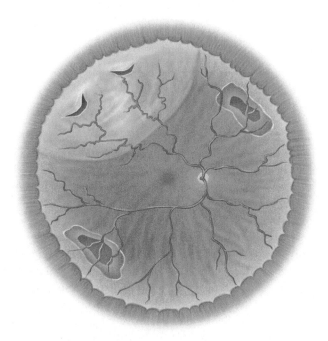

Fig. 23.4 Treated visible lattice lesions do not prevent additional retinal tears at sites of invisible vitreoretinal adhesion

Table 23.2 Grading of recommendations for prophylactic therapy [6]

Level	Recommendation	Type of case[a]
Level I "strong"	------------	------------------
--------	---	-------
Level II "substantial"	Treat promptly	Symptomatic flap tear
-------	------	----------
Level III "consensus"	No treatment	Asymptomatic lattice degeneration[a]
--------	-------	--------
--------	Rarely treat	Asymptomatic lattice[a] in aphakic eyes
----------	---------	Asymptomatic horseshoe tears
---------	-----------	Asymptomatic operculated tears
----------	------------	Asymptomatic atrophic holes
--------------	-----------------	-------------------------
--------------	Sometimes treat	Traumatic retinal breaks
----------------	-------------------	Symptomatic operculated tears
--------------------	-------------------	-------------------------
No level or consensus	------------------	Fellow eyes with horseshoe tears
--------------	------------------	Fellow eyes with lattice degeneration
--------------	-------------------	Asymptomatic dialyses

Modified from the American Academy of Ophthalmology PPP [6]
[a]All "lattice" includes lesions with and without holes

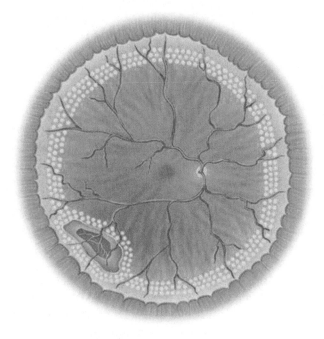

Fig. 23.5 Creation of 360° of prophylactic laser or cryotherapy has been recommended by some authors

ical forces leading to retinal detachment may be adversely affected by extensive preventative therapy. Since invisible vitreoretinal adhesions occur relatively posteriorly in highly myopic eyes [22], the theoretical problems of "barrage" therapy in these cases would appear to be particularly significant. A compelling case might be made for patients with Stickler 1 and a profound risk of retinal detachment. Three hundred sixty-degree cryotherapy straddling the ora serrata in such cases appears to some to be of value [25], although optimal prospective trials are yet to be performed.

23.4 Treatment of Rhegmatogenous Retinal Detachment in Myopia

As noted earlier, factors associated with myopia and RRD include increased vitreous liquefaction, frequency of PVD, lattice degeneration, and asymptomatic retinal breaks, with the prevalence of RRD directly related to the amount of myopia. In addition to peripheral retinal abnormalities, alterations of the vitreoretinal interface at the posterior pole play a role in the pathogenesis of RRD due to macular holes in highly myopic eyes. Less commonly, RRDs in highly myopic eyes are due to posterior retinal breaks that can easily escape diagnosis [26]. These typically have a linear shape, lie parallel to the adjacent retinal vessels of the posterior vascular arcades, and are almost exclusively located over areas of patchy chorioretinal atrophy. In addition to all types of retinal breaks, myopic atrophic and neovascular macular disorders, posterior pole staphylomas, and foveal retinoschisis can impact visual acuity in myopic patients.

Although controversy regarding the choice of surgical technique for RRD is widespread, surgeons generally agree on the three basic steps for closing retinal breaks and reattaching the retina:

1. Conducting thorough preoperative and intraoperative examinations with the goal of locating all retinal breaks and assessing vitreous traction on the retina
2. Creating a controlled injury to the retinal pigment epithelium and retina to produce a chorioretinal adhesion surrounding all retinal breaks so that intravitreal fluid can no longer reach the subretinal space
3. Employing a technique such as scleral buckling and/or intravitreal gas to approximate the retinal breaks to the underlying treated retinal pigment epithelium

If the surgeon follows these basics and applies modern surgical techniques, retinal reattachment may be expected following a single operation in more than 85% of uncomplicated primary detachments and in more than 95% following additional procedures. Following anatomically successful surgery, visual results in all eyes remain limited because of the profound influence of preoperative macular detachment and irreversible damage upon postoperative visual improvement, and additional posterior chorioretinal problems in high myopia result in visual acuity results that are relatively poor.

Traditional scleral buckling has served as a successful technique since the 1950s. However, more recent developments have produced a more comprehensive menu for retinal reattachment surgery from which the surgeon may select the appropriate procedure for each case (Table 23.3) [27]. Vitreous surgery has become the most popular method of repair, especially in pseudophakic eyes, whereas pneumatic retinopexy is favored by some surgeons for selected types of RD. Still, scleral buckling remains a valuable technique that is indicated in several situations, particularly in the repair of myopic retinal detachments associated with lattice degeneration or retinal dialyses, both of which are typically associated with limited PVDs. Nevertheless, opinions regarding the "best" operation for a given case will never be agreed upon universally, just as a single ice cream flavor will never be favored by all.

There are several relatively common types of uncomplicated myopic RRDs due to peripheral retinal breaks, and they are usually managed in one of three ways (Table 23.3). Those that are genuinely complicated are routinely managed with vitrectomy techniques. A large percentage of uncomplicated cases can be managed with scleral buckling and/or vitrectomy, and combinations are also employed by many surgeons. Regardless of technique, if all retinal breaks are surgically closed and PVR or other more unusual complications do not develop, the procedure will usually be anatomically successful.

23.4.1 Surgery for Uncomplicated Myopic RRDs with Peripheral Retinal Breaks

Scleral buckling, vitrectomy, and, in selected cases, pneumatic retinopexy (PR) have been employed in the repair of these relatively routine types of cases. Each procedure has its advantages and disadvantages.

Table 23.3 Surgical alternatives for repair of RRD

Scleral buckle with and without drainage of subretinal fluid
Encircling
Segmental
Vitrectomy
With gas injection
With silicone oil injection
With epiretinal membrane peeling
With ILM peeling
Pneumatic retinopexy
Combinations

23.4.2 Scleral Buckling

As the only popular method of managing RRDs until the 1980s, scleral buckling can be employed in the vast majority of uncomplicated cases in which the retina can be adequately visualized. Anatomic success rates do not appear to be significantly impacted by myopia [28]. The diminished popularity of this technique is not primarily due to limitations in anatomical success but rather to the development of alternative techniques that provide acceptable reattachment rates, fewer or different complications, and additional advantages in selected cases.

The most common complications of scleral buckling (other than anatomic failure) do not usually follow vitrectomy without buckling or PR. In addition, the latter alternative offers additional advantages of an office procedure and reduced postoperative discomfort, whereas vitreous surgery provides a remedy for the most common relative contraindications of buckling, significant vitreous opacification, and posterior retinal breaks.

23.4.3 Advantages

The primary advantage of scleral buckling is the fact that it has served as a standard of care for decades, and its success and complication rates are therefore relatively well understood and acceptable. An additional important advantage is the fact that buckling is usually an extraocular procedure except for the important frequently optional steps of draining subretinal fluid and/or injecting gas. It therefore usually does not cause direct changes in the vitreous gel that routinely follow pneumatic procedures and vitrectomy. The costs of equipment and accessory materials are considerably less than for vitrectomy although much more than for PR. It is not associated with progressive cataract formation following surgery.

23.4.4 Disadvantages

Compared to PR, important disadvantages of scleral buckling are the necessity of performing the operation in an operating room and the costs of this and additional equipment. More patient morbidity occurs following buckling than after PR and most vitrectomies without buckling. Compared to vitrectomy, significant disadvantages include increased difficulties in the management of very large and/or posterior retinal breaks and increased patient morbidity following repairs of relatively "difficult" cases. Postoperative muscle imbalance and altered refractive errors are important complications that are more commonly seen following scleral buckling than after PR or vitrectomy without buckling. Myopic cases are frequently associated with thin sclera, and this dis-advantage is associated with increased chances of sclera perforation during placement of sutures. A growing but relatively obscure disadvantage is that many vitreoretinal training programs appear to be providing less extensive scleral buckling educational experiences than was true in years past.

23.4.5 Vitrectomy

Retinal detachments that were initially managed with a "primary" vitrectomy were usually complicated by severe vitreous hemorrhage, PVR, PDR, giant tears, etc., and the technique was not employed for more routine cases until the mid-1980s. Since then this form of surgery has become tremendously popular, particularly in regard to the management of pseudophakic cases.

23.4.6 Advantages

The primary advantages of vitrectomy include the elimination of media opacities and transvitreal and periretinal membranous traction forces, improved visualization and localization of retinal breaks, internal intraoperative reattachment of the retina, and precise application of adhesive therapy. These steps can usually be accomplished without the complications that are relatively common following scleral buckling unless a buckling procedure is performed simultaneously with the vitrectomy. As noted above, highly myopic eyes are associated with an increased frequency of posterior retinal breaks and residual posterior vitreoretinal adhesions, and these realities favor vitreous surgery.

23.4.7 Disadvantages

In phakic eyes, the routine development of postoperative nuclear sclerotic cataracts represents a major disadvantage to vitrectomy, and there is some evidence that open angle glaucoma may develop in pseudophakic vitrectomized eyes over decades following surgery. The costs of this alternative are substantially higher than with PR or scleral buckling. Myopic RDs are associated with an increased incidence of posterior vitreoretinal adhesions, and separation of the vitreous and retina may be relatively difficult, especially in younger patients. Failure of vitrectomy may be associated with the development of relatively severe forms of PVR, although considerably more research is needed to evaluate this phenomenon. A hopefully transient disadvantage is the lack of information regarding precise causes of failure following vitrectomy, and as additional data accumulate in regard to this relatively new technique, more answers will hopefully be forthcoming.

23.4.8 Pneumatic Retinopexy

The classic and "ideal" uncomplicated RRD for a pneumatic procedure (PR) is one associated with a retinal break or group of breaks located between approximately 10:00 and 2:00 and extending no more than 1 clock hour in circumference. Although the technique can be employed successfully when breaks are not located either superiorly or close together, fewer surgeons would select the procedure in these instances. Additional features that add to the attractiveness of PR include an apparently total PVD, an absence of lattice degeneration and vitreous hemorrhage, and a phakic lens status.

PR is associated with approximately a 10% reduction in 1-operation anatomical success rate when compared to scleral buckling, but ultimate success following reoperation is not compromised. It therefore is a procedure that represents a legitimate standard of care as an option to other forms of reattachment surgery. Interestingly, this operation is considerably more popular in the USA than in Europe or the UK.

23.4.9 Advantages

The primary advantages of PR are that it can be performed quickly in an office setting with modest local anesthesia and that it has an acceptable success rate. Patient morbidity is usually less than with alternative operations, and costs are considerably lower with PR. Progressive cataract formation does not follow the procedure.

23.4.10 Disadvantages

The primary disadvantage of PR is that most surgeons limit its use to a relatively consistent subset of patients with single superior breaks and few signs of extensive vitreoretinal degenerative disorders, and there are many common types of cases in which it should not be employed. As noted, a total PVD is less common in myopic eyes, and lattice degeneration is relatively common, and these are two features that make PR less popular for highly myopic cases. Additionally, even in carefully selected cases, the 1-operation anatomic success rate is approximately 10% lower than for scleral buckling. Still, there is no evidence that a failed PR procedure lowers the ultimate anatomic or visual success rate.

23.4.11 Surgery for Myopic RRDs with Posterior Retinal Breaks

Posterior retinal breaks are significantly more common in myopic eyes, and there is a direct relationship between the incidence of macular hole RRDs and amount of myopia

[29]. The surgical management of these cases is particularly difficult in eyes with posterior staphylomas and extensive chorioretinal atrophy. As is the case with RDs due to peripheral breaks, treatment has been based upon either intraocular or extraocular approaches, with combinations being reserved for particularly complicated cases. Intraocular approaches can be as simple as a single injection of gas or as complex as a vitrectomy with silicone oil injection. Scleral buckling is theoretically straightforward but technically very difficult. All of these techniques have broad ranges of anatomical success, and visual results are frequently compromised because of posterior pole problems associated with high myopia. The relationships between the posterior cortical vitreous and retina are critical, and the presence of epiretinal membranes can complicate decision-making further.

23.4.12 Pneumatic Procedures for Myopic RRDs Due to Macular Holes

Several reports [29, 30] have described a simple gas injection as an appropriate first step in managing RRDs due to macular holes in myopia. An expanding gas bubble is injected with or without an attempt to remove fluid vitreous prior to injection. Other authors have drained subretinal fluid and treated the hole with laser therapy [31]. The advantages of a technique with only gas injection are its simplicity and the fact that it is an inexpensive office procedure. The major disadvantage is its unpredictability in permanently reattaching the retina, with anatomic results ranging from less than 20 to 90% [29]. The variable of a total PVD vs. persistent vitreous traction on the posterior retina would appear to be critical in predicting a successful outcome [29], although some reports do not support this premise [32].

23.4.13 Vitrectomy for Myopic RRDs Due to Macular Holes

Posterior vitreoretinal traction appears to be a major factor in the development of myopic RRDs associated with macular holes, and elimination of traction forces with vitrectomy has been discussed since 1982 [33]. This has been combined with injections of gas, perfluorocarbons, and both light and heavy silicone oil. Epiretinal membranes are removed by most authorities in an effort to reduce tangential traction forces [34], and there is increased interest in peeling internal limiting membranes (ILM) during the operation. Case selection and the wide variety of alternative accessory surgical techniques make a comparison of the advantages and disadvantages of vitrectomy for myopic RRDs due to macular holes most difficult.

Success rates with vitrectomy appear in general to be better than those following a simple pneumatic procedure, especially if all epiretinal membranes are successfully removed during the former operation [29]. The value of removing ILM remains somewhat uncertain [29], although a relatively recent report [35] in which "double peeling" of cortical vitreous and ILM with triamcinolone and trypan blue, respectively, demonstrated higher reattachment rates and better visual acuities in the cases managed in this fashion.

The main cause of anatomic failure is reopening of the macular hole, frequently apparently due to associated staphylomas, widespread chorioretinal atrophy, and a reduced natural adhesion between pigment epithelium and the sensory retina [20]. To improve anatomic success rates, some surgeons have favored a permanent intraocular tamponade with silicone oil. High-density silicone oils have more recently been employed in some countries, and improved success rates have been reported in some publications [36]. The principle of sealing responsible retinal breaks is frequently ignored in the repair of myopic RRDs due to macular holes because of the obvious effect upon postoperative vision. Still, laser therapy to treat the holes has been employed, especially in cases in which the break has reopened [36]. A evidence-based description of the genuine relative value of many accessory vitrectomy surgical techniques remains impossible at this time.

23.4.14 Scleral Buckling for Myopic RRDs Due to Macular Holes

Scleral buckling of macular holes provides a distinct advantage of changing the posterior sclera surface from concave to convex, relieving both vitreoretinal and tangential traction forces [36–38]. Some reports have demonstrated a superiority of this technique over vitrectomy procedures [35, 36]. The primary disadvantage of scleral buckling is its surgical difficulty.

As mentioned above, the absence of prospective randomized controlled trials, the small sample sizes in most reports, the differing methods of case selection, and the variations in follow-up periods result in major difficulties in comparing scleral buckling with other techniques [29].

23.5 Conclusions

RRDs are much more common in myopic eyes, particularly those with high degrees of myopia. Myopia is a major risk factor for retinal detachment because of vitreoretinal alterations associated with the refractive error as well as possible structural alterations in the myopic globe. Most retinal detachments are due to retinal flap tears or holes associated with persistent vitreoretinal traction upon sites of vitreoretinal adhesions that are near the respective retinal breaks. The most significant vitreoretinal traction forces occur following PVD, an event that occurs both earlier and more frequently in myopic eyes.

Vitreoretinal adhesions can be considered as forms of peripheral vitreoretinal degeneration. Most of these zones are invisible, but many such as lattice degeneration are quite apparent. To some degree, invisible vitreoretinal adhesions may be considered to be inversely age-related, as a relatively strong adhesion appears to exist in normal relatively youthful eyes [14]. Since vitreous liquefaction and detachment occur at a significantly younger age in highly myopic patients, this normal vitreoretinal adhesion may be considered "abnormal" if PVD occurs and the adhesion becomes the cause of a significant tear [13]. This combination of abnormal vitreous changes occurring in association with a relatively firm vitreoretinal adhesive force seems to be particularly common in myopic eyes.

Prevention of significant percentages of asymptomatic myopic retinal detachments does not appear to be possible unless [1] flap retinal tears are visualized at the time of symptomatic PVD or soon thereafter or [2] significant progression of "subclinical detachments" associated with atrophic holes in lattice lesions is identified [21]. Thus, the best current therapy for patients at increased risk for retinal detachment appears to be the following: to advise all patients of the critical importance of any symptoms suggesting the onset of PVD [21] and to periodically reexamine all patients with significant myopia and lattice degeneration, particularly if the lattice lesion is associated with atrophic holes and surrounded by minimal subretinal fluid.

Most RRDs that occur in myopic eyes are uncomplicated, and due to peripheral retinal breaks, they are repaired with methods that are identical to RRDs occurring in emmetropic cases. The choice of optimal surgical procedures remains controversial, although vitrectomy techniques are now clearly more popular than scleral buckling.

Myopic RRDs due to macular holes are an important subset of cases that are more common in certain geographic areas. The repair of these RRDs remains challenging in spite of numerous advances in vitreoretinal surgical techniques.

References

1. von Graefe A. Mittheilungen vermischten Inhalts. Arch f Ophthalmol. 1857;2:187–9.
2. The Eye Disease Case Control Study Group. Risk factors for idiopathic rhegmatogenous retinal detachment. Am J Epidemiol. 1993;137:749–57.
3. Austin KL, Palmer JR, Seddon JM, et al. Case–control study of idiopathic retinal detachment. Int J Epidemiol. 1990;19:1045–50.

4. Burton TC. The influence of refractive error and lattice degeneration on the incidence of retinal detachment. Trans Am Ophthalmol Soc. 1989;87:143–55.

5. Wilkinson CP. Evidence-based analysis of prophylactic treatment of asymptomatic retinal breaks and lattice degeneration. Ophthalmology. 2000;107:12–5.

6. American Academy of Ophthalmology. Management of posterior vitreous detachment, retinal breaks, and lattice degeneration. Preferred practice pattern. San Francisco: American Academy of Ophthalmology; 2008.

7. Byer NE. Rethinking prophylactic therapy of retinal detachment. In: Stirpe M, editor. Advances in vitreoretinal surgery. New York: Ophthalmic Communications Society; 1992. p. 399–411.

8. Sebag J. Myopia effects upon vitreous-significance in retinal detachments. In: Stirpe M, editor. Anterior and posterior segment surgery: mutual problems and common interests. New York: Ophthalmic Communications Society; 1998. p. 366–72.

9. Pierro L, Camesasca FI, Mischi M, Brancato R. Peripheral retinal changes and axial myopia. Retina. 1992;12:12–7.

10. Akiba J. Prevalence of posterior vitreous detachment in high myopia. Ophthalmology. 1993;100:1384–8.

11. Meskauskas J, Repetto R, Siggers J. Shape changes of the vitreous chamber influences retinal detachment and reattachment processes: is mechanical stress during eye rotations a factor? Invest Ophthalmol Vis Sci. 2012;53(10):6271–81.

12. Johnson MW, Brucker AJ, Chang S, et al. Vitreomacular disorders: pathogenesis and treatment. Retina. 2012;32 Suppl 2:S173–232.

13. Sebag J. Anomalous posterior vitreous detachment: a unifying concept in vitreo-retinal disease. Greaefes Arch Clin Exp Ophthalmol. 2004;242:690–8.

14. Sebag J. Age-related differences in the human vitreo-retinal interface. Arch Ophthalmol. 1991;109:966–71.

15. Ripandelli G, Coppe AM, Pavisi V, et al. Fellow eye findings of highly myopic subjects operated for retinal detachment associated with macular hole. Ophthalmology. 2008;115:1489–93.

16. Chan CK, Tarasewicz DG, Lin SG. Relation of pre-LASIK and post-LASIK retinal lesions and retinal examination for LASIK eyes. Br J Ophthalmol. 2005;89:299–301.

17. Mastropasqua L, Carpineto P, Ciancaglini M, et al. Treatment of retinal tears and lattice degeneration in fellow eyes in high risk patients suffering retinal detachment: a prospective study. Br J Ophthalmol. 1999;83:1046–9.

18. Mitry D, Fleck BW, Wright AF, et al. Pathogenesis of rhegmatogenous retinal detachment: predisposing anatomy and cell biology. Retina. 2010;30:1561–72.

19. Chen L, Wang K, Esmaili DD, Xu G. Rhegmatogenous retinal detachment due to paravascular linear retinal breaks over patchy chorioretinal atrophy in pathologic myopia. Arch Ophthalmol. 2010;128(12):1551–4.

20. Stirpe M, Heimann K. Vitreous changes and retinal detachment in highly myopic eyes. Eur J Ophthalmol. 1996;6:50–8.

21. Byer NE. Natural history of posterior vitreous detachment with early management as the premier line of defense against retinal detachment. Ophthalmology. 1994;101:1503–13.

22. Folk JC, Arrindell EL, Klugman MR. The fellow eye of patients with phakic lattice retinal detachment. Ophthalmology. 1989;96:72–9.

23. Koh HJ, Cheng L, Kosobucki B, et al. Prophylactic intraoperative 360-degree laser retinopexy for prevention of retinal detachment. Retina. 2007;27:744–9.

24. Chalam KV, Murthy RK, Gupta SK, et al. Prophylactic circumferential intraoperative laser retinopexy decreases the risk of retinal detachment after macular hole surgery. Eur J Ophthalmol. 2012;22:799–802.

25. And A, Poulson AV, Goodburn SF, et al. Retinal detachment and prophylaxis in type 1 stickler syndrome. Ophthalmology. 2008;115:164–8.

26. Chen L, Wang K, Esmaili DD, et al. Rhegmatogenous retinal detachment due to paravascular linear breaks over patchy chorioretinal atrophy in pathologic myopia. Arch Ophthalmol. 2012;128:1551–5.

27. Alyward GW. Optimal procedures for retinal detachment repair. In: Ryan SJ, Wilkinson CP, editors. Retina, vol. 3. 5th ed. New York: Elsevier; 2013. p. 1784–92.

28. Rodriguez FJ, Lewis H, Krieger AE, et al. Scleral buckling for rhegmatogenous retinal detachment associated with severe myopia. Am J Ophthalmol. 1991;111:595–600.

29. Ortisi E, Avitabile T, Bonfiglio V. Surgical management of retinal detachment because of macular hole in highly myopic eyes. Retina. 2012;32:1704–18.

30. Miyake Y. A simplified method of treating retinal detachment with macular hole. Long-term follow-up. Arch Ophthalmol. 1986;104:1234–6.

31. Ripandelli G, Parisi V, Friberg TR, et al. Retinal detachment associated with macular hole in high myopia: using the vitreous anatomy to optimize the surgical approach. Ophthalmology. 2004;111:726–31.

32. Chen FT, Yeh PT, Lin CP, et al. Intravitreal gas injection for macular hole with localized retinal detachment in highly myopic patients. Acta Ophthalmol. 2011;89:172–8.

33. Gonvers M, Machemer R. A new approach to treating retinal detachment with macular hole. Am J Ophthalmol. 1982;94:468–72.

34. Oshima Y, Ikuno Y, Motokura M, et al. Complete epiretinal membrane separation in high myopic eyes with retinal detachment resulting from a macular hole. Am J Ophthalmol. 1998;126:669–76.

35. Avitabile T, Bonfiglio V, Buccoliero D, et al. Heavy versus standard silicone oil in the management of retinal detachment with macular hole in myopic eyes. Retina. 2011;31:540–6.

36. Yu J, Wang F, Cao H, et al. Combination of internal limiting membrane peeling and endophotocoagulation for retinal detachment related to high myopia in patients with macular hole. Ophthalmic Surg Lasers Imaging. 2012;41:215–21.

37. Ripandelli G, Coppe AM, Fedeli R, et al. Evaluation of primary surgical procedures for retinal detachment with macular hole in highly myopic eyes: a randomized comparison of vitrectomy versus posterior episcleral buckling surgery. Ophthalmology. 2001;108:2258–64.

38. Ando F, Ohba N, Touura K, et al. Anatomical and visual outcomes after episcleral macular buckling compared with those after pars plana vitrectomy for retinal detachment caused by macular hole in highly myopic eyes. Retina. 2007;27:37–44.

Glaucoma in Myopia

24

Sung Chul (Sean) Park, Jeffrey M. Liebmann, and Robert Ritch

24.1 Introduction

Over the past few decades, the prevalence of myopia and also pathologic myopia has been increasing rapidly worldwide, especially in East Asia [1–3]. Increasing prevalence of myopia has a large public health impact because of the concomitant increase in potentially blinding diseases associated with it. This chapter focuses on glaucoma among the many myopia-associated pathologic conditions.

Glaucoma is a progressive optic neuropathy characterized by specific patterns of optic nerve head and visual field damage. Myopia increases the risk of open-angle glaucoma (OAG) independently of other risk factors including intraocular pressure (IOP) [4, 5], although the pathophysiologic mechanism underlying this association is unclear. Myopia adds significant complexity to the diagnosis, monitoring, and treatment of glaucoma. The diagnostic and therapeutic challenges in the myopic eye stem from similarities between glaucomatous and myopic optic discs and between glaucomatous visual field defects and those that are associated with myopia. Understanding the structural characteristics of myopic optic disc, retina, and sclera and the effects of myopia on ocular imaging and visual field tests is crucial for accurate diagnosis of glaucoma and proper management. Results of ocular imaging tests should be interpreted carefully not only because the normative data of imaging devices do not represent the myopic population but also because myopic eyes often cause imaging artifacts and false-positive or false-negative results. Diagnosis and monitoring of glaucoma become more difficult when myopic optic disc and retinal changes progress over time. Therapeutic challenges in glaucoma with myopia result mostly from thin sclera associated with axial elongation of the globe.

24.2 Myopia as a Risk Factor for Open-Angle Glaucoma

Myopia is a risk factor for OAG, increasing the risk of developing the disease approximately by two- to threefold [4, 5]. In a meta-analysis of 11 population-based cross-sectional studies [4], the pooled odds ratio of the association between any myopia and OAG was 1.92 (95% confidence interval [CI], 1.54–2.38). There was a moderate dose-response relationship between the degree of myopia and glaucoma with a pooled odds ratio of 2.46 (95% CI, 1.93–3.15) for high myopia and 1.77 (95% CI, 1.41–2.23) for low myopia, with a cutoff value of approximately −3.00 diopters (D). However, the range of refractive error (severity of myopia) that is important for OAG is unclear. In the 11 studies analyzed in this meta-analysis, the cutoff point between emmetropia and (low) myopia varied between −0.01 and −1.5 D (−0.5 or −1 D in most studies).

The pathophysiologic mechanism(s) underlying the association between myopia and OAG remains unclear, although several hypotheses have been made [6, 7]. IOP-induced stress and strain within the lamina cribrosa and peripapillary sclera may cause structural, cellular, or molecular changes in the connective tissue [8]. IOP-induced stress and strain may also impair blood flow in the laminar region, decreasing the delivery of oxygen and nutrients to the retinal ganglion cell axons [8]. Compared to non-myopic eyes, myopic eyes have greater peripapillary scleral tension, making them more susceptible to glaucomatous optic neuropathy [9]. The lamina cribrosa is thinner in myopic eyes than in non-myopic eyes,

S. C. (Sean) Park (✉)
Department of Ophthalmology, Manhattan Eye, Ear and Throat Hospital and Lenox Hill Hospital, New York, NY, USA

Department of Ophthalmology, Donald and Barbara Zucker School of Medicine at Hofstra/Northwell, Hempstead, NY, USA

J. M. Liebmann
Bernard and Shirlee Brown Glaucoma Research Laboratory, Edward S. Harkness Eye Institute, Columbia University Irving Medical Center, New York, NY, USA

R. Ritch
Einhorn Clinical Research Center, New York Eye and Ear Infirmary of Mount Sinai, New York, NY, USA

© Springer Nature Switzerland AG 2021
R. F. Spaide et al. (eds.), *Pathologic Myopia*, https://doi.org/10.1007/978-3-030-74334-5_24

contributing to a steeper translaminar pressure gradient [10, 11] which also increases the susceptibility to glaucomatous damage [12–14]. IOP was similar between myopic and non-myopic eyes in one population-based study [15], but other studies found significantly greater IOP in myopic eyes than in non-myopic eyes, making them more prone to development and progression of glaucoma [16, 17]. Additionally, ocular blood flow, which appears to play an important role in the pathophysiology of glaucoma, is decreased in myopia [18, 19], possibly leading to an increased vulnerability to the effects of IOP on the optic nerve head. Optic disc tilting is one of the features of myopic eyes [20–22]. A greater degree of disc tilting correlates with greater myopia and longer axial length [23]. The path of some retinal ganglion cell axons may be disturbed in tilted discs, interfering with axonal transport and contributing to the association between myopia and glaucoma [24].

Central corneal thickness is a predictor for the development of primary open-angle glaucoma [25] and a risk factor for advanced glaucomatous damage at the initial examination [26]. Axial elongation of the eyeball is a hallmark of myopia, but thinning of the outer ocular layer (cornea, sclera, and lamina cribrosa) occurs mainly in the posterior part of the eye [27, 28]. Previous studies demonstrated that central corneal thickness did not increase or decrease significantly with increasing axial length or myopic refractive error [29–32]. Similar studies on Korean and Indian populations reported a positive correlation between central corneal thickness and axial length, indicating a thicker cornea in more myopic subjects [33, 34]. These results suggest that corneal architecture and thickness may not contribute to the association between myopia and glaucoma.

24.3   Diagnosis and Monitoring of Glaucoma in Myopia: Optic Nerve Structure

Compared to non-myopic eyes, myopic eyes have more tilted discs [20–22, 35, 36], greater cup-to-disc ratio [7], larger disc area [35, 37, 38], and larger beta zone peripapillary atrophy (PPA) [21, 22, 37, 39, 40]. Because of these characteristics, accurate diagnosis and monitoring of glaucoma in myopic eyes are challenging.

When the optic disc is evaluated using ophthalmoscopy or stereo disc photography for glaucoma, the integrity of the neuroretinal rim is assessed among other parameters. Localized or diffuse neuroretinal rim narrowing and resultant increase in cup-to-disc ratio are characteristic features of glaucoma. Larger optic discs and greater cup-to-disc ratio in myopic eyes can mimic glaucomatous optic neuropathy and result in an erroneous diagnosis of glaucoma and unnecessary treatment. In addition, in myopic eyes, accurate evaluation of rim width is more difficult than in non-myopic eyes. Tilted discs in myopic eyes have a more gradually sloped rim surface in the direction of disc tilting (Fig. 24.1). Therefore, it is more difficult to delineate the rim margin in stereo disc photographs. Because evaluation of static rim structure is challenging, assessment of changes in the rim structure over time to determine glaucoma progression is also problematic.

A retinal nerve fiber layer (RNFL) defect, in which the circumpapillary RNFL is thinner than the adjacent areas, appears as a dark stripe or wedge during clinical examination. RNFL defects are more easily identified in eyes with darker retinal pigment epithelium (RPE), for example, in Asian eyes than in Caucasian eyes. Myopic eyes have less pigmentation in the fundus, and therefore it is more difficult to detect RNFL defects in those eyes. Circumpapillary RNFL thickness measurement using optical coherence tomography (OCT) is commonly used to diagnose and monitor glaucoma. RNFL thickness profile and RNFL thickness sector maps (e.g., quadrant or clock hour maps) are compared with those of the normative database to detect significant RNFL thinning. Because the RNFL is generally thinner in myopic eyes than in non-myopic eyes [41–45], myopic eyes are more likely to have false-positive RNFL thickness measurements that mimic glaucomatous optic neuropathy [46].

Correct OCT RNFL scan circle placement is important because the scan circle location affects the circumpapillary RNFL thickness profile and RNFL thickness measurements in sector maps. The RNFL thickness profile is more comparable to the normative database when the scan circle is placed based on the contour of the neural canal opening, rather than based on the clinical optic disc [47]. In non-myopic eyes with a non-tilted disc, the clinical optic disc forms an almost concentric circle or ellipse with the neural canal opening (Bruch's membrane opening). Therefore, the RNFL scan circle can be placed concentrically on the optic disc in eyes with non-tilted discs. However, in myopic eyes, the tilted disc forms an eccentric circle or ellipse with the neural canal opening. Consequently, for example, in a myopic eye with a temporally tilted disc, the temporal RNFL thickness will be overestimated, and nasal RNFL thickness will be underestimated if the scan circle is centered on the clinical optic disc (Fig. 24.2). Also, portions of the RNFL thickness profile may be statistically borderline (1–5% of the normative database) or outside normal limits (less than 1% of the normative database), and some circumpapillary sectors may be also be coded as borderline or outside normal limits if the scan circle is centered on the myopic tilted disc (Fig. 24.2). The typical OCT RNFL thickness profile has two peaks, at the superotemporal and inferotemporal RNFL bundles. With increasing axial length, the angle bounded by the superotemporal and inferotemporal RNFL bundles decreases, which means these RNFL bundles become closer to the macula in myopic eyes

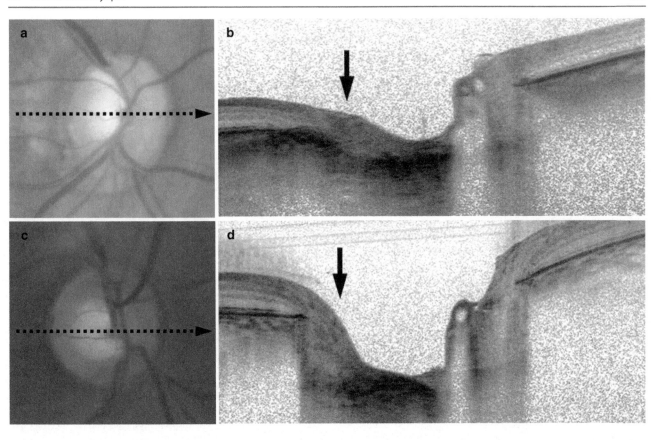

Fig. 24.1 Temporal neuroretinal rim surface (*black arrows*) is more gradually sloped in the myopic eye (**a, b**) than in the non-myopic eye (**c, d**). The *dotted lines* with *arrows* in (**a**) and (**c**) indicate the locations of the cross-sectional OCT scans in (**b**) and (**d**)

than in non-myopic eyes [48–50]. This is another reason why myopic eyes have false-positive or false-negative RNFL thickness results on OCT more frequently than non-myopic eyes (Fig. 24.2).

When part of the scan circle passes through the beta zone PPA area in myopic eyes, the quality of the OCT RNFL image decreases locally. In this situation, the OCT RNFL segmentation algorithm often fails, resulting in underestimation or overestimation of the RNFL thickness and a false-positive or false-negative result. This OCT imaging artifact and segmentation error can be avoided by using a larger scan circle (Fig. 24.3) [51].

In myopic eyes, the raw RNFL scan has greater undulation than in non-myopic eyes. Therefore, myopic eyes are more likely to have part of the RNFL scan located outside of the OCT scan range, which in turn results in erroneous RNFL segmentation and thickness results. Greater undulation of the raw RNFL scan also causes a focal area of poor quality, which also leads to erroneous RNFL thickness results (Fig. 24.4).

Based on clinical and histological characteristics, PPA is divided into alpha and beta zones. The alpha zone PPA is the outer area of the PPA distinguished by irregular hypo- and hyperpigmentation and thinning of the chorioretinal tissues,

and the beta zone PPA is the whitish area between the alpha zone and the scleral ring characterized by atrophy of the RPE and choriocapillaris. Studies have revealed the presence of beta zone PPA to be associated with both the occurrence of glaucoma [52–55] and progression of functional damage in glaucomatous eyes [56–59]. Enlargement of beta zone PPA was also related to glaucoma progression [60, 61]. In myopic eyes, however, the current clinical definition of beta zone PPA often includes the area of externalized scleral canal wall associated with axial elongation of the globe [62]. The area of externalized scleral canal wall is not true atrophy because there is no RPE or choriocapillaris on the scleral canal wall embryologically. Therefore, evaluation of the presence, size, and enlargement of beta zone PPA is often misleading in myopic eyes. The classic beta zone PPA has been divided further into a gamma zone and a new beta zone based on the presence or absence of Bruch's membrane (Fig. 24.5) [63, 64]. Gamma zone PPA was defined as the PPA area without Bruch's membrane or RPE and was associated with axial length but not with glaucoma. The newly defined beta zone PPA was defined as the PPA area with Bruch's membrane but no RPE and was associated with glaucoma, but not with axial length [63, 64]. These findings suggest that the newly defined beta zone PPA is

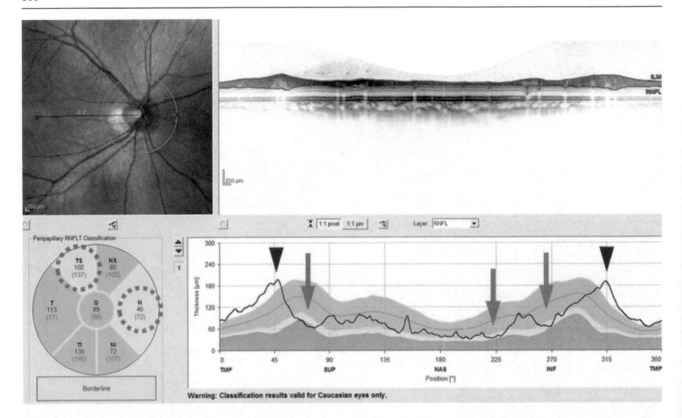

Fig. 24.2 Circumpapillary retinal nerve fiber layer (RNFL) thickness profile in a highly myopic eye with a temporally tilted disc when the OCT scan circle is placed on the clinical optic disc. Average RNFL thickness in the temporal quadrant is overestimated (113 μm) and that in the nasal quadrant is underestimated (46 μm) compared to the norma-

tive database (77 and 72 μm, respectively). Note that the superotemporal and inferotemporal RNFL bundles (*blue arrowheads*) are closer to the line connecting the disc center and the fovea than those in normative data. *Red arrows* and *dotted circles* indicate the areas with borderline or abnormal RNFL thickness

specifically related to glaucoma and should be evaluated in clinical practice. However, the new beta zone PPA is not readily identifiable ophthalmoscopically or in disc photographs and needs imaging technology such as spectral-domain OCT for accurate identification.

Macular ganglion cell layer thickness analysis using OCT improves the diagnostic accuracy of glaucoma especially in highly myopic eyes. The macular ganglion cell layer is sometimes measured together with inner plexiform layer as "ganglion cell-inner plexiform layer" or with both inner plexiform layer and RNFL as "ganglion cell complex," because it is difficult to demarcate between the ganglion cell layer and inner plexiform layer accurately. When compared to circumpapillary RNFL thickness, ganglion cell-inner plexiform layer or ganglion cell complex thickness had comparable [65, 66] or better [67, 68] diagnostic ability to detect glaucoma in high myopia. Considering that the ganglion cell layer mainly consists of the cell bodies of retinal ganglion cells and the RNFL mainly consists of their axons, they can be used as mutually complementary parameters for the diagnosis and monitoring of glaucoma.

Assessment of optic disc and peripapillary structures is challenging in highly myopic eyes. Clinicians should know

the structural characteristics of myopic optic discs and RNFL and how to avoid and correct false-positive and false-negative imaging test results. Careful monitoring will help clinicians confirm the diagnosis of glaucoma and make therapeutic decisions in highly myopic eyes.

24.4   Diagnosis and Monitoring of Glaucoma in Myopia: Optic Nerve Function

Automated perimetry is the most commonly used modality to evaluate visual function of glaucoma suspects or patients. Eyes with early glaucoma do not necessarily have detectable visual field defects (e.g., preperimetric glaucoma), but the presence of visual field defects corresponding to neuroretinal rim, RNFL, or retinal ganglion cell layer loss adds confidence to the diagnosis of glaucoma. When structural tests for glaucoma (optic disc photography and imaging tests) are inconclusive in myopic eyes, visual field testing becomes more important in the diagnosis and monitoring of glaucoma. However, it is often difficult to interpret the perimetric test results accurately in myopic eyes because many of them

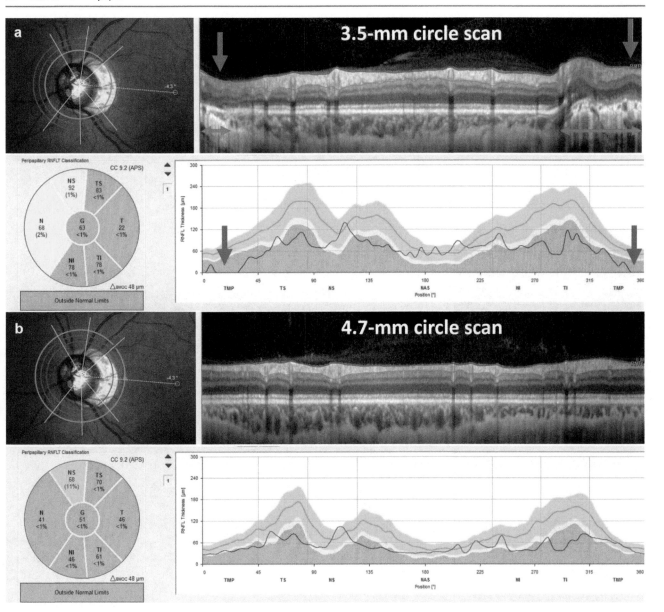

Fig. 24.3 Circumpapillary retinal nerve fiber layer (RNFL) thickness profile of a highly myopic eye with large beta zone peripapillary atrophy. (**a**) *Blue arrows* indicate RNFL segmentation error caused by imaging artifacts in the area of peripapillary atrophy (*red double arrows*), resulting in underestimation of RNFL thickness. (**b**) There is no imaging artifact or RNFL segmentation error in a larger circle scan. (Modified from Ghassibi MP, et al. [51])

have retinal or optic disc abnormalities that can lead to visual field defects mimicking glaucoma.

Visual field sensitivity decreases with an increasing degree of myopia in eyes with moderate to high myopia [69]. In 99 young myopic male soldiers with refractive error worse than −4 D, the visual field mean deviation decreased significantly as axial length increased and as refractive error became more myopic. This result was consistent when two methods of refractive error correction (trial lens and contact lens) were used. The authors postulated that the reduced sen-

sitivity in greater myopia may be attributed to ectasia of the fundus, structural changes in the retina and choroid, axial elongation of the eye with increased spacing or distortion of retinal photoreceptor matrix, and minification/distortion of the stimulus by the negative prescription of the lenses. Asymmetric and uneven posterior surface such as posterior staphyloma is also associated with visual field defects in highly myopic eyes.

Eyes with myopic tilted optic discs tend to have visual field defects more frequently than non-myopic eyes. In the

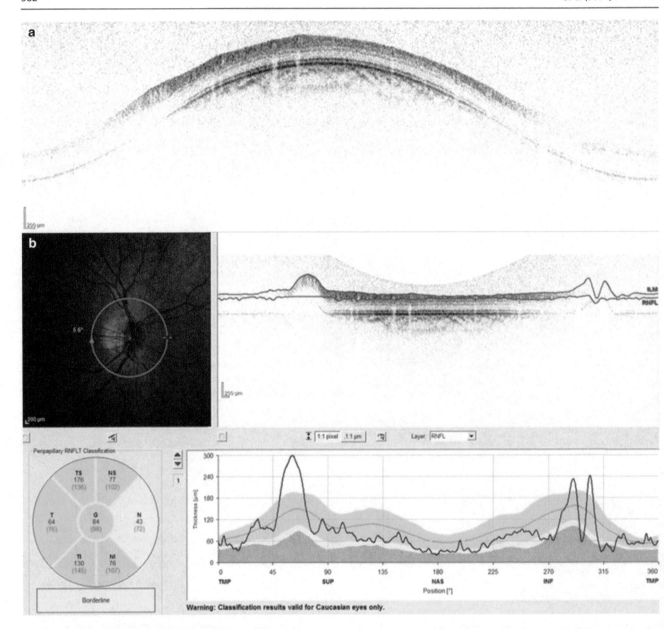

Fig. 24.4 Greater undulation of the raw retinal nerve fiber layer (RNFL) scan (**a**) in a highly myopic eye resulted in areas of poor image quality at both ends, which lead to erroneous RNFL thickness profile (**b**)

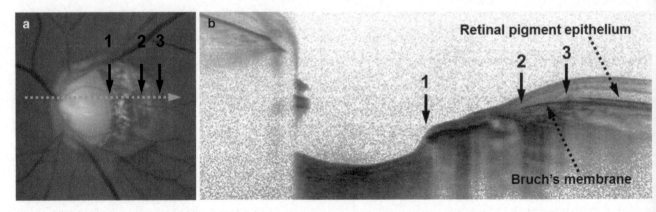

Fig. 24.5 The classic beta zone peripapillary atrophy (between *arrows 1* and *3*) can be divided into a gamma zone (between *arrows 1* and *2*) and a new beta zone (between arrows 2 and 3) based on the presence or absence of Bruch's membrane. The *dotted line* with an *arrow* in (**a**) indicates the location of the cross-sectional OCT scans in (**b**)

Blue Mountains Eye Study, a population-based study conducted in Australia, 12 of 62 eyes with a tilted disc (19.4%) had visual field defects, most commonly in the superotemporal quadrant of visual field [36]. This study only looked for inferiorly, infero-nasally, nasally, or superonasally tilted discs. Therefore, many of the eyes enrolled in this study likely had tilted disc syndrome. When 41 eyes with a tilted disc were examined after a mean period of 61 months, 11 had glaucoma or myopic retinopathy [36]. In a prospective study on 137 young men aged 19–24 years with myopia, 40.2% of subjects had tilted discs with a disc ovality index (a ratio of shortest disc diameter to longest disc diameter) of 0.8 or less [23]. In this study, four subjects had visual field defects with the trial lens but not with the contact lens. Only one subject had a reproducible visual field defect with both trial lens and contact lens optical correction. In a study on 38 eyes with tilted disc syndrome, small additional myopic correction improved visual field test results [70]. After initial visual field testing using the Goldmann perimetry, the defective isopters in 35 eyes were tested again with gradually increasing myopic correction until no further change was noted. The visual field defect partly or totally disappeared with increased myopic correction of 3.1 ± 1.5 D. A retrospective case series reported 16 patients with refractive error ranging from −11.25 to +0.25 D who had optic disc cupping and visual field defects stable for 7 years [24]. A tilted disc was present in 75% of the patients. In another retrospective study on 492 highly myopic eyes with a mean follow-up period of 11.6 years, visual field defects newly developed in 13.2% of the eyes [71]. The incidence of visual field defects was significantly higher in eyes with an oval disc than in eyes with a round disc. Based on the high proportion of temporal visual field defects, the authors of this study claimed that the visual field defects in highly myopic eyes were most likely not caused by the same mechanisms that caused glaucomatous visual field defects. However, about one third of the eyes had nasal visual field defects only [71].

Peripapillary intrachoroidal cavitation, which was previously known as peripapillary detachment in pathologic myopia, is associated with visual field defects. It appears clinically as a yellowish-orange lesion around the optic disc myopic conus [72]. OCT revealed an intrachoroidal cavity separating the RPE from the sclera [73]. In a study on 127 highly myopic eyes, glaucoma-like visual field defects were detected more frequently in eyes with peripapillary intrachoroidal cavitation than in eyes without (64.3% vs. 19.5%) [74]. In addition, one-quarter of eyes with peripapillary intrachoroidal cavitation had full-thickness defects in the retina which may cause visual field defects that mimic those found in glaucoma [75].

Considering these results, interpretation of visual field defects in myopic eyes remains a clinical dilemma. Visual field defects (relative scotomata) in myopic eyes may be associated with myopic retinal or optic disc abnormalities,

disappear with a proper correction of refractive error, be present with glaucoma-like disc cupping but stable for many years, and develop by glaucomatous damage. All of these should be taken into consideration in the interpretation of visual fields of myopic patients. Reproducible visual field defects and progression of such defects corresponding to structural changes in optic disc, RNFL, or ganglion cell layer will help confirm the diagnosis of glaucoma as the cause of visual dysfunction. Nonetheless, future studies are needed to see if the pathophysiologic mechanism(s) of visual field progression in myopic eyes is different from glaucomatous process, as well as to develop better functional tests or visual field algorithms that can confirm the diagnosis and progression of glaucoma in myopic eyes more easily.

24.5 Treatment of Glaucoma in Myopia

Miotic eye drops (parasympathomimetics, cholinergic agents) help open the trabecular meshwork and increase the aqueous outflow facility. These drugs may cause a variety of side effects and rarely result in retinal detachment. Because patients with high myopia are more prone to retinal detachment, thorough fundus examination for peripheral retinal evaluation should be performed before prescribing miotics. In addition, induced myopia is a common side effect of miotics. Myopic patients should be informed that they may become more nearsighted during the period of miotic use.

Myopia is a more important factor to consider during surgical treatment of glaucoma than during medical treatment. Highly myopic eyes have a greater risk of ocular trauma and globe perforation during retrobulbar anesthesia [76]. Preoperative measurement of axial length is helpful in estimating the size of the globe and managing the angle of the retrobulbar needle during anesthesia. For extremely long eyes, other types of anesthesia are recommended such as subtenon anesthesia.

Myopia is one of the risk factors for hypotony and choroidal detachment during or after glaucoma filtering surgery [77, 78]. Because of thinner-than-normal sclera [27, 28], myopic eyes can partially collapse and lose their original shape more easily than non-myopic eyes when they have intraocular surgery or penetrating trauma. Thinner sclera also makes it difficult to make an adequate partial-thickness scleral flap and suture during trabeculectomy, which is a guarded filtering procedure. Meticulous conjunctival closure to prevent wound leak, larger scleral flap and tighter scleral flap sutures to prevent overfiltration, and less exposure to antifibrotic agents will reduce the risk of hypotony in myopic eyes. Extra care should be taken in young male myopic patients because they have a higher risk of hypotony maculopathy [79]. Myopia is also one of the risk factors for intraoperative or postoperative suprachoroidal hemorrhage. In addition to the aforementioned procedures to prevent hypotony, tight control of blood pressure, maximal medical reduction of preoperative IOP, slow reduction of IOP intraoperatively, and maintenance of the anterior chamber during the entire surgery should be considered. In addition, myopic eyes are more prone to have late-onset scleral thinning or perforation and endophthalmitis associated with the use of adjunctive antifibrotic chemotherapy. This is another reason why the antifibrotic agents during filtering surgery should be used more prudently in myopic eyes. Nonpenetrating glaucoma surgery or minimally invasive glaucoma surgery, which uses less or no antimetabolites and decreases IOP more slowly with less IOP fluctuation during the procedure, may be safer with a reduced risk of complications for highly myopic eyes, but the IOP outcome may not be as good as with conventional filtering surgery [80, 81].

In highly myopic eyes with thin sclera, the tube of a glaucoma drainage device tends to have a position more anteriorly than intended in the anterior chamber, increasing the risk of corneal edema and decompensation. Oblique and longer intrascleral tube tract rather than the radial and shorter one and inserting the tube in the ciliary sulcus rather than in the anterior chamber will help reduce the risk of corneal damage. Myopic eyes with prior ocular surgery may have localized areas of scleral thinning, which warrants careful preoperative and intraoperative surveillance.

24.6 Conclusions

Although myopia may complicate the diagnosis and treatment of glaucoma, many of these challenges can be overcome with the knowledge of the structural characteristics of myopic optic disc and retina and correct interpretation of ocular imaging and visual field test results. Considering that a large proportion of myopic eyes may have clinical features compatible with glaucoma but never progress, a more conservative therapeutic approach with closer surveillance may be beneficial in myopic patients to avoid overtreatment until the diagnosis of glaucoma and its progression are confirmed, especially when the IOP is within normal limits. Severity of structural and functional damage, proximity of visual field defects to the fixation, history of disc hemorrhage, central corneal thickness, presence of secondary causes of glaucoma (e.g., pseudoexfoliation syndrome and pigment dispersion syndrome), and family history of glaucoma should be considered when deciding how closely patients should be monitored and how aggressively they should be treated. Because the rising rate of myopia will increase the burden of difficult glaucoma cases, diagnostic and therapeutic guidelines for glaucoma in myopic eyes should be established. Further investigation is warranted to define and manage nonglaucomatous optic neuropathy associated with myopia (myopic optic neuropathy).

References

1. Lin LL, Shih YF, Hsiao CK, Chen CJ. Prevalence of myopia in Taiwanese schoolchildren: 1983 to 2000. Ann Acad Med Singap. 2004;33(1):27–33.
2. Pan CW, Ramamurthy D, Saw SM. Worldwide prevalence and risk factors for myopia. Ophthalmic Physiol Opt. 2012;32(1):3–16.
3. Vitale S, Sperduto RD, Ferris FL 3rd. Increased prevalence of myopia in the United States between 1971-1972 and 1999-2004. Arch Ophthalmol. 2009;127(12):1632–9.
4. Marcus MW, de Vries MM, Junoy Montolio FG, Jansonius NM. Myopia as a risk factor for open-angle glaucoma: a systematic review and meta-analysis. Ophthalmology. 2011;118(10):1989–94. e1982
5. Mitchell P, Hourihan F, Sandbach J, Wang JJ. The relationship between glaucoma and myopia: the Blue Mountains eye study. Ophthalmology. 1999;106(10):2010–5.
6. Chang RT. Myopia and glaucoma. Int Ophthalmol Clin. 2011;51(3):53–63.
7. Fong DS, Epstein DL, Allingham RR. Glaucoma and myopia: are they related? Int Ophthalmol Clin. 1990;30(3):215–8.
8. Crawford Downs J, Roberts MD, Sigal IA. Glaucomatous cupping of the lamina cribrosa: a review of the evidence for active progressive remodeling as a mechanism. Exp Eye Res. 2011;93(2):133–40.
9. Cahane M, Bartov E. Axial length and scleral thickness effect on susceptibility to glaucomatous damage: a theoretical model implementing Laplace's law. Ophthalmic Res. 1992;24(5):280–4.
10. Jonas JB, Berenshtein E, Holbach L. Lamina cribrosa thickness and spatial relationships between intraocular space and cerebrospinal fluid space in highly myopic eyes. Invest Ophthalmol Vis Sci. 2004;45(8):2660–5.
11. Ren R, Wang N, Li B, et al. Lamina cribrosa and peripapillary sclera histomorphometry in normal and advanced glaucomatous Chinese eyes with various axial length. Invest Ophthalmol Vis Sci. 2009;50(5):2175–84.
12. Chihara E, Liu X, Dong J, et al. Severe myopia as a risk factor for progressive visual field loss in primary open-angle glaucoma. Ophthalmologica. 1997;211(2):66–71.
13. Jonas JB, Budde WM. Optic nerve damage in highly myopic eyes with chronic open-angle glaucoma. Eur J Ophthalmol. 2005;15(1):41–7.
14. Lotufo D, Ritch R, Szmyd L Jr, Burris JE. Juvenile glaucoma, race, and refraction. JAMA. 1989;261(2):249–52.
15. Xu L, Wang Y, Wang S, Jonas JB. High myopia and glaucoma susceptibility the Beijing eye study. Ophthalmology. 2007;114(2):216–20.
16. Abdalla MI, Hamdi M. Applanation ocular tension in myopia and emmetropia. Br J Ophthalmol. 1970;54(2):122–5.
17. Perkins ES, Phelps CD. Open angle glaucoma, ocular hypertension, low-tension glaucoma, and refraction. Arch Ophthalmol. 1982;100(9):1464–7.
18. Ravalico G, Pastori G, Croce M, Toffoli G. Pulsatile ocular blood flow variations with axial length and refractive error. Ophthalmologica. 1997;211(5):271–3.
19. Shimada N, Ohno-Matsui K, Harino S, et al. Reduction of retinal blood flow in high myopia. Graefes Arch Clin Exp Ophthalmol. 2004;242(4):284–8.
20. How AC, Tan GS, Chan YH, et al. Population prevalence of tilted and torted optic discs among an adult Chinese population: the Tanjong Pagar study. Arch Ophthalmol. 2009;127(7):894–9.
21. Hyung SM, Kim DM, Hong C, Youn DH. Optic disc of the myopic eye: relationship between refractive errors and morphometric characteristics. Korean J Ophthalmol. 1992;6(1):32–5.
22. Samarawickrama C, Mitchell P, Tong L, et al. Myopia-related optic disc and retinal changes in adolescent children from Singapore. Ophthalmology. 2011;118(10):2050–7.

23. Tay E, Seah SK, Chan SP, et al. Optic disk ovality as an index of tilt and its relationship to myopia and perimetry. Am J Ophthalmol. 2005;139(2):247–52.

24. Doshi A, Kreidl KO, Lombardi L, Sakamoto DK, Singh K. Nonprogressive glaucomatous cupping and visual field abnormalities in young Chinese males. Ophthalmology. 2007;114(3):472–9.

25. Gordon MO, Beiser JA, Brandt JD, et al. The Ocular Hypertension Treatment Study: baseline factors that predict the onset of primary open-angle glaucoma. Arch Ophthalmol. 2002;120(6):714–20. discussion 829-730

26. Herndon LW, Weizer JS, Stinnett SS. Central corneal thickness as a risk factor for advanced glaucoma damage. Arch Ophthalmol. 2004;122(1):17–21.

27. Norman RE, Flanagan JG, Rausch SM, et al. Dimensions of the human sclera: thickness measurement and regional changes with axial length. Exp Eye Res. 2010;90(2):277–84.

28. Vurgese S, Panda-Jonas S, Jonas JB. Scleral thickness in human eyes. PLoS One. 2012;7(1):e29692.

29. Fam HB, How AC, Baskaran M, Lim KL, Chan YH, Aung T. Central corneal thickness and its relationship to myopia in Chinese adults. Br J Ophthalmol. 2006;90(12):1451–3.

30. Oliveira C, Tello C, Liebmann J, Ritch R. Central corneal thickness is not related to anterior scleral thickness or axial length. J Glaucoma. 2006;15(3):190–4.

31. Garcia-Medina M, Garcia-Medina JJ, Garrido-Fernandez P, et al. Central corneal thickness, intraocular pressure, and degree of myopia in an adult myopic population aged 20 to 40 years in Southeast Spain: determination and relationships. Clin Ophthalmol. 2011;5:249–58.

32. Liu Z, Pflugfelder SC. The effects of long-term contact lens wear on corneal thickness, curvature, and surface regularity. Ophthalmology. 2000;107(1):105–11.

33. Lee S, Kim B, Oh TH, Kim HS. Correlations between magnitude of refractive error and other optical components in Korean myopes. Korean J Ophthalmol. 2012;26(5):324–30.

34. Kunert KS, Bhartiya P, Tandon R, Dada T, Christian H, Vajpayee RB. Central corneal thickness in Indian patients undergoing LASIK for myopia. J Refract Surg. 2003;19(3):378–9.

35. Chihara E, Chihara K. Covariation of optic disc measurements and ocular parameters in the healthy eye. Graefes Arch Clin Exp Ophthalmol. 1994;232(5):265–71.

36. Vongphanit J, Mitchell P, Wang JJ. Population prevalence of tilted optic disks and the relationship of this sign to refractive error. Am J Ophthalmol. 2002;133(5):679–85.

37. Jonas JB, Gusek GC, Naumann GO. Optic disk morphometry in high myopia. Graefes Arch Clin Exp Ophthalmol. 1988;226(6):587–90.

38. Wang TH, Lin SY, Shih YF, Huang JK, Lin LL, Hung PT. Evaluation of optic disc changes in severe myopia. J Formos Med Assoc. 2000;99(7):559–63.

39. Fulk GW, Goss DA, Christensen MT, Cline KB, Herrin-Lawson GA. Optic nerve crescents and refractive error. Optom Vis Sci. 1992;69(3):208–13.

40. Tong L, Saw SM, Chua WH, et al. Optic disk and retinal characteristics in myopic children. Am J Ophthalmol. 2004;138(1):160–2.

41. Hwang YH, Kim YY. Macular thickness and volume of myopic eyes measured using spectral-domain optical coherence tomography. Clin Exp Optom. 2012;95(5):492–8.

42. Kang SH, Hong SW, Im SK, Lee SH, Ahn MD. Effect of myopia on the thickness of the retinal nerve fiber layer measured by Cirrus HD optical coherence tomography. Invest Ophthalmol Vis Sci. 2010;51(8):4075–83.

43. Mohammad Salih PA. Evaluation of peripapillary retinal nerve fiber layer thickness in myopic eyes by spectral-domain optical coherence tomography. J Glaucoma. 2012;21(1):41–4.

44. Qiu KL, Zhang MZ, Leung CK, et al. Diagnostic classification of retinal nerve fiber layer measurement in myopic eyes: a compari-

son between time-domain and spectral-domain optical coherence tomography. Am J Ophthalmol. 2011;152(4):646–53. e642

45. Savini G, Barboni P, Parisi V, Carbonelli M. The influence of axial length on retinal nerve fibre layer thickness and optic-disc size measurements by spectral-domain OCT. Br J Ophthalmol. 2012;96(1):57–61.

46. Kim NR, Lim H, Kim JH, Rho SS, Seong GJ, Kim CY. Factors associated with false positives in retinal nerve fiber layer color codes from spectral-domain optical coherence tomography. Ophthalmology. 2011;118(9):1774–81.

47. Chung JK, Yoo YC. Correct calculation circle location of optical coherence tomography in measuring retinal nerve fiber layer thickness in eyes with myopic tilted discs. Invest Ophthalmol Vis Sci. 2011;52(11):7894–900.

48. Hwang YH, Yoo C, Kim YY. Myopic optic disc tilt and the characteristics of peripapillary retinal nerve fiber layer thickness measured by spectral-domain optical coherence tomography. J Glaucoma. 2012;21(4):260–5.

49. Hwang YH, Yoo C, Kim YY. Characteristics of peripapillary retinal nerve fiber layer thickness in eyes with myopic optic disc tilt and rotation. J Glaucoma. 2012;21(6):394–400.

50. Leung CK, Yu M, Weinreb RN, et al. Retinal nerve fiber layer imaging with spectral-domain optical coherence tomography: interpreting the RNFL maps in healthy myopic eyes. Invest Ophthalmol Vis Sci. 2012;53(11):7194–200.

51. Ghassibi MP, Chien JL, Patthanathamrongkasem T, et al. Glaucoma diagnostic capability of circumpapillary retinal nerve fiber layer thickness in circle scans with different diameters. J Glaucoma. 2017;26(4):335–42.

52. Jonas JB, Nguyen XN, Gusek GC, Naumann GO. Parapapillary chorioretinal atrophy in normal and glaucoma eyes. I. Morphometric data. Invest Ophthalmol Vis Sci. 1989;30(5):908–18.

53. Jonas JB, Naumann GO. Parapapillary chorioretinal atrophy in normal and glaucoma eyes. II Correlations. Invest Ophthalmol Vis Sci. 1989;30(5):919–26.

54. Kono Y, Zangwill L, Sample PA, et al. Relationship between parapapillary atrophy and visual field abnormality in primary open-angle glaucoma. Am J Ophthalmol. 1999;127(6):674–80.

55. Park SC, Lee DH, Lee HJ, Kee C. Risk factors for normal-tension glaucoma among subgroups of patients. Arch Ophthalmol. 2009;127(10):1275–83.

56. Araie M, Sekine M, Suzuki Y, Koseki N. Factors contributing to the progression of visual field damage in eyes with normal-tension glaucoma. Ophthalmology. 1994;101(8):1440–4.

57. Tezel G, Kolker AE, Kass MA, Wax MB, Gordon M, Siegmund KD. Parapapillary chorioretinal atrophy in patients with ocular hypertension. I. An evaluation as a predictive factor for the development of glaucomatous damage. Arch Ophthalmol. Dec 1997;115(12):1503–8.

58. Martus P, Stroux A, Budde WM, Mardin CY, Korth M, Jonas JB. Predictive factors for progressive optic nerve damage in various types of chronic open-angle glaucoma. Am J Ophthalmol. 2005;139(6):999–1009.

59. Teng CC, De Moraes CG, Prata TS, Tello C, Ritch R, Liebmann JM. Beta-Zone parapapillary atrophy and the velocity of glaucoma progression. Ophthalmology. 2010;117(5):909–15.

60. Uchida H, Ugurlu S, Caprioli J. Increasing peripapillary atrophy is associated with progressive glaucoma. Ophthalmology. 1998;105(8):1541–5.

61. Budde WM, Jonas JB. Enlargement of parapapillary atrophy in follow-up of chronic open-angle glaucoma. Am J Ophthalmol. 2004;137(4):646–54.

62. Kim TW, Kim M, Weinreb RN, Woo SJ, Park KH, Hwang JM. Optic disc change with incipient myopia of childhood. Ophthalmology. 2012;119(1):21–26 e21–23.

63. Dai Y, Jonas JB, Huang H, Wang M, Sun X. Microstructure of parapapillary atrophy: beta zone and gamma zone. Invest Ophthalmol Vis Sci. 2013;54(3):2013–8.

64. Jonas JB, Jonas SB, Jonas RA, et al. Parapapillary atrophy: histological gamma zone and delta zone. PLoS One. 2012;7(10):e47237.

65. Kim NR, Lee ES, Seong GJ, Kang SY, Kim JH, Hong S, Kim CY. Comparing the ganglion cell complex and retinal nerve fibre layer measurements by Fourier domain OCT to detect glaucoma in high myopia. Br J Ophthalmol. 2011;95(8):1115–21.

66. Choi YJ, Jeoung JW, Park KH, Kim DM. Glaucoma detection ability of ganglion cell-inner plexiform layer thickness by spectral-domain optical coherence tomography in high myopia. Invest Ophthalmol Vis Sci. 2013;54(3):2296–304.

67. Shoji T, Sato H, Ishida M, Takeuchi M, Chihara E. Assessment of glaucomatous changes in subjects with high myopia using spectral domain optical coherence tomography. Invest Ophthalmol Vis Sci. 2011;52(2):1098–102.

68. Shoji T, Nagaoka Y, Sato H, Chihara E. Impact of high myopia on the performance of SD-OCT parameters to detect glaucoma. Graefes Arch Clin Exp Ophthalmol. 2012;250(12):1843–9.

69. Aung T, Foster PJ, Seah SK, et al. Automated static perimetry: the influence of myopia and its method of correction. Ophthalmology. 2001;108(2):290–5.

70. Vuori ML, Mantyjarvi M. Tilted disc syndrome may mimic false visual field deterioration. Acta Ophthalmol. 2008;86(6):622–5.

71. Ohno-Matsui K, Shimada N, Yasuzumi K, et al. Long-term development of significant visual field defects in highly myopic eyes. Am J Ophthalmol. 2011;152(2):256–65. e251

72. Freund KB, Ciardella AP, Yannuzzi LA, et al. Peripapillary detachment in pathologic myopia. Arch Ophthalmol. 2003;121(2):197–204.

73. Toranzo J, Cohen SY, Erginay A, Gaudric A. Peripapillary intrachoroidal cavitation in myopia. Am J Ophthalmol. 2005;140(4):731–2.

74. Shimada N, Ohno-Matsui K, Nishimuta A, Tokoro T, Mochizuki M. Peripapillary changes detected by optical coherence tomography in eyes with high myopia. Ophthalmology. 2007;114(11):2070–6.

75. Spaide RF, Akiba M, Ohno-Matsui K. Evaluation of peripapillary intrachoroidal cavitation with swept source and enhanced depth imaging optical coherence tomography. Retina. 2012;32:1037–44.

76. Churchill A, James TE. Should myopes have routine axial length measurements before retrobulbar or peribulbar injections? Br J Ophthalmol. 1996;80(6):498.

77. Silva RA, Doshi A, Law SK, Singh K. Postfiltration hypotony maculopathy in young Chinese myopic women with glaucomatous appearing optic neuropathy. J Glaucoma. 2010;19(2):105–10.

78. Costa VP, Arcieri ES. Hypotony maculopathy. Acta Ophthalmol Scand. 2007;85(6):586–97.

79. Fannin LA, Schiffman JC, Budenz DL. Risk factors for hypotony maculopathy. Ophthalmology. 2003;110(6):1185–91.

80. Hamel M, Shaarawy T, Mermoud A. Deep sclerectomy with collagen implant in patients with glaucoma and high myopia. J Cataract Refract Surg. 2001;27(9):1410–7.

81. Ahmed IIK, Fea A, Au L, et al. A prospective randomized trial comparing Hydrus and iStent microinvasive Glaucoma surgery implants for standalone treatment of open-angle Glaucoma: the COMPARE study. Ophthalmology. 2019; [Epub ahead of print].

Myopic Optic Neuropathy

Richard F. Spaide and Kyoko Ohno-Matsui

Nearly every feature of the eye is influenced by the development of high myopia. For some structures, such as the sclera, there are well-established abnormalities that have been evaluated in humans, and our knowledge has been amplified by experiments using multiple animal models. For others, the changes associated with high myopia are less clear. The anatomic changes in the optic nerve head and surrounding structures are readily evident by imaging, but the functional changes induced, and the possible pathophysiologic mechanisms are not clearly understood or defined. Ocular imaging is improving rapidly and has provided clues suggesting there may be classes of abnormalities in optic nerve structure and function in high myopia. This chapter explores possible abnormalities of the optic nerve associated with high myopia. Considerations about the possible pathophysiology involved hinges on detailed knowledge of the anatomic and physiology of the optic nerve and associated structures and incorporates analysis of changes induced by high myopia.

25.1 Embryology of the Optic Nerve

The optic vesicle evaginates from the prosencephalon but remains connected by a short optic stalk. Invagination of the optic vesicle forms the optic cup, and the fetal fissure closes not only the optic cup but also the optic stalk. The hyaloid artery and vein enters the stalk medially and continues into the eye to come into contact with the primary vitreous. The hyaloid artery exits the hyaloid canal on the inner aspect of the disc. Between the sixth and seventh weeks, the fissure in the optic stalk, called the choroidal fissure, begins to close to form a tube. Failure of closure would lead to an optic nerve coloboma. The retinal nerve fibers converge on the optic disc through a complicated interaction between attractive and repulsive forces acting on their growth [1]. By the seventh week, axons line the inner wall of the lumen of the optic stalk, and by the eighth week, the stalk is filled with axons that extend back to a primitive chiasm. The cells on the inner side of the stalk are destined to form glial cells between the nerve fibers while the external cells form the glial mantle around the nerve. The scleral development is covered in more detail in Chaps. 5 and 8, but the collagen fibers in the sclera develop in a sequence from the front of the eye to back to eventually reach the already formed nerve. There is penetration of the nerve by collagen fibers starting in the fourth month. The lamina cribrosa then develops and is not fully formed until after birth [2]. The meningeal coverings of the optic nerve start to become evident as layers in the 12th week. Myelination of the nerve begins somewhat before the sixth month of gestation.

25.2 Anatomy of the Optic Nerve

In normal eyes, there are approximately 1.2 million non-myelinated nerve fibers converging on the optic canal to leave the eye through the lamina cribrosa. The aggregate of these nerve fibers and the associated glial cells make up the bulk of the optic nerve. These fibers make a nearly 90 degree turn to enter the optic nerve in emmetropes. The internal opening of the optic nerve is defined by the opening in Bruch's membrane and more posteriorly by the opening in the sclera called the optic canal. The portion of the optic nerve internal to the lamina cribrosa is the prelaminar portion of the nerve. Its internal surface is bounded by a layer of collagen and astrocytes called the inner limiting membrane of Elschnig, which is a distinct entity from the internal limiting membrane of the retina. The prelaminar portion of the nerve is composed of nerve fiber bundles separated by an

R. F. Spaide (✉)
Vitreous, Retina, Macula Consultants of New York,
New York, NY, USA

K. Ohno-Matsui
Department of Ophthalmology and Visual Science, Tokyo Medical and Dental University, Bunkyo-Ku, Tokyo, Japan
e-mail: k.ohno.oph@tmd.ac.jp

© Springer Nature Switzerland AG 2021
R. F. Spaide et al. (eds.), *Pathologic Myopia*, https://doi.org/10.1007/978-3-030-74334-5_25

almost equal volume of glial cells. At the outer border of the nerve, separating it from the surrounding retina is the intermediary tissue of Kuhnt, and separating it from the choroid is the border tissue of Jacoby. The laminar portion of the nerve is that section passing through the lamina cribrosa. The connective tissue and glial elements of the lamina cribrosa are more prominent in the nasal and temporal quadrants as compared with the inferior and superior ones [3]. The pores within the lamina cribrosa are larger in the inferior and superior quadrants [4]. There is a bow tie-shaped ridge in the lamina cribrosa that extends from the nasal to the temporal side of the optic canal near the horizontal meridian [5]. There appears to be more robust connective tissue support in the lamina in the horizontal meridians than along the inferosuperior axis. This raises interesting questions, since a greater expanse of the globe is exposed to trauma in the horizontal meridians than in the vertical ones. Posterior to the lamina, the optic nerve expands in diameter and becomes myelinated. Within the intraorbital optic nerve, there are also glial cells and blood vessels and connective tissue septae. The optic nerve is covered by pia mater. The subarachnoid space ends in a blind pouch at the scleral border of the eye. The dura mater is continuous with the outer 1/3 of the sclera.

The blood supply of the nerve varies by location and has been the source of disagreement. The nerve fiber layer derives its supply from the central retinal artery. Branches coursing in a centripetal direction may help supply the prelaminar portion of the nerve. The short posterior ciliary vessels supply a perineural arterial ring, often incomplete, called the circle of Zinn-Haller (first described by Zinn [6] in 1755) that is located in the sclera [6–11]. Branches from the circle of Zinn-Haller supply the prelaminar and laminar nerve and anastomose with the adjacent choroidal circulation. Past theories concerning blood flow have proposed direct communication between the choroid and the prelaminar optic nerve [7]. There is controversy about the circle of Zinn-Haller. Blood supply to the nerve (and the posterior choroid) is derived from many short posterior ciliary arteries that converge upon and anastomose around the nerve. This raises the question of whether the so-called circle of Zinn-Haller is a just the manifestation of a group of anastomoses or if it is a separate and distinct structure in its own right [12]. In this chapter the circle of Zinn-Haller will be considered a distinct anatomic structure. The blood drains from the nerve into branches of the central retinal vein.

25.3 Morphometric Characteristics of the Optic Disc in Normal Eyes

Ordinarily the optic nerve is a slightly ovoid structure that had a mean vertical measurement of 1.92 mm by 1.76 mm horizontally in a study of 319 subjects using magnification-corrected morphometry of optic disc photographs [13]. In a

study of 60 eye bank eyes, the measurements were 1.88 mm vertically by 1.76 horizontally [14]. These measurements should be viewed as being approximate because the size of the optic disc among studies has shown variation by study, race, and measurement method. The mean disc area in Caucasians ranged from 1.73 mm^2 to 2.63 mm^2, in African Americans 2.46 mm^2 to 2.67 mm^2, and a similarly large range of sizes among various Asian populations (extensively reviewed in reference [15]). Studies seem to indicate African Americans have larger optic disc areas than other races. The cup is a central depression in the optic nerve. A common metric used to gauge the morphology of the optic disc is the cup-to-disc ratio, or cup/disc, the proportion calculated by dividing the diameter of the depression by the diameter of the disc. Although in common usage there are several difficulties with this metric, the diameter of the disc varies by what feature is measured, that is, the color change, elevation change, or the actual canal diameter. The margin of the optic disc as seen by color photography or ophthalmoscopy does not appear to have a consistent anatomic correlate in OCT imaging [15]. The diameter of the depression is a function of what definition is used for "depression" and what the specified height or curve change used is open to contention. The cup/disc varies with age and race. Finally, the cup-to-disc ratio along the vertical axis usually is not the same as the horizontal axis. Using magnification adjusted planimetry, Jonas and coworkers found the mean horizontal cup/disc was 0.39, while the mean vertical ratio was 0.39 [13]. The Rotterdam study of subjects 55 years of age or older using stereoscopic simultaneous optic disc transparencies found a vertical cup/disc of 0.49 and a horizontal cup/disc of 0.40 [16].

Evaluation of the nerve generally starts with appraising the scleral ring to delineate the optic disc size. As they exit the eye, the retinal nerve fibers arch over and create the optic nerve rim. The substance of the prelaminar nerve comprises nerve fibers and glial cells. Although Anderson stated nerve has a large proportion of glial cells [17], the variability of the mix from one person to the next is not known. Monkeys with larger nerve heads were found to have a greater number of retinal nerve fibers [18]. Large optic disc sizes also generally have greater neural rim area, and the number of nerve fibers is increased in larger nerves in humans as well [19]. It is likely that large nerves are not necessarily scaled up versions of smaller ones. Even though the rim area may be larger in bigger optic discs, the cup generally increases in size as well. A normal optic nerve shows varying rim thickness in most eyes known as the ISNT rule in which the order of nerve fiber thickness is from greatest to least inferior, superior, nasal, and temporal. Loss of the rim to include notching is suspicious for associated nerve fiber loss. The optic nerve is a vascular structure and ordinarily has a pinkish-orange color. In a sense, the nerve fibers act like light pipes, and a healthy nerve shows a reflection that has a depth. Loss of neurons, such as in optic neuropathies, causes the nerve to become pallorous; the reflection is whiter with less depth.

25.4 Optic Nerve Hypoplasia

Optic nerve hypoplasia is the most common congenital abnormality of the optic nerve [20]. The optic nerve appears small, often misshapen, and can be surrounded by a ring of altered pigmentation that is called the double ring sign. The vessels on the nerve often show anomalies as well to include abnormal branching patterns, altered vascular density on the nerve head, and venous dilation. The retinal nerve fiber layer can show a generalized decrease, sector defects, or a combination of the two. Often there are sufficient nerve fibers in the maculopapillary bundle to support nearly normal visual acuity.

25.5 Glaucoma

Glaucoma, the most commonly acquired abnormality of the nerve, shows loss of the retinal nerve fiber layer to a greater extent than age alone would dictate and associated changes in the optic nerve head including changes in the collagen, elastic fibers, and extracellular matrix [21–29]. There is increased cupping of the nerve, tensile expansion, and distortion of load-bearing structures in the eye such as the peripapillary sclera, the scleral canal, and the lamina cribrosa [30–33]. Expansion of the scleral canal, compaction, and posterior displacement of the lamina cribrosa occur in glaucoma. The changes in the lamina cribrosa appear to be the result of more than simple stress-induced strain effects, as biologic remodeling of the lamina occurs [34]. These alterations appear to reverse somewhat following glaucoma surgery [35, 36]. There are lines of evidence that converge on the concept that retinal nerve fiber damage at the level of the lamina cribrosa is an important pathophysiologic mechanism in glaucoma. Since this is the site of biomechanical changes induced by glaucoma, a logical, biologically plausible assumption is that the mechanically induced effects ultimately lead to nerve fiber damage.

25.6 Optic Neuropathies Associated with High Myopia

25.6.1 Overview

The most common ocular finding associated with unilateral high myopia is optic nerve hypoplasia [37]. Conversely high myopia occurs frequently in eyes with optic nerve hypoplasia [38]. This is difficult to explain on the basis of current theories of the development of high myopia, which posits a local effect in the eye as the major cause of myopization. It is possible that yet unnamed syndromes exist to link optic nerve hypoplasia or even smaller-sized optic nerve heads with high myopia, as it does appear to be an association that may be more common than the joint probabilities would indicate [39]. Tilting of the optic nerve is more common in high myopia than among emmetropes [40–43]. Tilting of the nerve is associated with smaller optic discs and also visual field defects [40, 41] (Figs. 25.1 and 25.2). In general though, the size of the optic nerve head increases with the amount of myopic refractive error (after correction for image magnification differences) [16, 44] (Fig. 25.3). Expansion of the scleral canal and the lamina cribrosa occurs with enlargement of the optic nerve head. By Laplace's law, the scleral wall stress would be higher per unit cross-sectional area because of the increased radius of the myopic eye and the thinning of the sclera observed in high myopia. Some myopes develop extremely enlarged optic discs with stretching and flattening of the cup (Figs. 25.4 and 25.5). The course of the optic nerve often is skewed as it courses through the sclera in high myopes. Expansion of the posterior portion of the eye in myopia can be associated with acquired pits of the optic nerve, dehiscences of the lamina cribrosa, expansion of the dural attachment posteriorly with enlargement of the subarachnoid space immediately behind the eye (Figs. 25.6 and 25.7), and expansion of the circle of Zinn-Haller with potential compromise of circulation into the prelaminar portion of the nerve. Potential for both mechanical stressors and circulatory compromise exists in high myopia, and any or all of these factors may influence the health of the nerve. In the remaining portion of this chapter, these potential contributors to optic nerve dysfunction will be discussed.

Glaucoma can represent a particular set of difficulties in high myopia. Because of the induced anatomic changes in high myopia, enlargement of the disc in macrodiscs with flattening of the cup, or distortion of the disc with small cups seen in tilted optic discs being prominent examples, diagnosing glaucoma can be difficult. The problem frequently boils down to deciding if the observed abnormalities are due, at least in part, to glaucoma and then determining if the changes are progressive. If so, the eye is generally treated with modalities to reduce the intraocular pressure. It is possible that myopia may cause progressive abnormalities in the retinal nerve fiber by mechanisms not found in emmetropic eyes. What if these changes are lessened by reducing intraocular pressure? Should these conditions be lumped together with glaucoma? In an analysis of 5277 participants from the National Health and Nutrition Examination Survey data, high myopes were found to have a much higher prevalence of visual field defects than either emmetropes or low myopes even though the self-reported prevalence of glaucoma was the same [45]. Since high myopia is a significant risk factor for the development of glaucoma, Qui and coworkers concluded glaucoma surveillance should be intensified in high

Fig. 25.1 Schematic drawing of the optic nerve in an emmetrope. The numbered regions are as follows: (1a) inner limiting membrane of the retina, (1b) inner limiting membrane of Elschnig, (2) central meniscus of Kuhnt, (3) border tissue of Elschnig, (4) border tissue of Jacoby, (5) intermediary tissue of Kuhnt, (6) anterior portion of lamina cribrosa, and (7) posterior portion of lamina cribrosa. The abbreviations are as follows: Du, dura mater; Ar, arachnoid mater; Pia, pia mater; Gl.M., glial mantle of Fuchs; Gl.C, glial cell; Sep, septae. (From Anderson and Hoyt)

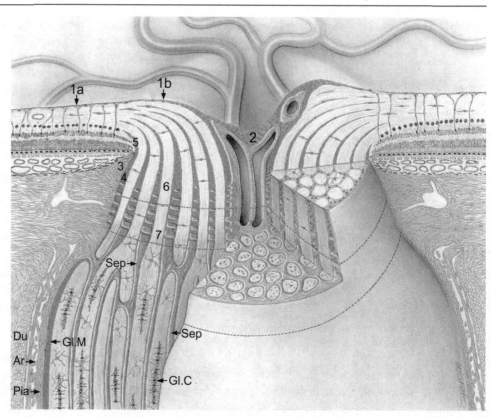

myopes because glaucoma is probably being underdiagnosed in patients with high myopia [45].

Peripapillary atrophy is common in highly myopic eyes. The atrophy is deceptively simple but occurs in zones around the nerve. The outermost region is the alpha zone, which is a region on the outer border of the beta zone and demonstrates irregular pigmentation. The beta zone is a region of loss of the retinal pigment epithelium (RPE). The underlying choroid and sclera are rendered increasingly visible by the absence of the RPE. Further investigation of these eyes with EDI-OCT showed Bruch's membrane stopped short of the optic disc border. The gap between Bruch's membrane and the optic disc border was called the gamma zone [46]. In a histologic evaluation of highly myopic eyes, an area within the gamma zone was identified in which there were no blood vessels >50 μm in diameter. This region was called the delta zone. Alternate terminology has been proposed. The beta zone without Bruch's membrane has been termed βPPA_{-BM}. The beta zone with Bruch's membrane is βPPA_{+BM} [47]. This meanings implied by the expanded nomenclature may be easier to remember.

Rudnicka and Edgar found that increasing size of peripapillary atrophy is associated with decreased global threshold visual field indices [48, 49]. Beta zone peripapillary atrophy, in particular, occurs more commonly in glaucomatous eyes. Glaucomatous visual field progression occurs more rapidly in eyes with a beta zone of peripapillary atrophy [50]. Size of beta zone peripapillary atrophy shows an inverse correlation with neuroretinal rim area and a spatial correlation to visual field loss in glaucoma patients [51].

25.7 Tilted Discs

There are three axes of rotation of an object, and current ophthalmic terminology describing the optic nerve only has terms for two of these. Tilting of the optic nerve refers to one of the horizontal borders of the nerve which are rotated in the transverse plane. Usually the temporal portion of the nerve is posterior to the nasal portion. The optic disc in eyes appears to be smaller than normal; the long axis of the nerve is typically larger, while the horizontal aspect is smaller than a normal disc. This may be related to the underlying structural support of the lamina in which the superior and inferior portions of the lamina appear less robust than the horizontal aspects. The true horizontal width is difficult to measure accurately, however. The visualized width is the true width of the nerve multiplied by the cosine of the angle of posterior rotation. By visual inspection, it is difficult to know what this angle is, but with the advent of optical coherence tomography (OCT), this angle potentially is measurable. However some recent authors estimate the amount of tilt by calculating the ratio between the minimum and maximum diameter of the nerve, a value they termed the index of tilt [52]. This ratio is certainly decreased in tilted optic nerves, but the

Fig. 25.2 Stylized drawing after Fig. 25.1 showing an emmetropic eye (**a**) and one with a tilted optic disc (**b**). Missing from the drawing in Fig. 25.1 is Bruch's membrane (BrM). The nerve fibers course through the opening in Bruch's membrane, which is centered over the scleral canal. In high myopes with a tilted disc, there is a shifting of the opening in Bruch's membrane temporally. There is a shifting of the inner sclera, which itself is thinned in high myopes. There are thinning of the choroid and absence of the temporal peripapillary choroid. The subarachnoid space (SAS) is expanded

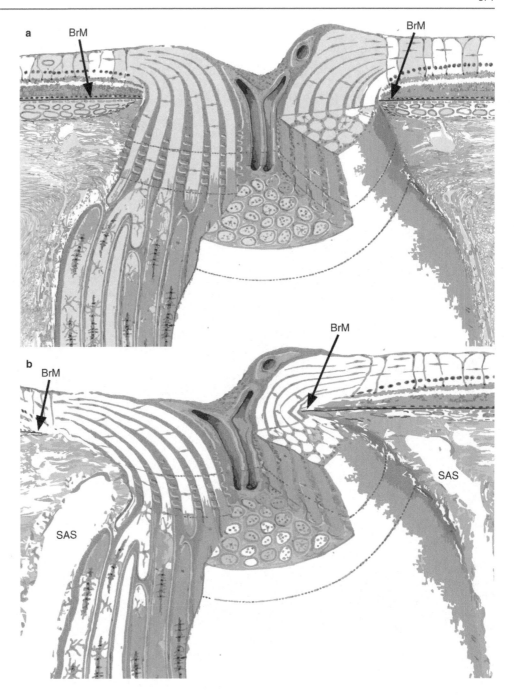

number is not comparable among patients because the minimum width observed in a color photograph is not the true horizontal width. One patient with a very narrow disc with little tilt may have the same index of tilt as another patient with a wider disc but more tilt. In addition, this ratio does not account for vertical elongation of the disc.

Tilted optic discs occur more commonly in myopic eyes but also occur in emmetropic and hyperopic eyes [40–43]. Tilted optic discs also are associated with higher cylindrical errors and longer axial lengths. Intraocular abnormalities associated with tilted optic nerves include smaller optic discs, small optic nerve cups, situs inversus of the retinal ves-

sels, abnormal vascularity on the nerve, and anomalous branching patterns of the retinal vessels in the retina. These associated abnormalities occur in some but not all eyes. Ordinarily a single central retinal artery branches into four arcade vessels, one each supplying the superotemporal, inferotemporal, inferonasal, and superonasal quadrants. In eyes with tilted optic discs, there are often fewer or more vessels branching on the nerve than what is normally seen, and these vessels do not necessarily follow the pattern of the four arcades. On occasions, larger vessels may branch in unusual patterns near the disc in the retina. Some authorities refer to tilted optic discs as congenital tilted optic disc; how-

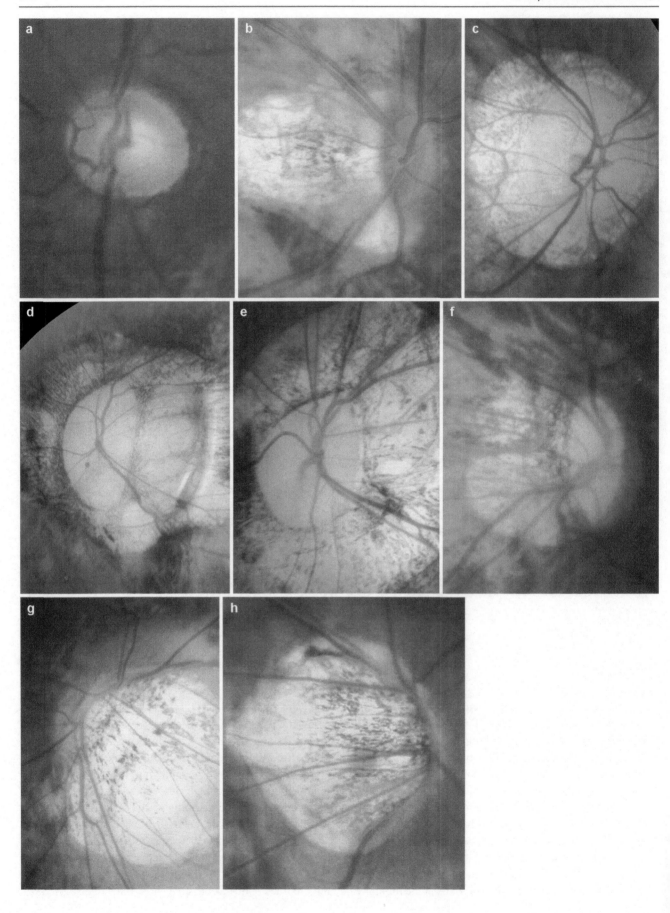

Fig. 25.3 Optic disc appearance in emmetropic eyes (**a**) and in eyes with pathologic myopia (**b–h**). (**a**) A round optic disc in an emmetropic eye (axial length; 23.3 mm) in a 43-year-old woman. The optic disc area is 2.49 mm². (**b**) Small optic disc in a highly myopic eye (axial length; 29.0 mm) in a 71-year-old woman. The optic disc area, 0.975 mm², was corrected for axial length and corneal curvature, as were all of the other disc areas shown. (**c–e**) Various patterns of megalodisc in eyes with pathologic myopia. (**c**) A large and round optic disc with little tilting, torsion, or ovality in the right fundus (axial length; 32.3 mm) of a 29-year-old man. The optic disc area adjusted by an axial length and corneal curvature is 9.57 mm². (**d**) A large and oval disc in the left fundus (axial length; 33.0 mm) of a 59-year-old woman. The optic disc area was 5.21 mm². (**e**) A large disc in the left fundus (axial length; 35.3 mm) of a 50-year-old woman. The optic disc area corrected for axial length and corneal curvature was 5.09 mm². (**f**) A vertically oval disc in the right fundus (axial length; 32.3 mm) of a 41-year-old woman. Ovality index (maximum diameter/minimum diameter of the optic disc) is 2.36. (**g, h**) Examples of extremely tilted optic discs

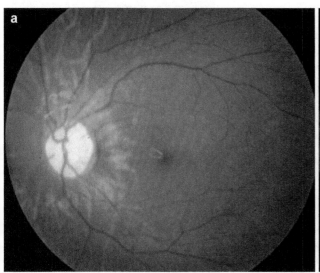
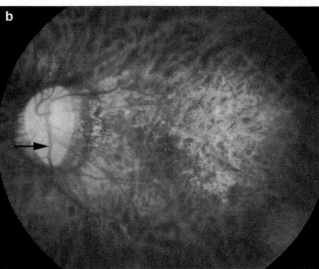

Fig. 25.4 Development of acquired megalodisc in a highly myopic patient with age. (**a**) The left fundus of an 8-year-old boy shows a slightly oval disc. Axial length is 27.96 mm. (**b**) Twenty-four years later, the optic disc is vertically elongated and becomes megalodisc like. Axial length increases to 31.11 mm. The optic disc area was 5.96 mm². Over the 24-year follow-up, there is vertical elongation of the disc. Note the retinal vein coursing on the optic disc (arrow) shows bifurcation at the disc border in (**a**) but is within the disc area in (**b**)

Fig. 25.5 (**a**) The right fundus of a 14-year-old boy shows almost round optic disc. (**b**) Twenty-two years later, the optic disc shows enlargement and torsion

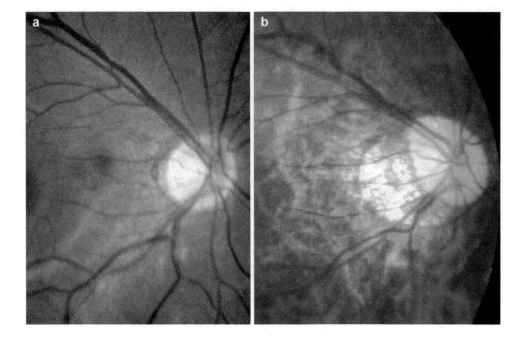

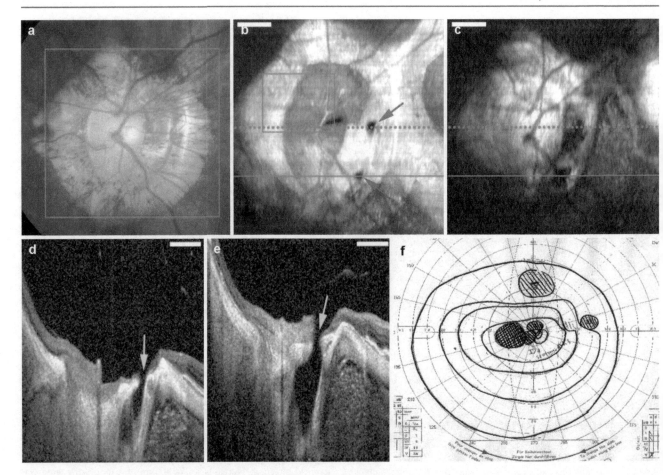

Fig. 25.6 Fundus photograph and swept-source OCT images showing deep pits extending toward the subarachnoid space (SAS). (**a**) Color fundus photograph of the optic disc showing a large annular conus. (**b**, **c**) En face cross-sectional images scanned in the area shown by the green square in (**a**). These en face images are from different levels and show that there are two pit-like pores (arrows) at the temporal border of the optic disc (**b**) and that these pores extend toward the SAS (**c**). (**d**, **e**) B-scan images acquired by 3D scan protocol showing the pits (arrows) extending toward the SAS; it is likely that there may be a direct communication with the SAS. (**f**) Visual fields from Goldmann perimetry show a central and a paracentral scotoma in addition to the nasal step. Scale bar, 1 mm

ever, there is not enough data at present to be certain of what proportion of tilted discs are congenital.

Samarawickrama and coworkers examined retinal images of 1765 children aged 6 years and found 20 (1.6%) had tilted discs [53]. In these children, there was no association with myopia. A similar study in adolescent children in Singapore found tilted optic discs in 454 (37%) of 1227 children with a mean age of 14 years, and there was a very strong association with myopia [54]. Except for 20 cases, all eyes with tilted optic nerve had beta zone peripapillary atrophy. In the Blue Mountains study, which some of the same authors participated [40], tilted discs were found in 56 subjects among 3583 adult participants, or 1.6%. The proportion of eyes with tilted discs was much greater among adult eyes with high myopia. The authors concluded the similar prevalence was evidence that tilted optic discs are really congenital. On the other hand, Kim and colleagues documented how the tilted appearance occurs over time in children [55], including the development of alteration in the shape of the optic disc.

Patients with unilateral myopia have tilted discs only or, more prominently, in the myopic eye. Therefore, some tilted discs may be a function of morphogenic changes of the eye wall contour that occur in the development of high myopia, such as staphyloma formation. Another interesting take on this data is some patients have identifiable traits early when they are not myopic that may be predictive of high myopia later in life. The true estimation of the proportion of congenital tilted discs would be obtained from examining babies.

The retinal nerve fibers in a highly myopic eye still converge on the optic canal, but the path taken by the fibers is different in a highly myopic eye with a tilted disc. The shifting of the layers, particularly of the opening in Bruch's membrane in relationship to the scleral opening, was readily known to ophthalmologists in the nineteenth century [56, 57]. With the advent of high-resolution OCT, the changes seen in gross specimens can now be seen in vivo. There is a shift of the Bruch's membrane opening over the scleral canal in the temporal direction, so the nasal aspect of Bruch's

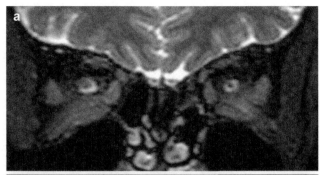

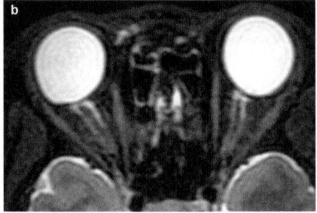

Fig. 25.7 Dilation of subarachnoid space (SAS) shown as ring sign in MRI images. (**a**) Coronal section of T_2-weighted MRI image showing a ring sign to show a dilated SAS around the optic nerve. (**b**) Horizontal section showing a tram track sign along the retrobulbar optic nerve

membrane appears to "slice" into the nasal aspect of the tilted nerve. The nasal border of the nerve, as defined by the Bruch's membrane opening, is often much more temporal than would be appreciated by cursory ophthalmoscopy. This causes the nasal retinal nerve fibers to make a sharp hairpin turn to enter the optic nerve. This was called "supertraktion" by German ophthalmologists and "supertraction" or "supertraction crescent" by the English [56–58]. On the temporal side of the nerve, the absence of tissue was called the "distraction crescent" [59], signifying the pulling away of tissue by shifting tissue planes. The temporal retinal nerve fibers enter the tilted nerve at an angle greater than 90 degrees. Tilted discs are often associated with inferior staphylomas, which are discussed in Chaps. 8 and 13.

Eyes with tilted discs commonly have visual field defects, which typically are arcuate. The most common is a bitemporal arcuate defect that does not respect the midline. This feature helps rule out the possibility of a chiasmal disorder. The arcuate-shaped defects also do not necessarily respect the horizontal midline, a finding uncommon in early glaucoma. Vongphanit and associates found the mean spherical refraction in eyes with tilted optic disc and visual field defects was −5.6 diopters [60], but visual field defects associated with tilted discs do not necessarily occur in eyes that are highly myopic or even myopic at all [60–62]. In agreement with the original article by Young [61], the most common location was superotemporal. The blind spot also may be enlarged and is usually proportional to the area of atrophy related to the conus. In the original description of tilted disc syndrome in 1976, one cause for the superior field defects was considered to be the "variable myopia" caused by "localized staphylomatous ectasia" [61]. Prior to being called tilted disc syndrome, earlier authors described similar eye configurations using terms such as situs inversus of the optic disc with inferior conus [62–66]. These authors noted the variable myopia and the ability to cause the visual field defect to disappear by changing the refraction [63, 65], an observation reported again decades later [67]. In inferior staphyloma, the eye wall bulges out posteriorly inferiorly, and as a consequence the image plane lies increasingly in front of the retina. The sensitivity of the retina is dependent on the illuminance, the luminous flux incident per unit area of the photoreceptors. A defocused image spreads the same number of photons of light over a larger area thus potentially reducing the sensitivity to threshold change. Altering the refraction in front of the eye can make visual field defects disappear in some eyes with inferior staphylomas. Even though this effect appears to be well known, as it was described repeatedly since the 1950s, reported studies in which the correction was actually done are rare. Therefore, it is likely many reported studies of visual field defects in tilted disc syndrome may be related to refractive abnormalities. However Young and coworkers stated not every patient had a staphyloma [61], and Hamada and coworkers found the visual field defects frequently did not correlate with the anatomic changes in the eye [68]. Odland et al. reported that stronger myopic correction could decrease the scotoma but in their patients did not cause it to completely disappear [65]. So there must be additional reasons for the field defects. These eyes can show alterations of the critical fusion frequency [69], and electroretinographic abnormalities to include the multifocal electroretinogram [68, 70, 71], and reduced visual evoked responses [68]. Nevertheless some of these abnormalities were attributed to locally defocused images by the respective authors. Some of the pathophysiologic causes have proposed and include hypoplasia of the retina and choroid with subsequent distortion of structures around the disc [63], altered retinal pigment epithelium, and choroidal atrophy [66].

The visual field defects in tilted disc syndrome are generally stable, which can be a help in ruling out a concurrent diagnosis of glaucoma. The visual fields are not stable in all high myopes. Carl Stellwag von Carion noted in the nineteenth century that staphylomas appeared to be acquired and they progressed, sometimes very slowly, over a period of many years [72]. To the extent the visual field defects are related to staphylomas, either because of refractive or physiologic reasons, there is a possibility with long-term follow-up the visual field may progress. In highly myopic patients who showed VF defects which are not explained by myopic fundus lesions, Ohno-Matsui and coworkers performed multiple regression analyses to determine the correlations between the visual field score and these possible factors: age at the initial examination, age at the last examination, axial length, initial IOP, mean IOP during the follow-up, maximum to minimum diameter measurements of the optic disc, and the presence of an abrupt change of scleral curvature temporal to the optic disc [73]. The results showed that the presence of an abrupt change of scleral curvature temporal to the optic disc was the only factor which correlated with a progression of visual field defects in highly myopic patients [73]. In addition to all of the previously mentioned theories for decreased sensitivity, the findings of this study raise new possibilities. One is that the sharp bend in the sclera may put mechanical stress on the nerve fiber to potentially cause injury. Second, there is the possibility of the Stiles-Crawford effect playing a role, since the tilted photoreceptors would be expected to have a reduced response. Akagi and coworkers found the retinal nerve fiber thickness was inversely related to the angle the fibers had to take to hug scleral protrusions near the optic disc [74]. This finding may be a proxy for the curvature of the associated staphyloma. When considering the possibility of glaucoma, confirmatory evidence from retinal nerve fiber thickness measurements can be helpful. The pattern of retinal nerve fiber distribution is altered in tilted disc syndrome with thinner average; superior, nasal, and inferior but thicker temporal nerve fiber thicknesses; and a temporal shift in the superior and inferior peak locations [75, 76]. Eyes with tilted optic nerves generally show more tilt with greater amounts of myopia, and eyes with more tilting have a greater temporal shift in nerve fiber thickness measurements. Nerve fiber measurements in these eyes can be difficult and unreliable because of defects in segmentation, peripapillary atrophy, and schisis within the nerve fiber layer.

Torsion of the disc occurs when the ovoid of the optic nerve head is rotated in the coronal plane. More commonly this rotation is counterclockwise when viewing the right eye such that the superior aspect of the long axis is rotated temporally. The direction of optic disc torsion is a strong predictor of visual field defect location in normal-tension glaucoma [77]. There is a correlation between the amount of torsion and the visual field defect severity [78]. The retinal nerve fibers from the temporal periphery course around the central macula, apparently so they do not pass directly over the fovea. This diverts fibers to the superior and inferior nerve head. The retinal nerve fibers from the superior and inferior macula follow the analogous routes, respectively. Therefore, a large number of nerve fibers converge on the optic canal either superiorly or inferiorly. Rotation of the nerve would be expected to cause a shift of nerve fibers entering the nerve. In the Chennai Glaucoma Study [79] nerves showing outward rotation of the superior aspect of the nerve had thicker superior optic rims. In a study by Park and coworkers myopes with normal tension glaucoma were much younger than nonmyopes and the biggest predictor of their visual field defects were the direction of optic nerve torsion [77]. Torsion of the nerve is much more common than is simple tilting. Some authors have used the term tilted to refer to both tilt and torsion. The remaining axis about which the optic disc potentially could rotate would cause deviation in the sagittal plane. This would produce a difference in elevation of the superior aspect of the disc in relation to the inferior portion. Given that inferior staphylomas are common, the inferior portion of the disc is commonly more posterior.

25.8 Optic Neuropathy Associated with Optic Nerve Abnormalities That May Not Be Progressive

Doshi and coworkers [80] described a group of young to middle-aged men of Chinese origin who had optic nerve cupping and visual field abnormalities suggestive of glaucoma, but they had stable ocular findings for up to 7 years. The authors hypothesized that during the ocular expansion and associated deformation of the lamina cribrosa and altered entry angles for retinal nerve fibers may have put undue stress on some of the nerve fibers. The authors hypothesized that loss of these nerve fibers would lead to cupping and field loss, but with stabilization of myopic expansion, the process may not be progressive. The follow-up period, even though it was up to 7 years, does not mean the subjects would not show visual field progression, particularly in later years when glaucoma is much more common. Of interest is that analysis of 26 eyes of 26 young myopic primary open-angle glaucoma patients with progressive optic disc tilting showed an associated visual field mean deviation worsening [81].

25.9 Optic Disc Abnormalities Associated with Generalized Expansion

While it would seem to be an easy research question to answer, the exact relationship between axial length, myopia, and disc size is still a matter of contention. A histogram of proportion of the population tested versus refractive error shows a nearly normal distribution, albeit one skewed to the right. For most eyes, that is those having a refractive error somewhere between low grades of hyperopia to moderate amounts of myopia, there is little to no significant relationship between refractive error (or the corresponding axial length) and disc area [82–89]. There is a clear relationship for eyes with high amounts of myopia and disc area. These eyes represent a small proportion of the general population and show values clearly different than the rest of the data. In a sense, highly myopic eyes are outliers and when included with the rest of the population can influence the overall correlation between refractive error and disc size. The Rotterdam Eye study reported a 0.033 mm² increase in disc area with each diopter of refractive error [16]. Even if this were applicable to lower grades of myopia, the increase in disc area is very small. However among highly myopic eyes, particularly those with a refractive error greater than − 8 diopters, the disc area increases substantially in size [85, 86]. Two groups of investigators using OCT thought there was an inverse correlation between optic disc size and either refractive error or axial length, but the authors did not appear to perform any image size corrections for magnification variations [90, 91].

Optic discs in normal eyes show significant variation is size, independent of refractive error. Discs much larger than typical are called macrodiscs. For the Beijing Eye study, the calculated threshold was 3.79mm² [85]. Eyes with macrodiscs generally fall into one of two classes. One is termed primary macrodisc in which the size of the disc does not appear to bear any relationship to refractive error. In secondary, or acquired, macrodisc, the optic nerve enlargement is associated with myopia, generally a refractive error of −8 or greater. Macrodiscs associated with myopia typically show generalized enlargement, but this enlargement may not necessarily be isotropic. As a consequence, it is possible to see discs that are distorted in shape as well as being large. Macrodiscs typically have a flattening of the cup with reduced optic disc rim thickness and consequently increased cup/disc metrics. These discs may also appear somewhat pallorous as compared with normal discs in emmetropes. The macrodiscs not related to myopia generally do not show pallor or flattening of the disc and they have deeper cups. Along with the generalized enlargement of the disc, there are associated thinning of the adjacent sclera and development of pits in the nerve and adjacent sclera.

The peripapillary region in eyes with megadiscs secondary to high myopia invariably have prominent peripapillary atrophy that involves the choroid, RPE, and outer retina. In some eyes, there can be marked thinning or even frank defects of the nerve fiber layer. In these eyes the segmentation routines used to detect retinal nerve fiber layer thickness break down and consequently do not accurately measure the thickness of the retinal nerve fiber layer. These are the patients that are among the most difficult to evaluate for glaucoma. Under the best of circumstances, the optic disc in high myopia with disc enlargement may have a smaller rim, the disc is usually pale, visual field testing shows at least an enlargement of the blind spot, and retinal nerve fiber layer measurements are not reliable. Patients with very high amounts of myopia have depressed threshold sensitivities.

There are potential difficulties with retinal nerve fiber layer analysis in high myopes; an alternative measurement could be to measure the cell bodies instead of the axons. The ganglion cell complex can be visualized, segmented, and measured in eyes and has been proposed as a method to help diagnose and follow glaucoma in highly myopic eyes [92–94]. The area under the curve for ganglion cell complex measurements appears as good as or better than nerve fiber layer measurements. There is disagreement about parameter variation and myopia with this newer modality. Shoji and coworkers [93] found no association between thickness and amount of myopia while Zhao and Jiang did [94].

25.9.1 Dilation of Perioptic Subarachnoid Space and Thinning of Peripapillary Sclera

Expansion of the subarachnoid space (SAS) near the exit of the optic nerve has been noted more than 100 years ago [95–100]. The terminology used then was a bit different than today. The subarachnoid space was seen to end in a blind pouch that was thought to be bounded by scleral fibers that were confluent with the termination of the arachnoid and the dura, which themselves merged together. The space was called the intervaginal space by many authorities, and others called it the subarachnoid space. The space was seen to be enlarged in cases of infection because of increased intracranial pressure, tumor, optic atrophy, and in myopia. First described by von Jaeger, early ideas were that the expansion of the space was due to ocular expansion during myopia development, Schnabel considered the enlargement a congenital abnormality that occurred in eyes that also commonly developed myopia, while Landolt thought the expansion of the dural insertion caused weakness of the posterior portion of the eye with staphyloma development as a consequence [100]. In myopic eyes with an enlarged intervaginal space, the sclera was seen to be exceedingly thin by a number of authorities of that age and was described by Parsons as leaving only a "few layers of scleral lamellae" [99]. Okisaka [101] reported that in emmetropic eyes, the perioptic SAS was narrow and the SAS blindly ended at the level of lamina cribrosa. The dura of the SAS was attached to the peripapillary sclera just around the lamina cribrosa. In contrary, in highly myopic eyes, the perioptic SAS was enlarged together with an increase of the axial length (Fig. 25.7).

Observations by investigators such as Okisaka and Jonas [102, 103] have helped refine concepts of the enlargement of the subarachnoid space and associated histologic changes in the posterior eye wall. Jonas found that the scleral flange, the distance between the optic nerve border, and the attachment of the dura to the sclera were correlated with increased axial length and inversely correlated with the scleral thickness

[102]. The scleral flange thickness was seen to be attenuated in myopic eyes, with some having thicknesses of less than 100 microns [103]. Over the course of more than a century, observations of the perioptic subarachnoid space were typically made on autopsy eyes.

In T_2 images of MRI, the dilated SAS around the optic nerve can be observed as a ring sign, which is somewhat similar to the findings seen in patients with increased intracranial pressure (Fig. 25.7). Enhanced depth imaging (EDI)-OCT and swept-source OCT provided deeper imaging capabilities as compared with conventional spectral domain (SD) OCT and made it possible to visualize the deeper structures in detail in vivo. Park et al. [104] used EDI-OCT and observed the SAS around the optic nerve in 25 of the 139 glaucomatous eyes (18%). Most of the 25 eyes had high myopia and extensive parapapillary atrophy. Ohno-Matsui and coworkers [105] used swept-source OCT and visualized a dilated SAS in 124 of 133 highly myopic eyes (93.2%) but could not visualize the SAS in the emmetropic eyes. The SAS was triangular, with the base toward the eye surrounding the optic nerve (Fig. 25.5) and it contained a branching internal structure. The attachment of the dura to the eye wall could be clearly seen offset from the immediate peripapillary area, and there was a change in the scleral curvature at the site of attachment. In one highly myopic eye, there appeared to be a direct communication between the intraocular cavity and SAS through pit-like pores (Fig. 25.6).

The expanded area of exposure to CSF pressure along with thinning of the posterior eye wall may influence staphyloma formation and the way in which diseases may be manifested. Marcus Gunn stated that he rarely saw optic nerve swelling in high myopes with brain tumors [106]. While he stated the joint probability of the two was low, he proposed the excessive cerebrospinal fluid pressure in the subarachnoid space may be spread out over a larger area of the posterior portion of the eye or may be locally dissipated by the thinned dura near the eye in highly myopic eyes. There may in fact be weakening of the ocular wall, as Landolt suggested [96], but the amount of staphyloma formation would be influenced by not only the thinning of the sclera but also by the alteration in trans-scleral forces caused by the wider region of exposure to the cerebrospinal fluid pressure. Many questions remain unanswered but potentially could be modeled now that imaging techniques are capable of visualizing these areas.

25.9.2 Formation of Acquired Pits in the Optic Disc and Conus Regions

Because of the expansion of the posterior portion of the globe, scleral emissaries can show remarkable expansion in size as shown in Chap. 8. Similar expansion of the region centered on the nerve can cause several broad classes of analogous abnormalities (Fig. 25.8). Pit-like changes can be seen in the region of the conus similar to those in the macular region [107]. There can be clefts at the border of the optic nerve, which may be secondary to expansion-induced stress at this junction. Finally tears in the lamina cribrosa, similar to those seen in glaucomatous eyes, have been seen in highly myopic eyes, and these dehiscences may be associated with depressions or pits in the optic nerve [108]. By using swept-source OCT, Ohno-Matsui and colleagues [107] found pit-like clefts at the outer border of the optic nerve or within the adjacent scleral crescent in 32 of 198 highly myopic eyes (16.2%) but in none of the emmetropic eyes. The pits were located in the optic disc in 11 of 32 eyes (Figs. 25.9 and 25.10) and in the area of the conus outside the optic disc (conus pits) in 22 of 32 eyes. The nerve fiber tissue was discontinuous overlying the pits, and this discontinuity may be yet another reason for visual field defects in highly myopic patients. In some cases, the retinal vessels herniated into the

Fig. 25.8 Deeply excavated pit-like structures within the optic disc area in a highly myopic eye suspected of having glaucoma. The refractive error was −18.0 D and the axial length was 29.4 mm. Bar, 1 mm. (**a**) Right fundus of a 45-year-old woman shows an atrophic glaucomatous optic disc and temporal conus. The green arrows show the scanned lines of the swept-source OCT images shown in D and E. (**b**) Magnified view shows the large optic disc with saucerization. Note how the vessels inferiorly dip out of view at the inferior border of the disc indicative of cupping. The green lines are the scanned lines of the swept-source OCT images shown in F and G. (**c**) En face view of the optic disc reconstructed from three-dimensional images of swept-source OCT shows two large pits at the upper and lower poles of the optic disc (arrows). These pits have a triangular shape, and their bases are directed to the edge of the optic disc. Multiple pit-like structures are also observed along the temporal margin of the optic disc (arrowheads). (**d**) B-scan swept-source OCT image of the scanned line shown in (**a**) shows a deep pit (arrow) in the inferior pole of the disc extending posteriorly beyond the lamina cribrosa. The inner surface of the lamina is indicated by arrowheads. The nerve fiber overlying the pit is disrupted. (**e**) B-scan swept-source OCT image of the scanned line shown in (**a**) shows an oval-shaped, deeply excavated pit (arrow) at the superior pole of the optic disc with a wide opening. The lamina is dehisced from the peripapillary sclera at the site of the pit, and the nerve fibers overlying the pit are discontinuous at the pit. The depth of the pit from its opening is 1,142 μm. (**f**) B-scan swept-source OCT image across the scanned line shown in (**b**) shows a shallow pit (arrow) along the temporal margin of the optic disc. (**g**) Section adjacent to that shown in (**f**) shows a discontinuity of the lamina (arrow). A hyporeflective space is observed posterior to the defect

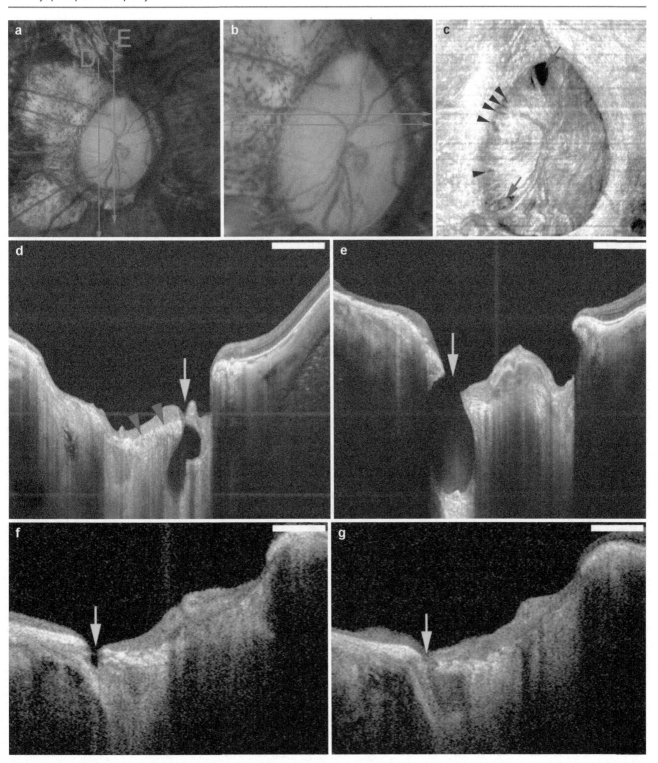

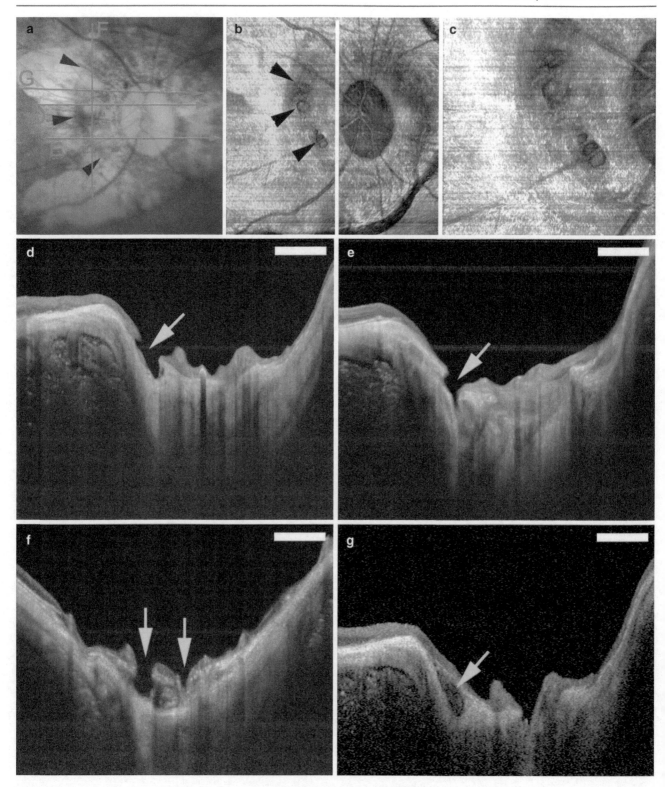

Fig. 25.9 Conus pits present on the temporal side of the scleral ridge in an eye with type IX staphyloma (Curtin's classification). The axial length of this eye was 32.8 mm with an intraocular lens implanted. Bar, 1 mm. (**a**) Photograph of right fundus of 64-year-old woman shows an oval disc with a large annular conus. A scleral ridge is shown by arrowheads. The green lines show the area scanned by swept-source optical coherence tomography (swept-source OCT) for the images shown in d through g. (**b**) En face image of the optic disc area reconstructed from three-dimensional swept-source OCT images shows multiple pits on the slope inside the ridge at approximately same distance from the optic

disc margin (arrowheads). (**c**) Magnified view of (**b**) shows a collection of pits just temporal to the scleral ridge. (**d**) B-scan swept-source OCT image shows that the pit is present on the inner slope of the ridge (arrow). The peripapillary sclera and overlying nerve fiber tissue is discontinuous at the pit site. (**e**) Another pit can be seen inferotemporal to the optic disc. (**f**) Vertical OCT scan temporal to the optic disc shows multiple pits (arrows), and the tissue around the pits appears like a sclera schisis. (**g**) Swept-source OCT section adjacent to the pits shows a hyporeflective space resembling a sclera schisis (arrow). The defects appear to be interruptions in the nerve fiber layer

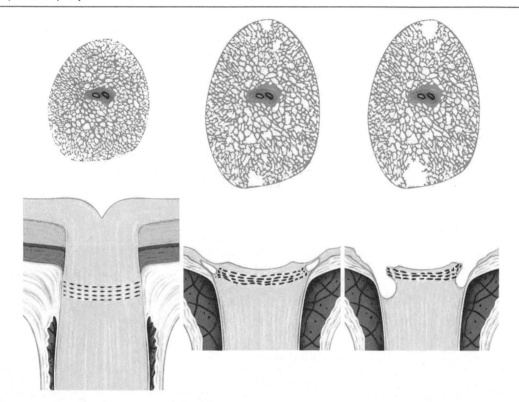

Fig. 25.10 Hypothetical scheme showing how optic disc pits develop. Upper panels show drawings of en face view of the optic disc and peripapillary area. Lower panels show cross-sectional images. The optic disc is first enlarged by a mechanical expansion of the papillary region (upper middle image). Because of the mechanical expansion, the lamina eventually dehisces from the peripapillary sclera particularly at the superior and inferior poles. This stage is observed by swept-source OCT as hyporeflective gap at the junction between the lamina cribrosa and the peripapillary sclera. With further increase of the size of the gap, the nerve fiber overlying this gap may be sunken, displaced, or disrupted, and this stage is observed as optic disc pits by swept-source OCT (lower right image)

conus pits. Schematic illustration of development of optic disc pits and conus pits are shown.

25.9.3 Separation of Circle of Zinn-Haller from the Optic Nerve

Because of its intrascleral location, it had been difficult to observe the circle of Zinn-Haller in situ. Thus, most of the studies of the circle of Zinn-Haller have been done using histological sections [10, 109] or vascular castings with methyl methacrylate [110–112] of human cadaver eyes. Expansion of the circle of Zinn-Haller and associated circulatory alterations were proposed to be a cause peripapillary choroidal atrophy in high myopia by Elmassri in 1971 [113]. Following identification of the circle of Zinn-Haller by angiography and Doppler ultrasonography [114], it was observed using fluorescein fundus angiography and indocyanine green (ICG) angiography in eyes with pathologic myopia with peripapillary atrophy (Fig. 25.11) [115–119]. EDI-OCT showed intrascleral cross sections of the vessels that were identified in ICG angiography images to correspond to the circle of Zinn-Haller. The filling of the circle of Zinn-Haller can be observed by ICG angiography to occur as would be expected by the known anatomy. In highly myopic eyes with large conus, the circle of Zinn-Haller had a horizontally long rhomboid shape, and the entry point of the lateral and/or medial short posterior ciliary arteries was at the most distant point from the optic disc margin. There are no currently known abnormalities correlated with the expansion of the circle of Zinn-Haller at present, but compromise in blood flow to the nerve may be a potential reason for the pallor sometimes seen in the optic disc of highly myopic eyes and also may be a contributing factor for the increased risk of glaucoma in highly myopic eyes. The increased radial distance between the expanded circle of Zinn-Haller in high myopes may decrease the blood perfusion into the nerve and may contribute to optic neuropathies such as glaucoma.

25.10 Eye Shape Abnormalities

Klein and Curtin, in their original description of lacquer cracks, sound a uniform constriction of the central fields, with a greater constriction to blue as compared with red test objects [120]. They thought the field defects were related to staphyloma formation and not the lacquer cracks. They also stated the increased constriction of the blue as compared

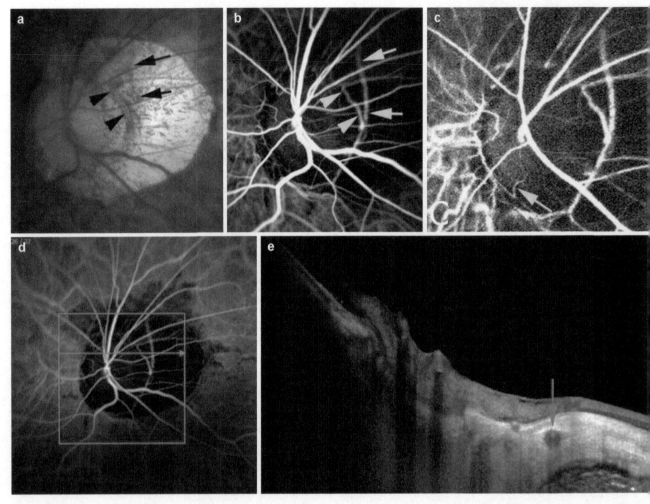

Fig. 25.11 Detection of Zinn-Haller arterial ring in a highly myopic patient by both indocyanine green (ICG) angiography and optical coherence tomography (OCT). (**a**) Fundus photograph of the left eye of a 60-year-old man with a refractive error of −11.25 D (spherical equivalent) and axial length of 28.4 mm. A large temporal conus is seen. Blood vessels suggesting the Zinn-Haller ring are seen within the conus (arrowheads). The vessels originating from short posterior ciliary arteries can also be seen (arrows). (**b**) ICG angiographic finding at 1 min after dye injection showing the Zinn-Haller ring (arrowheads) surrounding the optic disc in almost a circular shape. Vessels originating from the short posterior ciliary arteries can also be seen (arrows). (**c**)

ICG angiographic image 12 s after the ICG injection showing the centripetal branch (arrow) running toward the optic nerve from the Zinn-Haller ring. (**d**) The scanned line by OCT (in bottom-right image) is shown on the ICG angiographic image. (**e**) Horizontal OCT scan shown as green line in bottom-left figure shows a cross section of the vessel of the Zinn-Haller ring as a small hyporeflective circle (arrowhead) near the inner surface of the peripapillary sclera. The vessel connecting the Zinn-Haller ring and retrobulbar SPCA is seen as a hyporeflective circle (arrow), which is wider and is situated deeper than the vessels of the Zinn-Haller ring

with the red test was a sign of retinal dysfunction [120]. Fledelius and Goldschmidt evaluated the eye shape and visual field abnormalities of the eyes with high myopia and found that abnormalities of both eye shape and visual field defects were more common with increasing myopia [121]. Moriyama and colleagues analyzed the shape of the human eye by using 3D MRI (see the "Staphyloma" chapter for details) [122]. The ocular shape as viewed from the inferior aspect of the eye was divided into distinct types, nasally distorted, temporally distorted, cylindrical, and barrel shaped. Statistical comparisons of the eyes showed that significant VF defects were found significantly more fre-

quently in eyes with a temporally distorted shape. The area where the optic nerve is implanted in the globe was at the nasal edge of a temporal protrusion in these eyes. Thus, these eyes showed the presence of a change of the ocular shape just temporal to the optic disc. This corresponded to the stereoscopic fundus observation that eyes with a ridge-like protrusion just temporal to the optic disc tend to have VF defects significantly more frequently than eyes without the temporal ridge [74]. Using swept-source OCT to examine highly myopic eyes, Ohno-Matsui and coworkers analyzed the shape of sclera [123], which could be seen in its entire thickness. The curvatures of the inner scleral surface of highly myopic eyes could be divided into those that were sloped toward the optic nerve, were symmetrical and centered on the fovea, were asymmetrical, and finally were irregular. Patients with irregular curvature were significantly older and had longer axial lengths than those with other curvatures. The subfoveal scleral thickness was significantly thinner in eyes with irregular curvature than the eyes with other curvatures. Myopic fundus lesions as well as visual field defects were present significantly more frequently in the eyes with irregular curvature. By comparison between OCT images and 3D MRI images, all of the eyes with temporally distorted shape by 3D MRI had irregular curvature by swept-source OCT. Combining these studies, the eye shape shown as temporally dislocated type by 3D MRI, irregular curvature by swept-source OCT, and steeply curved staphyloma visualized by stereoscopic fundus observation may be the same. While these changes in eye shape may induce local refractive variations, the same distortions also have the potential to put abnormal stresses on the retinal nerve fiber layer, and thus there could be a neurologic component. Future research will aim to clarify these questions. If eyes with these characteristics are found to have visual field defects, the likelihood is that visual field defects are due to local effects and not any type of optic neuropathy.

25.11 Myopic Optic Neuropathy

Since its earliest description, there has been controversy about the pathophysiology of glaucoma. Intraocular pressure may cause stress to the nerve fibers, particularly with elevated pressure. Intraocular pressure also appears to participate in remodeling of tissues such as the lamina cribrosa, which may compound the mechanical stress on nerve fibers. Another major group of hypotheses for glaucoma posits abnormalities in tissue perfusion as a cause of nerve fiber loss. Glaucoma is a neurodegenerative disease associated with specific ocular findings. Cupping in emmetropic eyes in relation to glaucoma is the result of loss of the nerve fibers and associated glial cells in the optic nerve head and to deformation of the lamina [124]. In pathologic myopia, the optic nerve head can show expansion, tilting, torsion, and effacement. All of these factors may put mechanical stress on the nerve fibers. Expansion of the circle of Zinn-Haller may also affect the perfusion into the nerve tissue. Pathologic myopes may develop an optic neuropathy that results in saucerization of the disc and visual field defects that resemble those seen in emmetropes with glaucoma. In a series of 155 patients in Korea [125] with normal tension glaucoma and asymmetric field loss, the eye with higher pressure in emmetropes showed more visual field loss. In myopes, refractive error, ovality index of the optic disc, and peripapillary atrophy were the predictors of visual field loss. This suggests there may be different pathophysiological reasons for visual field loss in emmetropes versus myopes in the eyes that do not demonstrate overtly elevated intraocular pressure, but both are the result of loss of nerve fibers. Is the diagnosis of glaucoma appropriate for all of these cases?

When evaluating a patient who may have glaucoma, one valuable test is visual field testing. In a study of 1434 visual field tests of 487 high myopes from a myopia registry, "arcuate-like" scotomata were found in 16.1%, advanced arcuate scotomata in 3.4%, nasal step in 5.1%, and enlarged blind spots in 25.6% [126]. Another common test is measuring the thickness of the retinal nerve fiber layer. This is often done in the parapapillary region with a circular scan. The distortion in pathologically myopic eyes places this circle at varying distances from the border of the optic nerve as compared with emmetropes. Therefore, the nomograms derived for emmetropic eyes does not apply to highly myopic eyes. A useful test in evaluating for possible glaucoma is the ganglion cell volume. This involves performing a volume scan of the macula followed by segmentation of the ganglion cell layer. This second step presents a challenge in highly myopic eyes. The distortion caused by staphylomata can lead to incorrect segmentation and image folding. Many image segmentation algorithms do not work if the eye has patchy atrophy. The lack of expected retinal layers obfuscates correct recognition of the remaining layers, yielding an incorrect result.

While tests used to diagnose glaucoma have a large variability, this is particularly true in pathologic myopia. A practical response is to examine repeated testing for signs of nerve fiber, ganglion cell, or visual field loss. If this can be demonstrated with certainty, the patient is often said to have glaucoma. This axiomatically leads to the only treatment for glaucoma, reduction in intraocular pressure. It may be possible that the numerous alterations in pathologic myopia have an unfavorable impact on retinal nerve fiber health by mechanisms that may overlap, but not be entirely the same as in "glaucoma," an admittedly nebulously defined disease. This second condition could be labeled myopic optic neuropathy. Under current levels of technology and understanding, this myopic optic neuropathy would be treated with reduction of intraocular pressure, even though we do not have good efficacy data.

25.12 The Need for Future Research

Patients with high myopia may have visual field defects, but how certain are we these defects are due specifically to the nerve and not to other coexistent abnormalities? We know that glaucoma is more common in eyes with myopia; it may be more difficult to diagnose glaucoma, particularly in highly myopic eyes; and there may be changes in high myopia that emulate those occurring in glaucoma that may not, strictly speaking, be true glaucoma. There are undoubtedly altered mechanical stress on the nerve fibers and potential compromises in prelaminar perfusion. These considerations support the general idea that there may be types of optic neuropathy related to or accentuated by high myopia. There are many confounding factors that have not been fully evaluated. The interactions between expansion of the SAS, the myopic changes induced in the circle of Zinn-Haller, thinning sclera, and translaminar pressure are all variables that need closer examination. Many if not most of the visual field abnormalities also are associated with shape changes in the eye that directly or indirectly may cause decreased visual field performance independent of actual optic nerve abnormalities. The eye in myopia is longer, and as a consequence any test object of a given size will produce a larger image size on the retina, even if focused correctly. Since many eyes with abnormal visual fields also have abnormal shapes, there is a high likelihood of regionally varying focus. There is a complex aberration induced not necessarily by the dioptric mechanism of the eye, but by fluctuating deviations in distance of the retina from the image plane. This same expansion has the potential to cause regional variations in photoreceptor packing densities, as has been determined with adaptive optics imaging [127, 128]. The peripheral visual acuity is decreased in the periphery in myopes [129]. Deviation of the peripheral refraction from the measured central refractive error is much more pronounced in eyes with high myopia as compared with emmetropic eyes [130], and these alterations in peripheral refraction have potential to change the visual field test results. Coexistent with stretching of the wall of the eye is thinning of the choroid. Trying to determine the root cause of visual field defects in high myopia represents a significant challenge because of the many simultaneously changing variables, some known, some unknown, which coexist with any observed variable. Control, or at least measurement, of these simultaneously changing variables will be the only way to fully evaluate the contributions each of them make to visual field abnormalities in high myopia.

References

1. Stuermer CA, Bastmeyer M. The retinal axon's pathfinding to the optic disk. Prog Neurobiol. 2000;62(2):197–214.
2. Wang J, Liu G, Wang D, Yuan G, Hou Y, Wang J. The embryonic development of the human lamina cribrosa. Chin Med J. 1997;110(12):946–9.
3. Radius RL, Gonzales M. Anatomy of the lamina cribrosa in human eyes. Arch Ophthalmol. 1981;99(12):2159–62.
4. Quigley HA, Addicks EM. Regional differences in the structure of the lamina cribrosa and their relation to glaucomatous optic nerve damage. Arch Ophthalmol. 1981;99(1):137–43.
5. Park SC, Kiumehr S, Teng CC, Tello C, Liebmann JM, Ritch R. Horizontal central ridge of the lamina cribrosa and regional differences in laminar insertion in healthy subjects. Invest Ophthalmol Vis Sci. 2012;53(3):1610–6.
6. Zinn IG. Descripto Anatomica Oculi Humani. 1st ed. Gottingen: Abrami Vandenhoeck; 1755. p. 216–7.
7. Hayreh SS. Blood supply of the optic nerve head and its role in optic atrophy, glaucoma, and oedema of the optic disc. Br J Ophthalmol. 1969;53(11):721–48.
8. Lieberman MF, Maumenee AE, Green WR. Histologic studies of the vasculature of the anterior optic nerve. Am J Ophthalmol. 1976;82:405.
9. Jonas JB, Jonas SB. Histomorphometry of the circular peripapillary arterial ring of Zinn-Haller in normal eyes and eyes with secondary angle-closure glaucoma. Acta Ophthalmol. 2010;88(8):e317–22.
10. Ko MK, Kim DS, Ahn YK. Morphological variations of the peripapillary circle of Zinn-Haller by flat section. Br J Ophthalmol. 1999;83(7):862–6.
11. Zhao Y, Li F. Microangioarchitecture of the optic papilla. Jap J Ophthalmol. 1987;31:147–59.
12. Ruskell G. Blood flow in the Zinn-Haller circle. Br J Ophthalmol. 1998;82(12):1351.
13. Jonas JB, Gusek GC, Naumann GO. Optic disc, cup and neuroretinal rim size, configuration and correlations in normal eyes. Invest Ophthalmol Vis Sci. 1988;29(7):1151–8.
14. Quigley HA, Brown AE, Morrison JD, Drance SM. The size and shape of the optic disc in normal human eyes. Arch Ophthalmol. 1990;108(1):51–7.
15. Reis AS, Sharpe GP, Yang H, et al. Optic disc margin anatomy in patients with glaucoma and normal controls with spectral domain optical coherence tomography. Ophthalmology. 2012;119(4):738–47.
16. Ramrattan RS, Wolfs RC, Jonas JB, Hofman A, de Jong PT. Determinants of optic disc characteristics in a general population: the Rotterdam Study. Ophthalmology. 1999;106(8):1588–96.
17. Anderson DR. Ultrastructure of human and monkey lamina cribrosa and optic nerve head. Arch Ophthalmol. 1969;82(6):800–14.
18. Quigley HA, Coleman AL, Dorman-Pease ME. Larger optic nerve heads have more nerve fibers in normal monkey eyes. Arch Ophthalmol. 1991;109(10):1441–3.
19. Jonas JB, Schmidt AM, Müller-Bergh JA, Schlötzer-Schrehardt UM, Naumann GO. Human optic nerve fiber count and optic disc size. Invest Ophthalmol Vis Sci. 1992;33(6):2012–8.
20. Brodsky MC. Congenital Optic Disc Anomalies in Pediatric Neuro-Ophthalmology. New York: Springer; 2010. p. 59–67.
21. Quigley HA, Green WR. The histology of human glaucoma cupping and optic nerve damage: clinicopathologic correlation in 21 eyes. Ophthalmology. 1979;86:1803–30.
22. Quigley HA, Addicks EM, Green WR, et al. Optic nerve damage in human glaucoma. II. The site of injury and susceptibility to damage. Arch Ophthalmol. 1981;99:635–49.
23. Quigley HA, Hohman RM, Addicks EM, Massof RW, Green WR. Morphologic changes in the lamina cribrosa correlated with neural loss in open-angle glaucoma. Am J Ophthalmol. 1983;95(5):673–91.
24. Hernandez MR. Ultrastructural immunocytochemical analysis of elastin in the human lamina cribrosa. Changes in elastic fibers in primary open-angle glaucoma. Invest Ophthalmol Vis Sci. 1992;33(10):2891–903.
25. Fukuchi T, Sawaguchi S, Hara H, Shirakashi M, Iwata K. Extracellular matrix changes of the optic nerve lamina cribrosa in monkey eyes with experimentally chronic glaucoma. Graefes Arch Clin Exp Ophthalmol. 1992;230(5):421–7.
26. Fukuchi T, Sawaguchi S, Yue BY, Iwata K, Hara H, Kaiya T. Sulfated proteoglycans in the lamina cribrosa of normal mon-

key eyes and monkey eyes with laser-induced glaucoma. Exp Eye Res. 1994;58(2):231–43.

27. Hernandez MR, Yang J, Ye H. Activation of elastin mRNA expression in human optic nerve heads with primary open-angle glaucoma. J Glaucoma. 1994;3(3):214–25.

28. Park HY, Jeon SH, Park CK. Enhanced depth imaging detects lamina cribrosa thickness differences in normal tension glaucoma and primary open-angle glaucoma. Ophthalmology. 2012;119(1):10–20.

29. Quigley HA, Dorman-Pease ME, Brown AE. Quantitative study of collagen and elastin of the optic nerve head and sclera in human and experimental monkey glaucoma. Curr Eye Res. 1991;10(9):877–88.

30. Burgoyne CF, Downs JC, Bellezza AJ, et al. Three-dimensional reconstruction of normal and early glaucoma monkey optic nerve head connective tissues. Invest Ophthalmol Vis Sci. 2004;45:4388–99.

31. Downs JC, Yang H, Girkin C, et al. Three Dimensional histomorphometry of the normal and early glaucomatous monkey optic nerve head: neural canal and subarachnoid space architecture. Invest Ophthalmol Vis Sci. 2007;48:3195–208.

32. Yang H, Downs JC, Girkin C, et al. 3-D Histomorphometry of the normal and early glaucomatous monkey optic nerve head: lamina cribrosa and peripapillary scleral position and thickness. Invest Ophthalmol Vis Sci. 2007;48:4597–607.

33. Yang H, Downs JC, Bellezza AJ, et al. 3-D Histomorphometry of the normal and early glaucomatous monkey optic nerve head: prelaminar neural tissues and cupping. Invest Ophthalmol Vis Sci. 2007;48:5068–84.

34. Crawford Downs J, Roberts MD, Sigal IA. Glaucomatous cupping of the lamina cribrosa: a review of the evidence for active progressive remodeling as a mechanism. Exp Eye Res. 2011;93(2):133–40.

35. Mochizuki H, Lesley AG, Brandt JD. Shrinkage of the scleral canal during cupping reversal in children. Ophthalmology. 2011;118(10):2008–13.

36. Lee EJ, Kim TW, Weinreb RN. Reversal of lamina cribrosa displacement and thickness after trabeculectomy in glaucoma. Ophthalmology. 2012;119(7):1359–66.

37. Weiss AH. Unilateral high myopia: optical components, associated factors, and visual outcomes. Br J Ophthalmol. 2003;87(8):1025–31.

38. Weiss AH, Ross EA. Axial myopia in eyes with optic nerve hypoplasia. Graefes Arch Clin Exp Ophthalmol. 1992;230(4):372–7.

39. Fledelius HC, Goldschmidt E. Optic disc appearance and retinal temporal vessel arcade geometry in high myopia, as based on follow-up data over 38 years. Acta Ophthalmol. 2010;88(5):514–20.

40. Vongphanit J, Mitchell P, Wang JJ. Population prevalence of tilted optic disks and the relationship of this sign to refractive error. Am J Ophthalmol. 2002;133(5):679–85.

41. You QS, Xu L, Jonas JB. Tilted optic discs: the Beijing eye study. Eye (Lond). 2008;22(5):728–9.

42. How AC, Tan GS, Chan YH, Wong TT, Seah SK, Foster PJ, Aung T. Population prevalence of tilted and torted optic discs among an adult Chinese population in Singapore: the Tanjong Pagar study. Arch Ophthalmol. 2009;127(7):894–9.

43. Witmer MT, Margo CE, Drucker M. Tilted optic disks. Surv Ophthalmol. 2010;55(5):403–28.

44. Jonas JB, Gusek GC, Naumann GO. Optic disk morphometry in high myopia. Graefes Arch Clin Exp Ophthalmol. 1988;226(6):587–90.

45. Qiu M, Wang SY, Singh K, Lin SC. Association between myopia and glaucoma in the United States population. Invest Ophthalmol Vis Sci. 2013;54(1):830–5.

46. Dai Y, Jonas JB, Huang H, Wang M, Sun X. Microstructure of parapapillary atrophy: beta zone and gamma zone. Invest Ophthalmol Vis Sci. 2013;54(3):2013–8.

47. Suh MH, Na JH, Zangwill LM, et al. Deep-layer microvasculature dropout in preperimetric glaucoma patients. J Glaucoma. 2020;29(6):423–8.

48. Rudnicka AR, Edgar DF. Automated static perimetry in myopes with peripapillary crescents–part I. Ophthalmic Physiol Opt. 1995;15(5):409–12.

49. Rudnicka AR, Edgar DF. Automated static perimetry in myopes with peripapillary crescents–part II. Ophthalmic Physiol Opt. 1996;16(5):416–29.

50. Teng CC, De Moraes CG, Prata TS, Tello C, Ritch R, Liebmann JM. Beta-zone parapapillary atrophy and the velocity of glaucoma progression. Ophthalmology. 2010;117(5):909–15.

51. Jonas JB, Fernández MC, Naumann GO. Glaucomatous parapapillary atrophy. Occurrence and correlations. Arch Ophthalmol. 1992;110(2):214–22.

52. Tay E, Seah SK, Chan SP, Lim AT, Chew SJ, Foster PJ, Aung T. Optic disk ovality as an index of tilt and its relationship to myopia and perimetry. Am J Ophthalmol. 2005;139(2):247–52.

53. Samarawickrama C, Pai A, Tariq Y, Healey PR, Wong TY, Mitchell P. Characteristics and appearance of the normal optic nerve head in 6-year-old children. Br J Ophthalmol. 2012;96(1):68–72.

54. Samarawickrama C, Mitchell P, Tong L, et al. Myopia-related optic disc and retinal changes in adolescent children from Singapore. Ophthalmology. 2011;118(10):2050–7.

55. Kim TW, Kim M, Weinreb RN, Woo SJ, Park KH, Hwang JM. Optic disc change with incipient myopia of childhood. Ophthalmology. 2012;119(1):21–6.e1–3.

56. Jaeger E. Beiträge zur Pathologie des Auges 1870 Wien, Kaiserlich-Königliche Hof- und Staatsdruckerei, p202.

57. Heine L. Beiträge zur Anatomie des myopischen Auges. Arch f Augenheilk. 1899;36:277–90.

58. Siegrist A. Refraktion und akkomodation des menschlichen auges. Berlin, J. Springer 1925, p 111.

59. Collins ET, Mayou MS. An International System of Ophthalmic Practice. Pathology and Bacteriology. Philadelphia: P. Blakiston's Sone and Co; 1912. p. 505–7.

60. Vongphanit J, Mitchell P, Wang JJ. Prevalence and progression of myopic retinopathy in an older population. Ophthalmology. 2002;109(4):704–11.

61. Young SE, Walsh FB, Knox DL. The tilted disk syndrome. Am J Ophthalmol. 1976;82(1):16–23.

62. Caccamise WC. Situs inversus of the optic disc with inferior conus and variable myopia: a case report. Am J Ophthalmol. 1954;38(6):854–6.

63. Fuchs E. Uber den anatomischen Befund einiger angeborener Anomalien der Netzhaut und des Sehnerven. v. Graefes Arch. Ophthal. 1917;93:1–48.

64. Schmidt T. Perimetrie relativer Skotome. Ophthalmologica. 1955;129:303–15.

65. Odland M. Bitemporal defects of the visual fields due to anomalies of the optic discs. Acta Neurol Scand. 1967;43(5):630–9.

66. Traquair HM. Choroidal changes in myopia. In: Scott GI, editor. Traquair's clinical perimetry. 7th ed. London: Kimpton; 1957. p. 105–6.

67. Vuori ML, Mäntyjärvi M. Tilted disc syndrome may mimic false visual field deterioration. Acta Ophthalmol. 2008;86(6):622–5.

68. Hamada T, Tsukada T, Hirose T. Clinical and electrophysiological features of tilted disc syndrome. Jpn J Ophthalmol. 1987;31(2):265–73.

69. Feigl B, Zele AJ. Macular function in tilted disc syndrome. Doc Ophthalmol. 2010;120(2):201–3.

70. Giuffrè G, Anastasi M. Electrofunctional features of the tilted disc syndrome. Doc Ophthalmol. 1986;62(3):223–30.

71. Moschos MM, Triglianos A, Rotsos T, Papadimitriou S, Margetis I, Minogiannis P, Moschos M. Tilted disc syndrome: an OCT and mfERG study. Doc Ophthalmol. 2009;119(1):23–8.

72. Carl Stellwag von Carion. Treatise on the diseases of the eye, including the anatomy of the organ. [Translated by Roosa J, Bull CS, Hackley CE.] New York: William Wood and Co. 1873, pp 354–355.

73. Ohno-Matsui K, Shimada N, Yasuzumi K, Hayashi K, Yoshida T, Kojima A, Moriyama M, Tokoro T. Long-term development of significant visual field defects in highly myopic eyes. Am J Ophthalmol. 2011;152(2):256–265.e1.

74. Akagi T, Hangai M, Kimura Y, Ikeda HO, Nonaka A, Matsumoto A, Akiba M, Yoshimura N. Peripapillary scleral deformation and retinal nerve fiber damage in high myopia assessed with swept-source optical coherence tomography. Am J Ophthalmol. 2013;155(5):927–36.

75. Hwang YH, Yoo C, Kim YY. Myopic optic disc tilt and the characteristics of peripapillary retinal nerve fiber layer thickness measured by spectral-domain optical coherence tomography. J Glaucoma. 2012;21(4):260–5.

76. Hwang YH, Yoo C, Kim YY. Characteristics of peripapillary retinal nerve fiber layer thickness in eyes with myopic optic disc tilt and rotation. J Glaucoma. 2012;21(6):394–400.

77. Park HY, Lee K, Park CK. Optic disc torsion direction predicts the location of glaucomatous damage in normal-tension glaucoma patients with myopia. Ophthalmology. 2012;119(9):1844–51.

78. Lee KS, Lee JR, Kook MS. Optic disc torsion presenting as unilateral glaucomatous-appearing visual field defect in young myopic Korean eyes. Ophthalmology. 2014;121(5):1013–9.

79. Arvind H, George R, Raju P, Ve RS, Mani B, Kannan P, Vijaya L. Neural rim characteristics of healthy South Indians: the Chennai Glaucoma Study. Invest Ophthalmol Vis Sci. 2008;49(8):3457–64.

80. Doshi A, Kreidl KO, Lombardi L, Sakamoto DK, Singh K. Nonprogressive glaucomatous cupping and visual field abnormalities in young Chinese males. Ophthalmology. 2007;114(3):472–9.

81. Yoon JY, Sung KR, Yun SC, et al. Progressive optic disc tilt in young myopic glaucomatous eyes. Korean J Ophthalmol. 2019;33(6):520–7.

82. Britton RJ, Drance SM, Schulzer M, Douglas GR, Mawson DK. The area of the neuroretinal rim of the optic nerve in normal eyes. Am J Ophthalmol. 1987;103(4):497–504.

83. Varma R, Tielsch JM, Quigley HA, Hilton SC, Katz J, Spaeth GL, Sommer A. Race-, age-, gender-, and refractive error-related differences in the normal optic disc. Arch Ophthalmol. 1994;112(8):1068–76.

84. Rudnicka AR, Frost C, Owen CG, Edgar DF. Nonlinear behavior of certain optic nerve head parameters and their determinants in normal subjects. Ophthalmology. 2001;108(12):2358–68.

85. Wang Y, Xu L, Zhang L, Yang H, Ma Y, Jonas JB. Optic disc size in a population based study in northern China: the Beijing Eye Study. Br J Ophthalmol. 2006;90(3):353–6.

86. Xu L, Li Y, Wang S, Wang Y, Wang Y, Jonas JB. Characteristics of highly myopic eyes: the Beijing Eye Study. Ophthalmology. 2007;114(1):121–6.

87. Samarawickrama C, Wang XY, Huynh SC, Burlutsky G, Stapleton F, Mitchell P. Effects of refraction and axial length on childhood optic disk parameters measured by optical coherence tomography. Am J Ophthalmol. 2007;144(3):459–61.

88. Nangia V, Matin A, Bhojwani K, Kulkarni M, Yadav M, Jonas JB. Optic disc size in a population-based study in central India: the Central India Eye and Medical Study (CIEMS). Acta Ophthalmol. 2008;86(1):103–4.

89. Fledelius HC. Optic disc size: are methodological factors taken into account? Acta Ophthalmol. 2008;86(7):813–4.

90. Cheung CY, Chen D, Wong TY, Tham YC, Wu R, Zheng Y, Cheng CY, Saw SM, Baskaran M, Leung CK, Aung T. Determinants of quantitative optic nerve measurements using spectral domain optical coherence tomography in a population-based sample of non-glaucomatous subjects. Invest Ophthalmol Vis Sci. 2011;52(13):9629–35.

91. Knight OJ, Girkin CA, Budenz DL, Durbin MK, Feuer WJ, Cirrus OCT Normative Database Study Group. Effect of race, age, and axial length on optic nerve head parameters and retinal nerve fiber layer thickness measured by Cirrus HD-OCT. Arch Ophthalmol. 2012;130(3):312–8.

92. Kim NR, Lee ES, Seong GJ, Kang SY, Kim JH, Hong S, Kim CY. Comparing the ganglion cell complex and retinal nerve fibre layer measurements by Fourier domain OCT to detect glaucoma in high myopia. Br J Ophthalmol. 2011;95(8):1115–21.

93. Shoji T, Nagaoka Y, Sato H, Chihara E. Impact of high myopia on the performance of SD-OCT parameters to detect glaucoma. Graefes Arch Clin Exp Ophthalmol. 2012;250(12):1843–9.

94. Zhao Z, Jiang C. Effect of myopia on ganglion cell complex and peripapillary retinal nerve fibre layer measurements: a Fourier domain optical coherence tomography study of young Chinese persons. Clin Exp Ophthalmol. 2013;41(6):561–6. https://doi.org/10.1111/ceo.12045.

95. Donders FC. Die Anomalien der Refraction und Accommodation des Auges. Wein: Wilhelm Braumuller; 1866. p. 316.

96. Landolt E. Refraction and Accommodation of the Eye and their anomalies. [Translated by Culver CM]. Philadelphia: J. B. Lippincott Company. 1886; 432.

97. De Wecker L. Ocular Therapeutics. [Translated by Forbes L]. London, Smith Elder & Co. 1879, pp 413, 419.

98. Terrien F. Contribution a l'anatomie de loeil myope. Arch Ophtalmol. 1906:737–61.

99. Parsons JH. The pathology of the eye, vol. III. New York: G.P. Putnam's Sons; 1906.

100. Schnabel I (translated by Reed CH). The anatomy of staphyloma posticum, and the relationship of the condition to myopia. In, Norris WF, Oliver CA System of Diseases of the Eye. Part III. Local Diseases, Glaucoma, Wounds and Injuries, Operations. Philadelphia, J. B. Lippincott, 1900.

101. Okisaka S. Myopia. Tokyo: Kanehara Shuppan; 1987. p. 110–21.

102. Jonas JB, Berenshtein E, Holbach L. Lamina cribrosa thickness and spatial relationships between intraocular space and cerebrospinal fluid space in highly myopic eyes. Invest Ophthalmol Vis Sci. 2004;45:2660–5.

103. Jonas JB, Jonas SB, Jonas RA, Holbach L, Dai Y, Sun X, Panda-Jonas S. Parapapillary atrophy: histological gamma zone and delta zone. PLoS One. 2012;7(10):e47237. https://doi.org/10.1371/journal.pone.0047237.

104. Park SC, De Moraes CG, Teng CC, et al. Enhanced depth imaging optical coherence tomography of deep optic nerve complex structures in glaucoma. Ophthalmology. 2012;119:3–9.

105. Ohno-Matsui K, Akiba M, Moriyama M, et al. Imaging the retrobulbar subarachnoid space around the optic nerve by swept source optical coherence tomography in eyes with pathologic myopia. Invest Ophthalmol Vis Sci. 2011;52:9644–50.

106. Marcus Gunn R. Certain affections of the optic nerve. In, Ophthalmology. Essays, Abstracts and Reviews. Volume III. 1907(4): 253–269.

107. Ohno-Matsui K, Akiba M, Moriyama M, et al. Acquired optic nerve and peripapillary pits in pathologic myopia. Ophthalmology. 2012;119(8):1685–92.

108. Kiumehr S, Park SC, Syril D, et al. In vivo evaluation of focal lamina cribrosa defects in glaucoma. Arch Ophthalmol. 2012;130(5):552–9.

109. Jonas JB, Jonas SB. Histomorphometry of the circular peripapillary arterial ring of Zinn-Haller in normal eyes and eyes

with secondary angle-closure glaucoma. Acta Ophthalmol. 2010;88(8):1755–3768.
110. Olver JM, Spalton DJ, McCartney AC. Quantitative morphology of human retrolaminar optic nerve vasculature. Invest Ophthalmol Vis Sci. 1994;35(11):3858–66.
111. Olver JM, Spalton DJ, McCartney AC. Microvascular study of the retrolaminar optic nerve in man: the possible significance in anterior ischaemic optic neuropathy. Eye. 1990;4(Pt 1):7–24.
112. Morrison JC, Johnson EC, Cepurna WO, Funk RH. Microvasculature of the rat optic nerve head. Invest Ophthalmol Vis Sci. 1999;40(8):1702–9.
113. Elmassri A. Ophthalmoscopic appearances after injury to the circle of Zinn. Br J Ophthalmol. 1971;55(1):12–8.
114. Park KH, Tomita G, Onda E, Kitazawa Y, Cioffi GA. In vivo detection of perineural circular arterial anastomosis (circle of Zinn-Haller) in a patient with large peripapillary chorioretinal atrophy. Am J Ophthalmol. 1996;122(6):905–7.
115. Ohno-Matsui K, Morishima N, Ito M, et al. Indocyanine green angiography of retrobulbar vascular structures in severe myopia. Am J Ophthalmol. 1997;123(4):494–505.
116. Hollo G. Peripapillary circle of Zinn-Haller revealed by fundus fluorescein angiography. Br J Ophthalmol. 1998;82(3):332–3.
117. Ko MK, Kim DS, Ahn YK. Peripapillary circle of Zinn-Haller revealed by fundus fluorescein angiography. Br J Ophthalmol. 1997;81(8):663–7.
118. Ohno-Matsui K, Futagami S, Yamashita S, Tokoro T. Zinn-Haller arterial ring observed by ICG angiography in high myopia. Br J Ophthalmol. 1998;82(12):1357–62.
119. Yasuzumi K, Ohno-Matsui K, Yoshida T, et al. Peripapillary crescent enlargement in highly myopic eyes evaluated by fluorescein and indocyanine green angiography. Br J Ophthalmol. 2003;87(9):1088–90.
120. Klein RM, Curtin BJ. Lacquer crack lesions in pathologic myopia. Am J Ophthalmol. 1975;79(3):386–92.

121. Fledelius HC, Goldschmidt E. Eye shape and peripheral visual field recording in high myopia at approximately 54 years of age, as based on ultrasonography and Goldmann kinetic perimetry. Acta Ophthalmol. 2010;88(5):521–6.
122. Moriyama M, Ohno-Matsui K, Hayashi K, et al. Topographical analyses of shape of eyes with pathologic myopia by high resolution three dimensional magnetic resonance imaging. Ophthalmology. 2011;118(8):1626–37.
123. Ohno-Matsui K, Akiba M, Modegi T, et al. Association between shape of sclera and myopic retinochoroidal lesions in patients with pathologic myopia. Invest Ophthalmol Vis Sci. 2012;9:9.
124. Burgoyne C. The morphological difference between glaucoma and other optic neuropathies. J Neuroophthalmol. 2015;35 Suppl 1(0 1):S8–S21.
125. Lee EJ, Han JC, Kee C. Intereye comparison of ocular factors in normal tension glaucoma with asymmetric visual field loss in Korean population. PLoS One. 2017;12(10):e0186236.
126. Ding X, Chang RT, Guo X, et al. Visual field defect classification in the Zhongshan Ophthalmic Center-Brien Holden Vision Institute High Myopia Registry Study. Br J Ophthalmol. 2016;100(12):1697–702.
127. Kitaguchi Y, Bessho K, Yamaguchi T, et al. In vivo measurements of cone photoreceptor spacing in myopic eyes from images obtained by an adaptive optics fundus camera. Jpn J Ophthalmol. 2007;51:456–61.
128. Chui TY, Song H, Burns SA. Individual variations in human cone photoreceptor packing density: variations with refractive error. Invest Ophthalmol Vis Sci. 2008;49:4679–87.
129. Chui TY, Yap MK, Chan HH, Thibos LN. Retinal stretching limits peripheral visual acuity in myopia. Vis Res. 2005;45:593–605.
130. Atchison DA, Pritchard N, Schmid KL. Peripheral refraction along the horizontal and vertical visual fields in myopia. Vis Res. 2006;46(8–9):1450–8.

Special Considerations for Cataract Surgery in the Face of Pathologic Myopia

26

Jack M. Dodick and Jonathan B. Kahn

26.1 Introduction

Modern-day, small-incision cataract surgery by phacoemulsification enjoys a high success rate and safety profile. Eyes with axial myopia present unique considerations in cataract surgery that require careful planning and management by the cataract surgeon. All aspects of the cataract surgery require special attention, including preoperative planning and risk assessment, surgical technique, and postoperative care.

26.2 Epidemiology

Population-based studies have attempted to generate a link associating myopia and cataract. The cross-sectional association between myopia and nuclear cataract was supported by data from the Beaver Dam Eye Study. In that study, myopia was not directly linked to cataract formation but rather, to incident cataract surgery (Odds Ratio, OR 1.99) [1]. The Blue Mountains Eye Study found a statistically significant association between high myopia (-6.0 D or less) and incident nuclear cataract (OR 3.3). Moderate and high myopia (-3.5 D or less) was also associated with posterior subcapsular cataract (OR 4.4). The high myopia group had the highest incidence of cataract surgery (OR 3.4) among all groups. Furthermore, it was found that early-onset myopia (before age 20 years) was a strong and independent risk factor for posterior subcapsular cataract. A dose response relationship was suggested between levels of myopia and posterior subcapsular cataract. High myopia was associated with all types of cataract [2, 3].

26.3 Pathogenesis

Biochemical studies on antioxidants and free radicals have demonstrated that retinal lipid peroxidation may play a key role in cataractogenesis. Higher concentrations of malondialdehyde, a final product of the lipid peroxidation process, have been observed in diabetic and myopic cataracts [4, 5]. In a rabbit model, injection of peroxidative products in the vitreous resulted in posterior subcapsular cataract formation [6]. A follow-up study showed that reduced levels of the antioxidant glutathione and higher levels of oxidized glutathione have been found in myopic cataracts as compared to senile cataracts [7], supporting the role of antioxidants in myopic cataract formation.

26.4 Preoperative Planning

The cataract surgeon must perform a careful preoperative assessment, often in conjunction with the vitreoretinal specialist. The preoperative evaluation should be meticulous and methodical to ensure completeness and appropriate preparedness.

The first step in the preoperative evaluation is a careful ophthalmic history. Previous surgery of either eye should be identified. Patients may have undergone cataract surgery in the fellow eye, in which case any surgical or postoperative complications, such as retinal detachment or refractive surprise, should be discovered. Appropriate precautions or modifications in calculations and technique could then be undertaken to reduce the chances of future surgical complications.

Patients who have had refractive surgery in one or both eyes should describe their previous refractive status and current refractive goals. For example, some patients may strongly prefer monovision or wish to avoid it completely, depending on previous experiences and the outcomes of refractive surgery. Other patients may report a history of refractive re-treatments, which are not uncommon in high

J. M. Dodick (✉) · J. B. Kahn
Department of Ophthalmology, NYU Langone Health, New York, NY, USA

© Springer Nature Switzerland AG 2021
R. F. Spaide et al. (eds.), *Pathologic Myopia*, https://doi.org/10.1007/978-3-030-74334-5_26

myopia. The full refractive records must be sought and evaluated prior to cataract surgery, especially to aid in intraocular lens calculations [8].

It must also be discerned if the patient has undergone previous retinal surgery for retinal breaks, tears, or detachments of one or both eyes, as this may portend an increased risk of future retinal detachments after cataract surgery [9]. Patients should specifically be asked about prior laser treatments for retinal breaks or tears, as many patients may not consider laser treatments as prior surgery.

Any history of refractive amblyopia or patching should also be uncovered, as amblyopia may be common in eyes with high myopia and/or astigmatism [10] and may ultimately limit the best-corrected postoperative visual acuity.

Next, the surgeon must perform a careful refraction. This will identify the extent of refractive myopia, astigmatism, and anisometropia, if present. The lenticular status and refraction of the fellow eye must be considered. Younger patients with rapidly progressing myopia and astigmatism should be carefully evaluated for keratoconus and post-refractive ectasia, as these patients may require medical or surgical treatment, such as collagen cross-linking, prior to undertaking cataract surgery [11].

A comprehensive examination by biomicroscopy, including a detailed dilated fundus examination, is performed. Often, the cataract surgeon will perform a careful retinal examination in conjunction with a vitreoretinal specialist to thoroughly search for peripheral breaks, holes, or weaknesses. Myopic maculopathy may also be present that could ultimately limit visual outcomes from surgery. These retinal disorders must be treated and stabilized prior to undertaking cataract surgery so as to reduce the risk of intraoperative or

postoperative retinal detachment and to maximize postoperative visual potential [12, 13].

The surgeon must then have a detailed discussion with the patient about the purpose, expectations, and risks of surgery and obtain appropriate informed consent. In particular, the patient must be educated about the increased risks of retinal detachment and refractive surprise in cataract surgery of highly myopic eyes. Retinal detachment rates in uncomplicated eyes with high myopia have been recently reported as 0.8% [12], an increased risk as compared to eyes without axial myopia (0.4%) [13].

26.4.1 Axial Length and Keratometry

Preoperative planning also includes careful measurement of corneal keratometry as well as axial length. Assessment of axial length may be particularly difficult in eyes with pathologic myopia, as there may be posterior staphylomata that result in artificially high axial length measurements [14] (see Fig. 26.1). In particular, eyes with tilted discs and/or staphyloma edges that pass across the fovea can have poor quality and inaccurate A-scan readings. It has been reported that posterior staphylomata may be found in 70% of eyes with axial lengths of greater than 33.5 mm, but in reality, nearly all eyes with pathologic myopia have some degree of posterior staphylomata [15].

Automated biometry is an excellent tool to accurately assess biometry using coherence interferometry [16]. Instruments such as the IOL Master and Lenstar (Haag-Streit) may increase the accuracy of measuring refractive axial lengths, the distance from the corneal vertex to the fovea, by

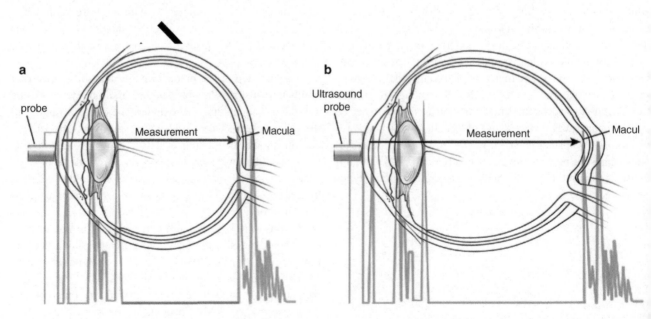

Fig. 26.1 (**a**) Contact A-scan measurements in an average-sized eye. (**b**) Contact A-scan measurements in an eye with a posterior staphyloma

allowing the patient to fixate on a visual target. In recent models, visualization of the fovea pit in cross section is possible, helping assure more accurate measurement of the axial length to the foveola. It is possible to visualize the measured optical axis of the eye as part of the workflow. Anatomic axial length (the distance from the corneal vertex to the posterior pole) as measured by A-scan contact and immersion biometry may provide a falsely high axial length in the presence of staphylomata [15]. Additional variables, such as the anterior chamber depth, white-to-white distance, and lens thickness, can be measured routinely. These variables may assist axial length and keratometry-based biometry in estimating a proper effective lens position, increasing the accuracy of refractive outcomes. Topography (both Placido disc and Scheimpflug) may be additionally useful in identifying irregular astigmatism and ectasia in eyes with high myopia and astigmatism [17].

As an alternative, in cases of poor fixation, immersion echography (using both B-scan and A-scan) can be used to achieve proper axial length measurements. In this technique, a horizontal axial B-scan is used to center the cornea and lens echoes. Then, an A-scan vector is adjusted so as to pass directly through the middle of the cornea and the anterior and posterior lens echoes. Such alignment assures that the vector will intersect the retina in the region of the fovea [18].

26.4.2 Intraocular Lens Power Calculation

When calculating an appropriate intraocular lens (IOL) power, attention should be placed on the formulae used for calculation. Earlier generations of formulae (such as the SRK formula) are not designed for eyes with high axial lengths [14]. Several advanced formulae, such as Barrett (or variants in post-myopic LASIK eyes) and Hill-RBF (based on artificial intelligence), may incorporate additional variables to recommend an IOL power which are not included in traditional formulae. Specifically, anterior and posterior corneal curvatures together with corneal thickness, white-to-white, lens thickness, anterior chamber depth, age, and preoperative refraction are incorporated in many advanced formulae, which allow adjustments appropriate for high axial lengths [8, 14].

There are an increasing number of patients presenting for cataract surgery who have previously undergone refractive surgery. This creates a difficult situation for determining the average keratometry for IOL calculations, since the corneal stroma undergoes reshaping in refractive surgery. Many formulae for IOL calculation exist for these complex refractive situations. The American Society of Cataract and Refractive Surgery provides an online tool for the calculation of IOL powers in these cases [19, 20]. If prior refractive data are available, the simple clinical history method may be quite elegant and successful. In this calculation, the change in refractive error resulting from LASIK or PRK is subtracted (or added, if a hyperopic correction was performed) from/to the pre-refractive average keratometry readings. (That is, $K_2 = K_1 - [R_2 - R_1]$, where K_2 is the post-refractive "theoretical" keratometry, K_1 is the pre-refractive average keratometry, R_2 is the pre-refractive spherical equivalent, and R_1 is the post-refractive spherical equivalent. R_1 should be taken from a post-refractive visit within 12 months; later refractions may be affected by development of cataractous myopic shift.) This yields a "theoretical" average keratometry value that can be used in IOL calculations. The rigid contact lens overrefraction technique may also be employed, where a contact lens of known curvature and power is used to determine post-refractive average keratometry. Some surgeons also use estimated total corneal power measurements from Scheimpflug topography and tomography devices. Intraoperative aphakic aberrometry also adds to the landscape of options for IOL calculations in post-refractive patients. Many advanced automated biometers include formulas for calculating IOL powers automatically in eyes having previous refractive surgery in their software. It should be cautioned that manual keratometry, automated keratometry, and traditional topography are not sufficient means to measure the appropriate average keratometry in these patients. An expected hyperopic result may occur, along with a rather unhappy patient.

IOL power calculation is dependent on the patient's desired postoperative refractive outcome. Many patients with high myopia will be eager about the potential to reduce myopia with the use of lower IOL powers. A detailed discussion should be had about options in postoperative refractive outcomes. Some patients may request monovision, but we suggest that they undergo a monovision trial with glasses or contact lenses prior to committing to this choice. Patients should also be prepared for the possibility of mild refractive surprise. One study has shown that 69% of highly myopic patients were within 1 diopter of the desired refractive outcome after cataract surgery [21]. The surgeon should be prepared to address refractive surprises with a full toolbox of medical and surgical options, including spectacles or contact lenses, intraocular lens exchanges, and excimer corneal refractive surgery.

The refractive status of the fellow eye should be considered in determining postoperative refractive targets. If the fellow eye also has a visually significant cataract, then the surgeon may consider a target refractive outcome of plano to slight myopia (−0.75 sphere) if the fellow eye will also undergo cataract surgery soon. We tend to err on the side of slight myopia, which is a more desirable outcome to most patients than slight hyperopia. If the fellow eye does not have a visually significant cataract, then a target refractive outcome of plano to slight myopia for the operated eye will induce high anisometropia that may be intolerable for the patient. In those cases, the surgeon may consider a target refraction similar to that of the phakic fellow eye to achieve refractive balance. Alternatively, clear lens extraction, phakic IOLs, contact lenses, or refractive surgery may be considered for the fellow eye to balance both eyes and to counteract surgically induced anisometropia.

26.4.3 Intraocular Lens Options

The majority of patients undergoing cataract surgery choose monofocal IOLs. For eyes with high myopia, acrylic three-piece IOLs exist in powers as low as −5.0 D (MA60MA and MN60MA Alcon, Fort Worth, TX). In addition, silicone IOLs exist in powers as low as −10.0 D (MZ60PD, Alcon, Fort Worth, TX), although we tend to avoid silicone IOLs in eyes that may potentially require future retina surgery.

Specialty and premium IOLs may also be considered. If high astigmatism is present, the use of a toric IOL may be appropriate. Furthermore, the use of multifocal and accommodating IOLs may be considered in the appropriate patient population. These IOLs may be particularly useful in young, accommodating individuals. Multifocal and accommodating IOLs have limitations and tend to result in some reduction of contrast sensitivity postoperatively. High myopes, who may be accustomed to reading close-up without spectacles, might be disappointed if they need spectacles to read fine print after surgery. They may also require spectacles for intermediate vision, depending on their refractive outcome from the multifocal or accommodating IOL.

IOL choice should also take into consideration posterior capsular opacification (PCO) rates. An IOL with a lower PCO rate is ideal in order to avoid future Nd:YAG capsulotomy, which carries increased risks of retinal detachment in eyes with high myopia [12, 14].

26.4.4 Expectations

Lastly, appropriate expectations must be identified and set for both the surgeon and patient. The patient must understand that cataract surgery in high myopia carries increased perioperative risks and that she may require further surgery or treatment for possible postoperative retinal detachment or refractive surprise.

Pseudoexfoliation, if present, increases the risk of zonular instability and IOL dislocation. Patients should also be warned of the rare possibility of loss of vision, blindness, or even loss of the eye from retinal detachment or endophthalmitis. While the patient may have high expectations of post-

operative outcomes, it should be explained that it is unlikely that the patient will see 20/20 at all distances, even with the use of a multifocal or accommodating IOL. Further, if the presence of myopic maculopathy exists, the patient should understand that their best-corrected visual outcome might be limited by this pre-existing retinal condition.

26.5 Timing Considerations

Some cataract surgeons may recommend waiting until the cataract becomes of high functional impairment before asking the patient to undertake the increased risks of surgery in high myopia. However, the patient and surgeon must not wait too long; otherwise, the cataract's high density may make the surgery more technically difficult and further increase the possibility of surgical complications.

If any exudative maculopathy is present, the surgeon should await its stabilization prior to embarking on surgery. In a similar fashion, any active intraocular conditions, such as proliferative retinopathy, intraocular inflammation, and glaucoma, must be stabilized prior to cataract surgery. Retinopathy, inflammation, and intraocular pressure may be difficult to control in the immediate postoperative period if not previously stabilized. Ocular surface disease and external conditions such as ectropion and entropion should also await stabilization prior to undertaking cataract surgery; otherwise, corneal healing may be impaired in the postoperative period.

In some cases, the density of the cataract may limit the vitreoretinal specialist's view of the posterior pole, and the surgeon may proceed with cataract extraction prior to the ideal stabilization of maculopathy or retinopathy in order to enhance the vitreoretinal specialist's diagnostic and management capabilities.

In some regions, bilateral, immediate-sequential cataract surgery is gaining prevalence, although this technique may not be ideal for cases of high myopia given the increased risks of perioperative complications.

26.6 Anesthesia

The surgeon should develop an anesthesia plan that optimizes patient comfort and cooperability but that also minimizes perioperative risks. If the patient is cooperative, topical anesthesia should be considered. Patients whom the surgeon suspects may be less cooperative in the operating room should be considered for local (retrobulbar, peribulbar, or sub-Tenon's) or general anesthesia.

Classically, retrobulbar anesthesia has been avoided in this patient group due to the increased risk of globe perforation in high axial length eyes. If local anesthesia is to be undertaken, peribulbar or sub-Tenon's injections are preferred. The Greenbaum cannula (see Fig. 26.2) has been shown to be effective in providing a sub-Tenon's block to achieve adequate akinesia, anesthesia, and reduction of lid movements during surgery [22, 23]. This short, flexible, plastic, non-traumatic cannula may be preferred to other metallic commercially available cannulas due to its ease of use and disposability.

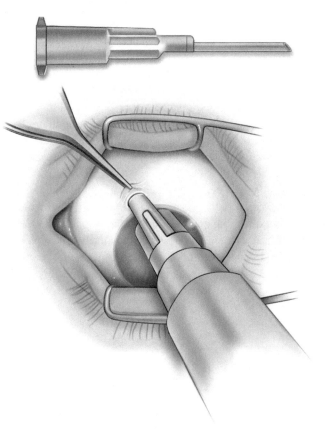

Fig. 26.2 (*Top*) Greenbaum cannula for anesthesia. (*Bottom*) Proper placement of the Greenbaum cannula for sub-Tenon's anesthesia

26.7 Surgical Considerations

Intraocular surgery in eyes with high myopia is made more difficult by the eye's long axial length. The anterior chamber tends to be deeper in these eyes. In addition, the lens-iris diaphragm and position of the posterior lens capsule often fluctuate in position due to a syneretic vitreous and elastic sclera (see Fig. 26.3). The surgeon may make several adjustments in surgical technique to address these anatomic findings.

In wound construction, if a clear-corneal incision is fashioned, a short, rather than long, tunnel is preferred. A short tunnel helps to avoid corneal striae that may result from instrument manipulation in a deep anterior chamber.

When performing the capsulorrhexis, the surgeon may consider a slightly larger rather than smaller size of anterior capsulorrhexis. This may facilitate movement of the lens out of the capsular bag and into the anterior chamber for supranuclear phacoemulsification, a technique that may reduce the difficulty of phacoemulsification handpiece manipulation in very deep anterior chambers (see Fig. 26.4). However, the surgeon must consider that eyes with high myopia often have pupils that dilate very well and that the capsulorrhexis should not be made too large in the setting of a large pupil.

After the capsulorrhexis, the surgeon should perform gentle hydrodissection of the lens. Many surgeons will also opt to perform hydrodelineation to separate the lens nucleus from the surrounding epinucleus and cortex. The epinucleus may provide a necessary protective buffer between the nucleus and the posterior capsule in the setting of a steep phacoemulsification angle.

The surgeon should avoid rapid changes in anterior chamber depth that may manifest in eyes with high axial lengths. Rapid movement of the vitreous anteriorly may increase the risk of retinal breaks and tears. Instruments, especially irrigating instruments such as the phacoemulsification hand-

a   b

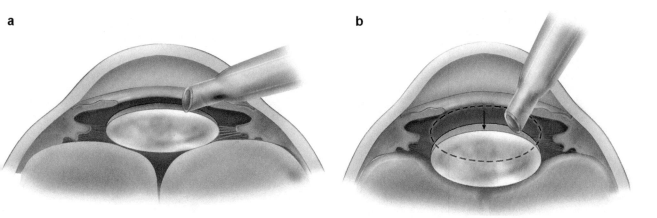

Fig. 26.3 (**a**) Phacoemulsification handpiece approaching a cataract in an average-sized eye. (**b**) Phacoemulsification handpiece attempting to approach a cataract in an eye with axial myopia; the steep angle of approach and deepened anterior chamber make the approach difficult

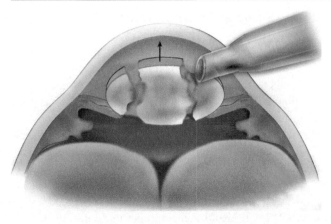

Fig. 26.4 Cataract being phacoemulsified using the supracapsular technique in the anterior chamber

piece and irrigation/aspiration handpieces, should not be removed and inserted multiple times in order to avoid excessive anterior-posterior movement of the lens-iris diaphragm. The irrigation bottle height may be lowered to reduce posterior push on the lens-iris diaphragm, but a bottle height that is too low may also increase the risk of post-occlusion surge during phacoemulsification. If sculpting the lens, a second instrument may be inserted in the paracentesis port to induce slow egress of irrigation fluid and avoid extreme deepening of the chamber. In addition, inflation of the anterior chamber

with a cohesive viscoelastic prior to removal of irrigation handpieces may avoid rapid shallowing of the anterior chamber.

Some surgeons advocate that introducing the phacoemulsification handpiece without irrigation to just below the iris plane can reduce fluctuations in anterior chamber depth. Once the handpiece is below the iris plane, irrigation can be initiated. Fluid will fill the posterior chamber, rather than the anterior chamber, and the lens-iris diaphragm may undergo less anterior-posterior movement. A more stable lens position makes for more predictable surgical maneuvers.

There are various choices of technique in nuclear disassembly. Among the most straightforward and basic techniques is divide-and-conquer (see Fig. 26.5). In this technique, the phacoemulsification handpiece is used to sculpt two initial grooves in a cruciate pattern; the nucleus is subsequently cracked into four quadrants. Each quadrant is lifted and emulsified in turn.

Techniques of chopping, such as horizontal chop or vertical chop, may reduce total ultrasound energy by avoiding sculpting the initial grooves. In vertical chop (see Fig. 26.6), also called quick chop, the phacoemulsification handpiece is embedded into the center of the nucleus while the chopper is placed just adjacent to or in front of the phaco handpiece; the handpiece is used to aspirate and pull upward, while the

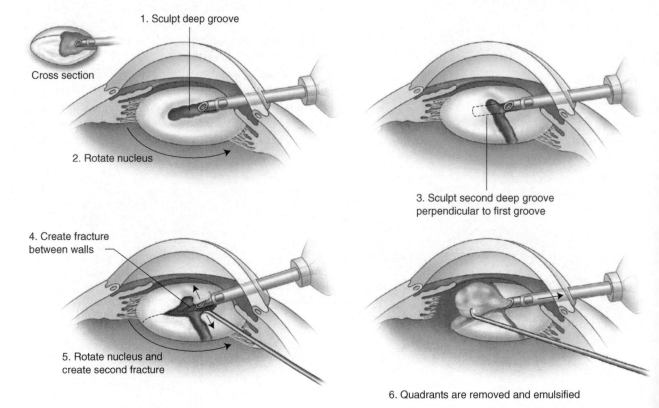

Fig. 26.5 Divide-and-conquer technique for nuclear disassembly

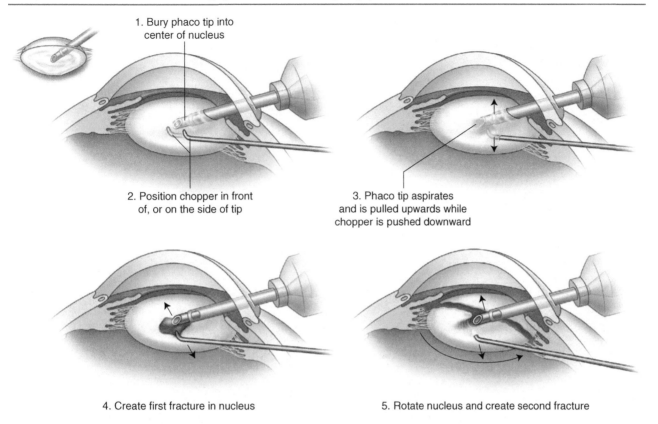

1. Bury phaco tip into center of nucleus

2. Position chopper in front of, or on the side of tip

3. Phaco tip aspirates and is pulled upwards while chopper is pushed downward

4. Create first fracture in nucleus

5. Rotate nucleus and create second fracture

Fig. 26.6 Quick-chop (vertical chop) technique for nuclear disassembly

chopper is drawn downward to create a fracture line in the lens. The resulting nuclear pieces may be chopped further, lifted, and emulsified.

Techniques of pre-slicing the nucleus (see Fig. 26.7) may reduce stress on the zonules and may allow initial nuclear deconstruction without the use of ultrasound power. Pre-slicing may be accomplished with the use of two right-angled choppers aligned 180 degrees apart, drawn centripetally toward one another, such that quadrants are created that may be lifted and emulsified as in previously described methods. miLOOP is a disposable device using a flexible nitinol ring to achieve a similar mechanical nuclear fragmentation of dense lenses (Iantech, Reno NV). Additional acceptable techniques may also include stop-and-chop, pop-and-chop, and flip-and-chop, among others.

The advent of femtosecond laser-assisted cataract surgery has provided surgeons with the ability to fashion reproducible and predictable anterior capsulotomies and arcuate incisions for treating astigmatism. A well-centered, perfectly circular capsulotomy may aid the surgeon in achieving evenly distributed forces on the zones during nuclear disassembly as well as proper IOL centration at the conclusion of the procedure. The femtosecond laser may also assist with fashioning the main and side port incisions and softening the crystalline lens. Studies regarding the safety, efficacy, and efficiency of femtosecond laser-assisted cataract surgery are ongoing.

After removal of the nucleus, epinucleus, and cortex, an adequate volume of viscoelastic must be injected to fill the anterior chamber and capsular bag prior to lens insertion. In the extremes of axial length, IOL calculations may result in the choice of very low or negative power IOLs. These low or negative powered IOLs may only be available in three-piece models, which may be either folded or injected prior to insertion. Even if a one-piece IOL is available in the power desired, some surgeons may still opt for a three-piece IOL due to its stabilizing effects in large capsular bags. The surgical wound may require enlargement to 3.0 mm to accommodate the insertion of a three-piece IOL. When the IOL calculation results in a planned IOL power of zero or close to zero diopters, we nonetheless recommend insertion of an IOL, rather than leaving the patient aphakic. The presence of an IOL offers stabilization of the capsular bag and lens-iris diaphragm and creates an important barrier between the posterior and anterior segments of the eye [14, 21].

Among the most devastating potential complications during cataract surgery is expulsive suprachoroidal hemorrhage. Previously, longer axial length was a known risk factor for acute intraoperative suprachoroidal hemorrhage [24]. This was a significant risk factor in extracapsular cataract extraction, but with a large shift toward phacoemulsification, the overall rates of acute intraoperative suprachoroidal hemorrhage have declined. In a more recent report by Ling et al.,

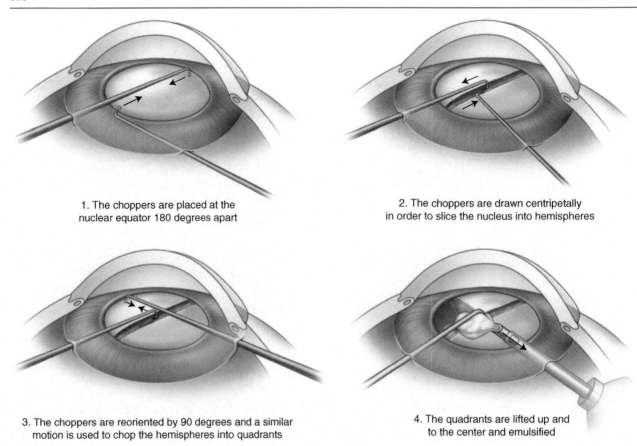

1. The choppers are placed at the
nuclear equator 180 degrees apart

2. The choppers are drawn centripetally
in order to slice the nucleus into hemispheres

3. The choppers are reoriented by 90 degrees and a similar
motion is used to chop the hemispheres into quadrants

4. The quadrants are lifted up and
to the center and emulsified

Fig. 26.7 Preslicing technique for nuclear disassembly

the estimated incidence of suprachoroidal hemorrhage during cataract surgery was 0.04% [25]. Given such a low rate
and small number of cases, the role of high myopia in the
risk of suprachoroidal hemorrhage is not established in
phacoemulsification.

26.8   Postoperative Management

The postoperative management is overall similar to cataract
surgery in a non-myope. Postoperative antibiotic, steroid,
and non-steroidal anti-inflammatory agents may be delivered
topically, typically four times daily, or intracamerally at the
conclusion of cataract surgery. In the United States, there is
no FDA-approved, commercially available intracameral
antibiotic, but many surgeons have trended toward using
moxifloxacin as an off-label intracameral agent. The use of a
non-steroidal anti-inflammatory agent is recommended to
aid in analgesia, reduction of inflammation, and prevention
of postoperative cystoid macular edema (CME).

Intraocular pressure must be closely monitored. Younger
myopes have a significantly increased risk of steroid response
(increase in intraocular pressure in response to steroid medi-

cation) after cataract surgery. In a study by Chang et al.,
patients younger than 65 years and with an axial length of
greater than 29.0 mm had a 35- to 39-fold increased risk for
steroid response than their counterparts over age 65 years
and with a normal axial length [26]. If intraocular pressure is
difficult to manage, steroid formulations of low potency,
such as loteprednol or fluorometholone, may be considered
to reduce the intensity of the steroid response. Intraocular
pressure lowering agents, such as timolol, dorzolamide, and
brimonidine, may also help to treat an acute pressure rise
postoperatively.

The postoperative refraction may take weeks or even
months to stabilize due to the variation of effective lens position as the capsular bag shrinks around the IOL. If refractive
surprise is present after surgery, the surgeon should wait
until this stabilization before embarking on refractive adjustments. If the refractive surprise is very large, IOL exchange
or piggyback IOLs may be considered. Alternatively, the
patient may consider the use of glasses, contact lenses, or
refractive surgery to counteract refractive surprise.

Posterior capsular opacification (PCO) may involve
approximately 8% of all cataract surgeries using acrylic
IOLs [27, 28]. The standard treatment of Nd-YAG laser cap-

sulotomy carries a higher risk of retinal detachment in eyes with axial myopia [12, 14]. Ranta et al. found a retinal detachment hazard ratio of 1.51 for each mm increase above 25.0 mm in axial length [28]. Some surgeons may preemptively avoid this risk by performing capsular polishing techniques at the time of surgery. Another option is to perform a posterior continuous, curvilinear capsulorrhexis during surgery, although a liquefied vitreous may be difficult to control if the posterior capsule is intentionally violated. As previously mentioned, some IOLs are designed to reduce the rate of PCO; preoperative choice of these IOLs may be a wise option.

Postoperative care should be conducted in conjunction with a vitreoretinal specialist who may be more adept in detecting subtle retinal breaks and tears and cystoid macular edema. In cases of intraoperative vitreous loss or retained lenticular fragments, prompt evaluation by a vitreoretinal surgeon is particularly important so that surgical vitrectomy and posterior lensectomy may be undertaken when appropriate.

26.9   Conclusion

Cataract surgery in eyes with high axial myopia may be safe and successful if appropriate perioperative measures are undertaken to reduce the risks of complications. There may be a high likelihood of favorable outcomes with careful operative planning and management.

References

1. Klein BE, Klein R, Moss SE. Incident cataract surgery: the Beaver Dam Eye Study. Ophthalmology. 1997;104(4):573–80.
2. Lim R, Mitchell P, Cumming RG. Refractive associations with cataract: the Blue Mountains Eye Study. Invest Ophthalmol Vis Sci. 1999;40(12):3021–6.
3. Younan C, Mitchell P, Cumming RG, et al. Myopia and incident cataract surgery: the Blue Mountains Eye Study. Invest Ophthalmol Vis Sci. 2002;43(12):3625–32.
4. Shah NV, Chow J, Yoo SH. Cataract Surgery after Refractive Surgery. In Henderson BA, Pineda IR, Chen SH (eds) Essentials of Cataract Surgery, Second Edition. Slack Inc., Thorofare, NJ, pp 341–50.
5. Simonelli F, Nesti A, Pensa M, Romano L, Savastano S, Rinaldi E. Lipid peroxidation and human cataratogenesis in diabetes and severe myopia. Exp Eye Res. 1989;49:181–7.
6. Goosey JD, Tuan WM, Garcia CH. A lipid peroxidative mechanism for posterior subcapsular cataract formation in the rabbit. A possible model for cataract formation in tapetoretinal disease. Invest Ophthalmol Vis Sci. 1984;25:608–12.

7. Micelli-Ferrari T, Vendemiale G, Grattagliano I, Boscia F, Arnese L, Altomare E, Cardia L. Role of lipid peroxidation in the pathogenesis of myopic and senile cataract. Br J Ophthalmol. 1996;80:840–3.
8. Mifflin MD, Wolsey DH. Chapter 31: Cataract surgery after refractive surgery. In: Essentials of cataract surgery. p. 271–82.
9. Williams MA, et al. The incidence and rate of rhegmatogenous retinal detachment seven years after cataract surgery in patients with high myopia. Ulster Med J. 2009;78(2):99–104.
10. Attebo K, et al. Prevalence and causes of amblyopia in an adult population. Ophthalmology. 1998;105(1):154–9.
11. Chiou AG, et al. Management of corneal ectasia and cataract following photorefractive keratectomy. J Cataract Refract Surg. 2006;32(4):679–80.
12. Jacobi FK, Hessemer V. Pseudophakic retinal detachment in high axial myopia. J Cataract Refract Surg. 1997;23(7):1095–102.
13. Szijarto Z, et al. Pseudophakic retinal detachment after phacoemulsification. Ann Ophthalmol. 2007;39(2):13409.
14. Seward H, et al. Management of cataract surgery in a high myope. Br J Ophthalmol. 2001;85:1372–8.
15. Hill W. www.doctor-hill.com/iol-main/iol_main.htm.
16. Roessler GF, et al. Accuracy of intraocular lens power calculation using partial coherence interferometry in patients with high myopia. Ophthalmic Physiol Opt. 2012;32:228–33.
17. Wolf A, et al. Mild topographic abnormalities that become more suspicious on Scheimpflug imaging. Eur J Ophthalmol. 2009;19(1):10–7.
18. Byrne SF, Green RL. Ultrasound of the eye and orbit. 2nd ed. St. Louis: Mosby; 2002.
19. Wang L, et al.. Evaluation of intraocular lens power prediction methods using the American Society of Cataract and Refractive Surgeons Post-Refractive Surgery IOL Calculator. ASCRS.org.
20. Keratorefractive intraocular lens power calculator. J Cataract Refract Surg. 2010;36(9):1466–73.
21. Kohnen S, Brauweiler PJ. First results of cataract surgery and implantation of negative power intraocular lenses in highly myopic eyes. J Cataract Refract Surg. 1996;22:416–20.
22. Greenbaum S. Parabulbar anesthesia. Am J Ophthalmol. 1992;114:776.
23. Kumar CM, Dodds D. Evaluation of the Greenbaum sub-Tenon's block. Br J Anaesth. 2001;87(4):631–3.
24. Beatty S, Lotery A, Kent D, et al. Acute intraoperative suprachoroidal hemorrhage in ocular surgery. Eye(Lond). 1998;12(Pt 5):815–20.
25. Ling R, Cole M, James C, et al. Suprachoroidal hemorrhage complicating cataract surgery in the UK: epidemiology, clinical features, management, and outcomes. Br J Ophthalmol. 2004;88(4):478–80.
26. Chang DF, Tan JJ, Tripodis Y. Risk factors for steroid response among cataract patients. J Cataract Refract Surg. 2011;37(4):675–81.
27. Wejde G, et al. Posterior capsular opacification: comparison of 3 intraocular lenses of different material and design. J Cataract Refract Surg. 2003;29(8):1556–9.
28. Ranta P, Tomilla P, Kivela T. Retinal breaks and detachment after neodymium:YAG laser posterior capsulotomy: five-year incidence in a prospective cohort. J Cataract Refract Surg. 2004;30(1):58–66.

Ocular Motility Abnormalities

27

Tsuranu Yokoyama

27.1 Highly Myopic Strabismus

Pathological myopia is sometimes responsible for a characteristic strabismus with distinct ocular motility abnormalities. The eye movement is mechanically restricted in both abduction and supraduction, resulting in esotropia and hypotropia [1, 2]. *Strabismus fixus* is the most advanced stage of this type of strabismus, in which the affected eye is so tightly fixed in an esotropic and hypotropic position that even passive movement in any other direction is impossible [3–5]. This extreme condition has also been called *convergent strabismus fixus* [3] or *myopic strabismus fixus* [6]. However, strabismus in high myopia does not always take the form of *strabismus fixus*. Severity varies from small-angle esotropia with mild restriction in abduction [6, 7], in which the eye can be moved past the midline, to *strabismus fixus*. In addition, the strabismus is not always esotropic, with even exotropia and hypotropia reported [8]. What these conditions have in common are axial high myopia and restrictive ocular motility. I therefore propose the term *highly myopic strabismus* for this entity.

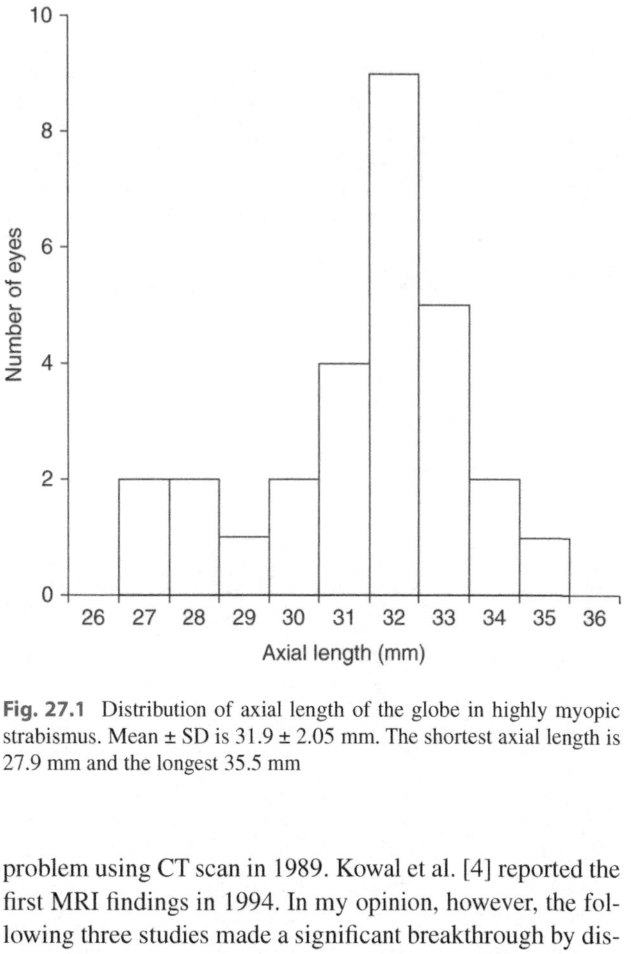

Fig. 27.1 Distribution of axial length of the globe in highly myopic strabismus. Mean ± SD is 31.9 ± 2.05 mm. The shortest axial length is 27.9 mm and the longest 35.5 mm

27.1.1 Etiology

Highly myopic strabismus is an acquired strabismus affecting highly myopic adults. The axial length of the eye often exceeds 30 mm [9]. Figure 27.1 is the distribution of axial length of eyes with *highly myopic strabismus*, ranging from 19.9 to 35.5 mm (mean ± SD, 31.9 ± 2.05 mm).

Several authors have proposed a variety of etiologies [10–13], but its mechanisms of development remained unknown until substantial progress was made in imaging technologies such as computed tomography or MRI. Demer and von Noorden [12] were the first to try to find an answer to this

problem using CT scan in 1989. Kowal et al. [4] reported the first MRI findings in 1994. In my opinion, however, the following three studies made a significant breakthrough by discovering inferior displacement of the lateral rectus (LR) muscle using different methods: axial CT scanning by Ohta et al. [14], intraoperative observation by Herzau and Ioannakis [15], and coronal MRI by Krzizok et al. [8]. Both Ohta et al. and Herzau and Ioannakis as well as Krzizok and Schroeder [16] speculated that downward displacement of the LR might disturb abduction. However, while downward shift of the LR may weaken the abducting force, this does not itself explain how both abduction and supraduction are simultaneously restricted, particularly in *strabismus fixus*.

T. Yokoyama (✉)
Department of Pediatric Ophthamology, Osaka City General
Hospital Children's Medical Center, Miyakojima-ku, Osaka, Japan

R. F. Spaide et al. (eds.), *Pathologic Myopia*, https://doi.org/10.1007/978-3-030-74334-5_27

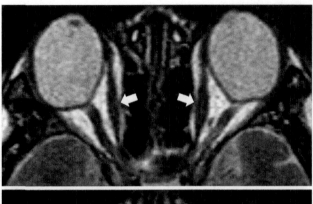

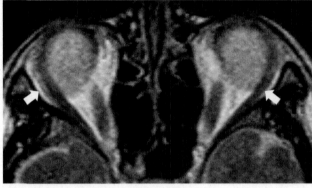

Fig. 27.2 Axial MRI of a patient with bilateral strabismus fixus. The medial rectus muscles (*top, arrows*) are not present in the same plane as the lateral rectus (*bottom, arrows*). The *bottom image* shows a slice 6 mm lower than the *top*. In strabismus fixus, the LR generally takes a longer path than it does under normal conditions, running along the under surface of the globe

Furthermore, no clear explanation was provided on how the LR becomes displaced.

As reported by Yokoyama et al. [17, 18], the globe of *highly myopic strabismus* is dislocated from the muscle cone through the space between the superior rectus (SR) and LR muscles, and this dislocation may be the direct cause of this disease. Their findings can also explain how the LR is inferiorly displaced.

Figure 27.2 shows axial MRI images of a patient with bilateral *strabismus fixus*. In axial scans, the medial and lateral rectus muscles are sometimes not present at the same level due to a downward shift of the LR. The top image shows the slice that includes the largest cross section of the globe. This slice also includes the medial rectus (MR) muscle. However, the LR is depicted at a lower level, 6 mm below the MR as in the bottom image. This is exactly what Ohta et al. [14] reported using CT scan. Nevertheless, it is not a common finding in *highly myopic strabismus* in general but only seen when dislocation of the globe is unusually severe, namely, as in *strabismus fixus*.

Coronal scanning is the most useful means for the diagnosis of *highly myopic strabismus*. The coronal MRI in Fig. 27.3 is recorded from another patient with bilateral *strabismus fixus*. The globe is abnormally displaced superiorly and temporally, with its large part being outside the muscle cone. Figure 27.4 is a three-dimensional reconstruction created from the same MRI. As shown in the dorsal view, the posterior part of the globe is obviously dislocated from the

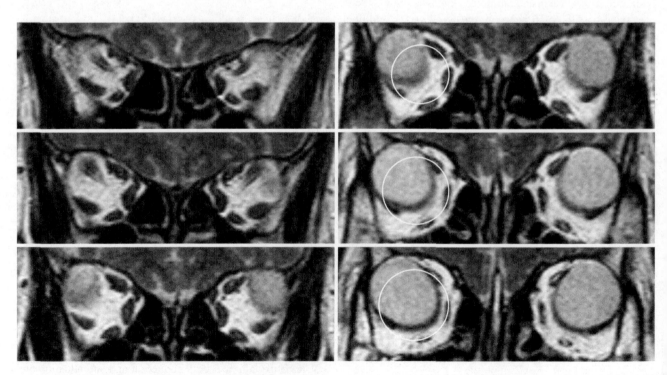

Fig. 27.3 Coronal MRI of a patient with bilateral strabismus fixus. Images are laid out sequentially from posterior to anterior with a slice thickness of 3 mm. *Circles* indicate cross sections of the muscle cone

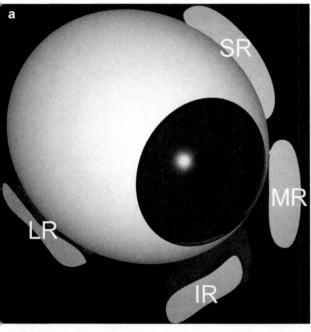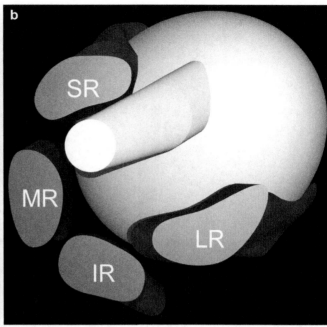

Fig. 27.4 Three-dimensional reconstruction. (**a**) Frontal view, (**b**) dorsal view, SR superior rectus, MR medial rectus, IR inferior rectus, LR lateral rectus. This is created from the MRI in Fig. 27.3. The four rectus muscles and the optic nerve are traced along their path on each slice. The globe is a spheroid superimposed to fit exactly the shape of the real globe

muscle cone and held between the SR and LR muscles. In this situation, the posterior pole of the globe cannot move nasally because the SR muscle is in its way, resulting in restriction in abduction. Supraduction is prevented similarly by the LR muscle, which suspends the posterior portion of the globe from below. Herzau and Ioannakis [15] described exactly the same observation about the LR during surgery. This is how the eye is mechanically immobilized.

Figure 27.5 compares orbits of a control subject and a patient with *strabismus fixus*. The control is a high myope without strabismus or any abnormal ocular movement. In the control subject, the SR is located slightly temporal to the inferior rectus (IR), and the MR and LR muscles are almost at the same level. In the patient, however, the SR is displaced nasally and the LR inferiorly. Some might consider that both these muscles have largely changed their positions, but in actual fact they are displaced only fractionally. It is the superior temporal displacement of the globe that creates the illusion of the SR and LR having been substantially displaced.

27.1.2 Angle of Dislocation

Some indicator to measure the severity of globe dislocation is vital to quantitative investigation of the relationship between the degree of globe dislocation and severity of restriction in ocular movement.

Small white circles in Fig. 27.6 represent the centers of the globe (G), SR (S), and LR (L). Their coordinates are obtained with computer software, Scion Image® (Scion Corporation, Frederick, Maryland, USA). Angle LGS, including the superior temporal quadrant of the orbit, is indicated with a curved line. Since this angle can be a useful indicator denoting the severity of globe dislocation, I call it the angle of dislocation. If this angle is larger than 180°, more than half of the cross section of the globe lies outside the muscle cone. Angle of dislocation has a significant correlation with the maximum angle of abduction and that of supraduction [9]. The mean angle of dislocation in 36 eyes with *highly myopic strabismus* is 179.9 ± 30.8°, whereas that in 27 normal controls is 102.9 ± 6.8°.

27.1.3 Surgical Treatment

A surgical procedure uniting the muscle bellies of the SR and LR muscles is effective on restoration of globe dislocation in *highly myopic strabismus*. It can improve not only abnormal eye position but defective ocular movement.

Figure 27.7 illustrates how to unite the SR and LR muscles. The purpose of this procedure is to push the globe back into its normal position, i.e., within the muscle cone. One single-armed suture is inserted into the two rectus muscles and ligated. Nonabsorbable 5-0 polyester is best suited for this procedure since it is strong enough to unite the muscles and does not produce any undesirable tissue reaction. The suture is inserted twice into each muscle at different distances from the muscle margin. In this way, the friction of

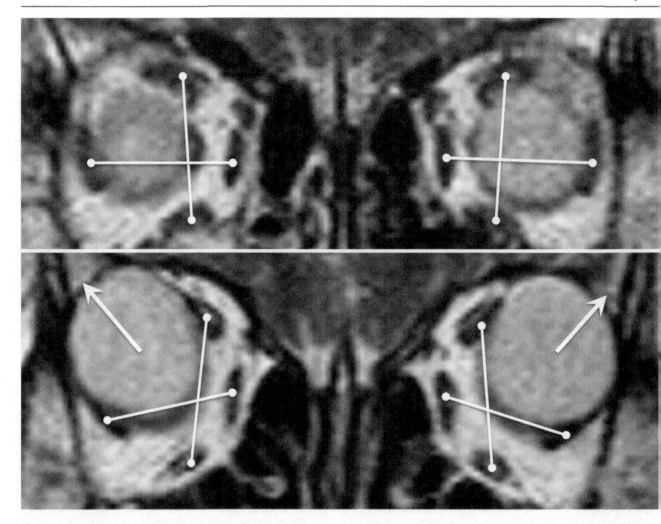

Fig. 27.5 Comparison of normal control and strabismus fixus. The *top image* is the orbits of a high myope without strabismus or ocular motility abnormality. The *bottom* is those of a patient with strabismus fixus. In the patient's scan, the SR is displaced nasally and the LR inferiorly because the dislocated globe (*arrows*) is pushing them aside

the suture can be utilized to firmly fix the muscles. The suture should not be locked until the two muscles securely get in close contact with each other. There must not be any gap left between them because, if any, the bare thread in the gap might slice into the sclera and eventually puncture the globe. The position of suture placement is approximately 15 mm behind the insertion for both the SR and LR. Because this position is sometimes hard to reach, a preplaced silk suture is often needed at about 10 mm behind the rectus muscle insertion in order to pull out the necessary part of the muscle (Fig. 27.8). Whenever the muscle is found to be too tight to manipulate with only muscle hooks, a preplaced suture should be used because, especially in elderly patients, rectus muscles are often so vulnerable to forcible manipulations that they can easily be torn up. This is particularly true for the SR because its insertion lies farthest from the corneal limbus among the four rectus muscles and also because it is covered with the upper lid. On the contrary, the LR is much easier to expose only with muscle hooks than the SR, and a

preplaced suture is not generally needed. During exposure of the muscles, intermuscular membranes should thoroughly and carefully be dissected so as to enable smooth sideways movements of the muscles, but the Tenon's capsule that covers the muscle itself must not be removed to prevent the muscles from splitting apart. Where to place the suture in the muscle is also important. Half the width of a muscle should at least be spared to avoid ischemia. However, if a suture is inserted too marginally, the muscle may well fail to be secured, and the result will end up being unsatisfactory.

There are some other minor but important points to be emphasized about the union procedure. In *strabismus fixus*, the insertion of the inferior oblique muscle frequently lies abnormally higher than the upper margin of the LR (Fig. 27.9a), although this insertion should normally be located around the lower margin of the LR. Similarly, the insertion of the superior oblique is found to be temporal to the temporal margin of the SR (Fig. 27.9b). This is because the courses of the two rectus muscles have shifted due to globe dislocation. One should be careful not to suture the oblique muscles together with the rectus muscles. That makes it impossible to move the rectus muscles.

There are two possibilities by which the muscle union surgery may take effect. First, this surgery can normalize the vectors of muscle force of the SR and LR. Second, the procedure can make the globe move freely within the muscle cone by eliminating the mechanical disturbance of eye movement. Myopexy of the LR at the equator of the globe [19] or muscle transposition aimed at correcting the displacement of the extraocular muscle path [15] are effective in some patients, but they also can work through the restoration of globe dislocation.

Figure 27.10 is coronal MR images recorded before and after union surgery. In the preoperative image, approximately half of the globe lies outside the muscle cone. The SR and LR muscles are pushed aside by the dislocated globe. Then in the postoperative scan, the globe has successfully returned within the muscle cone. Angle of dislocation improved from preoperative 181.1 to postoperative 103.6°.

27.1.4 Surgical Options

Union of the SR and LR muscles is sometimes insufficient to fully normalize the abnormal ocular movement of *highly myopic strabismus*. One reason for this is that the MR muscle is likely to become contractured due to long-standing convergent strabismus. If esotropia and mechanical restriction in abduction remain after union surgery even though restoration of globe dislocation is confirmed with postoperative MRI, recession of the MR muscle will be the next step to

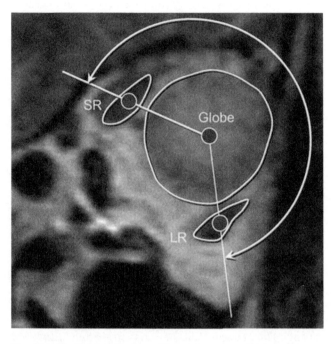

Fig. 27.6 Angle of dislocation. SR superior rectus, LR lateral rectus. The angle of dislocation is formed by connecting three points, the area centroids (*circles*) of the SR, globe, and LR, facing the superior temporal wall of the orbit (*curved line*). This angle has a significant correlation with the maximum angle of abduction and that of supraduction

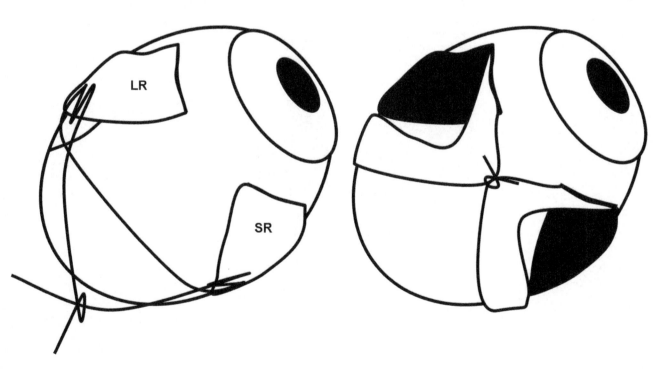

Fig. 27.7 Schematic illustrations of SR-LR union procedure. LR lateral recus, SR superior rectus (surgeon's view). A suture is placed in each rectus muscle approximately 15 mm behind the insertions

take. However, an excessive amount of MR recession prior to union surgery is not recommended, because it may lead to overcorrection and produce uncontrollable large-angle exotropia (Fig. 27.11). Resection of the LR before union procedure can aggravate dislocation of the globe, because when the angle of dislocation is greater than 180°, the shortened LR further pushes the globe out from the muscle cone, thus making it difficult to do an SR-LR union. Even if muscle

union successfully restores globe dislocation, the LR resection performed before the union surgery may cause overcorrection.

In my experience, 4 out of 23 eyes, which had not had previous strabismus surgery, did not need additional MR recession, and abnormal ocular movement was sufficiently corrected only with a union procedure. This fact implies that MR recession is not an essential part for the treatment of *highly myopic strabismus*. It should be planned only when contracture of the MR is confirmed after muscle union.

Here are improvements of several parameters after union procedure and MR recession (if necessary) in my hand: angle of dislocation from preoperative 184.0° ± 31.5° to postoperative 101.1° ± 21.7°, maximum angle of abduction from −14.0° ± 42.1° to 46.3° ± 22.1°, maximum angle of supraduction from −10.8° ± 30.6° to 38.5° ± 15.7°, and angle of deviation from 56.8° ± 36.0° to 0.7° ± 9.0°. The negative values for abduction and supraduction indicate that the eye cannot reach the midline.

27.1.5 Dynamic Changes of Globe Dislocation

All the images in Fig. 27.12 are obtained from the same patient. This patient had bilateral *strabismus fixus* and received SR-LR union surgery in both eyes. In the left column, the patient is instructed to look in the lower right direction. The right eye is infraducting because it cannot abduct past the midline. In the right column, the patient is looking in the lower left direction with the right eye infra-adducting. Note that globe dislocation in the right eye is much more pronounced when the eye is infra-adducting than is infraducting. In other words, the severity of globe dislocation can dynami-

Fig. 27.8 Preplaced suture to the superior rectus muscle. A silk suture (*arrow*) is placed about 10 mm behind the insertion to pull out the muscle. This suture makes it safer to expose the necessary part of the muscle than using only muscle hooks

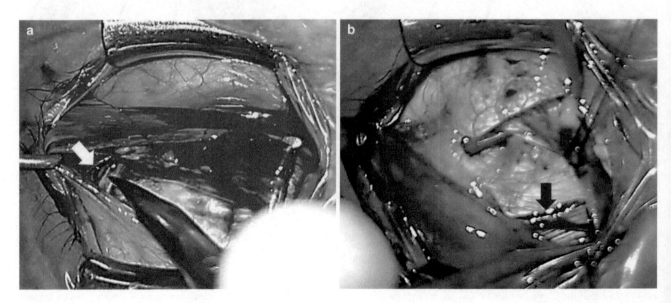

Fig. 27.9 Abnormal positions of the inferior and superior oblique muscles in strabismus fixus. (**a**) Inferior oblique (*arrow*), (**b**) superior oblique (*arrow*)

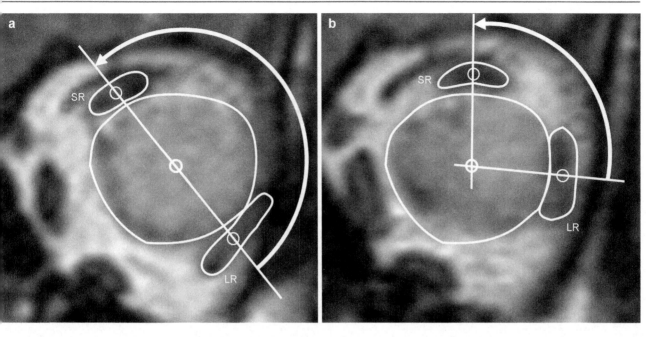

Fig. 27.10 Improvement of the angle of dislocation after union procedure. (**a**) Preoperative MRI, (**b**) MRI after union surgery. SR superior rectus, LR lateral rectus. Angle of dislocation improved from preoperative 181.1 to postoperative 103.6°

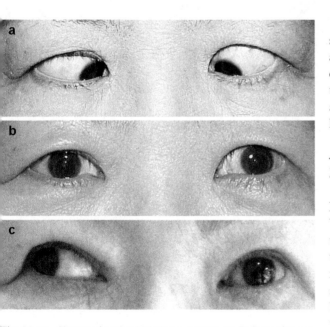

Fig. 27.11 Change of ocular deviation over time. (**a**) Before union surgery, (**b**) 52 days after bilateral union surgery, (**c**) 14 years later. This patient had received multiple recession-resection procedures in both eyes prior to the union surgery

cally change according to different eye positions. When evaluating MRI, therefore, it must be recorded in several different eye positions, at least in infra-adduction and infra-abduction, not to miss such dynamic changes. This is a case in which muscle union procedure is insufficient to correct abnormal ocular motility. I have not been able to find any other way to improve the ocular movement of this patient.

This instability of globe dislocation was also demonstrated by Ohba et al. [20] in a different way. They reported a case of unilateral *strabismus fixus* in which the patient could manually reposition the dislocated globe. By pushing the eye with the finger tips over the eyelid, the patient was able to normalize the abduction deficit temporarily by herself.

27.2 Myopia and Concomitant Strabismus

Myopia can be associated with both esotropia and exotropia. With the presence of uncorrected myopia in children, binocular visual function is not likely to develop properly because the eyes are constantly stimulated with blurred retinal images. Unilateral high myopia is more likely to give rise to strabismus, *sensory heterotropia*, than bilateral myopia because impairment of binocular vision is more profound in unilateral cases. If the onset of unilateral visual loss is at birth or between birth and 5 years of age, almost equal frequency of esotropia and exotropia is observed, although exotropia predominates in older children and adults [21]. Up to the present there has been no evidence of myopia-specific mechanism leading to concomitant esotropia. Some authors say that most clinical characteristics of nonaccommodative esotropia in myopia are no different from those associated with emmetropia or hypermetropia [22].

Curtin found that exodeviations (574) were more prevalent than esodeviations (303) in a consecutive series of 1017 myopes [23]. One might consider that those exodeviations

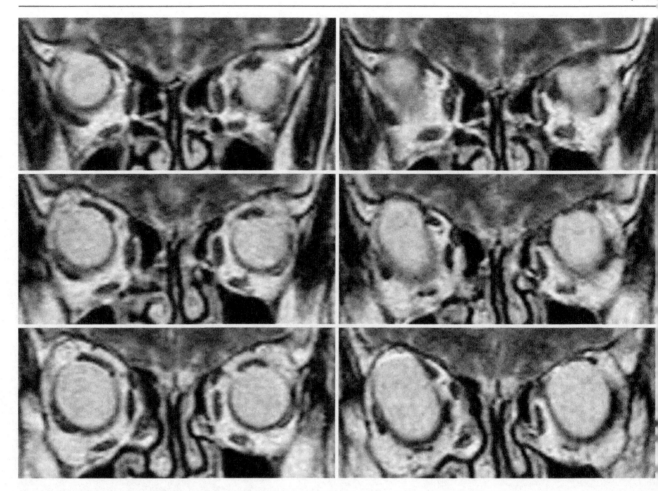

Fig. 27.12 Dynamic changes of globe dislocation. In the *left column*, the patient is instructed to look in the lower right direction and in the *right column*, to look in the lower left. Globe dislocation of the right eye is much more pronounced when the eye is infra-adducting than is infraducting

are caused by reduced accommodative convergence resulting from lesser demand for accommodation in uncorrected myopia. However, distribution of refractive errors in exotropes resembles that in the nonstrabismic population [22]. It is true that some adult exotropes try to achieve orthotropia by exerting an excessive amount of accommodative convergence at the cost of clear image [24]. They often prefer to wear overcorrected myopic spectacles to get both ocular alignment and clear vision. This pseudomyopia disappears immediately after surgical correction of the exotropia. Recently Ekdawi et al. reported that in children with intermittent exotropia, myopia occurred in over 90% of patients by 20 years of age [25]. This is quite intriguing in that there might be a possibility that exotropia is a cause of myopia.

Angle kappa is the angle formed by the pupillary axis and the visual axis. It is generally smaller or occasionally even negative in myopic eyes. Damms et al. reported negative angle kappa and macular dislocation in the direction of the optic disc in highly myopic children [26]. When angle kappa is negative, corneal light reflection is observed on the temporal side of the pupillary center as opposed to the nasal in eyes with a positive angle. It gives a false impression of esotropia, but the cover test should generally reveal the true position of eyes. For example, when there is no strabismus, an eye with negative angle kappa remains in the same apparent esotropic position even if the other eye is occluded. However, attention must be paid in conducting the corneal light reflection test to determine the presence of strabismus in infants or uncooperative patients, in which accurate cover testing is not always possible.

References

1. Mansour AM, Wang F, El-Baba F, Henkind P. Ocular complications in strabismus fixus convergens. Ophthalmologica. 1987;195:161–6.
2. Kaynak S, Durak I, Ozaksoy D, Canda T. Restrictive myopic myopathy: computed tomography, magnetic resonance imaging, echography, and histological findings. Br J Ophthalmol. 1994;78:414–5.
3. Bagolini B, Tamburrelli C, Dickmann A, Colosimo C. Convergent strabismus fixus in high myopic patients. Doc Ophthalmol. 1990;74:309–20.
4. Kowal L, Troski M, Gilford E. MRI in the heavy eye phenomenon. Aust N Z J Ophthalmol. 1994;22:125–6.

5. Taylor R, Whale K, Raines M. The heavy eye phenomenon: orthoptic and ophthalmic characteristics. Ger J Ophthalmol. 1995;4:252–5.

6. Sturm V, Menke MN, Chaloupka K, Landau K. Surgical treatment of myopic strabismus fixus: a graded approach. Graefes Arch Clin Exp Ophthalmol. 2008;246:1323–9.

7. Hayashi T, Iwashige H, Maruo T. Clinical features and surgery for acquired progressive esotropia associated with severe myopia. Acta Ophthalmol Scand. 1999;77:66–71.

8. Krzizok TH, Kaufmann H, Traupe H. Elucidation of restrictive motility in high myopia by magnetic resonance imaging. Arch Ophthalmol. 1997;115:1019–27.

9. Yamaguchi M, Yokoyama T, Shiraki K. Surgical procedure for correcting globe dislocation in highly myopic strabismus. Am J Ophthalmol. 2010;149:341–6.

10. Hugonnier R, Magnard P. Oculomotor disequilibrium observed in cases of severe myopia. Ann Ocul (Paris). 1969;202:713–24.

11. Duke-Elder S, Wybar KC. Strabismus fixus. In: Duke-Elder S, editor. System of ophthalmology, vol. 6. London: Henry Kimpton; 1973. p. 607–8.

12. Demer JL, von Noorden GK. High myopia as an unusual cause of restrictive motility disturbance. Surv Ophthalmol. 1989;33:281–4.

13. Aydin P, Kansu T, Sanac AS. High myopia causing bilateral abduction deficiency. J Clin Neuroophthalmol. 1992;12:163–5; discussion 166.

14. Ohta M, Iwashige H, Hayash T, Maruo T. Computed tomography findings in convergent strabismus fixus. Nippon Ganka Gakkai Zasshi Soc. 1995;99:980–5.

15. Herzau V, Ioannakis K. Pathogenesis of eso- and hypotropia in high myopia. Klin Monatsbl Augenheilkd. 1996;208:33–6.

16. Krzizok TH, Schroeder BU. Measurement of recti eye muscle paths by magnetic resonance imaging in highly myopic and normal subjects. Invest Ophthalmol Vis Sci. 1999;40:2554–60.

17. Yokoyama T, Tabuchi H, Ataka S, Shiraki K, Miki T, Mochizuki K. The mechanism of development in progressive esotropia with high myopia. In: de Faber JTHN, editor. Transactions of the 26th meeting, European Strabismological Association, Barcelona, Spain, September 2000. Lisse: Swets & Zeitlinger Publishers; 2001. p. 218–21.

18. Yokoyama T, Ataka S, Tabuchi H, Shiraki K, Miki T. Treatment of progressive esotropia caused by high myopia – a new surgical procedure based on its pathogenesis. In: de Faber JTHN, editor. Transactions of the 27th meeting, European Strabismological Association, Florence, Italy, June 2001. Lisse: Swets & Zeitlinger Publishers; 2002. p. 145–8.

19. Krzizok TH, Kaufmann H, Traupe H. New approach in strabismus surgery in high myopia. Br J Ophthalmol. 1997;81:625–30.

20. Ohba M, Kawata H, Ohguro H, Fukushi N. An unusual case of adult progressive esotropia caused by high myopia. Binocul Vis Strabismus Q. 2008;23:31–5.

21. Sidikaro Y, von Noorden GK. Observations in sensory heterotropia. J Pediatr Ophthalmol Strabismus. 1982;19:12–9.

22. von Noorden GK, Campos EC. Binocular vision and ocular motility. Theory and management of strabismus. 6th ed. St. Louis: Mosby; 2002.

23. Curtin BJ. Motility. In: The myopias. Basic science and clinical management. Philadelphia: Harper & Row; 1985. p. 292–7.

24. Shimojyo H, Kitaguchi Y, Asonuma S, Matsushita K, Fujikado T. Age-related changes of phoria myopia in patients with intermittent exotropia. Jpn J Ophthalmol. 2009;53:12–7.

25. Ekdawi NS, Nusz KJ, Diehl NN, Mohney BG. The development of myopia among children with intermittent exotropia. Am J Ophthalmol. 2010;149:503–7.

26. Damms T, Damms C, Schulz E, Haase W. Pseudo-esotropia caused by nasal dislocation of the macula in patients with high infantile myopia. Ophthalmologe. 1994;91:77–80.

Myopia: Ocular and Systemic Disease

28

Daryle Jason G. Yu and Quan V. Hoang

28.1 Introduction

Ocular conditions, systemic disease, syndromic disorders, and adverse effects from certain drugs may predispose development of myopia (Fig. 28.1). In-depth study of this topic may further our understanding of the pathogenesis of myopia and associated factors for its progression and may even set the occasion for the development of possible treatment. Although early recognition of mild myopic changes that commonly arise with certain ocular and systemic factors may limit the burden of vision loss with simple refractive correction, the recognition of high and pathologic axial myopia is important since there is a risk of permanent vision loss from vision-threatening sequelae. Therefore, the study of cases of high axial myopia, and specifically those cases in which there may be a causal relationship, is of particular interest and discussed in this chapter. Additionally, some syndromic causes may develop ocular problems solely on the basis of high myopia. Recognition of the tendency of some syndromes to be associated with myopia heightens the clinical suspicion for detection of severe refractive errors in patients who may be preverbal or unable to effectively communicate.

Clinical studies and basic scientific discoveries oftentimes mirror and motivate each other. In this chapter we detail clinical observations and studies that have been proven, or may in the future prove themselves, relevant to current thoughts on emmetropization and animal models of myopia

discussed more thoroughly elsewhere in this book. Specifically, concepts provided by research in specific gene defects or syndromes may provide clues to understanding the pathogenesis of myopia. Conversely recognition of high myopia may provide a clue that there is a recognizable syndromic cause. Additionally, uncovering gene defects that are associated with myopia in syndromes may provide clues in the search for candidate genes in population-based studies.

28.2 Myopia in Association with Ocular Diseases

Form-deprivation myopia and lens-induced myopia are two commonly employed techniques in establishing myopia animal models [1–7]. Additionally, studies have suggested that a change in the component scleral collagen in the eye wall or its turnover may contribute to pathologic eye elongation [8–12]. Not surprisingly, most clinical reports and studies of ocular disease that may have a causal relationship with myopia development tend to be related to conditions with visual deprivation or connective tissue disorders. This is most evident in cases of unilateral axial high myopia [13] and twin studies [14]. However, there are many ocular diseases associated with myopia in which a causal relationship is not clear, for example, diseases that occur simultaneously with axial eye elongation (such as microcornea and congenital stationary night blindness) or those that tend to occur later on in highly myopic patients.

28.2.1 High Myopia Associated with Form-Depriving Ocular Conditions

Form deprivation that may lead to high axial myopia can occur at any point along the visual axis anterior to the photoreceptive retina. This ranges from eyelid and orbital disorders to changes in the nerve fiber layer. These situations support the idea that a focus sensor may exists in the retina,

D. J. G. Yu
Singapore Eye Research Institute, Singapore, Singapore

Q. V. Hoang (✉)
Singapore Eye Research Institute, Singapore, Singapore

Department of Ophthalmology, Duke-NUS, Singapore, Singapore

Singapore National Eye Centre, Singapore, Singapore

Department of Ophthalmology, Edward S. Harkness Eye Institute, Columbia University Medical Center, New York, NY, USA
e-mail: qvh2001@columbia.edu

© Springer Nature Switzerland AG 2021
R. F. Spaide et al. (eds.), *Pathologic Myopia*, https://doi.org/10.1007/978-3-030-74334-5_28

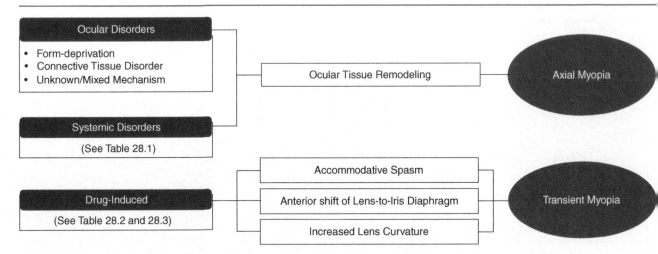

Fig. 28.1 Etiology and mechanisms of the pathogenesis of myopia

often thought to reside in the peripheral retina, which transmits signals that regulate scleral remodeling. Whether this signal is self-contained within the retina-choroid-sclera complex or requires communication via the optic nerve is still unknown [15].

Monocular axial myopia development was reported to be associated with unilateral infantile blepharoptosis. This was consistent with the experimental model of neonatal lid fusion [16, 17]. Additionally, myopic and astigmatic refractive errors that persist in patients with infantile capillary hemangiomas of the upper eyelids, even after resolution of the vascular tumors, may support a contributing role of form deprivation [18, 19].

Eyes with early unilateral corneal opacities have been associated with axial lengths of >26 mm due to lengthening of the posterior segment [20, 21], which was thought to be consistent with similar observations in the macaque monkey [22]. Moreover, it is important to note that bilateral form deprivation in the macaque also resulted in bilateral axial myopia [1]. Congenital cataracts are also associated with high myopia, exemplified in a pair of identical twins, one of which had a congenital lens opacity [14]. In terms of posterior segment disorders associated with high myopia, a small case series among infants younger than 2.5 years old with unilateral vitreous hemorrhage obscuring the posterior pole exhibited myopic anisometropia ranging from 1.37 to 12.00 diopters [23].

28.2.2 High Myopia Associated with Ocular Disorders of Connective Tissue

Axial myopia is likely influenced by the component structural elements of the sclera: collagen. Several ocular conditions in which there may be alteration in connective tissue have been reported to develop high myopia. In congenital

scleral ectasia, thinning and bulging of the posterior sclera occur, usually in the peripapillary area, that is associated with axial myopia [24]. Myopia has also been associated with systemic connective tissue disorders, which are discussed later in this chapter.

Of note, keratoconus is a corneal collagen disorder characterized by progressive central or paracentral thinning and anterior bulging of the cornea. Keratoconus may occur in isolation or concurrent with numerous congenital abnormalities of the eye and malformative syndromes. Notwithstanding the fact that virtually all keratoconus eyes are myopic, a vast majority are refractive in nature. There have been reports of concurrent axial length elongation in keratoconus eyes, but only to the 24.40 mm range (with the main contribution from posterior segment elongation) [25–27]. If keratoconus were related to a more global connective tissue disorder (that involved scleral collagen as well), one would expect the level of corneal ectasia to correlate with the axial length of the eye. No such correlation has been found in studies thus far [25, 26].

28.2.3 Other Ocular Disorders That Associate with Myopia

There are also a variety of other ocular disorders that are associated with high axial myopia (some that may develop simultaneously with myopia or that tend to develop later in myopic eyes). In the anterior segment, one such disorder is microcornea, characterized by a horizontal corneal diameter of <11 mm, a flatter corneal surface, normal pachymetry, and degenerated endothelium, is rarely reported to associate with high axial myopia, despite a generally shallower anterior chamber depth [28, 29]. Aniridia is a congenital bilateral ocular disorder that is associated with hypoplasia of the iris with variable foveal and optic nerve hypoplasia, nystagmus, cataracts, glaucoma, and corneal opacification. High myopia may be present, presumably due to iridocorneal junction abnormalities, and PAX6 mutations have been associated with high myopia [30, 31]. This is consistent with animal experiments that showed changes in retinal PAX6 gene expression in chick and primate myopia models [32, 33].

Several posterior segment disorders also fall into this category. Congenital stationary night blindness (CSNB) is a nonprogressive rod dystrophy typically associated with high myopia. The types of CSNB that are highly myopic are inherited as an X-linked recessive, but CSNB can also be an autosomal recessive or autosomal dominant trait [34, 35]. CSNB is often associated with a negative electroretinography (ERG) in the maximal response, where there is selective loss of the b-wave [36]. The more complete the CSNB is, the more likely for it to be associated with higher amounts of myopia [37]. Intriguingly, X-linked transmission of high axial myopia has also been reported in cone-rod dystrophy [38], achromatopsia [39], and retinitis pigmentosa [40, 41]. This connection helped direct genetic studies, revealing the first identified locus for high myopia on chromosome X (MYP1, OMIM 310460) [42] and associated TEX28 copy number variations [43].

In retinopathy of prematurity (ROP), there is abnormal retinal vascular development in premature infants with subsequent peripheral neovascularization and eventually traction retinal detachment in untreated cases. Myopia is seen commonly with ROP. Although this may be attributed to the changes in the anterior segment, there is a positive correlation between the degree of myopia and the severity of cicatricial retinal vascular disease [44]. Approximately 70% of high-risk pre-threshold retinopathy of prematurity (ROP) eyes are myopic in early childhood, with the proportion with high myopia increased steadily between ages 6 months and 3 years [45]. These cases are generally not high axial myopes and have been associated with a shallow anterior chamber depth and a thicker lens [45]. Cryotherapy treatment for ROP is associated with high refractive myopia development [46], more so than laser treatment. However, it is important to note that anti-VEGF treatment of ROP may be associated with less myopia than laser treatment [47]. Additionally, a retrospective observational case series among patients with Vogt-Koyanagi-Harada disease, reported that increased axial lengths were associated with the severity of sunset glow fundus as well as thinner choroidal thickness among patients who experienced acquired myopia [48].

28.3 Myopia Associated with Systemic Diseases and Syndromes

A large number of systemic diseases and syndromes have been reported to be associated with myopia. Table 28.1 summarizes the main systemic and ocular characteristics of some

of these syndromes. The most frequent and relevant entities will be described in this section.

As mentioned in Sect. 28.2.2, systemic diseases of connective tissue have been associated with high myopia. Mutations in the FBN1 gene on chromosome 15 in Marfan syndrome (MFS), a common inherited connective tissue disorder, result in defective fibrillin-1 connective tissue proteins [112]. Patients with MFS typically present with tall stature, dolichostenomelia, arachnodactyly, scoliosis, mitral valve prolapse, aortic aneurysm, and recurrent pneumothorax. Ocular findings of MFS include superotemporal lens subluxation, glaucoma, retinal pigmentary degeneration, retinal detachment, and high axial myopia [113]. Adult MFS patients display longer ocular axial lengths versus age-matched controls [114]. Although the spherical equivalents were more myopic among patients with MFS, it is interesting to note that children and adolescents with MFS do not typically have longer ocular axial lengths as compared to their age-matched control group [114, 115]. This may be due to non-axial length changes in MFS eyes. The role of FBN1 mutation in ocular involvement is still poorly elucidated. It has been associated with an increased active form of TGF-ß. However, the more important effect of FBN1 mutation is the resulting fibrillin deficiency in the zonules and capsules that leads to structural incompetence rather than the interaction with TGF-ß [116]. In both children and adults, higher degrees of axial myopia and its complications are more commonly found among MFS patients with ectopia lentis [114, 115, 117]. Despite increased axial lengths, a myopic shift in refractive error might be mitigated by flatter corneas [114, 115, 117, 118]. It is therefore important for clinicians to consider performing biometry among MFS patients in addition to assessment of refractive error. Loeys-Dietz syndrome, another rare autosomal dominant connective tissue disorder caused by mutations in transforming growth factor beta receptor 1 or 2, presents with typical features of bifid/broad uvula, cleft palate, and hypertelorism and has been associated with development of high myopia, blue or dusk sclera, cataract, retinal detachment, retinal tortuosity, strabismus, and amblyopia [85].

Ehlers-Danlos syndrome is a heterogeneous group of soft connective tissue diseases which have also been reported to develop high myopia and staphyloma [119]. It is associated with mutations affecting collagen (ADAMTS2, COL1A1, COL1A2, COL3A1, COL5A1, COL5A2, PLOD1, and TNXB [119, 120]), resulting in widespread fragility of collagen in the skin, ligaments, joints, blood vessels, and organs including the eye [120]. Stickler syndrome, characterized by a defect in the type II procollagen gene, has been associated with high myopia, glaucoma, cortical cataracts, high risk of retinal detachment with giant or large retinal breaks, high incidence of bilaterality, and proliferative vitreoretinopathy. The vitreous gel abnormalities in Stickler syndrome may

Table 28.1 Myopia syndromes

Syndrome	Systemic features	Ocular features
Aberfeld syndrome (Schwartz-Jampel-Aberfeld syndrome) [49]	Myotonic myopathy, bone dysplasia, joint contractures, dwarfism	Blepharophimosis, long eyelashes, myopia
Achard syndrome [50]	Dysostoses, joint laxity limited to hands and feet, arachnodactyly, short mandibular rami	Strabismus, spherophakia, ectopia lentis, coloboma, and cataract
Beals-Hecht syndrome [51–53]	Contractual arachnodactyly, marfanoid habit, scoliosis, crumpled ears	Blue sclera, lens coloboma, ciliary body, hypoplasia, glaucoma, high myopia
Chromosome 18 partial deletion syndrome (de Grouchy syndrome) [54]	Retardation, dwarfism, hypotonia, hearing impairment, foot deformities, microcephaly	Myopia
Cohen syndrome [55, 56]	Dwarfism, delayed puberty, mental retardation, microcephaly, obesity, hypotony	Microphthalmia, pigmentary chorioretinal dystrophy, myopia
Congenital external ophthalmoplegia [57, 58]	None	Congenital nonprogressive restrictive external ophthalmoplegia and ptosis
Cornelia de Lange syndrome [59, 60]	Delayed growth and dwarfism, mental retardation, microcephaly, limb abnormalities, hirsutism with typical synophrys, hypoplastic genitalia	Ptosis, nystagmus, high myopia
Donnai-Barrow syndrome [61]	Craniofacial anomalies, deafness, low molecular weight proteinuria, congenital diaphragmatic hernia, omphalocele, brain anomalies	High myopia, hypertelorism, coloboma, cataracts, retinal detachment
Emanuel syndrome [62]	Craniofacial dysmorphism, intellectual disability, facial asymmetry, ear abnormalities, micrognathia, kidney abnormalities, congenital heart defects, male genital abnormalities,	High myopia, juvenile open angle glaucoma, hypertelorism, strabismus, unilateral ptosis, Duane syndrome, optic atrophy, cataract, nystagmus
Fabry disease [63–65]	Acroparesthesia, proteinuria and renal failure, angiokeratomas, hypertension, cardiomyopathy	Cornea verticillate, posterior spoke-like cataract, papilledema or optic atrophy, and retinal vascular dilation, conjunctival ampulliform vessel dilatations, myopia
Fetal alcohol syndrome [66, 67]	Growth deficiency, smooth philtrum, thin vermilion and blepharophimosis, neurologic damage	Strabismus, optic nerve hypoplasia, myopia
Forsius-Eriksson syndrome (Aland island disease) [68]	None	Hypopigmentation of the ocular fundus, progressive axial myopia, nystagmus, and dyschromatopsia
Gillum-Anderson syndrome [69]	None	Ptosis, high myopia, and ectopia lentis
Haney-Falls syndrome [70]	Mental retardation, delayed growth, brachydactyly	Posterior keratoconus posticus circumscriptus, myopia
Hereditary ectodermal dysplasia syndrome [71–73]	Abnormalities of two or more ectodermal structures (hairs, nails, teeth, skin)	Xerophthalmia, madarosis, increased periorbital pigmentation, cataracts, myopia
Kartagener syndrome [74–76]	Situs inversus (dextrocardia), chronic sinusitis, bronchiectasis and hypoacousia due to primary ciliary dyskinesia	Retinitis pigmentosa
Kenny syndrome [77, 78]	Dwarfism, cortical thickening of tubular bones, variable anomalies of the calvaria, prominent forehead, midfacial dysplasia, anemia, transient hypoparathyroidism	Microphthalmia, high myopia or hyperopia
Kniest's disease [79, 80]	Dwarfism, enlarged joints with pain and restricted movement, kyphoscoliosis, platyspondyly, round flat face, hypoacousia	Myopia
Laurence-Moon-Bardet-Biedl syndrome [81–84]	Mental retardation, obesity, polydactyly, hypogenitalism, diabetes insipidus, renal dysfunction, seizures	Retinitis pigmentosa, coloboma, nystagmus, and myopia
Loeys-Dietz syndrome [85]	Cerebral, thoracic, and abdominal arterial aneurysm and dissection, craniofacial dysmorphologies, skeletal abnormalities	Myopia, ectopia lentis, thin central corneal thickness, cataract, retinal detachment, blue or dusk sclera
Marchesani syndrome (Weill-Marchesani syndrome) [86, 87]	Brachycephaly, brachydactyly, stiff joints	Microspherophakia and ectopia lentis, myopia
Marshall syndrome [88]	Micrognathia, cleft palate, joint hyperelasticity and arthritis, hypoacousia	Myopia, cataract

(continued)

Table 28.1 (continued)

Syndrome	Systemic features	Ocular features
Matsoukas syndrome (Matsoukas-Liarikos-Giannika syndrome) [89]	Dwarfism, mental retardation, joint hyperelasticity, micrognathia	Myopia
McCune-Albright syndrome [90, 91]	Polyostotic fibrous dysplasia of the legs, arms and skull, precocious puberty, unilateral café au lait spots	Myopia, compressive optic neuropathy
Meyer-Schwickerath and Weyers (oculodentodigital) syndrome [92, 93]	Microdontia and anodontia, syndactyly, brittle nails, hypoplastic alae nasi, microcephaly, dysarthria, spastic paraparesis, seizures, hypotrichosis, hypoacousia	Microphthalmos, microcornea, fine, porous spongy abnormalities of the iris, cataract, glaucoma, optic atrophy, high myopia
Noonan syndrome [94–96]	Dwarfism, mental retardation, pterygium coli, pulmonary valvular stenosis, posterior cervical hygroma, amegakaryocytic thrombocytopenia, Arnold-Chiari malformation, scoliosis	High myopia
Obesity-cerebral-ocular-skeletal anomalies syndrome [97]	Obesity, hypotonia, mental retardation, microcephaly, hyperextensibility at elbows and proximal interphalangeal joints and syndactyly	Microphthalmia, strabismus, coloboma, prominent choroidal vessels, high myopia
Pierre Robin syndrome [98, 99]	Micrognathia, glossoptosis, cleft palate	Association with Sticker's syndrome, myopia, strabismus, Möbius syndrome, nasolacrimal duct obstruction, glaucoma, cataract, microphthalmos, choroidal coloboma, retinal detachment
Prader-Willi syndrome [100, 101]	Hypotonia, hypogonadism, lethargy, scoliosis, obesity, mental retardation	Esotropic strabismus, myopia
Riley-Day syndrome (familial dysautonomia) [102, 103]	Global failure in autonomic functions with anhidrosis, hypotension, decreased lacrimation, hypoesthesia, dysphagia, dysarthria, scoliosis	Xerophthalmia, myopia
Rubinstein-Taybi syndrome (broad thumb-hallux syndrome) [80, 104, 105]	Short stature, broad thumbs and broad first toes, mental retardation, increased risk for cancer	Lacrimal duct obstruction, corneal abnormalities, myopia, glaucoma, cataract
Schwartz syndrome (Schwartz-Jampel syndrome) [106, 107]	Short stature, myotonic dystrophy, blepharophimosis, puckered facial appearance, skeletal dysplasia and joint rigidity	Myopia
Tuomaala-Haapanen syndrome [108]	Dwarfism, short fingers and toes, wide nose bridge, small maxilla, oxycephaly, cutaneous depigmentation alopecia, micrognathia, anodontia	Antimongoloid lid fissures, distichiasis, nystagmus, strabismus, myopia, cataract, foveal hypoplasia
Van Bogaert-Hozay syndrome [109]	Mental retardation, atrophic skin, micrognathia, ear abnormalities, arrested growth of extremities and acrocyanosis, aplastic fingers and toes	High myopia, ptosis, strabismus
Wrinkly skin syndrome [110, 111]	Mental retardation, dwarfism, wrinkled skin, hypotonia, microcephaly	Cataract, myopia, and strabismus

exhibit particular characteristics classified as type 1 (in which vitreous is not properly produced resulting in an empty appearance with a retrolental vestigial remnant) and type 2 in which the vitreous gel appears beaded and fibrous [121]. Stickler syndrome has four main identified mutations: COL2A1 (75%), COL11A1, COL11A2 (non-ocular Stickler), and COL9A1 (autosomal recessive variant) [122]. Systemic features of Stickler syndrome include flattened facial appearance (with a frequent association with the Pierre-Robin sequence), joint hyperelasticity and arthritis, micrognathia, and hypoacusia [99, 123]. A closely related variant is Wagner syndrome, which is typically characterized by an "empty" vitreous gel that lacks the normal structure. This is due to a defect in chondroitin sulfate proteoglycan-2, a component of the vitreous, resulting from a defect in the versican gene. In contrast to Stickler syndrome, Wagner syn-

drome does not exhibit systemic manifestations and has a lower incidence of retinal detachment; however, high myopia is a common finding [123]. Since the described mutations resulting in Wagner syndrome alter different vitreous components as compared to Stickler syndrome, their effect on adhesions at the vitreoretinal interface may differ and partly explain the differing incidence of retinal detachment. In Stickler and Wagner syndromes, the abnormal vitreous likely plays a large role in the associated high refractive myopia, in contrast to the high axial myopia that can be seen with Ehlers-Danlos syndrome. Furthermore, Van der Hoeve syndrome, a subtype of osteogenesis imperfecta characterized by blue sclera, brittle bones, and conductive deafness, is associated with high axial myopia [124, 125]. A strong association was also reported (as high as 43% [126]) between juvenile idiopathic arthritis and myopia. Chronic inflammation has been hypothesized to weaken the scleral connective tissue and predispose eyes to a myopic state [126, 127]. Also, in tilted disc syndrome, posterior ectasia at the conus is thought to contribute to the moderate and high axial myopia found in these patients [128–130].

Myopia has also been associated with inborn errors of metabolism. Gyrate atrophy, due to autosomal recessive inherited mutations in the OAT gene resulting in hyperornithinemia, is characterized by nyctalopia, high axial myopia (>26 mm), capsular cataract, and typical chorioretinal atrophic patches in the midperipheral retina [131–135]. Homocystinuria syndrome, also known as cystathionine beta synthase deficiency, is an inherited disorder of methionine metabolism resulting in increased serum and urine levels of homocysteine that results in mental retardation, seizures, dolichostenomelia, and extensive atheroma. High refractive error may be a presenting sign of homocystinuria, allowing earlier diagnosis, implementation of appropriate management and avoidance of thromboembolic complications in patients with homocystinuria syndrome. In contrast to the axial myopia that may be seen with gyrate atrophy, the high myopia in homocystinuria is usually associated with a typical downward subluxation or luxation of the lens [136, 137].

Approximately 25% of Down syndrome patients develop myopia [138–141]. Due to a trisomy, systemic features typically include mental retardation, delayed growth, microgenia, epicanthus, hypotonia, flat nasal bridge, macroglossia, and atrioventricular septal defects. Other associated ocular findings include strabismus, cataract, glaucoma, keratoconus, and iris peripheral brushfield spots. Additionally, animal studies suggest albino subjects are predisposed to induced form-deprivation myopia [142, 143], and a few case reports and series support this link [144].

28.4　Drug-Induced Myopia

Drug-induced myopia has been reported throughout the years and, fortunately, tends to be almost uniformly transient. The clinical picture stereotypically includes the onset of symptoms 1–2 days following initiation of the drug and lasts for 2–8 days after discontinuation of the inciting medication [145]. Sulfonamides, sulfonamide-derivatives, and anti-epileptics are the most commonly cited drugs, with the level of induced myopia ranging from −0.75 to −8 diopters (D) [146]. Moreover, in most cases, shallowing of the anterior chamber has been observed, leading to acute, angle-closure glaucoma, requiring emergent intervention to prevent permanent vision loss, including immediate discontinuation of the offending drug, instillation of intraocular pressure-lowering drugs, and consideration of peripheral iridotomy.

Retinal edema and central radial folds have also been observed [146], as have choroidal detachments [147].

28.4.1　Proposed Mechanisms of Drug-Induced Myopia

The mechanism of drug-induced myopia is still under debate [148, 149] and may differ depending on the particular inciting drug. There is growing evidence that supports choroidal effusion as the postulated mechanism based on ultrasound studies that demonstrate choroidal effusions [150] and ciliochoroidal effusions with resultant anterior shift of the lens and only minimal thickening of the crystalline lens [151–154]. Spasm of accommodation and anterior shift of the lens-iris diaphragm (from ciliary body swelling or choroidal effusion) and increased curvature of the lens surface (due to ciliary body swelling or lenticular swelling) have also been reported [149, 155, 156].

Ciliary, or accommodative, spasm was hypothesized to be the cause in a case of equine anti-lymphocytic globulin-induced myopia. This was based on the fact that there was complete resolution with cycloplegia [157, 158]. However, some authors noted that instillation of cycloplegics oftentimes does not completely abolish the refractive error change in drug-induced myopia, suggesting additional mechanisms are involved [159–161]. Ciliary body edema has been theorized to be the cause of anterior ciliary body rotation with exaggerated zonule relaxation leading to lenticular thickening and anterior lens movement [145, 161, 162]. It is postulated to arise from either allergic [162–166] or non-allergic mechanisms (such as from supraciliary effusion) [145]. Specifically, Krieg and Schipper proposed that an imbalance in eicosanoids (prostaglandin-thromboxane-leukotriene) metabolism [145] can lead to ciliary body edema in the absence of a systemic allergic response [150, 166].

Alternatively, choroidal effusion is a postulated mechanism based on ultrasound studies that showed choroidal effusions [167] and ciliochoroidal effusions with resultant anterior shift of the lens and only minimal thickening of the crystalline lens [151–154]. Jampolsky and Flom estimated that a reduction in anterior chamber depth from 3.0 to 0.5 mm is capable of effecting a −3.3 D change in refraction [151]. Some authors support the role of lens thickening in drug-induced myopia, especially in the cases where diuretics are the inciting agent, since osmotic movements could potentially play a major role [148, 152, 161, 168]. Jampolsky and Flom also suggested possible mechanisms in addition to those focused on changes in the crystalline lens and ciliary body [151]. They postulated that transient drug-induced myopia might be due to changes to the media and sclera, such as changes to refractive index of media, differential changes in the refractive index of the vitreous and aqueous (due to varying sugar levels), and stretching of the sclera.

28.4.2 Differentiating Between Mechanisms

The mechanism of drug-induced myopia has been explored in the past via several methods. A test of cycloplegia has been employed to determine if myopia is corrected in cases where accommodative or ciliary spasm is the suspected etiologic mechanism. Imaging also plays an important role in teasing out possible etiologic mechanisms. Ultrasound biomicroscopy (UBM, Fig. 28.2) and anterior-segment optical coherence tomography (AS-OCT, Fig. 28.3) can allow for higher resolution imaging, focused more anteriorly than B-scan ultrasound, which is useful when examining for ciliary body edema, anterior rotation of the ciliary body, or ciliochoroidal effusion. These mechanisms usually occur to various degrees simultaneously.

28.4.3 Drugs Reported to Induce Myopia

Transient myopia from drugs was reported as early as 1952 by Mattsson, who reported over 50 references due to sulfon-

amides [169]. In 1960, Muirhead and Scheie reported eight cases of transient myopia from sulfonamide acetazolamide [170]. This was shortly followed by reports of transient myopia from carbonic anhydrase inhibitors such as ethoxolamide [171], sulfonamide-derived antihypertensive diuretics such as hydrochlorothiazide [172], chlorthalidone [173], and prochlorperazine [174]. Although transient drug-induced myopia is rare, the list of drugs that have been reported to induce myopia is extensive. Some of these drugs are listed below in Table 28.2, with their corresponding references.

Among the drugs reported in the literature, the most frequently cited family of drugs include the sulfonamides (including sulfonamide derivatives (Table 28.3) found in carbonic anhydrase inhibitors [147, 170, 171, 175, 176, 201], antihypertensives particularly diuretics [150, 166, 186, 193], diabetic drugs [191], and trimethoprim-sulfamethoxazole antibiotics [161, 183]) and anti-epileptics (especially topiramate) [155, 167, 211, 216–221]. Autonomic blocking agents (beta-blockers [184] and adrenergic agents [177]) and nonsteroidal anti-inflammatory drugs [181, 182, 200, 203] have also been reported to induce myopia. Nitrates, such as isosorbide dinitrate, are commonly reported to cause transient myopia [194]. A selective serotonin agonist, zolmitriptan, has been recently reported to cause transient myopia through ciliochoroidal effusion that has been postulated to induce

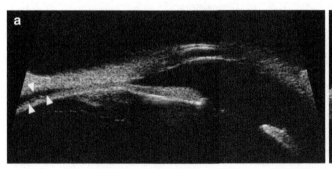
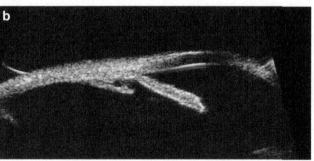

Fig. 28.2 Ultrasound biomicroscopy (UBM) image showing choroidal effusion (arrowheads) with ciliary body edema and anterior rotation of the iris in a 29-year-old, male complaining of blurring of vision after phentermine-topiramate intake (**a**). UBM image 2 weeks after discon-

tinuation of drug shows resolution of the choroidal effusion (**b**). (Courtesy of Dr. Thasarat S. Vajaranant, M.D. and Dr. Ronald H. Silverman, Ph.D.)

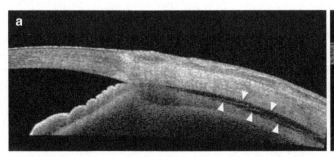
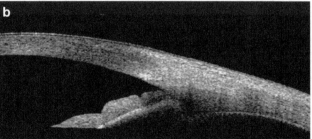

Fig. 28.3 Anterior segment optical coherence tomography (AS-OCT) image showing choroidal effusion (arrowheads) (**a**). AS-OCT image showing the absence of choroidal effusion (**b**). (Courtesy of Dr. Shamira Perera, MBBS, FRCOphth)

Table 28.2 Drugs reported to induce myopia

Drug	Reference
Acetazolamide	[147, 170, 175, 176]
Adrenergic blockers (hydralazine, hexamethonium)	[177]
Amisulpride	[178]
Aripiprazole	[179, 180]
Aspirin	[181, 182]
Bactrim (trimethoprim-sulfonamide)	[163, 164, 183]
Beta-blockers (betaxolol, timolol)	[184]
Bimatoprost	[158]
Bromocriptine	[185]
Carbachol	[148]
Chlorthalidone	[145, 173, 186, 187]
Corticosteroids	[188]
Cyclophosphamide	[189]
Ethoxzolamide	[171]
Flecainide	[190]
Glibenclamide	[191]
Hydrochlorothiazide	[150, 172, 192]
Indapamide	[193]
Isosorbide dinitrate	[194]
Isotretinoin, etretinate	[195–197]
Lamotrigine	[198]
Levomepromazine	[199]
Mefenamic acid (and other NSAIDs, i.e., ibuprofen)	[200]
Methazolamide	[201]
Metronidazole	[202]
Olsalazine	[203]
Opioids (codeine, morphine)	[204]
Oral contraceptives	[205]
Penicillamine	[206]
Phenformin	[207]
Phenothiazines	[165, 199]
Physostigmine	[208]
Pilocarpine	[161]
Prochlorperazine	[174]
Promethazine	[165, 168]
Quinine	[209]
Spironolactone	[168, 210]
Succinimide anti-epileptics (ethosuximide, methsuximide, phensuximide)	[211]
Sulfonamides (sulfasalazine)	[152, 155, 156, 161, 162, 164, 169, 212, 213]
Tetracyclines	[214]
Timolol	[215]
Topiramate	[149, 167, 216–221]
Zanamivir	[222]
Zolmitriptan	[153]

anterior displacement of the ciliary processes, forward rotation of the lens-iris diaphragm, and concomitant angle closure [153]. Another antipsychotic medication, aripiprazole, a quinolone derivative agonist of dopamine and serotonin, has been reported to cause transient myopic shift with shallowing of the anterior chamber [179, 180]. Zanamivir, an inhaled neuraminidase inhibitor, has also been reported to cause a

transient myopic shift that resolves spontaneously after discontinuation of the drug [222]. Moreover, isotretinoin, a first-generation non-aromatic retinoid beta-carotene, has also been reported to cause angle closure and transient myopic shift, which was documented by ultrasound biomicroscopy showing a supraciliary effusion with shallow anterior chamber [195]. Bimatoprost, a prostaglandin analogue used as an ocular hypotensive, has been reported to cause pseudomyopia due to accommodative spasm and its direct effect on the ciliary body [158].

28.4.3.1 Sulfonamides

The functional group of sulfonamide is $-S(=O)2-NH2$, a sulfonyl group connected to an amine group. Sulfonamides are commonly used in medicine for a variety of purposes, such as sulfasalazine, which has been reported to induce myopia when used for rheumatoid arthritis [212, 226]. This class of drugs has been reported to cause uveoscleral effusion with anterior rotation of the ciliary body resulting to transient myopia and angle closure [226]. However, it is oftentimes not apparent that a drug is a sulfonamide or a sulfonamide-derived chemical based on the drug name, especially when present as a component of a combination drug [225]. Table 28.3 lists the generic and brand name of commonly encountered sulfonamide and sulfonamide-derived drugs.

28.4.3.2 Anti-epileptics

Anti-epileptics have been cited as inducing myopia, in particular topiramate, but also others (i.e., succinimides: ethosuximide, methsuximide, and phensuximide) [148, 167, 211, 216–221]. Topiramate is a sulfamate-substituted monosaccharide containing a $-O-S(=O)2-NH2$ group that is used for partial-onset seizures. Since there is an adjacent oxygen atom, instead of a carbon atom (as is the case in a sulfonamide, see above), the sulfur is in a different oxidation state. The sulfamates and sulfonamides are still bioisosteres of each other and therefore function similarly as drugs. Fraunfelder et al. reported a case series of 115 patients with ocular affects from topiramate that included abnormal vision, acute intraocular pressure elevation, acute myopia, diplopia at high doses, nystagmus at high doses, and shallow anterior chamber with angle closure [148]. They also noted probable associations with blepharospasm, myokymia, oculogyric crisis, and suprachoroidal effusions. Specifically, they noted 17 cases of acute bilateral myopia up to −8.75 diopters, 9 cases of suprachoroidal effusion, and 86 cases of acute-onset glaucoma. Acute myopia occurred from a matter of hours after starting topiramate but could take weeks to fully resolve on or off medication. The mechanism of topiramate-induced myopia is under debate but has been suggested to include lenticular swelling [221], forward rotation of the lens-iris diaphragm [167, 219, 220], ciliary body swelling causing increased curva-

Table 28.3 Examples of sulfonamide and sulfonamide-derived medications

Drug	Generic	Brand name
Anti-epileptics	Topiramate [148, 149, 167, 216–221] Zonisamide	Topamax Zonegran
Antihypertensives		
Thiazide diuretics	Hydrochlorothiazide (HCTZ) [150, 172, 192] Metolazone	Zaroxolyn
Combination antihypertensives		
Diuretic combo	Triamterene [150] and HCTZ [150, 172, 192] Spironolactone and HCTZ [150, 172, 192]	Dyazide, Maxzide, Aldactazide
B-blocker and diuretic	Atenolol and chlorthalidone [145, 173, 186, 187] Bisoprolol and HCTZ [150, 172, 192]	Tenoretic Ziac
ACE inhibitor and diuretic	Lisinopril and HCTZ [150, 172, 192] Enalapril and HCTZ [150, 172, 192]	Zestoretic Vaseretic
Angiotensin II receptor	Losartan and HCTZ [150, 172, 192]	Hyzaar
Antagonist and diuretic	Valsartan and HCTZ [150, 172, 192] Irbesartan and HCTZ [150, 172, 192]	Diovan Avalide
Loop diuretics	Furosemide [223]	Lasix
Carbonic anhydrase inhibitor	Acetazolamide [147, 170, 175, 176] Methazolamide [201]	Diamox Neptazane
Diabetic medications		
Sulfonylureas [191]	Glipizide Glimepiride Glyburide	Glucotrol Amaryl Diabeta
Antimicrobials	Sulfadiazine [213] Sulfamethoxazole/trimethoprim [163, 164, 183]	Bactrim
Anti-inflammatory	Sulfasalazine [212]	Azulfidine
Other medications	Celecoxib [224] Valdecoxib [224]	Celebrex Bextra

Adapted from Lee et al. [225]

ture of the lens surfaces [216], and spasm of accommodation [148]. Additionally, recent reports using imaging (UBM, AS-OCT, and MRI) demonstrate that topiramate can cause ciliochoroidal effusion resulting in anterior displacement of the lens-iris diaphragm with concomitant angle closure [154, 227].

References

1. Wiesel TE, Raviola E. Myopia and eye enlargement after neonatal lid fusion in monkeys. Nature. 1977;266:66–8.
2. Sherman SM, Norton TT, Casagrande VA. Myopia in the lid sutured tree shrew (Tupaia glis). Brain Res. 1977;124:154–7.
3. Kirby AW, Sutton L, Weiss AH. Elongation of cat eyes following neonatal lid suture. Invest Ophthalmol Vis Sci. 1982;22:274–7.
4. Raviola E, Wiesel TN. An animal model of myopia. N Engl J Med. 1985;312:1609–16.
5. Lauber JK, Oishi T. Lid suture myopia in chicks. Invest Ophthalmol Vis Sci. 1987;28:1851–8.
6. Diether S, Schaeffel F. Local changes in eye growth induced by imposed local refractive error despite active accommodation. Vis Res. 1997;37(6):659–68.
7. Kaufman L Jr. Pediatric tumors of the eye and orbit. Pediatr Clin N Am. 2003;50(1):149–72.
8. McBrien NA, Cornell LM, Gentle A. Structural and ultrastructural changes to the sclera in a mammalian model of high myopia. Invest Ophthalmol Vis Sci. 2001;42(10):2179–87.
9. Avetisov ES, Savitskaya NF, Vinetskaya MI, Iomdina EN. A study of biochemical and biomechanical qualities of normal and myopic eye sclera in humans of different age groups. Metab Pediatr Syst Ophthalmol. 1983;7(4):183–8.
10. Wollensak G, Iomdina E. Crosslinking of scleral collagen in the rabbit using glyceraldehyde. J Cataract Refract Surg. 2008;34(4):651–6.
11. McBrien NA, Lawlor P, Gentle A. Scleral remodeling during the development of and recovery from axial myopia in the tree shrew. Invest Ophthalmol Vis Sci. 2000;41:3713–9.
12. Norton TT, Rada JA. Reduced extracellular matrix in mammalian sclera with induced myopia. Vis Res. 1995;35(9):1271–81.
13. Weiss AH. Unilateral high myopia: optical components, associated factors, and visual outcomes. Br J Ophthalmol. 2003;87(8):1025–31.
14. Johnson CA, Post RB, Chalupa LM, Lee TJ. Monocular deprivation in humans: a study of identical twins. Invest Ophthalmol Vis Sci. 1982;23(1):135–8.
15. Wildsoet CF, Schmid KL. Optical correction of form deprivation myopia inhibits refractive recovery in chick eyes with intact or sectioned optic nerves. Vis Res. 2000;40(23):3273–82.
16. Hoyt CS, Stone RD, Fromer C, Billson FA. Monocular axial myopia associated with neonatal eyelid closure in human infants. Am J Ophthalmol. 1981;91(2):197–200.
17. von Noorden GK, Lewis RA. Ocular axial length in unilateral congenital cataracts and blepharoptosis. Invest Ophthalmol Vis Sci. 1987;28(4):750–2.
18. Castillo BV Jr, Kaufman L. Pediatric tumors of the eye and orbit. Pediatr Clin N Am. 2003;50(1):149–72.
19. Robb RM. Refractive errors associated with hemangiomas of the eyelids and orbit in infancy. Am J Ophthalmol. 1977;83(1):52–8.

20. Gee SS, Tabbara KF. Increase in ocular axial length in patients with corneal opacification. Ophthalmology. 1988;95(9):1276–8.
21. Mahler O, Hoffman P, Pollack A, Marcovich A. Increase in posterior segment depth in eyes with corneal opacities. Harefuah. 2006;145(3):202–4, 245.
22. Wiesel TN, Raviola E. Increase in axial length of the macaque monkey after corneal opacification. Invest Ophthalmol Vis Sci. 1979;18:1232–6.
23. Miller-Meeks MJ, Bennett SR, Keech RV, Blodi CF. Myopia induced by vitreous hemorrhage. Am J Ophthalmol. 1990;109(2):199–203.
24. Yesou C, Poletti J. Posterior scleral ectasis. Bull Soc Ophtalmol Fr. 1990;90(3):349–52.
25. Ernst BJ, Hsu HY. Keratoconus association with axial myopia: a prospective biometric study. Eye Contact Lens. 2011;37(1):2–5.
26. Tuft SJ, Fitzke FW, Buckley RJ. Myopia following penetrating keratoplasty for keratoconus. Br J Ophthalmol. 1992;76(11):642–5.
27. Touzeau O, Scheer S, Allouch C, Borderie V, Laroche L. The relationship between keratoconus and axial myopia. J Fr Ophtalmol. 2004;27(7):765–71.
28. Sohajda Z, Holló D, Berta A, Módis L. Microcornea associated with myopia. Graefes Arch Clin Exp Ophthalmol. 2006;244(9):1211–3.
29. Batra DV, Paul SD. Microcornea with myopia. Br J Ophthalmol. 1967;51(1):57–60.
30. Hewitt AW, Kearns LS, Jamieson RV, Williamson KA, van Heyningen V, Mackey DA. PAX6 mutations may be associated with high myopia. Ophthalmic Genet. 2007;28(3):179–82.
31. Valenzuela A, Cline RA. Ocular and nonocular findings in patients with aniridia. Can J Ophthalmol. 2004;39(6):632–8.
32. Zhong XW, Ge J, Deng WG, Chen XL, Huang J. Expression of pax-6 in rhesus monkey of optical defocus induced myopia and form deprivation myopia. Chin Med J. 2004;117(5):722–6.
33. Ashby RS, Megaw PL, Morgan IG. Changes in the expression of Pax6 RNA transcripts in the retina during periods of altered ocular growth in chickens. Exp Eye Res. 2009;89(3):392–7.
34. Price MJ, Judisch GF, Thompson HS. X-linked congenital stationary night blindness with myopia and nystagmus without clinical complaints of nyctalopia. J Pediatr Ophthalmol Strabismus. 1988;25(1):33–6.
35. Haim M, Fledelius HC, Skarsholm. X-linked myopia in Danish family. Acta Ophthalmol. 1988;66(4):450–6.
36. Schubert G, Bornschein H. Analysis of the human electroretinogram. Ophthalmologica. 1952;123(6):396–413.
37. Miyake Y, Yagasaki K, Horiguchi M, et al. Congenital stationary night blindness with negative electroretinogram: a new classification. Arch Ophthalmol. 1986;104(7):1013–20.
38. Mäntyjärvi M, Tuppurainen K. Progressive cone-rod dystrophy and high myopia in a Finnish family. Acta Ophthalmol. 1989;67(3):234–42.
39. François J, Verriest G, Matton-Van Leuven T, De Rouck A, Manavian D. Atypical achromatopia of sex-linked recessive inheritance. Am J Ophthalmol. 1966;61(5 Pt 2):1101–8.
40. Kaplan J, Bonneau D, Frézal J, Munnich A, Dufier JL. Clinical and genetic heterogeneity in retinitis pigmentosa. Hum Genet. 1990;85(6):635–42.
41. Bende P, Natarajan K, Marudhamuthu T, Madhavan J. Severity of familial isolated retinitis pigmentosa across different inheritance patterns among an Asian Indian cohort. J Pediatr Ophthalmol Strabismus. 2013;50(1):34–6.
42. Schwartz M, Haim M, Skarsholm D. X-linked myopia: Bornholm eye disease. Linkage to DNA markers on the distal part of Xq. Clin Genet. 1990;38(4):281–6.
43. Metlapally R, Michaelides M, Bulusu A, Li YJ, Schwartz M, Rosenberg T, Hunt DM, Moore AT, Züchner S, Rickman CB, Young TL. Evaluation of the X-linked high-grade myopia locus

(MYP1) with cone dysfunction and color vision deficiencies. Invest Ophthalmol Vis Sci. 2009;50(4):1552–8.
44. Nissenkorn I, Yassur Y, Mashkowski D, Sherf I, Ben-Sira I. Myopia in premature babies with and without retinopathy of prematurity. Br J Ophthalmol. 1983;67(3):170–3.
45. Quinn GE, Dobson V, Davitt BV, Hardy RJ, Tung B, Pedroza C, Good WV, Early Treatment for Retinopathy of Prematurity Cooperative Group. Progression of myopia and high myopia in the early treatment for retinopathy of prematurity study: findings to 3 years of age. Ophthalmology. 2008;115(6):1058–64.e1.
46. Quinn GE, Dobson V, Siatkowski R, Hardy RJ, Kivlin J, Palmer EA, Phelps DL, Repka MX, Summers CG, Tung B, Chan W, Cryotherapy for Retinopathy of Prematurity Cooperative Group. Does cryotherapy affect refractive error? Results from treated versus control eyes in the cryotherapy for retinopathy of prematurity trial. Ophthalmology. 2001;108(2):343–7.
47. Harder BC, Schlichtenbrede FC, von Baltz S, Jendritza W, Jendritza B, Jonas JB. Intravitreal bevacizumab for retinopathy of prematurity: refractive error results. Am J Ophthalmol. 2013;155(6):1119–24.e1.
48. Takahashi H, Takase H, Terada Y, Mochizuki M, Ohno-Matsui K. Acquired myopia in Vogt-Koyanagi-Harada disease. Int Ophthalmol. 2019;39(3):521–31.
49. Nessler M, Puchala J, Kwiatkowski S, Kobylarz K, Mojsa I, Chrapusta-Klimeczek A. Multidisciplinary approach to the treatment of a patient with chondrodystrophic myotonia (Schwartz-Jampel vel Aberfeld syndrome): case report and literature review. Ann Plast Surg. 2011;67(3):315–9.
50. Duncan PA. The Achard syndrome. Birth Defects Orig Artic Ser. 1975;11(6):69–73.
51. Jones JL, Lane JE, Logan JJ, Vanegas ME. Beals-Hecht syndrome. South Med J. 2002;95(7):753–5.
52. Tunçbilek E, Alanay Y. Congenital contractural arachnodactyly (Beals syndrome). Orphanet J Rare Dis. 2006;1:20.
53. Gallego-Pinazo R, López-Lizcano R, Millán JM, Arevalo JF, Mullor JL, Díaz-Llopis M. Beals-Hecht syndrome and choroidal neovascularization. Clin Ophthalmol. 2010;4:845–7.
54. Izquierdo NJ, Maumenee IH, Traboulsi EI. Anterior segment malformations in 18q- (de Grouchy) syndrome. Ophthalmic Paediatr Genet. 1993;14(2):91–4.
55. Kivitie-Kallio S, Norio R. Cohen syndrome: essential features, natural history, and heterogeneity. Am J Med Genet. 2001;102(2):125–35.
56. Douzgou S, Petersen MB. Clinical variability of genetic isolates of Cohen syndrome. Clin Genet. 2011;79(6):501–6.
57. Mace JW, Sponaugle HD, Mitsunaga RY, Schanberger JE. Congenital hereditary nonprogressive external ophthalmoplegia. Am J Dis Child. 1971;122(3):261–3.
58. Houtman WA, van Weerden TW, Robinson PH, de Vries B, Hoogenraad TU. Hereditary congenital external ophthalmoplegia. Ophthalmologica. 1986;193(4):207–18.
59. Levin AV, Seidman DJ, Nelson LB, Jackson LG. Ophthalmologic findings in the Cornelia de Lange syndrome. J Pediatr Ophthalmol Strabismus. 1990;27(2):94–102.
60. Liu J, Baynam G. Cornelia de Lange syndrome. Adv Exp Med Biol. 2010;685:111–23.
61. Khalifa O, Al-Sahlawi Z, Imtiaz F, et al. Variable expression pattern in Donnai-Barrow syndrome – report of two novel LRP2 mutations and review of the literature. Eur J Med Genet. 2015;58(5):293–9.
62. Saffren BD, Capasso JE, Zanolli M, Levin AV. Ocular manifestations of Emanuel syndrome. Am J Med Genet A. 2018;176(9):1964–7.
63. Galanos J, Nicholls K, Grigg L, Kiers L, Crawford A, Becker G. Clinical features of Fabry's disease in Australian patients. Intern Med J. 2002;32(12):575–84.

64. Orssaud C, Dufier J, Germain D. Ocular manifestations in Fabry disease: a survey of 32 hemizygous male patients. Ophthalmic Genet. 2003;24(3):129–39.

65. Nguyen TT, Gin T, Nicholls K, Low M, Galanos J, Crawford A. Ophthalmological manifestations of Fabry disease: a survey of patients at the Royal Melbourne Fabry Disease Treatment Centre. Clin Exp Ophthalmol. 2005;33(2):164–8.

66. Strömland K, Pinazo-Durán MD. Ophthalmic involvement in the fetal alcohol syndrome: clinical and animal model studies. Alcohol Alcohol. 2002;37(1):2–8.

67. Hiratsuka Y, Li G. Alcohol and eye diseases: a review of epidemiologic studies. J Stud Alcohol. 2001;62(3):397–402.

68. O'Donnell FE, Green WR, McKusick VA, Forsius H, Eriksson AW. Forsius-Eriksson syndrome: its relation to the Nettleship-Falls X-linked ocular albinism. Clin Genet. 1980;17(6):403–8.

69. Gillum WN, Anderson RL. Dominantly inherited blepharoptosis, high myopia, and ectopia lentis. Arch Ophthalmol. 1982;100(2):282–4.

70. Haney WP, Falls HF. The occurrence of congenital keratoconus posticus circumscriptus in two siblings presenting a previously unrecognized syndrome. Am J Ophthalmol. 1961;52:53.

71. Gündüz K, Shields CL, Doych Y, Schnall B, Shields JA. Ocular ectodermal syndrome of epibulbar dermoid and cutaneous myxovascular hamartoma. Br J Ophthalmol. 2000;84(6):669–70.

72. Ekins MB, Waring GO III. Absent Meibomian glands and reduced corneal sensation in hypohidrotic ectodermal dysplasia. J Pediatr Ophthalmol Strabismus. 1981;18:44–7.

73. Freire MN, et al. A syndrome of hypohidrotic ectodermal dysplasia with normal teeth, peculiar facies, pigmentary disturbances, psychomotor and growth retardation, bilateral nuclear cataract, and other signs. J Med Genet. 1975;12:308–10.

74. Mossberg R. Immotile-cilia syndrome: clinical features. Eur J Respir Dis Suppl. 1982;118:111–5.

75. Davenport JR, Yoder BK. An incredible decade for the primary cilium: a look at a once-forgotten organelle. Am J Physiol Renal Physiol. 2005;289(6):F1159–69.

76. Krawczyński MR, Dmeńska H, Witt M. Apparent X-linked primary ciliary dyskinesia associated with retinitis pigmentosa and a hearing loss. J Appl Genet. 2004;45(1):107–10.

77. Majewski F, Rosendahl W, Ranke M, Nolte K. The Kenny syndrome, a rare type of growth deficiency with tubular stenosis, transient hypoparathyroidism and anomalies of refraction. Eur J Pediatr. 1981;136(1):21–30.

78. Tsai CE, Chiu PC, Lee ML. Kenny syndrome: case report and literature review. J Formos Med Assoc. 1996;95(10):793–7.

79. Maumenee IH, Traboulsi EI. The ocular findings in Kniest dysplasia. Am J Ophthalmol. 1985;100(1):155–60.

80. Bardelli AM, Lasorella G, Barberi L, Vanni M. Ocular manifestations in Kniest syndrome, Smith-Lemli-Opitz syndrome, Hallermann-Streiff-François syndrome, Rubinstein-Taybi syndrome and median cleft face syndrome. Ophthalmic Paediatr Genet. 1985;6(1–2):343–7.

81. Héon E, Westall C, Carmi R, Elbedour K, Panton C, Mackeen L, Stone EM, Sheffield VC. Ocular phenotypes of three genetic variants of Bardet-Biedl syndrome. Am J Med Genet A. 2005;132A(3):283–7.

82. Abd-El-Barr MM, Sykoudis K, Andrabi S, Eichers ER, Pennesi ME, Tan PL, Wilson JH, Katsanis N, Lupski JR, Wu SM. Impaired photoreceptor protein transport and synaptic transmission in a mouse model of Bardet–Biedl syndrome. Vis Res. 2007;47(27):3394–407.

83. Zaldivar RA, Neale MD, Evans WE, Pulido JS. Asymptomatic renal cell carcinoma as a finding of Bardet Biedl syndrome. Ophthalmic Genet. 2008;29(1):33–5.

84. Heon E, Kim G, Qin S, Garrison JE, Tavares E, Vincent A, Nuangchamnong N, Scott CA, Slusarski DC, Sheffield VC. Mutations in C8ORF37 cause Bardet Biedl syndrome (BBS21). Hum Mol Genet. 2016;25(11):2283–94.

85. Busch C, Voitl R, Goergen B, Zemojtel T, Gehle P, Salchow DJ. Ocular findings in Loeys-Dietz syndrome. Br J Ophthalmol. 2018;102(8):1036–40.

86. Evereklioglu C, Hepsen IF, Er H. Weill-Marchesani syndrome in three generations. Eye (Lond). 1999;13(Pt 6):773–7.

87. Faivre L, Dollfus H, Lyonnet S, Alembik Y, Mégarbané A, Samples J, Gorlin RJ, Alswaid A, Feingold J, Le Merrer M, Munnich A, Cormier-Daire V. Clinical homogeneity and genetic heterogeneity in Weill-Marchesani syndrome. Am J Med Genet A. 2003;123A(2):204–7.

88. Shanske AL, Bogdanow A, Shprintzen RJ, Marion RW. The Marshall syndrome: report of a new family and review of the literature. Am J Med Genet. 1997;70(1):52–7.

89. Matsoukas J, Liarikos S, Giannikas A, Agoropoulos Z, Papachristou G, Soukakos P. A newly recognized dominantly inherited syndrome: short stature, ocular and articular anomalies, mental retardation. Helv Paediatr Acta. 1973;28(5):383–6.

90. Bocca G, de Vries J, Cruysberg JR, Boers GH, Monnens LA. Optic neuropathy in McCune-Albright syndrome: an indication for aggressive treatment. Acta Paediatr. 1998;87(5):599–600.

91. Niwald A, Budzińska-Mikurenda M, Rogozińska-Zawiślak A, Mikołajczyk W, Niwald M, Grałek M. Visual symptoms in McCune-Albright syndrome--case report. Klin Ocz. 2006;108(1–3):131–3.

92. Braun M, Seitz B, Naumann GO. Juvenile open angle glaucoma with microcornea in oculo-dento-digital dysplasia (Meyer-Schwickerath-Weyers syndrome). Klin Monatsbl Augenheilkd. 1996;208(4):262–3.

93. Reich H. Meyer-Schwickerath-Weyers syndrome (oculo-dento-digital syndrome). Hautarzt. 1980;31(9):515.

94. Tartaglia M, Mehler EL, Goldberg R, Zampino G, Brunner HG, Kremer H, van der Burgt I, Crosby AH, Ion A, Jeffery S, Kalidas K, Patton MA, Kucherlapati RS, Gelb BD. Mutations in PTPN11, encoding the protein tyrosine phosphatase SHP-2, cause Noonan syndrome. Nat Genet. 2001;29(4):465–8.

95. Tartaglia M, Gelb BD, Zenker M. Noonan syndrome and clinically related disorders. Best Pract Res Clin Endocrinol Metab. 2011;25(1):161–79.

96. Marin Lda R, da Silva FT, de Sá LC, Brasil AS, Pereira A, Furquim IM, Kim CA, Bertola DR. Ocular manifestations of Noonan syndrome. Ophthalmic Genet. 2012;33(1):1–5.

97. Cohen MM Jr, Hall BD, Smith DW, Graham CB, Lampert KJ. A new syndrome with hypotonia, obesity, mental deficiency, and facial, oral, ocular, and limb anomalies. J Pediatr. 1973;83(2):280–4.

98. Huang F, Kuo HK, Hsieh CH, Lai JP, Chen PK. Visual complications of Stickler syndrome in paediatric patients with Robin sequence. J Craniomaxillofac Surg. 2007;35(2):76–80.

99. Witmer MT, Vasan R, Levy R, Davis J, Chan RV. Bilateral maculopathy associated with Pierre Robin sequence. J AAPOS. 2012;16(4):409–10.

100. Hered RW, Rogers S, Zang YF, Biglan AW. Ophthalmologic features of Prader-Willi syndrome. J Pediatr Ophthalmol Strabismus. 1988;25(3):145–50.

101. Wang XC, Norose K, Kiyosawa K, Segawa K. Ocular findings in a patient with Prader-Willi syndrome. Jpn J Ophthalmol. 1995;39(3):284–9.

102. Josaitis CA, Matisoff M. Familial dysautonomia in review: diagnosis and treatment of ocular manifestations. Adv Exp Med Biol. 2002;506(Pt A):71–80.

103. Mendoza-Santiesteban CE, Hedges TR 3rd, Norcliffe-Kaufmann L, Warren F, Reddy S, Axelrod FB. Clinical neuro-ophthalmic findings in familial dysautonomia. J Neuroophthalmol. 2012;32(1):23–6.

104. van Genderen MM, Kinds GF, Riemslag FC, Hennekam RC. Ocular features in Rubinstein-Taybi syndrome: investigation of 24 patients and review of the literature. Br J Ophthalmol. 2000;84(10):1177–84.

105. Kumar S, Suthar R, Panigrahi I, Marwaha RK. Rubinstein-Taybi syndrome: clinical profile of 11 patients and review of literature. Indian J Hum Genet. 2012;18(2):161–6.

106. Mallineni SK, Yiu CK, King NM. Schwartz-Jampel syndrome: a review of the literature and case report. Spec Care Dentist. 2012;32(3):105–11.

107. Arya R, Sharma S, Gupta N, Kumar S, Kabra M, Gulati S. Schwartz Jampel syndrome in children. J Clin Neurosci. 2013;20(2):313–7.

108. Tuomaala P, Haapanen E. Three siblings with similar anomalies in the eyes, bones and skin. Acta Ophthalmol. 1968;46(3):365–71.

109. Durner W. Van Bogaert-Hozay-syndrome. A case demonstration. Klin Monatsbl Augenheilkd. 1973;162(5):658–60.

110. Zlotgora J. Wrinkly skin syndrome and the syndrome of cutis laxa with growth and developmental delay represent the same disorder. Am J Med Genet. 1999;85(2):194.

111. Hamamy H, Masri A, Ajlouni K. Wrinkly skin syndrome. Clin Exp Dermatol. 2005;30(5):590–2.

112. Dietz HC, Saraiva JM, Pyeritz RE, Cutting GR, Francomano CA. Clustering of fibrillin (FBN1) missense mutations in Marfan syndrome patients at cysteine residues in EGF-like domains. Hum Mutat. 1992;1(5):366–74.

113. Nahum Y, Spierer A. Ocular features of Marfan syndrome: diagnosis and management. Isr Med Assoc J. 2008;10(3):179–81.

114. Gehle P, Goergen B, Pilger D, Ruokonen P, Robinson PN, Salchow DJ. Biometric and structural ocular manifestations of Marfan syndrome. PLoS One. 2017;12(9):e0183370.

115. Salchow DJ, Gehle P. Ocular manifestations of Marfan syndrome in children and adolescents. Eur J Ophthalmol. 2019;29(1):38–43.

116. Latasiewicz M, Fontecilla C, Millá E, Sánchez A. Marfan syndrome – ocular findings and novel mutations-in pursuit of genotype-phenotype associations. Can J Ophthalmol. 2016;51(2):113–8.

117. Drolsum L, Rand-Hendriksen S, Paus B, Geiran OR, Semb SO. Ocular findings in 87 adults with Ghent-1 verified Marfan syndrome. Acta Ophthalmol. 2015;93(1):46–53.

118. Konradsen TR, Zetterström C. A descriptive study of ocular characteristics in Marfan syndrome. Acta Ophthalmol. 2013;91(8):751–5.

119. De Paepe A, Malfait F. The Ehlers-Danlos syndrome, a disorder with many faces. Clin Genet. 2012;82(1):1–11.

120. Pemberton JW, Freeman HM, Schepens CL. Familial retinal detachment and the Ehlers-Danlos syndrome. Arch Ophthalmol. 1966;76(6):817–24.

121. Snead MP, Yates JR. Clinical and molecular genetics of Stickler syndrome. J Med Genet. 1999;36(5):353–9.

122. Snead MP, McNinch AM, Poulson AV, Bearcroft P, Silverman B, Gomersall P, Parfect V, Richards AJ. Stickler syndrome, ocular-only variants and a key diagnostic role for the ophthalmologist. Eye (Lond). 2011;25(11):1389–400.

123. Godel V, Nemet P, Lazar M. The Wagner-Stickler syndrome complex. Doc Ophthalmol. 1981;52(2):179–88.

124. Van der Hoeve J, de Kleyn A. Blaue Scleren, Knochenbrüchigkeit und Schwerhörigkeit. Arch Ophthalmol. 1918;95:81–93.

125. Alikadić-Husović A, Merhemić Z. The blue sclera syndrome (Van der Heave syndrome). Med Arh. 2000;54(5–6):325–6.

126. Fedelius H, Zak M, Pedersen FK. Refraction in juvenile chronic arthritis: a long-term follow-up study, with emphasis on myopia. Acta Ophthalmol Scand. 2001;79:237–9.

127. Herbort CP, Papadia M, Neri P. Myopia and inflammation. J Ophthalmic Vis Res. 2011;6(4):270–83.

128. Alexander LJ. The tilted disc syndrome. J Am Optom Assoc. 1978;49(9):1060–2.

129. Sowka J, Aoun P. Tilted disc syndrome. Optom Vis Sci. 1999;76(9):618–23.

130. Manor RS. Temporal field defects due to nasal tilting of discs. Ophthalmologica. 1974;168(4):269–81.

131. Bangal S, Bhandari A, Dhaytadak P, Gogri P. Gyrate atrophy of choroid and retina with myopia, cataract and systemic proximal myopathy: a rare case report from rural India. Australas Med J. 2012;5(12):639–42.

132. Shenoi A. L N, Christopher R. Hyperornithinemia associated with gyrate atrophy of the choroid and retina in a child with myopia. Indian Pediatr. 2001;38(8):914–8.

133. Valle D, Kaiser-Kupfer M. Gyrate atrophy of the choroid and retina. Prog Clin Biol Res. 1982;82:123–34.

134. Sergouniotis PI, Davidson AE, Lenassi E, Devery SR, Moore AT, Webster AR. Retinal structure, function, and molecular pathologic features in gyrate atrophy. Ophthalmology. 2012;119(3):596–605.

135. Renner AB, Walter A, Fiebig BS, Jägle H. Gyrate atrophy: clinical and genetic findings in a female without arginine-restricted diet during her first 39 years of life and report of a new OAT gene mutation. Doc Ophthalmol. 2012;125(1):81–9.

136. François J. Ocular manifestations in aminoacidopathies. Adv Ophthalmol. 1972;25:28–103.

137. Zaidi SH, Faiyaz-Ul-Haque M, Shuaib T, Balobaid A, Rahbeeni Z, Abalkhail H, Al-Abdullatif A, Al-Hassnan Z, Peltekova I, Al-Owain M. Clinical and molecular findings of 13 families from Saudi Arabia and a family from Sudan with homocystinuria. Clin Genet. 2012;81(6):563–70.

138. Scherbenske JM, Benson PM, Rotchford JP, James WD. Cutaneous and ocular manifestations of Down syndrome. J Am Acad Dermatol. 1990;22(5 Pt 2):933–8.

139. Creavin AL, Brown RD. Ophthalmic abnormalities in children with Down syndrome. J Pediatr Ophthalmol Strabismus. 2009;46(2):76–82.

140. Ljubic A, Trajkovski V. Refractive errors in children and young adults with Down's syndrome. Acta Ophthalmol. 2011;89(4):324–7.

141. Stirn Kranjc B. Ocular abnormalities and systemic disease in Down syndrome. Strabismus. 2012;20(2):74–7.

142. Jiang L, Long K, Schaeffel F, Zhang S, Zhou X, Lu F, Qu J. Disruption of emmetropization and high susceptibility to deprivation myopia in albino guinea pigs. Invest Ophthalmol Vis Sci. 2011;52(9):6124–32.

143. Rymer J, Choh V, Bharadwaj S, Padmanabhan V, Modilevsky L, Jovanovich E, Yeh B, Zhang Z, Guan H, Payne W, Wildsoet CF. The albino chick as a model for studying ocular developmental abnormalities, including refractive errors, associated with albinism. Exp Eye Res. 2007;85(4):431–42.

144. Fonda G, Thomas H, Gore GV 3rd. Educational and vocational placement, and low-vision corrections in albinism. A report bases on 235 patients. Sight Sav Rev. 1971;41(7):29–36.

145. Krieg PH, Schipper I. Drug-induced ciliary body oedema: a new theory. Eye (Lond). 1996;10(Pt 1):121–6.

146. Ryan EH Jr, Jampol LM. Drug-induced acute transient myopia with retinal folds. Retina. 1986;6(4):220–3.

147. Fan JT, Johnson DH, Burk RR. Transient myopia, angle-closure glaucoma, and choroidal detachment after oral acetazolamide. Am J Ophthalmol. 1993;115(6):813–4.

148. Fraunfelder FT, Fraunfelder FW. Drug-induced ocular side effects. 5th ed. Boston: Butterworth-Heinemann; 2001.

149. Fraunfelder FW, Fraunfelder FT, Keates EU. Topiramate-associated acute, bilateral, secondary angle-closure glaucoma. Ophthalmology. 2004;111(1):109–11.

150. Söylev MF, Green RL, Feldon SE. Choroidal effusion as a mechanism for transient myopia induced by hydrochlorothiazide and triamterene. Am J Ophthalmol. 1995;120(3):395–7.

151. Jampolsky A, Flom B. Transient myopia associated with anterior displacement of the crystalline lens. Am J Ophthalmol. 1953;36(1):81–5.

152. Alvaro ME. Effects other than anti-infectious of sulfonamide compounds on the eye. Arch Ophthalmol. 1960;63:315–8.

153. Lee JTL, Skalicky SE, Lin ML. Drug-induced myopia and bilateral angle closure secondary to zolmitriptan. J Glaucoma. 2017;26(10):954–6.

154. Lan YW, Hsieh JW. Bilateral acute angle closure glaucoma and myopic shift by topiramate-induced ciliochoroidal effusion/ case report and literature review. Int Ophthalmol. 2018;38(6):2639–48.

155. Bovino JA, Marcus DF. The mechanism of transient myopia induced by sulfonamide therapy. Am J Ophthalmol. 1982;94(1):99–102.

156. Hook SR, Holladay JT, Prager TC, Goosey JD. Transient myopia induced by sulfonamides. Am J Ophthalmol. 1986;101(4):495–6.

157. Milea D, Zech C, Dumontet C, Coiffier B, Trepsat C. Transient acute myopia induced by antilymphocyte globulins. Ophthalmologica. 1999;213(2):133–4.

158. Padhy D, Rao A. Bimatoprost (0.03%)-induced accommodative spasm and pseudomyopia. BMJ Case Rep. 2015;2015:pii: bcr2015211820.

159. Ramos-Esteban JC, Goldberg S, Danias J. Drug induced acute myopia with supraciliary choroidal effusion in a patient with Wegener's granulomatosis. Br J Ophthalmol. 2002;86(5):594–6.

160. Kimura R, Kasai M, Shoji K, Kanno C. Swollen ciliary processes as an initial symptom in Vogt-Koyanagi-Harada syndrome. Am J Ophthalmol. 1983;95(3):402–3.

161. Drug-induced myopia. Rev Prescr. 2002;22(226):200–2.

162. Maddalena MA. Transient myopia associated with acute glaucoma and retinal edema following vaginal administration of sulfanilamide. Arch Ophthalmol. 1968;80(2):186–8.

163. Chirls IA, Norris JW. Transient myopia associated with vaginal sulfanilamide suppositories. Am J Ophthalmol. 1984;98(1):120–1.

164. Grinbaum A, Ashkenazi I, Gutman I, Blumenthal M. Suggested mechanism for acute transient myopia after sulfonamide treatment. Ann Ophthalmol. 1993;25(6):224–6.

165. Bard LA. Transient myopia associated with promethazine (Phenergan) therapy: report of a case. Am J Ophthalmol. 1964;58:682–6.

166. Ericson LA. Hygroton-induced myopia and retinal edema. Acta Ophthalmol (Copenh). 1963;41:538–43.

167. Craig JE, Ong TJ, Louis DL, Wells JM. Mechanism of topiramate-induced acute-onset myopia and angle closure glaucoma. Am J Ophthalmol. 2004;137(1):193–5.

168. Harrison RJ. Ocular adverse reactions to systemic drug therapy. Adv Drug React Bull. 1996;180:683–6.

169. Mattsson R. Transient myopia following the use of sulphonamides. Acta Ophthalmol. 1952;30(4):385–98.

170. Muirhead JF, Scheie HG. Transient myopia after acetazolamide. Arch Ophthalmol. 1960;63:315–8.

171. Beasley FJ. Transient myopia and retinal edema during ethoxzolamide (Cardrase) therapy. Arch Ophthalmol. 1962;68:490–1.

172. Beasley FJ. Transient myopia and retinal edema during hydrochlorothiazide (Hydrodiuril) therapy. Arch Ophthalmol. 1961;65:212–3.

173. Michaelson JJ. Transient myopia due to hygroton. Am J Ophthalmol. 1962;54:1146–7.

174. Yasuna E. Acute myopia associated with prochlorperazine (Compazine) therapy. Am J Ophthalmol. 1962;54:793–6.

175. Galin MA, Baras I, Zweifach P. Diamox-induced myopia. Am J Ophthalmol. 1962;54:237–40.

176. Garland MA, Sholk A, Guenter KE. Acetazolamide-induced myopia. Am J Obstet Gynecol. 1962;84:69–71.

177. Grossman EE, Hanley W. Transient myopia during treatment for hypertension with autonomic blocking agents. Arch Ophthalmol. 1960;63:853–5.

178. Stratos AA, Peponis VG, Portaliou DM, Stroubini TE, Skouriotis S, Kymionis GD. Secondary pseudomyopia induced by amisulpride. Optom Vis Sci. 2011;88(11):1380–2.

179. Praveen Kumar KV, Chiranjeevi P, Alam MS. Aripiprazole-induced transient myopia – a rare entity. Indian J Ophthalmol. 2018;66(1):130–1.

180. Nair AG, Nair AG, George RJ, Biswas J, Gandhi RA. Aripiprazole induced transient myopia - a case report and review of literature. Cutan Ocul Toxicol. 2012;31(1):74–6.

181. Sandford-Smith JH. Transient myopia after aspirin. Br J Ophthalmol. 1974;58(7):698–700.

182. Korol EA. Transitory myopia in combination with transitory glaucoma. Zdravookhr Beloruss. 1962;8:66–7.

183. Postel EA, Assalian A, Epstein DL. Drug-induced transient myopia and angle-closure glaucoma associated with supraciliary choroidal effusion. Am J Ophthalmol. 1996;122(1):110–2.

184. Gilmartin B, Winfield NR. The effect of topical beta-adrenoceptor antagonists on accommodation in emmetropia and myopia. Vis Res. 1995;35(9):1305–12.

185. Manor RS, Dickerman Z, Llaron Z. Myopia during bromocriptine treatment. Lancet. 1981;1(8211):102.

186. Pallin O, Ericsson R. Ultrasound studies in a case of hygroton-induced myopia. Acta Ophthalmol. 1965;43(5):692–6.

187. Mahesh G, Giridhar A, Saikumar SJ, Fegde S. Drug-induced acute myopia following chlorthalidone treatment. Indian J Ophthalmol. 2007;55(5):386–8.

188. Stern JJ. Transient myopia in case of dermatitis treated with corticotropin. AMA Arch Ophthalmol. 1955;54(5):762.

189. Arranz JA, Jiménez R, Alvarez-Mon M. Cyclophosphamide-induced myopia. Ann Intern Med. 1992;116(1):92–3.

190. Flecinide Orale LP-Flecaine LP. L'evaluation n'a pas progresse. Rev Prescr. 2006;26(269):96.

191. Teller J, Rasin M, Abraham FA. Accommodation insufficiency induced by glybenclamide. Ann Ophthalmol. 1989;21(7):275–6.

192. Roh YR, Woo SJ, Park KH. Acute-onset bilateral myopia and ciliochoroidal effusion induced by hydrochlorothiazide. Korean J Ophthalmol. 2011;25(3):214–7.

193. Blain P, Paques M, Massin P, Erginay A, Santiago P, Gaudric A. Acute transient myopia induced by indapamide. Am J Ophthalmol. 2000;129(4):538–40.

194. Dangel ME, Weber PA, Leier CB. Transient myopia following isosorbide dinitrate. Ann Ophthalmol. 1983;15(12):1156–8.

195. Park YM, Lee TE. Isotretinoin-induced angle closure and myopic shift. J Glaucoma. 2017;26(11):e252–4.

196. Fraunfelder FT, Fraunfelder FW, Edwards R. Ocular side effects possibly associated with isotretinoin usage. Am J Ophthalmol. 2001;132(3):299–305.

197. Palestine AG. Transient acute myopia resulting from isotretinoin (Accutane) therapy. Ann Ophthalmol. 1984;16(7):660–2.

198. Woodcock IR, Taylor LE, Ruddle JB, Freeman JL, Dabscheck G. Acute bilateral myopia caused by lamotrigine-induced uveal effusions. J Paediatr Child Health. 2017;53(10):1013–4.

199. Kashani S, Barclay D, Lee E, Hollick E. A case of transient myopia in a patient with multiple myeloma secondary to levomepromazine. Palliat Med. 2005;19(3):261–2.

200. Vishwakarma P, Raman GV, Sathyan P. Mefenamic acid-induced bilateral transient myopia, secondary angle closure glaucoma and choroidal detachment. Indian J Ophthalmol. 2009;57(5):398–400.

201. Kwon SJ, Park DH, Shin JP. Bilateral transient myopia, angle-closure glaucoma, and choroidal detachment induced by methazolamide. Jpn J Ophthalmol. 2012;56(5):515–7.

202. Grinbaum A, Ashkenazi I, Avni I, Blumenthal M. Transient myopia following metronidazole treatment for Trichomonas vaginalis. JAMA. 1992;267(4):511–2.

203. Doman DB, Baum MD. Olsalazine sodium can cause myopia that can be clinically confused with the uveitis of inflammatory bowel disease. Am J Gastroenterol. 1992;87(11):1684–5.

204. Zeyneloglu P, Karaaslan P, Kizilkan A, Durmaz L, Arslan G. An unusual adverse effect of an accidental epidural morphine overdose. Eur J Anaesthesiol. 2006;23(12):1061–2.

205. Corcelle L. The eye and oral contraceptives. Annee Ther Clin Ophtalmol. 1971;22:157–63. French.

206. Michiels J, Laterre C, Dumoulin D. Ocular manifestations of Wilson's disease treated by penicillamine. Bull Soc Belge Ophtalmol. 1963;132:552–61. French.

207. Johnston L. Ocular toxicity-of systemic drugs. Contin Pract. 1988;15(3):2–6.

208. Rengstorff RH. Myopia induced by ocular instillation of physostigmine. Am J Optom Arch Am Acad Optom. 1970;47(3):221–7.

209. Segal A, Aisemberg A, Ducasse A. Quinine, transient myopia and angle-closure glaucoma. Bull Soc Ophtalmol Fr. 1983;83(2):247–9.

210. Belci C. Transitory myopia in the course of therapy with diuretics. Boll Ocul. 1968;47(1):24–31. Italian.

211. Hilton EJ, Hosking SL, Betts T. The effect of antiepileptic drugs on visual performance. Seizure. 2004;13(2):113–28. Review.

212. Santodomingo-Rubido J, Gilmartin B, Wolffsohn JS. Drug-induced bilateral transient myopia with the sulphonamide sulphasalazine. Ophthalmic Physiol Opt. 2003;23(6):567–70.

213. Panday VA, Rhee DJ. Review of sulfonamide-induced acute myopia and acute bilateral angle-closure glaucoma. Compr Ophthalmol Updat. 2007;8(5):271–6. Review.

214. Edwards TS. Transient myopia due to tetracycline. JAMA. 1963;186:69–70.

215. Worthen DM. Patient compliance and the "usefulness product" of timolol. Surv Ophthalmol. 1979;23(6):403–6.

216. Banta JT, Hoffman K, Budenz DL, Ceballos E, Greenfield DS. Presumed topiramate-induced bilateral acute angle-closure glaucoma. Am J Ophthalmol. 2001;132(1):112–4.

217. Dorronzoro E, Santos-Bueso E, Vico-Ruiz E, Sáenz-Frances F, Argaya J, Gegúndez-Fernández JA. Myopia and retinal striae induced by topiramate. Arch Soc Esp Oftalmol. 2011;86(1):24–6.

218. Gualtieri W, Janula J. Topiramate maculopathy. Int Ophthalmol. 2013;33(1):103–6.

219. Ikeda N, Ikeda T, Nagata M, Mimura O. Ciliochoroidal effusion syndrome induced by sulfa derivatives. Arch Ophthalmol. 2002;120(12):1775.

220. Rhee DJ, Goldberg MJ, Parrish RK. Bilateral angle-closure glaucoma and ciliary body swelling from topiramate. Arch Ophthalmol. 2001;119(11):1721–3.

221. Sen HA, O'Halloran HS, Lee WB. Case reports and small case series: topiramate-induced acute myopia and retinal striae. Arch Ophthalmol. 2001;119(5):775–7.

222. Weng TH, Lin SM, Pao SI, Chiang SY. Relenza-induced acute myopia change. Optom Vis Sci. 2016;93(3):307–9.

223. Kirchner KA, Martin CJ, Bower JD. Prostaglandin E2 but not I2 restores furosemide response in indomethacin-treated rats. Am J Phys. 1986;250(6 Pt 2):F980–5.

224. Fraunfelder FW, Solomon J, Mehelas TJ. Ocular adverse effects associated with cyclooxygenase-2 inhibitors. Arch Ophthalmol. 2006;124(2):277–9.

225. Lee GC, Tam CP, Danesh-Meyer HV, Myers JS, Katz LJ. Bilateral angle closure glaucoma induced by sulphonamide-derived medications. Clin Exp Ophthalmol. 2007;35(1):55–8.

226. Paz T, Rappoport D, Hilely A, Leiba H. Bilateral transient myopia with sulfasalazine treatment. Clin Med Insights Case Rep. 2019;12:1179547619855388.

227. Saffra N, Smith SN, Seidman CJ. Topiramate-induced refractive change and angle closure glaucoma and its ultrasound biomicroscopy findings. BMJ Case Rep. 2012;2012:pii: bcr2012006509.

Part IV

Treatment of Pathologic Myopia

Takashi Fujikado

29.1 Introduction

Myopia in children and adolescents is principally caused by an elongation of the axial length after the emmetropization process [1]. Once myopia develops, it can continue to progress throughout childhood. Because pathological processes tend to develop more frequently in eyes with higher myopia [2], even a partial prevention of the progression of myopia can provide important protection from the development of the pathological processes. The strategies that have been used to prevent axial elongation are based on three different concepts. The first concept is controlling the environmental conditions such as increasing the outdoor activities and reducing near visual tasks. The second concept is that of altering the optical properties of the eye such as the prescription of bifocal spectacles. And the third concept is the use of pharmacological agents such as atropine eye drops.

In this review, I shall discuss each of these concepts in more detail with emphasis on their effectiveness in preventing or reducing the degree of myopia.

29.2 Emmetropization

We must first discuss the normal development of the refractive power of the eye. At birth, the axial length of the eye is approximately 17 mm, and it increases rapidly during infancy. The rate begins to slow by the age of 2–3 years, and no significant increase is observed after 10 years of age [3] (Fig. 29.1a). The axial length at this time is approximately 23 mm, and thus during this period, there is an average increase in the axial length of 6 mm. An increase in the axial length would make the eye more myopic if other factors remained unchanged.

Serial keratometric measurements of the dioptric power of the anterior surface of the cornea showed that there is a rapid decrease in the corneal power from neonates to 6-months-of-age but no significant changes thereafter [3] (Fig. 29.1b). A recent study reported that the average corneal power at birth is about 47–48 diopters (D), and it decreased to about 43–44 D at 3 to 9 months of age [4]. Thus, there is a hyperopic shift of about 4.0–5.0 D during this period.

The power of the crystalline lens changes the most during the first year of life, and the rate slows thereafter. After 6 to 7 years of age, no significant change in the power of the crystalline lens is observed through adulthood [3] (Fig. 29.1c). A recent study reported that the average power of the crystalline lens is age-related and changes from 41 D in infancy to 22–23 D by age 14 years. The average radius of curvature of the anterior surface of the lens is 7.2 mm in early infancy, and it flattens by 4.5 mm to reach 11–12 mm by the age of 14 years. The radius of curvature of the posterior surface follows a similar time course.

The average depth of the vitreous chamber is 10–11 mm at birth and increases to 16–17 mm by age 14 years [4].

The refractive power of the eye at birth is widely distributed with a range from +1.00 to +2.50 D with standard deviations of 1.50–2.50 D [5]. The refractive power of the eye decreases with increasing age, and the changes in the refractive power stabilize and remain fairly constant throughout life under normal conditions. The refractive power of the eye is normally distributed but with a positive kurtosis and a peak at 0 to +1 D in adolescents.

Thus, in spite of the relatively large changes in the refractive power of the cornea, crystalline lens, and vitreous during the development of the eye, the refractive error of the eye stabilizes close to 0 or emmetropia in more than that expected if the refractive power was normally distributed. This indicates that there must be mechanisms in the visual system that

T. Fujikado (✉)
Osaka University Graduate School of Frontier Bioscience, Osaka, Japan
e-mail: fujikado@ophthal.med.osaka-u.ac.jp

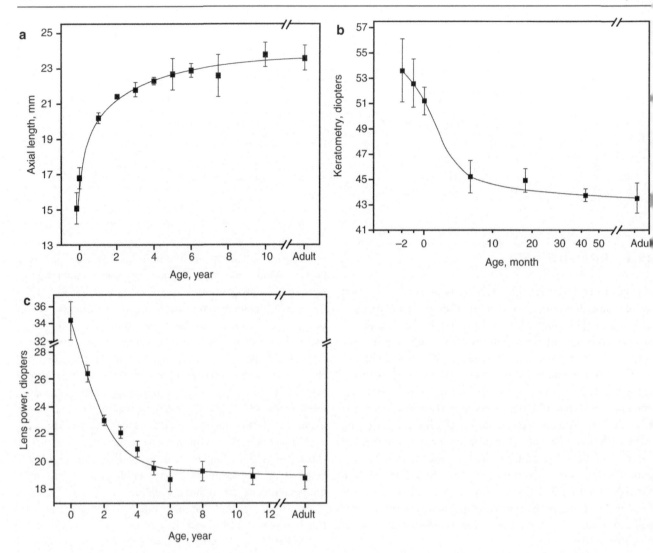

Fig. 29.1 Changes of ocular biometric parameters in relation to age. (**a**) Axial length in relation to age. (**b**) Corneal power in relation to age. (**c**) Lens power in relation to age

controls the developmental process of these very different organs so that the refractive errors stabilize close to emmetropia. This process is called emmetropization [6]. Importantly, these findings indicate that the optical system of the eye is undergoing dynamic change during the normal development of the refractive power of the eye. Thus, the question arises whether it is possible to affect the course of the dynamic changes in the eye.

In general, myopia develops after 10 years of age [7] after the alterations of the different dioptric components have stopped changing (Fig. 29.2). However, there is evidence that the axial length of some of the eyes does not stop increasing but continues to elongate. This axial elongation after the dioptric components have stopped changing has been the cause of myopia. Assuming this is correct, experiments have been designed to determine the factors that control the growth of the axial length of the eye.

29.3 Environmental Risk Factors for Axial Elongation

The importance of environmental risk factors is supported by the rapid increase in the prevalence of myopia. The prevalence of myopia between 1999 and 2004 was 41.6%, which is higher than the 25% it was between 1971 and 1972 in the USA [8].

The Sydney Myopia Study showed that near work was a weak factor significantly associated with myopia and that children who read continuously or at close distances were more likely to be myopic [9]. Other myopia study also showed that near work is associated with myopia in young children [10]. A meta-analysis comparing 12 cohort studies and 15 cross-sectional studies showed the odds of myopia increase by 2% for every diopter-hour more of near work per week [11].

Fig. 29.2 Change of refraction in relation to age. Myopia progresses mostly at ages between 10 and 16 years

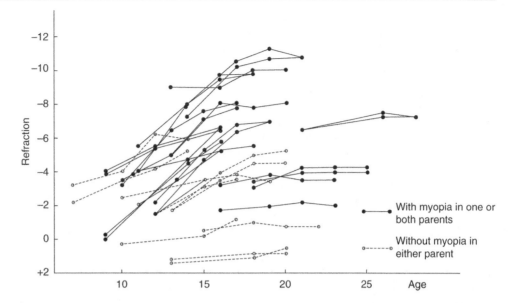

In contrast, a 2011 study involving 1318 children, some of whom were myopes and others were emmetropes, did not show a difference in near work activity before the onset or advancement of myopia [12]. Other studies also raise some doubts about the association between near work and myopia [13]. These findings suggested that near work may not play an important role in the onset of myopia; however, those who became myopic were less involved in sports and outdoor activity both before and after the onset of myopia.

Significant associations between lifestyle, educational activity, and parental refractive history in relation to the development of myopia in children have been demonstrated in recent studies [14].

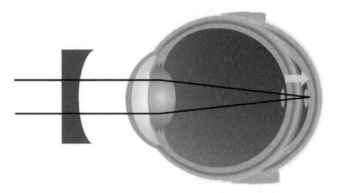

Fig. 29.3 Defocus of retinal image and axial elongation. Retinal hyperopic blur causes axial elongation

29.4 Outdoor Activities

A meta-analysis showed a 2% reduced odds of myopia per additional hour of time spent outdoors/week. This is equivalent to a 13% reduced odds for each additional hour of time spent outdoors each day [15]. Other studies support that outdoor activity reduces the myopia onset or prevalence of myopia in children [16, 17]. These results suggested that increasing time outdoors is protectively against myopia to a modest degree.

A school-based trial of outdoor activity at a school in Beijing [18] showed that less outdoor sports time was significantly associated with myopia (OR: 0.32). A recent school-based trial in Taiwan showed that children who spent 11 hours or more outdoors a week had 54% lower risk of myopia progression than children who did not, and this effect was achieved with moderate light intensities such as under the tree [19].

29.5 Optical Intervention

29.5.1 Undercorrection

The literature on myopigenesis suggests that there is an active emmetropization mechanism regulated by optical defocus. Strong evidence was found for compensatory ocular growth in response to lens-induced defocus in different species of animals [20, 21]. A hyperopic defocus where the optical image is formed behind the retina results in a growth response toward myopia in animals (Fig. 29.3). A myopic defocus, where the optical image is formed in front of the retina, results in a growth response toward hyperopia in animals.

Chung et al. conducted a randomized clinical trial involving 94 children to determine the effect of a 0.75 D undercorrection to that of a full correction with single vision lenses.

At the 2-year examination, the refractive error of the fully corrected group was 0.77 D which was significantly less than the 1.0 D in the under corrected group ($P < 0.01$) [22]. Adler et al. have conducted a randomized clinical trial involving 48 children comparing the effect of undercorrection by 0.50 D to that of full correction with single vision lenses. After 18 months, the refractive error changed by −0.82 D in the fully corrected group and by −0.99 D in the under corrected group. This difference was not statistically significant [23]. However, Sun Y-Y et al. reported that children with uncorrected myopia showed slower myopic progression compared with full-corrected children [24].

These conflicting results show that undercorrection of myopic refractive error as an intervention for slowing myopia is still controversial. It should also be taken into account that undercorrection of myopia is associated with poor overall visual functioning [25].

In animal studies, induced myopic defocus led to hyperopic changes especially in chicks [20]. The effect of myopic defocus was not strong in monkeys (Fig. 29.4) [21]. Thus, the effect of myopic defocus on axial elongation might be different between chicks and primates.

29.5.2 Part-Time Full Correction

The schedule of lens wear in myopic patients can vary from (1) full-time wearers, (2) myopes who switched from distance only to full-time wear, (3) distance only wearers, and (4) non-wearers. Preliminary data of 43 subjects suggested that there was no effect of the schedule of lens wear on the progression of myopia [26]. Even after 3 years, the refractive shifts were not significantly different among the four groups with different schedules. A randomized clinical trial using a large sample of children is needed.

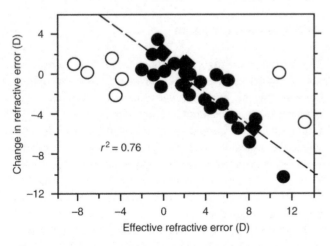

Fig. 29.4 Effective emmetropization range in monkeys. Filled circle represents emmetropized eyes and open circle represent eyes without emmetropization

29.5.3 Progressive Addition Lenses

The results of animal experiments showed that hyperopic defocus triggers an elongation of the axial length of the eye [21] (Fig. 29.3), and clinical results showed that myopic children had a lag of accommodation [27]. These observations stimulated several prospective randomized studies using progressive addition lenses (PALs) to be conducted [28–31]. The findings indicated that the use of progressive addition lenses has relatively small effects.

The correction of myopia evaluation trial (COMET), a multicenter, randomized, double-masked clinical trial using progressive addition lenses, concluded that the overall adjusted 3-year treatment effect of 0.20 ± 0.08 D was small but statistically significant ($P = 0.004$) [30]. All of the treatment effects occurred in the first year. Additional analyses showed that there were more significant effects in children with larger lags of accommodation in combination with near esophoria (0.64 ± 0.21 D), shorter reading distances (0.44 ± 0.20 D), or lower baseline myopia (0.48 ± 0.15 D).

In the Okayama study, a randomized, double-masked clinical trial using progressive addition lenses, a treatment effect of 0.17 D (95%; CI: 0.07–0.26 D) per 18 months was statistically significant ($P = 0.004$) [31]. The Cochrane Review showed that children wearing multifocal lenses, either PALs or bifocals, had an average change of 0.16 D (95% CI: 0.07–0.25) less than in children wearing monofocal lenses in 1-year follow-up [32]. Clinically, the treatment effect was not large. However, bifocal lenses, both with and without base-in prism, have been reported to slow myopia progression by 39–51% over 3 years [33]. Bifocal lens have a distinct larger area for near viewing, which may help children to reduce accommodation lag during near work.

Recent experiments in animals suggested that the peripheral retina can control eye growth at least in eyes without a fovea [34]. Peripheral hyperopia may contribute to the progression of myopia, and the use of localized manipulation of defocus could control myopia. The finding has led to the design of spectacles and contact lenses that try to reduce the progression of myopia (Fig. 29.5).

The results of a 1-year trial of spectacle lenses designed to correct central vision and reduce or eliminate peripheral hyperopic defocus [35] showed a statistically significant protection in the progression of myopia in a subgroup of younger children (6–12 years) with parental history of myopia (−0.68 ± 0.47 D with a new type of spectacle lenses vs. −0.97 ± 0.48 D with control spectacle lenses, $P = 0.038$). However, a randomized controlled trial of peripheral defocus spectacle lenses found no effect on myopia reduction in Japanese children [36].

Recently, the defocus incorporated multiple segments (DIMS) spectacle lens has developed. This lens has multiple, small segments incorporating relatively positive power

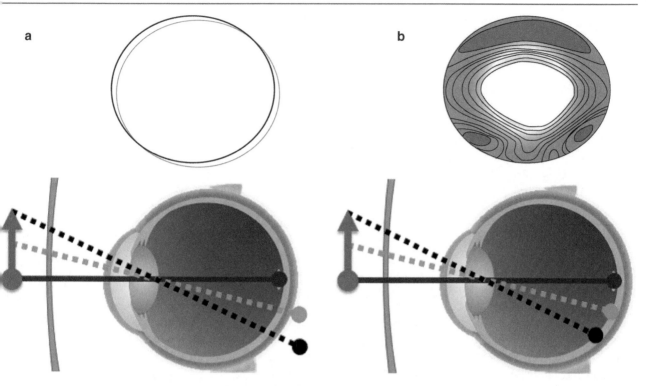

Fig. 29.5 Schema of retinal image in myopic eyes corrected by monofocal glasses (**a**) or by glasses with a concept to reduce peripheral defocus (**b**). With monofocal glasses, retinal image is blurred at the peripheral retina, but with glasses of new design, retinal image is less blurred at the peripheral retina

peripherally while providing clear vision centrally and has been reported to slow myopia progression by nearly 60% in children compared with single vision lenses [37]. The result is promising but requires validation in further studies.

29.5.4 Contact Lenses (CLs)

Soft contact lenses and rigid gas permeable (RGP) lenses have been shown not to be effective in retarding the progression of myopia [38–40]. In the Contact Lens and Myopia Progression study, subjects were randomized to wear either RGP or soft contact lenses for 3 years. The results showed a statistically significant difference in the progression of myopia in the RGP versus soft lens group with most of the treatment effect found in the first year. The corneal curvature steepened significantly less in the RGP group than in the soft lens group [41]. After 3 years, the axial elongation was not significantly different between the treatment groups. These results suggested that the slowing in the progression of myopia was mainly due to corneal flattening which may be reversible with a discontinuation of RGP lens wear. In the absence of significant differences in the axial elongation, the authors concluded that RGP lenses were not effective for myopia control [41].

The use of spectacle lenses for the correction of peripheral refractive errors can be limited by the changes in the gaze of fixation, i.e., viewing objects through a peripheral part of the lens. The results on contact lenses designed on the same principles as for the spectacles showed a 34% reduction (−0.57 D with new CL vs. −0.86 D with spectacle lenses) in the progression of myopia and a 33% reduction of the axial length (0.27 mm with new CL vs. 0.40 mm with spectacles) [42]. These findings suggested that a possibility exists that CLs designed to reduce the peripheral hyperopic blur may be useful in preventing the progression of myopia. CLs have been designed so that there is simultaneously a well-focused image and a myopically defocused image based on experiments in chicks [43].

Currently, three different types of multifocal soft contact lenses (MFSCL) for myopia control in children have been studied: bifocal concentric lenses [44–46], peripheral gradient lenses [47, 48], and extended depth of focus (EDOF) CLs [49]. The first two designs incorporate a central zone to correct myopic refractive error, but bifocal concentric lenses use a concentric zone of rings with plus power addition to simultaneously deliver peripheral myopic defocus, whereas peripheral gradient lenses simultaneously produce constant peripheral myopic defocus that increases gradually from the central optic axis toward the periphery. The third type of CL for controlling myopia progression is based on EDOF mechanism and the optical effect is similar to the concentric lenses. These MFSCL were shown to slow myopia by 25–50% in terms of spherical equivalent and 27–32% for axial length in children aged 8–16 of various ethnicities over a period of 24 months. The Food and Drug Administration (FDA) has recently granted regulatory approval for the use of the bifocal concentric lenses, MiSight dual focus contact lens (CooperVision, Pleasanton, CA, USA), for slowing myopia progression in children. A randomized clinical trial on MiSight contact lenses compared to single vision spectacles was reported. The study showed MiSight contact lenses provided a 59% reduction in myopic progression compared with control [50]. More randomized clinical trials (RCTs) are needed to prove their efficacy.

29.6   Orthokeratology

Orthokeratology (Ortho-K) is the use of rigid gas permeable contact lenses, generally worn only at night, to improve vision through the reshaping of the cornea. In myopic patients, Ortho-K lenses are worn overnight to temporarily flatten the cornea and provide clear vision during the day without any glasses or lower power contact lenses. The reduction in the refractive power of the eye of up to −6 D is achieved by a thinning of the central corneal epithelium and a midperipheral thickening of the epithelium and stroma. Recent reports have suggested that overnight orthokeratology with contact lenses might also convert relative peripheral hyperopia to relative peripheral myopia and could protect against myopic progression [51].

Walline showed that the annual rate of change in the axial length was 0.16 mm/year less ($P = 0.00004$) after wearing corneal reshaping lenses than soft contact lenses [52]. Hiraoka conducted a prospective 5-year study on the effect of Ortho-K on the growth of the axial length and showed that the increase in axial length during a 5-year period was 0.99 ± 0.47 mm for the Ortho-K group and 1.41 ± 0.68 mm for the spectacle group ($P = 0.0236$) [53].

A recent meta-analysis included seven studies (two RCTs and five NRCTs) and found a −0.26 mm (95% CI, −0.31 to −0.21) weighted mean difference for AL between the Ortho-K group and the control group in a 2-year period follow-up [54]. However, a meta-analysis described the association between Ortho-K lens wear and infectious keratitis [55]. Therefore the adoption of Ortho-K lenses to slow myopia progression in children should be carefully considered.

29.7   Pharmacological Interventions

29.7.1 Atropine Eye Drops

The use of atropine eye drops inhibited the development of myopia in tree shrews and monkeys, and atropine also blocked the form-deprivation myopia and lens-induced myopia in chicks [56]. Studies have shown that atropine did not

block the progression through blocking accommodation [57], and the authors suggested that atropine acted mainly through the M4 subtype of muscarinic receptors [58]. The Atropine in the Treatment of Myopia (ATOM) study was a randomized, double-masked, placebo-controlled trial involving 400 Singapore children [59]. The results showed that 1% atropine eye drops instilled nightly in one eye over a 2-year period reduce the myopic progression significantly in children by 77% (0.28 D in the atropine group vs. 1.2 D in the control group). The atropine group's mean axial length remained essentially unchanged, whereas the placebo group's mean axial length increased by 0.38 mm. The topical atropine was well tolerated by the children.

The side effects of atropine include photophobia due to mydriasis and decreased near vision due to cycloplegia. As a result, if atropine is used in both eyes, the patient needs progressive lenses for near vision. The ATOM study [59] reported no systemic side effects of atropine eye drops, although the potential side effects included dry eyes, dry mouth, dry throat, flushed skin, and constipation. In addition, there was an initial increase in the rate of myopia progression following the cessation of atropine treatment in the ATOM study. Thus, the myopia progressed by -1.14 ± 0.8 D in the atropine group and -0.38 ± 0.39 D in the control group, $P = 0.0001$) [60]. This rebound phenomenon is probably related to the strong cycloplegic effects of atropine.

In the Atropine 2 Treatment of Childhood Myopia (ATOM 2) study, atropine 0.01%, displayed myopia progression (-0.49 D ± 0.63 D/2 years) with smaller differences in spherical equivalent value with the higher-dose atropine 0.5% group (-0.30 D ± 0.60 D/2 years). In addition, atropine 0.01% provided a better ocular side effect profile than the higher-dose groups, with the accommodation remaining at 11.8 D (compared with 6.8 D and 4 D in the 0.1% and 0.5% atropine groups, respectively) and a mean photopic pupil size change after 2 years of 0.74 mm (2.25 mm and 3.11 mm in the 0.1% and 0.5% groups, respectively) [61]. After washing out, the atropine 0.01% drops caused the least rebound effect and showed a long-term clinical efficacy in slowing down myopia progression with tolerable side effects [62].

Recently, Yam et al. evaluated the efficacy and safety of low-concentration atropine eye drops at 0.05%, 0.025%, and 0.01% compared with placebo over a 1-year period by randomized placebo-controlled study [63]. The results were that 0.05%, 0.025%, and 0.01% atropine eye drops reduced myopia progression along a concentration-dependent response. All concentrations were well tolerated without an adverse effect on vision-related quality of life. Of the three concentrations used, 0.05% atropine was most effective in reducing SE progression (67%) and AL elongation (51%) compared with placebo group over a period of 1 year. The optimal concentration and the desired duration of drug application need to be established.

Table 29.1 Methods and effects to prevent myopia progression

Methods	Control	Degree of prevention
Atropine eye drop 1%	Placebo eye drop	1.0 D/year [32]
Atropine eye drop 0.05%, 0.01%	Placebo eye drop	0.54 D/year (0.05%) [63] 0.22 D/year (0.01%) [63]
Pirenzepine gel 2%	Placebo eye drop	0.31 D/year [32]
Progressive additional or bifocal glasses	Monofocal glasses	0.14 D/year [32]
Concentric bifocal contact lenses	Monofocal glasses	0.24 D/year [50]
Orthokeratology	Monofocal glasses	Axial length 0.13 mm/year [54]

29.8 Pirenzepine 2% Gel

Pirenzepine 2% gel is a selective M1 antagonist with a long history of oral use to treat dyspepsia and pediatric endocrine disorders. Unlike atropine, which is equipotent in binding to M3 (accommodation and mydriasis) and M1 muscarinic receptors, pirenzepine is relatively selective for the M1 muscarinic receptor and thus is less likely than atropine to produce mydriasis and cycloplegia. In the USA, pirenzepine 2% gel applied twice a day slowed the progression of myopia for over 2 years (0.58 D vs. 0.99 D) [64]. In Asia, the mean increase in myopia was 0.47 D, 0.70 D, and 0.84 D in twice daily, once nightly, and control groups over 1 year [65]. Pirenzepine 2% gel applied twice/day and nightly reduced myopia progression by 50% and 44%, respectively (Table 29.1). Currently, the development of pirenzepine as an anti-myopia therapeutic agent has ceased due to regulatory and financial obstacles.

29.9 Conclusion

The current strategies to prevent axial elongation are based on three different concepts. The first concept is controlling the environmental conditions such as increasing the outdoor activities. The second concept is that of altering the optical properties of the eye such as the prescribing of multifocal contact lenses to reduce the hyperopic defocus on the retina. And the third concept is the use of pharmacological agents such as low-dose atropine eye drops. The treatment effects to reduce myopia based on the abovementioned strategies are modest but it would be worth analyzing the potential additive effects of low-dose atropine combined with other therapies in larger-scale randomized control study (Table 29.2).

Table 29.2 Strategies to prevent myopia progression

Target	Methods
Environment	Increase of outdoor activity
Retinal image	Bifocal or progressive additional lenses
	Correcting peripheral defocus (Glasses, CLs, Ortho K)
Retinal information processing or sclera	Muscarinic antagonist (Atropine, Pirenzepine)

References

1. Mutti DO, Mitchell GL, Sinnott LT, Jones-Jordan LA, Moeschberger ML, Cotter SA, Kleinstein RN, Manny RE, Twelker JD, Zadnik K. Corneal and crystalline lens dimensions before and after myopia onset. Optom Vis Sci. 2012;89(3):251–62.
2. Morgan IG, Ohno-Matsui K, Saw SM. Myopia. Lancet. 2012;379(9827):1739–48.
3. Gordon RA, Donzis PB. Refractive development of the human eye. Arch Ophthalmol. 1985;103(6):785–9.
4. Mutti DO, Mitchell GL, Jones LA, Friedman NE, Frane SL, Lin WK, Moeschberger ML, Zadnik K. Axial growth and changes in lenticular and corneal power during emmetropization in infants. Invest Ophthalmol Vis Sci. 2005;46(9):3074–80.
5. Cook RC, Glasscock RE. Refractive and ocular findings in the newborn. Am J Ophthalmol. 1951;34(10):1407–13.
6. Young TL. Myopia. In: Levin LA, Albert DM, editors. Ocular disease: mechanisms and management. Saunders, Philadelphia; 2010. p. 424–32.
7. Tokoro T, Suzuki K. Changes in ocular refractive components and development of myopia during seven years. Jpn J Ophthalmol. 1969;13:27–34.
8. Vitale S, Sperduto RD, Ferris FL 3rd. Increased prevalence of myopia in the United States between 1971–1972 and 1999–2004. Arch Ophthalmol. 2009;127(12):1632–9.
9. Ip JM, Saw SM, Rose KA, Morgan IG, Kifley A, Wang JJ, Mitchell P. Role of near work in myopia: findings in a sample of Australian school children. Invest Ophthalmol Vis Sci. 2008;49(7):2903–10.
10. Saw SM, Chua WH, Hong CY, Wu HM, Chan WY, Chia KS, et al. Nearwork in early-onset myopia. Invest Ophthalmol Vis Sci. 2002;43(2):332–9.
11. Huang HM, Chang DS, Wu PC. The association between near work activities and myopia in children-a systematic review and meta-analysis. PLoS One. 2015;10:e0140419.
12. Jones-Jordan LA, Mitchell GL, Cotter SA, Kleinstein RN, Manny RE, Mutti DO, Twelker JD, Sims JR, Zadnik K. Visual activity before and after the onset of juvenile myopia. Invest Ophthalmol Vis Sci. 2011;52(3):1841–50.
13. Lu B, Congdon N, Liu X, Choi K, Lam DS, Zhang M, et al. Associations between near work, outdoor activity, and myopia among adolescent students in rural China: the Xichang Pediatric Refractive Error Study report no. 2. Arch Ophthalmol. 2009;127(6):769–75.
14. Rose KA, Morgan IG, Smith W, Burlutsky G, Mitchell P, Saw SM. Myopia, lifestyle, and schooling in students of Chinese ethnicity in Singapore and Sydney. Arch Ophthalmol. 2008;126(4):527–30.
15. Sherwin JC, Reacher MH, Keogh RH, Khawaja AP, Mackey DA, Foster PJ. The association between time spent outdoors and myopia

in children and adolescents: a systematic review and meta-analysis. Ophthalmology. 2012;119(10):2141–51.

16. Rose KA, Morgan IG, Ip J, Kifley A, Huynh S, Smith W, Mitchell P. Outdoor activity reduces the prevalence of myopia in children. Ophthalmology. 2008;115(8):1279–85.

17. Wu PC, Tsai CL, Wu HL, Yang YH, Kuo HK. Outdoor activity during class recess reduces myopia onset and progression in school children. Ophthalmology. 2013;120(5):1080–5.

18. Guo Y, Liu LJ, Xu L, Lv YY, Tang P, Feng Y, Meng M, Jonas JB. Outdoor activity and myopia among primary students in rural and urban regions of Beijing. Ophthalmology. 2013;120(2):277–83.

19. Pei-Chang Wu 1, Chueh-Tan Chen 1, Ken-Kuo Lin 2, Chi-Chin Sun 3, Chien-Neng Kuo 4, Hsiu-Mei Huang 1, Yi-Chieh Poon 1, Meng-Ling Yang 2, Chau-Yin Chen 4, Jou-Chen Huang 4, Pei-Chen Wu 4, I-Hui Yang 1, Hun-Ju Yu 1, Po-Chiung Fang 1, Chia-Ling Tsai 5, Shu-Ti Chiou 6, Yi-Hsin Yang 7 Myopia Prevention and Outdoor Light Intensity in a School-Based Cluster Randomized Trial Ophthalmology 2018;125(8):1239–50.

20. Schaeffel F, Glasser A, Howland HC. Accommodation, refractive error and eye growth in chickens. Vis Res. 1988;28(5):639–57.

21. Smith EL 3rd, Hung LF. The role of optical defocus in regulating refractive development in infant monkeys. Vis Res. 1999;39(8):1415–35.

22. Chung K, Mohidin N, O'Leary DJ. Undercorrection of myopia enhances rather than inhibits myopia progression. Vis Res. 2002;42(22):2555–9.

23. Adler D, Millodot M. The possible effect of undercorrection on myopic progression in children. Clin Exp Optom. 2006;89(5):315–21.

24. Sun YY, Li SM, Li SY, Kang MT, Liu LR, Meng B, Zhang FJ, Millodot M, Wang N. Effect of uncorrection versus full correction on myopia progression in 12-year-old children. Graefes Arch Clin Exp Ophthalmol. 2017;255(1):189–95.

25. Lamoureux EL, Saw SM, Thumboo J, Wee HL, Aung T, Mitchell P, Wong TY. The impact of corrected and uncorrected refractive error on visual functioning: the Singapore Malay Eye Study. Invest Ophthalmol Vis Sci. 2009;50(6):2614–20.

26. Ong E, Grice K, Held R, Thorn F, Gwiazda J. Effects of spectacle intervention on the progression of myopia in children. Optom Vis Sci. 1999;76(6):363–9.

27. Gwiazda J, Thorn F, Bauer J, Held R. Myopic children show insufficient accommodative response to blur. Invest Ophthalmol Vis Sci. 1993;34(3):690–4.

28. Leung JT, Brown B. Progression of myopia in Hong Kong Chinese schoolchildren is slowed by wearing progressive lenses. Optom Vis Sci. 1999;76(6):346–54.

29. Edwards MH, Li RW, Lam CS, Lew JK, Yu BS. The Hong Kong progressive lens myopia control study: study design and main findings. Invest Ophthalmol Vis Sci. 2002;43(9):2852–8.

30. Gwiazda J, Hyman L, Hussein M, Everett D, Norton TT, Kurtz D, Leske MC, Manny R, Marsh-Tootle W, Scheiman M. A randomized clinical trial of progressive addition lenses versus single vision lenses on the progression of myopia in children. Invest Ophthalmol Vis Sci. 2003;44(4):1492–500.

31. Hasebe S, Ohtsuki H, Nonaka T, Nakatsuka C, Miyata M, Hamasaki I, Kimura S. Effect of progressive addition lenses on myopia progression in Japanese children: a prospective, randomized, double-masked, crossover trial. Invest Ophthalmol Vis Sci. 2008;49(7):2781–9.

32. Walline JJ, Lindsley K, Vedula SS, Cotter SA, Mutti DO, Twelker JD. Interventions to slow progression of myopia in children. Cochrane Database Syst Rev. 2020;1(1):CD004916.

33. Cheng D, Woo GC, Drobe B, Schmid KL. Effect of bifocal and prismatic bifocal spectacles on myopia progression in children: three-year results of a randomized clinical trial. JAMA Ophthalmol. 2014;132:258–64.

34. Smith EL 3rd, Kee CS, Ramamirtham R, Qiao-Grider Y, Hung LF. Peripheral vision can influence eye growth and refractive development in infant monkeys. Invest Ophthalmol Vis Sci. 2005;46(11):3965–72.

35. Sankaridurg P, Donovan L, Varnas S, Ho A, Chen X, Martinez A, Fisher S, Lin Z, Smith EL 3rd, Ge J, Holden B. Spectacle lenses designed to reduce progression of myopia: 12-month results. Optom Vis Sci. 2010;87(9):631–41.

36. Kanda H, Oshika T, Hiraoka T, et al. Effect of spectacle lenses designed to reduce relative peripheral hyperopia on myopia progression in Japanese children: a 2-year multicenter randomized controlled trial. Jpn J Ophthalmol. 2018;62:537–43.

37. Lam CSY, Tang WC, Tse DY, et al. Defocus incorporated multiple segments (DIMS) spectacle lenses slow myopia progression: a 2-year randomised clinical trial. Br J Ophthalmol. 2020;104(3):363–8.

38. Horner DG, Soni PS, Salmon TO, Swartz TS. Myopia progression in adolescent wearers of soft contact lenses and spectacles. Optom Vis Sci. 1999;76(7):474–9.

39. Walline JJ, Jones LA, Sinnott L, Manny RE, Gaume A, Rah MJ, Chitkara M, Lyons S. A randomized trial of the effect of soft contact lenses on myopia progression in children. Invest Ophthalmol Vis Sci. 2008;49(11):4702–6.

40. Katz J, Schein OD, Levy B, Cruiscullo T, Saw SM, Rajan U, Chan TK, Yew Khoo C, Chew SJ. A randomized trial of rigid gas permeable contact lenses to reduce progression of children's myopia. Am J Ophthalmol. 2003;136(1):82–90.

41. Walline JJ, Jones LA, Mutti DO, Zadnik K. A randomized trial of the effects of rigid contact lenses on myopia progression. Arch Ophthalmol. 2004;122(12):1760–6.

42. Sankaridurg P, Holden B, Smith E 3rd, Naduvilath T, Chen X, de la Jara PL, Martinez A, Kwan J, Ho A, Frick K, Ge J. Decrease in rate of myopia progression with a contact lens designed to reduce relative peripheral hyperopia: one-year results. Invest Ophthalmol Vis Sci. 2011;52(13):9362–7.

43. Liu Y, Wildsoet C. The effect of two-zone concentric bifocal spectacle lenses on refractive error development and eye growth in young chicks. Invest Ophthalmol Vis Sci. 2011;52(2):1078–86.

44. Aller TA, Liu M, Wildsoet CF. Myopia control with bifocal contact lenses: a randomized clinical trial. Optom Vis Sci. 2016;93(4):344–52.

45. Anstice NS, Phillips JR. Effect of dual-focus soft contact lens wear on axial myopia progression in children. Ophthalmology. 2011;118(6):1152–61.

46. Lam CSY, Tang WC, Tse DY-Y, Tang YY, To CH. Defocus incorporated soft contact (DISC) lens slows myopia progression in Hong Kong Chinese schoolchildren: a 2-year randomised clinical trial. Br J Ophthalmol. 2014;98(1):40–5.

47. Sankaridurg P, Holden B, Smith E, et al. Decrease in rate of myopia progression with a contact lens designed to reduce relative peripheral hyperopia: one-year results. Invest Ophthalmol Vis Sci. 2011;52(13):9362–7.

48. Fujikado T, Ninomiya S, Kobayashi T, Suzaki A, Nakada M, Nishida K. Effect of low-addition soft contact lenses with decentered optical design on myopia progression in children: a pilot study. Clin Ophthalmol. 2014;8:1947–56.

49. Sankaridurg P, Bakaraju RC, Naduvilath T, et al. Myopia control with novel central and peripheral plus contact lenses and extended depth of focus contact lenses: 2 year results from a randomized clinical trial. Ophthalmic Physiol Opt. 2019;39(4):294–307.

50. Chamberlain P, Peixoto-De-Matos SC, Logan NS, Ngo C, Jones D, Young G. A 3-year randomized clinical trial of MiSight lenses for myopia control. Optom Vis Sci. 2019;96(8):556–67.

51. Charman WN, Mountford J, Atchison DA, Markwell EL. Peripheral refraction in orthokeratology patients. Optom Vis Sci. 2006;83(9):641–8.

52. Walline JJ, Jones LA, Sinnott LT. Corneal reshaping and myopia progression. Br J Ophthalmol. 2009;93(9):1181–5.

53. Hiraoka T, Kakita T, Okamoto F, Takahashi H, Oshika T. Long-term effect of overnight orthokeratology on axial length elongation in childhood myopia: a 5-year follow-up study. Invest Ophthalmol Vis Sci. 2012;53(7):3913–9.

54. Si JK, Tang K, Bi HS, Guo DD, Guo JG, Wang XR. Orthokeratology for myopia control: a meta-analysis. Optom Vis Sci. 2015;92:252–7.

55. Kam KW, Yung W, Li GKH, Chen LJ, Young AL. Infectious keratitis and orthokeratology lens use: a systematic review. Infection. 2017;45:727–35.

56. Stone RA, Lin T, Laties AM. Muscarinic antagonist effects on experimental chick myopia. Exp Eye Res. 1991;52(6):755–8.

57. McBrien NA, Moghaddam HO, Reeder AP. Atropine reduces experimental myopia and eye enlargement via a nonaccommodative mechanism. Invest Ophthalmol Vis Sci. 1993;34(1):205–15.

58. McBrien NA, Arumugam B, Gentle A, Chow A, Sahebjada S. The M4 muscarinic antagonist MT-3 inhibits myopia in chick: evidence for site of action. Ophthalmic Physiol Opt. 2011;31(5):529–39.

59. Chua WH, Balakrishnan V, Chan YH, Tong L, Ling Y, Quah BL, Tan D. Atropine for the treatment of childhood myopia. Ophthalmology. 2006;113(12):2285–91.

60. Tong L, Huang XL, Koh AL, Zhang X, Tan DT, Chua WH. Atropine for the treatment of childhood myopia: effect on myopia progression after cessation of atropine. Ophthalmology. 2009;116(3):572–9.

61. Chia A, Chua WH, Cheung YB, Wong WL, Lingham A, Fong A, Tan D. Atropine for the treatment of childhood myopia: safety and efficacy of 0.5%, 0.1%, and 0.01% doses (atropine for the treatment of myopia 2). Ophthalmology. 2012;119(2):347–54.

62. Chia A, Chua WH, Wen L, Fong A, Goon YY, Tan D. Atropine for the treatment of childhood myopia: changes after stopping atropine 0.01%, 0.1% and 0.5%. Am J Ophthalmol. 2014;157:451–7.

63. Yam JC, Jiang Y, Tang SM, Law AKP, Chan JJ, Wong E, Ko ST, Young AL, Tham CC, Chen LJ, Pang CP. Low-concentration atropine for myopia progression (LAMP) study: a randomized, double-blinded, placebo-controlled trial of 0.05%, 0.025%, and 0.01% atropine eye drops in myopia control. Ophthalmology. 2019;126(1):113–24.

64. Siatkowski RM, Cotter SA, Crockett RS, Miller JM, Novack GD, Zadnik K, U.S. Pirenzepine Study Group. Two-year multicenter, randomized, double-masked, placebo-controlled, parallel safety and efficacy study of 2% pirenzepine ophthalmic gel in children with myopia. J AAPOS. 2008;12(4):332–9.

65. Tan DT, Lam DS, Chua WH, Shu-Ping DF, Crockett RS, Asian Pirenzepine Study Group. One-year multicenter, double-masked, placebo-controlled, parallel safety and efficacy study of 2% pirenzepine ophthalmic gel in children with myopia. Ophthalmology. 2005;112(1):84–91.

Optical Methods to Slow the Progression of Myopia

30

Jeffrey Cooper

30.1 Introduction

Myopia, the 6th leading cause of loss of vision, is increasing at epidemic rates; by 2050, almost half of the world's population will be myopic [1–3]. Thus, slowing the progression of myopia, specifically axial length, has been assumed to decrease associated myopia-related diseases that cause vision loss. Current methods of slowing progressive myopia are based upon light (spectral composition, brightness, contrast, and/or accommodative demand), optical defocus (either lag of accommodation or relative hyperopia in the retina periphery as a result of the shape of the eye), and/or pharmacological intervention [4, 5]. This chapter will deal with optical interventions.

30.2 Spectacle Correction

Historically, myopia has been associated with people who live in urban areas; who are more educated; and who are more intelligent [6–10]. It has been assumed that myopia is related to excessive near work, thus implicating accommodation as the cause [11–17]. Thus, bifocal lenses have been prescribed, based upon the assumption that prolonged accommodation or spasm of accommodation causes myopia [18–21]. Treatment, according to this theory, uses either bifocal or progressive spectacle lenses (PALs) to reduce the accommodative demand. Retrospective studies have showed that bifocals or progressive addition lenses (PALs) slow the progression of myopia by approximately 40% [22–24]. These studies have been historically criticized for being retrospective, unmasked, etc. The COMET (the Correction of Myopia Evaluation Trial) was a prospective clinical trial to determine if a +2.00 D PAL slowed the progression of myopia more than a single-vision correcting spectacle lens [25].

In the first year, PALs slowed the progression of myopia by 20%. However, after 4 years the net myopic reduction was only 0.2 D. This amount was clinically insignificant but statistically significant. Analysis of the data revealed that progressive lenses were the most effective when both parents were myopic, there was a large lag of accommodation, and/or the children had esophoria at near [20, 26].

Cheng et al. [27] evaluated the use of high fitting executive bifocal spectacle lenses with base-in prism in Canadian Asians vs. using single-vision lenses. They reported that the prismatic bifocal lenses slowed the progression of myopia by 40%. They believed that superior performance was due to the use of high fitting bifocals vs. PALs and base-in prism. Unfortunately, this study has not been replicated. In 2011, Shi-Ming Li et al. [28] performed a meta-analysis of nine clinical trials which evaluated PALs (+1.5 to +2.0 D). They reported that overall the PALs slowed myopic progression by 0.25 D/year as compared to SV lenses. This reduction in myopia was approximately 20% and was greater in Asian children vs. Caucasians. Those with a higher level of myopia at baseline progressed more rapidly [28]. In summary, the results of these studies suggest that lenses with near vision adds are only mildly successful in slowing the progression of myopia (see Fig. 30.1). The additive effect of PALs and atropine is unknown.

Numerous animal studies have shown that animal growth is regulated by blur on the retina [29]. Young animals will adjust the length of their eye to eliminate error created by lens-induced blur in a linear fashion, i.e., elongation when a minus lens is placed in front of the eye and shortening if a plus lens is placed in front of an eye [30]. This response to blur occurs even if the optic nerve is cut [31]. If a lens is placed in front of half the eye, then half of the eye will change in length. If a lens is placed in front of a monkey's eye which has two opposite powers (one plus and the other minus), the length of the eye will change to eliminate the peripherally induced refractive error (see Fig. 30.2). This occurs across species including those without a macula. In other words, the eye tries to eliminate the larger defocused

J. Cooper (✉)
SUNY-State College of Optometry, New York, NY, USA

a   Refraction

	Favours MLs			Favours SVLs				Mean Difference	Mean Difference
	Mean	SD	Total	Mean	SD	Total	Weight	IV. Random. 95% CI	IV. Random. 95% CI
Cheng 2010	-0.96	0.62	48	-1.55	0.62	38	9.7%	0.59 [0.33,0.85]	
Edwards 2002	-1.12	0.67	121	-1.26	0.74	133	13.0%	0.14 [-0.03, 0.31]	
Fulk 2000	-0.99	0.68	36	-1.24	0.65	39	8.5%	0.25 [-0.05, 0.55]	
Gwiazds 2003	-1.28	0.91	229	-1.48	0.92	233	13.2%	0.20 [0.03, 0.37]	
Hasebe 2008	-0.89	0.41	46	-1.2	0.51	44	12.3%	0.31 [0.12, 0.50]	
Leung 1999	-0.72	0.43	36	-1.23	0.51	32	11.0%	0.51 [0.28, 0.74]	
Parssinen 1989	-1.67	0.9	79	-1.48	0.9	79	9.2%	-0.19 [-0.47, 0.09]	
Shin 2001	-1.19	0.55	61	-1.4	0.7	61	11.1%	0.21 [-0.01, 0.43]	
Yang 2009	-1.24	0.56	74	-1.5	0.67	75	12.0%	0.26 [0.06, 0.46]	
Total (95% CI)			730			734	100.0%	0.25 [0.13, 0.38]	

Heterogeneity: Tau^2= 0.02; Chi^2= 23.32; df= 8 (P = 0.003); I^2= 66%
Test for overall effect: Z = 4.03 (P < 0.001)

-1   -0.5   0   0.5   1
Favours MLs   Favours SVLs

b   Axial length

	Favours MLs			Favours SVLs				Mean Difference	Mean Difference
	Mean	SD	Total	Mean	SD	Total	Weight	IV. Random. 95% CI	IV. Random. 95% CI
Cheng 2010	0.41	0.28	48	0.62	0.26	38	14.7%	-0.21 [-0.32, -0.10]	
Edwards 2002	0.61	0.24	121	0.63	0.28	133	21.9%	-0.02 [-0.08, 0.04]	
Fulk 2000	0.4	0.36	36	0.49	0.29	39	11.1%	-0.09 [-0.24, 0.06]	
Gwiazds 2003	0.64	0.3	229	0.75	0.31	233	23.1%	-0.11 [-0.17, -0.05]	
Leung 1999	0.46	0.27	36	0.74	0.39	32	10.0%	-0.28 [-0.44, -0.12]	
Shin 2001	0.49	0.23	61	0.59	0.23	61	19.2%	-0.10 [-0.18, -0.02]	
Total (95% CI)			531			536	100.0%	-0.12 [-0.18, -0.05]	

Heterogeneity: Tau^2= 0.00; Chi^2= 14.46; df= 5 (P = 0.01); I^2= 65%
Test for overall effect: Z = 3.63 (P = 0.0003)

-0.5   -0.25   0   0.25   0.5
Favours MLs   Favours SVLs

Fig. 30.1 Meta-analysis of spectacle lenses slowing myopic progression. Meta-analysis of nine clinical trials which compared progressive addition or bifocal spectacle lenses (MFL) to single-vision lenses (SVL) using the spherical equivalent (**a**) and axial length (**b**). The mean difference between SVL and MFL was 0.25D/year, and for those that reported axial length, the difference was .012 mm/year. MFL were more beneficial in Asian vs. Caucasian eyes (0.32D vs. 0.10D) and/or those that patients who were initially more myopic. (Reprinted with permission from Li et al. [28])

Fig. 30.2 Regional blur results in axial elongation. Regional retinal blur created by diffusion or lenses projected on half of the retina results in regional elongation of the eye. This occurs even when the optic nerve is cut, but not if atropine is injected into the eye. The eye responds appropriately to the direction of the blur, i.e., plus or minus lenses. (Reprinted with permission from Cooper et al. [18])

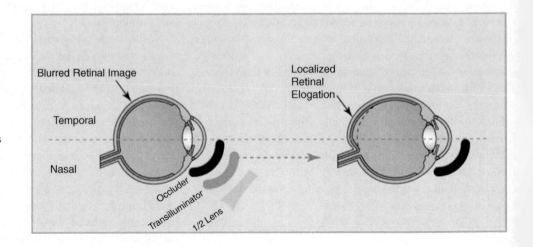

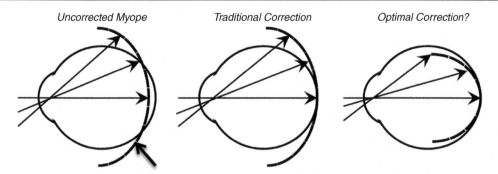

Uncorrected Myope   Traditional Correction   Optimal Correction?

Fig. 30.3 Image shell of a myopic eye with and without correction. Once the eye elongates secondary to the development of myopia, optical images from spherical lenses no longer fall on the retinal plane. The peripheral images which are out of focus fall on a plane behind the retina; this creates relative hyperopic error which is the stimulus for axial elongation. Current optical treatments move the peripheral focus in front of the retina. (Reprinted with permission from Cooper et al. [18])

Fig. 30.4 DIMS lens (*Defocus Incorporated Multiple Segments*). The center of the lens only has the distance Rx; this 9 mm zone is surrounded by a honeycomb pattern consisting of two focal powers (distance prescription and +3.50 D of defocus). This is cosmetically acceptable and results in minimal blur. (Reprinted with permission Lam et al. [34])

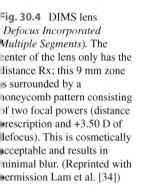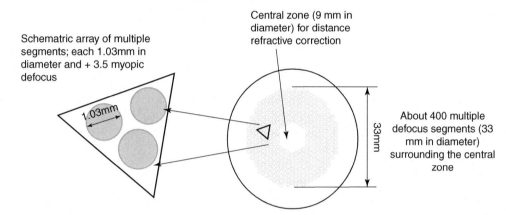

Schematic array of multiple segments; each 1.03mm in diameter and + 3.5 myopic defocus

1.03mm

Central zone (9 mm in diameter) for distance refractive correction

33mm

About 400 multiple defocus segments (33 mm in diameter) surrounding the central zone

error in the peripheral retina. Since the myopic eye is elongated, optical correction with spherical lenses creates relative hyperopia in the periphery (see Fig. 30.3). Current strategies to optically slow the progression of myopia impose myopic defocus by providing simultaneous competing defocus over all or part of the retina. Thus, understanding how the eye responds to simultaneous competing signals is important for designing lenses that slow myopic progression.

Various novel spectacle lenses have been designed to reduce peripheral hyperopic defocus [32]. In one study, none of the spectacle lenses had any significant effect in slowing the progression of myopia. Failure to achieve a significant result might be related to the constant changing of eye position when viewing through these lenses. At least in animals when the peripheral portion of the lenses is proportionally decreased in size by using alternating concentric rings, the peripheral hyperopic defocus is still dominant in regulating the length of the eyes during growth. This concept has been incorporated into a novel optical design known as DIMS (Defocus Incorporated Multiple Segments) [33]. The DIMS™ spectacles have a central area which uniformly corrects the distance myopic error and a surrounding zone that has a honeycomb composed of small +3.50 droplets [34]

(see Fig. 30.4). In between the "droplets" is the distance correction. Lam et al. have shown that their DIMS™ lens design slows both axial elongation and myopia progression by approximately 60% over 2 years of time. These lenses are currently available in countries outside the USA. Another spectacle lens which shows promise is the DOT™ lens [35]. This lens manufactured by SightGlass Vision has a central clear zone, surrounded by a diffusing annulus. It uses contrast modulation to reduce the contrast in the periphery. In an ongoing, randomized controlled clinical trial, they report a reduction in myopia progression as measured by a cycloplegic refraction of 59 percent and 74 percent at 12-months for two different designs. For the same period of time, there was a reduction in axial length by 33 percent and 50 percent at 12 months for each treatment design. Glasses are an important tool since they are the primary modality of correction in the younger population.

Many eye care professionals under-correct myopia in the belief that the myopic progression will slow down as a result of reduced accommodation. Two studies have demonstrated that under-correction actually results in a mild acceleration of myopia progression [36, 37]. Thus, under-correction should not be discouraged for the treatment of myopia.

30.3 Contact Lenses

For years, it was believed that gas permeable contact lenses slowed the progression of myopia. In two clinical trials, it was shown that neither conventional soft nor gas permeable contact lenses slow the progression of myopia [38, 39].

Orthokeratology (OK) was originally developed and FDA approved in 2002 as a nonsurgical procedure to reshape the cornea to eliminate the needs for glasses or contact lenses during the day. The lenses are designed with three principal sections: (1) a central zone which uses hydraulic forces to reshape the cornea and thereby eliminate the patient's refractive error, (2) a second concentric zone known as the return zone which is much steeper than the central flattening zone (see Fig. 30.5). This creates a strong plus lens in the mid-periphery of the eye, i.e., induced plus = 2× the refractive error, which is being corrected (3) an alignment zone which supports and aligns the contact lens. It should be noted that FDA approval for OK is only for reshaping the cornea to eliminate daytime need for contact lenses or glasses. The use of orthokeratology to slow myopic progression is off label. In 2003, Reim published a retrospective study of 253 children (ages 6–18). He reported that the rate of myopic progression was slowed from 0.5 diopters/year to 0.13 diopters/year.

Since then there have been a number of prospective clinical trials, which have demonstrated that OK slows the progression of myopia by approximately 40% [40–48].

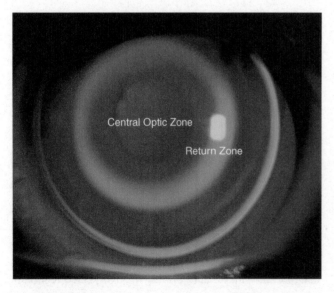

Fig. 30.5 Ortho-K lens with description. A typical ortho-K contact lens with its fluorescein pattern is shown. The central darker area eliminates the refractive error by flattening the central area of the cornea (optic zone OZ); the second bright curve is the return zone which creates a plus lens relative to the refractive error; the third dark ring is the alignment zone which is important in fitting the lens and maintaining stability of the fit. The last curve is the peripheral curve, which is important for tear exchange

Swarbrick et al. [46] studied 26 myopic children (11–17 years of age) of East Asian ethnicity using an A-B reversal design. Each child was fitted with an overnight OK lens in one eye and a conventional rigid gas permeable (RGP) lens for daytime wear in the other eye. After 6 months, the lens-eye combinations were crossed over for another 6 months. After the first 6 months of lens wear, the average axial length of the RGP eye had increased by an average of 0.04 mm, while the OK eye showed no change. After the second 6-month phase of lens wear, the OK eye showed no change from baseline in axial length, while the conventional RGP eye demonstrated a significant increase in mean axial length, i.e., 0.09 mm. In summary, the conventional RGP lens wearing eye showed progressive axial length growth (myopic progression) throughout the study while the OK eye did not.

Two OK studies (see Fig. 30.5) have provided long-term results (5 years and 7 years); they concluded that OK slows the rate of progression at the same rate as the first years [47, 48]. OK provides patients with a "wow" factor and eliminates the need for daily contact lenses or glasses. This is beneficial for athletic children. Generally, visual acuity is generally 20/20 with over 90% achieving 20/30 [49].

The true risk of infection for OK is unknown [50]. Any risk of infection in a voluntary treatment program that involves children must be weighed against the potential benefit of future reduction of ocular complications such as retinal detachment, macular degeneration, and glaucoma. The risk of microbial keratitis (MK) from OK is less than from extended wear of contact lenses. The rate of microbial OK infection appears to be 7.7 per 10,000 years of wear [51]. This compares to 1.4 per 10,000 patient years of wear in non-wearers, 11.9 per 10,000 patient years of wear in silicone hydrogel daily wearers, and 20 per 10,000 patient years of wear in soft contact lens extended wear [52]. It should be noted that OK is worn for 8–10 h per day which is far less than the 24 h. Of extended wear contacts, OK lenses have more oxygen permeably than soft lenses, and the surface of OK lenses is smoother or slipperier than soft lenses, so that a biofilm does not stick to the lens as easily. The incidence of MK is higher in children than adults [53]. The rare cases of *Acanthamoeba* or *Fusarium* infection often results in permanent destruction of the cornea; thus, it is important to maintain proper hygiene and cleaning [54]. Since wearing OK is at night, there is greater opportunity for the parents to supervise the wearing of these lenses vs. regular soft lenses.

OK is the most effective in children who have moderate myopia (between 1.25 and 4.0 diopters) and large pupils; thus, good results occur less frequently with lower or higher myopia [48, 55–57]. The poorer results are believed to be due to less relative peripheral hyperopia. Dropout rates are around 20% [42].

Cho et al. [58] had their patients discontinue OK lens wear to evaluate the rebound effect. There was a more rapid increase in axial length as compared to those wearing spectacles. When OK treatment was resumed axial elongation slowed again. They concluded that the rebound effect with OK lenses was similar to that found with atropine.

Recently, there has been increased interest in the use of soft lenses to mimic the effects of OK [59–65]. To design an optically similar lens as OK, one would need to manufacture a multifocal lens with a small, distance-centered optic zone. Walline et al. [64] evaluated 40 children with a Proclear Multifocal "D" (CooperVision, Fairport, NY) +2.00 D add power. He compared their results to a historical age-matched control group of single-vision distance lens wearers. The adjusted mean increase of myopia at 2 years was −1.03 ± 0.06 D for the single-vision contact lens wearers and −0.51 ± 0.06 D for the soft multifocal contact lens wearers. The adjusted mean axial elongation was 0.41 ± 0.03 mm and 0.29 ± 0.03 mm for the single-vision and soft multifocal contact lens wearers, respectively ($p < 0.0016$). Walline et al. concluded that soft multifocal contact lens wear results in a 50% reduction in the progression of myopia and a 29% reduction in axial elongation over a 2-year treatment period. There seems to be a disconnection between the AL and refractive data.

In a recent study, progressive myopic children were placed in one of three groups: soft radial refractive gradient (SRRG) contact lenses (same as the current MiSight™), orthokeratology (OK), or a single-vision glasses (SV) [65]. The SRRG was an experimental soft contact lens with a distance center and high plus in the mid-periphery. After 2 years, the mean myopia progression values for the SRRG were −0.56 D or 43%, OK was −0.32 D or 67%, and SV was −0.98 D. Measurement of axial length increase was less by 27% and 38% in the SRRG and OK groups as compared to the SV group. Aller et al. [66] used an Acuvue® Bifocal (Johnson & Johnson, Jacksonville, FL) center distance bifocal soft contact lens in a group of myopic esophoric patients and achieved almost a 70% reduction of myopia after 1 year. A meta-analysis, which included 587 subjects from 8 studies, found that concentric ring and distance-centered multifocal designs slowed myopia progression by 30–38% and axial elongation by 31–51% over 24 months [67]. Turnbull et al. [68] performed a retrospective case series analysis of 110 myopic children and reported that multifocal soft lens and OK slowed myopic progression equally.

As compared to OK, most of the designs have a maximum of a 2-diopter difference between the distance and peripheral portion of the lens. OK provides a larger differential, e.g., 4 diopters for a −2.00 and 6 diopters for a −3.00. In a recent experiment, Irving and Yakobchuk-

Stanger [69] used a −6.00 diopter lens in front of a young chick's eye to induce axial elongation followed by treatment of a control lens or various experimental multifocal lenses. One of the lens designs was effective in reversing the induced myopia. This lens design is currently used in the VTI/NaturalVue™ lens, which is FDA approved for the correction of presbyopia. Cooper et al. [70] published a retrospective case series analysis on 32 myopic children fit with this lens design. They reported that a center distance extended depth of focus soft multifocal contact lens design (NaturalVue™ by VTI) slowed myopic progression from X = −0.85D before treatment to 0.04D/year after, almost a 90% decrease in the progression of myopia. These findings suggest that both OK and multifocal lenses slow the progression of myopia by similar mechanisms and that the greater the plus over the largest retinal area has the greatest effect. Subsequent 5-year long-term data support the initial findings of this study.

Recently, a 3-year study comparing a single-vision contact lens with MiSight™ (CooperVision) demonstrated a 51% reduction in progression of myopia with the MiSight™ contact lens [71, 72]. The MiSight contact lens, which is approved for the reduction of progression of myopia in Europe, Canada, and the USA, is made up of a center distance vision segment and surrounding alternate plus and distance concentric rings. Figure 30.6 depicts the mean spherical equivalent progression of myopia with both the control, i.e., single-vision distance correcting lens and MiSight, while Fig. 30.7 depicts the axial length measurements. It is readily apparent that the MiSight slows the progression of myopia, improving over time. Though the study did not include a cessation phase, the results are compelling in demonstrating the optical effect of slowing myopia.

The most recent study, the BLINK study used a commercially available silicone-hydrogel lens to evaluate the effect of various amounts of the plus power in the periphery to slow the progression of myopia. The three lenses used were a single-vision lens and two different multifocals with the center distance ("D") and a +1.50 add and +2.50 add. They reported progression rates of 1.05 D for the SV group; 0.89 D for the +1.50 group; and 0.60 D for the +2.50 group. Similar findings were noted on axial length measurements. This NIH/NEI study clearly demonstrates that the stronger the add in the multifocal, the better the lens in controlling the progression of myopia [73]. In addition, this lens provides the opportunity to provide myopia management to patients having higher amounts of myopia with astigmatism.

Currently there are three center distance contact lenses with an appropriate design to slow the progression of myopia. A review of the current multifocal studies is presented in Table 30.1. There are no studies comparing each lens design.

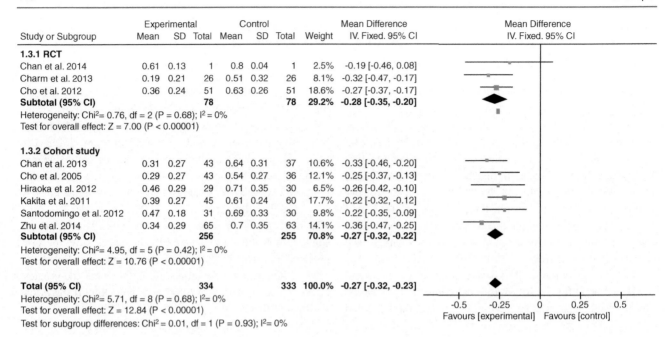

Study or Subgroup	Experimental			Control			Weight	Mean Difference IV. Fixed. 95% CI
	Mean	SD	Total	Mean	SD	Total		
1.3.1 RCT								
Chan et al. 2014	0.61	0.13	1	0.8	0.04	1	2.5%	-0.19 [-0.46, 0.08]
Charm et al. 2013	0.19	0.21	26	0.51	0.32	26	8.1%	-0.32 [-0.47, -0.17]
Cho et al. 2012	0.36	0.24	51	0.63	0.26	51	18.6%	-0.27 [-0.37, -0.17]
Subtotal (95% CI)			**78**			**78**	**29.2%**	**-0.28 [-0.35, -0.20]**

Heterogeneity: Chi² = 0.76, df = 2 (P = 0.68); I² = 0%
Test for overall effect: Z = 7.00 (P < 0.00001)

1.3.2 Cohort study								
Chan et al. 2013	0.31	0.27	43	0.64	0.31	37	10.6%	-0.33 [-0.46, -0.20]
Cho et al. 2005	0.29	0.27	43	0.54	0.27	36	12.1%	-0.25 [-0.37, -0.13]
Hiraoka et al. 2012	0.46	0.29	29	0.71	0.35	30	6.5%	-0.26 [-0.42, -0.10]
Kakita et al. 2011	0.39	0.27	45	0.61	0.24	60	17.7%	-0.22 [-0.32, -0.12]
Santodomingo et al. 2012	0.47	0.18	31	0.69	0.33	30	9.8%	-0.22 [-0.35, -0.09]
Zhu et al. 2014	0.34	0.29	65	0.7	0.35	63	14.1%	-0.36 [-0.47, -0.25]
Subtotal (95% CI)			**256**			**255**	**70.8%**	**-0.27 [-0.32, -0.22]**

Heterogeneity: Chi² = 4.95, df = 5 (P = 0.42); I² = 0%
Test for overall effect: Z = 10.76 (P < 0.00001)

| **Total (95% CI)** | | | **334** | | | **333** | **100.0%** | **-0.27 [-0.32, -0.23]** |

Heterogeneity: Chi² = 5.71, df = 8 (P = 0.68); I² = 0%
Test for overall effect: Z = 12.84 (P < 0.00001)
Test for subgroup differences: Chi² = 0.01, df = 1 (P = 0.93); I² = 0%

Fig. 30.6 Meta-analysis of ortho-K. Meta-analysis of 7 OK studies of 435 subjects between the ages 6 and 16 years and a mean difference between controls and OK patients of 0.26 mm over 2 years. This is a 40% reduction in the progression of myopia. (Reprinted with permission from Si et al. [104])

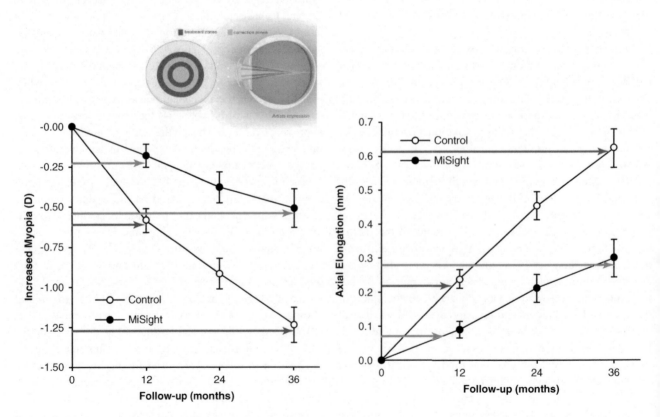

Fig. 30.7 MiSight data. A 3-year prospective, randomized clinical trial of progressive myopic children between the ages of 8–12 yrs was performed comparing two soft contact lenses: (**a**) single-vision control lens and (**b**) the experimental lens a soft lens with a 4 mm central distance zone surrounding by alternating concentric plus rings of +3.00 of power. The group wearing the experimental lens had a reduction in progression in myopia by as measured by 59% in refractive error and by 53% in measuring axial length. (Reprinted with permission Chamberlain et al. [72]. Reprinted with permission)

Table 30.1   Soft lens results. There are 13 studies using soft contact lenses to slow the progression of myopia. There are only three which include commercially available soft lenses. Two have relatively moderate adds (under 3 diopters) while one has a high add (VTI NaturalVue), i.e., +6.00. The higher the add, generally the more effective the lenses are in controlling myopic progression. Only the MiSight study is a well-designed prospective, masked clinical trial measuring both refractive error and axial length for over a year of time, i.e., 3 years

	Year	Lens name	Type of lens	Amount of add	No of subjects	Length	Control	Change in control (D)	Change in exp group (D)	Change in exp. group (AL)		Comparison to control	Progression AL/year
Aller, Liu, Widoso et al.	2016	Acuvue presbyopia	Gradient	2	86	12	SV soft	0.79	0.22	0.24	0.05	79%	0.19
Anstice NS, Phillips	2011	Custom	Dual focus	2	40	10	Other eye	0.69	0.44	0.22	0.11	49%	0.11
Lam CSY, Tang WC,	2014	Custom	Concentric	2.5	221	24	Random CL	-0.3	-0.4	0.18	0.13	32%	0.12
Fujikado	2014	Custom	Gradient	Low	24	12	Crossover		0.09	0.17		25%	0.05
Walline JJ, Greiner KL	2013	Proclear	Gradient	2	27	24	Historical	-0.52	-0.26	0.21	-0.15	29%	0.12
Sankaridurg P, Holden	2011	Custom	Gradient	?	95	12	Spectacle	-0.86	-0.45	0.4	0.27	38%	0.15
Pauné J, Morales	2015	Custom	Radial ref gradient		40		Spectacle	-98	-0.56			27%	0.14
Cooper	2018	VTI NaturalVue	Gradient	6	32	6-25	Historical	0.85	0.04				
Cheng	2015	Custom	Positive sph ab	?	82	24	Random CL	0.14	0.14	0.14	0.11	39%	0.14
Allen et al	2013	Custom	Aberration control	?	96	24	Random CL					-1%	-0.01
ruiz-pomeda	2018	MiSight	Dual focus	3.5	74	24	Spectacle	0.74	0.45	0.44	0.28	36%	0.16
Chamberlian et al	2019	MiSight	Dual focus	3.5	109	36	Random CL	-0.41	-0.17	0.21	0.11	52%	0.32
Sankaridurg P, Bakaraju	2019	Custom	Different designs	1.5–2.5	508	24		-0.575	-0.4	0.29	0.205	30%	0.09

30.4 Outside Exposure

Several recent studies suggest that time spent outdoors slows both onset and progression of myopia in children [74–83]. It is well known that myopia increases more during the winter than the summer. The effect of outdoor activities on myopia is not necessarily related to physical activity; rather, the amount of exposure to outdoor environment has the therapeutic effect [76]. The results of these studies are not surprising when the results of animal studies are considered. For example, it is well known that when animals are raised in a high ambient light (25,000 lux), form-deprivation myopia does not develop, but myopia does develop if the ambient light is reduced to 350 lux which is a normal room. It is believed that the dopamine antagonist blocks the protective effect of high levels of ambient light in developing form-deprivation myopia. However, dopamine antagonists have a minimum effect with lens-induced myopia. To add to the confusion, there are studies in which monkeys raised with lenses to create myopia were unaffected by the ambient light. These animal studies suggest that defocus has a greater effect on emmetropization than ambient light. Several other studies have suggested that exposure to brighter light, increased levels of vitamin D, increased levels of dopamine, or UV light by itself is responsible for the effect of outdoors on myopia onset and progression [84–93]. While other studies have ruled out the role of vitamin D and UV light in the inhibition of myopia development by exposure to outdoors [94, 95]. Flitcroft [96] has suggested that in addition there are dioptic and spectral composition factors that might explain the effect of outdoors to slow myopia progression. For example, distance viewing has a different spectral composition, outside being dominated by blue light (short) and inside dominated by red light (long). Distance viewing has minimal accommodative cues within the field of vision, and near vision requires accommodation, induces a lag of accommodation (a form of defocus), has a large field filled with objects that are out of focus, and induces relative hyperopia. Reading and computer use have even different demands, i.e., sustained accommodation with minimal ability to change. This variable has not been studied, but it is readily apparent that people who are in their 20s and 30s still progress in their myopia, while supporting staff (cleaning people, elevator operators, etc.) do not.

Recently Torii et al. [93] demonstrated that violet light (VL) (360–400 nm wavelength) suppresses myopia progression in chicks and humans. They retrospectively measured the AL elongation among myopic children, who wore either VL blocked eyeglasses or one of two types of contact lenses (partially VL blocking and VL transmitting). They reported that the VL transmitting contact lenses suppressed myopia progression more than VL blocking lenses. They suggested that since VL exposure is limited by UV protection from being indoors, filtered out UV by panel window glass, and filtered out by UV filtering glasses, some contact lenses and sunglasses that increased VL exposure may be a preventive strategy against myopia progression.

There is, also, evidence that increasing the illumination in classrooms decreases the incidence of myopia [97]. Bright light has been shown to inhibit form-deprivation myopia and reduce lens-induced (defocus-induced) myopia in animal studies [86–90]. However, there is no information whether bright light might have caused animals to close their eyes due to photophobia or did not take into account the use of sunglasses in bright light, which might account for substantial differences in the visual environment between indoors and outdoors [98]. Indoor activities create far more peripheral hyperopic defocus (causing myopia) than any outdoor activities. Outdoor activities decrease peripheral defocus that serves as a stop signal for the eye growth (thus inhibiting development of myopia). Brighter light intensity leads to pupil constriction and increased depth of focus, which reduces optical blur and increases contrast. Change in contrast, in turn, would affect the function of amacrine cells, which might explain the role of dopamine in myopia development in animal models. Although the exact mechanism responsible for the effect of outdoor activities on myopia is unknown, spending more time outdoors clearly has a therapeutic effect on myopia onset and is associated with 11–33% reduction in myopic progression. Thus, children, especially those who have two myopic parents and/or show signs of myopia development or progression, should spend more time outdoors to help prevent myopia from developing.

30.5 Combined Treatment

Different therapies work different ways. It is an obvious clinical question to determine if the effects are synergistic, i.e. does using atropine along with a contact lens slow the progression more. There have been three studies looking at the synergist effects of atropine and OK [99–101]. Kinoshita et al. [100] reported an AL increase in an OK group was 0.19 ± 0.12 mm/year and 0.09 ± 0.12 mm/year in the combination group. Chen et al. [102] reported that in rapidly progressing myopes where the mean axial elongation rate was 0.46 ± 0.16 mm/ when atropine was added, axial elongation decreased to 0.14 ± 0.14 mm/year. Wan et al. [101] performed a retrospective study, which compared the effects of OK and OK with supplemental atropine of either 0.025% or 0.125%; they reported that the addition of atropine was clinically significant for patients above and below 6 diopters of myopia. However, inspection of their data does not support a strong clinical difference. In summary, all of the studies comparing the use of OK or OK with atropine have concluded that the effects are additive.

30.6 Clinical Guidelines

The ability to control myopia has changed in the last 20 years. Both our understanding of how the eye uses visual feedback to control axial length and the effectiveness of both atropine and optical correction to slow the progression of myopia is better understood. The understandings have come with a concomitant increase in utilization of myopia control techniques. When parents ask if one can slow the progression of myopia, the answer should no longer be "no." Eye doctors need to be aware and prescribe the most appropriate treatment. Pediatric ophthalmologist who does not provide care which includes spectacles, multifocal contact lenses, and pharmaceutical agents should refer these patients to someone who provides the care measuring both refractive error and axial length. Retinal specialists who are seeing patients with myopic induced retinal complications should advise these patients, if they are of child-rearing age, to have their child watched for the development of myopia. Early treatment should be instituted when possible. Along with instituting myopia control therapy, we also advocate an increase in the amount of time a child should spend outdoors. We recommend at least 3 h per day of outside play.

Currently, Taiwan and Singapore eye doctors advocate the use of atropine, while China, New Zealand, and Australia are big proponents of ortho-K; the USA is more mixed with optometrists more commonly recommending OK, while ophthalmologists prescribe atropine. I believe that every modality should be used, the appropriate one being somewhat determined by the child-parent interaction. OK is great for the athletic child who has a refraction between 2D and 5D, while soft multifocal lenses are better for the lower myopes (1–2 diopters) and the higher myopes (above 5D). Some parents are concerned about microbial infection with overnight lenses and should be prescribed a treatment that they are comfortable with. Soft multifocal contacts should be daily when possible. Our protocol uses either atropine 0.02% or contact lenses as a starting point. Success rates are presented in Fig. 30.8. We measure refraction and axial length 3 months after prescribing the initial treatment. Our AL measurements are taken 20 times to eliminate measurement variability [103]. If there is no progression, then we re-examine the patient in 4 months and again in 6 months. However, if there is evidence of progression, we add or increase the dosage of atropine sequentially 0.02% to 0.05% to 0.1% to 0.25% to 1.00%. Progressive addition lenses which are photosensitive are prescribed to reduce photophobia and blur. The addition power is determined after a week of using the lower concentration of atropine. Either cross cylinder or accommodative balancing techniques can be used.

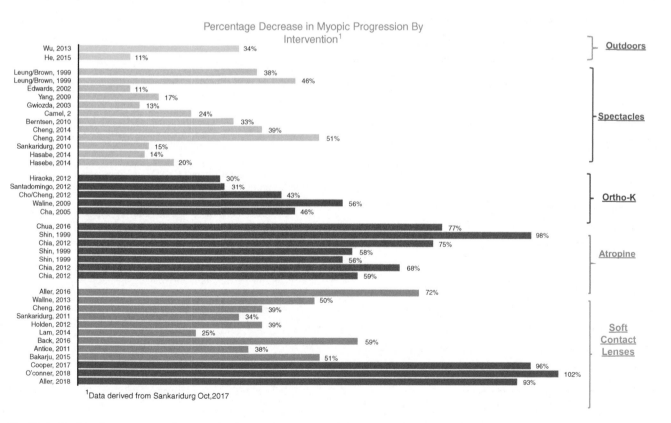

Fig. 30.8 Combined success rates. Commutative data provides a sense of the relative effectiveness of each treatment. It should be remembered that comparing studies must be put in perspective since populations studied differed in makeup in regard to race, age, initial refractive, etc

Combination therapies are the most effective. Even with this regiment, some myopes are not responsive. More research is needed to determine the exact optical characteristics in glasses and contact lenses to slow the progression of myopia; until that is done, in our opinion both optometrists and ophthalmologists need to use the available tools to slow the progression of myopia and hopefully reduce the morbidity associated with it. The risk is small and the benefit is great, despite the FDA not approving current methodologies.

References

1. Holden B, Sankaridurg P, Smith E, Aller T, Jong M, He M. Myopia, an underrated global challenge to vision: where the current data takes us on myopia control. Eye (Lond). 2014;28(2):142–6.
2. Holden BA, Fricke TR, Wilson DA, et al. Global prevalence of myopia and high myopia and temporal trends from 2000 through 2050. Ophthalmology. 2016;123(5):1036–42.
3. Cooper J, Weibel K, Borukhov G. Use of atropine to slow the progression of myopia: a literature review and guidelines for clinical use. Vision Dev & Rehab. 2018;4(1):12–28.
4. Cooper J, Tkatchenko AV. A review of current concepts of the etiology and treatment of myopia. Eye Contact Lens. 2018;44(4):231–47.
5. Huang J, Wen D, Wang Q, et al. Efficacy comparison of 16 interventions for myopia control in children: a network Meta-analysis. Ophthalmology. 2016;123(4):697–708.
6. Uzma N, Kumar BS, et al. A comparative clinical survey of the prevalence of refractive errors and eye diseases in urban and rural school children. Can J Ophthalmol. 2009;44(3):328–33.
7. Verhoeven VJ, Buitendijk GH, Consortium for Refractive Error and Myopia (CREAM), et al. Education influences the role of genetics in myopia. Eur J Epidemiol. 2013;28(12):973–80.
8. Dirani M, Shekar SN, Baird PN. The role of educational attainment in refraction: the Genes in Myopia (GEM) twin study. Invest Ophthalmol Vis Sci. 2008;49(2):534–8.
9. Al-Bdour MD, Odat TA, Tahat AA. Myopia and level of education. Eur J Ophthalmol. 2001;11(1):1–5.
10. Teasdale TW, Fuchs J, Goldschmidt E. Degree of myopia in relation to intelligence and educational level. Lancet. 1988;2(8624):1351–4.
11. Parssinen O, Lyyra AL. Myopia and myopic progression among schoolchildren: a three-year follow-up study. Invest Ophthalmol Vis Sci. 1993;34(9):2794–802.
12. Goss DA. Nearwork and myopia. Lancet. 2000;356(9240):1456–7.
13. Hepsen IF, Evereklioglu C, Bayramlar H. The effect of reading and near-work on the development of myopia in emmetropic boys: a prospective, controlled, three-year follow-up study. Vis Res. 2001;41(19):2511–20.
14. Saw SM, Chua WH, Hong CY, et al. Nearwork in early-onset myopia. Invest Ophthalmol Vis Sci. 2002;43(2):332–9.
15. Wong L, Coggon D, Cruddas M, Hwang CH. Education, reading, and familial tendency as risk factors for myopia in Hong Kong fishermen. J Epidemiol Community Health. 1993;47(1):50–3.
16. Saw SM, Wu HM, Seet B, et al. Academic achievement, close up work parameters, and myopia in Singapore military conscripts. Br J Ophthalmol. 2001;85(7):855–60.
17. Li SM, Li SY, Kang MT, et al. Near work related parameters and myopia in Chinese children: the Anyang Childhood Eye Study. PLoS One. 2015;10(8):e0134514.
18. Cooper J, Schulman E, Jamal N. Current status on the development and treatment of myopia. Optometry. 2012;83(5):179–99.
19. Rosenfield M, Gilmartin B. Accommodative error, adaptation and myopia. Ophthalmic Physiol Opt. 1999;19(2):159–64.
20. Gwiazda JE, Hyman L, Norton TT, et al. Accommodation and related risk factors associated with myopia progression and their interaction with treatment in COMET children. Invest Ophthalmol Vis Sci. 2004;45(7):2143–51.
21. Gwiazda J, Thorn F, Held R. Accommodation, accommodative convergence, and response AC/A ratios before and at the onset of myopia in children. Optom Vis Sci. 2005;82(4):273–8.
22. Goss DA. Variables related to the rate of childhood myopia progression. Optom Vis Sci. 1990;67(8):631–6.
23. Parssinen O, Hemminki E. Spectacle-use, bifocals and prevention of myopic progression. The two-years results of a randomized trial among schoolchildren. Acta Ophthalmol Suppl. 1988;185:156–61.
24. Goss DA, Grosvenor T. Rates of childhood myopia progression with bifocals as a function of nearpoint phoria: consistency of three studies. Optom Vis Sci. 1990;67(8):637–40.
25. Gwiazda JE, Hyman L, Everett D, Norton T, Kurtz D, Manny R. Five-year results from the correction of myopia evaluation trial (COMET). Invest Ophthalmol Vis Sci. 2006;47:1166.
26. Kurtz D, Hyman L, Gwiazda JE, et al. Role of parental myopia in the progression of myopia and its interaction with treatment in COMET children. Invest Ophthalmol Vis Sci. 2007;48(2):562–70.
27. Cheng D, Schmid KL, Woo GC, Drobe B. Randomized trial of effect of bifocal and prismatic bifocal spectacles on myopic progression: two-year results. Arch Ophthalmol. 2010;128(1):12–9.
28. Li SM, Ji YZ, Wu SS, et al. Multifocal versus single vision lenses intervention to slow progression of myopia in school-age children: a meta-analysis. Surv Ophthalmol. 2011;56(5):451–60.
29. Smith EL 3rd. Optical treatment strategies to slow myopia progression: effects of the visual extent of the optical treatment zone. Exp Eye Res. 2013;114:77–88.
30. Diether S, Schaeffel F. Local changes in eye growth induced by imposed local refractive error despite active accommodation. Vis Res. 1997;37(6):659–68.
31. Troilo D, Gottlieb MD, Wallman J. Visual deprivation causes myopia in chicks with optic nerve section. Curr Eye Res. 1987;6(8):993–9.
32. Sankaridurg P, Donovan L, Varnas S, et al. Spectacle lenses designed to reduce progression of myopia: 12-month results. Optom Vis Sci. 2010;87(9):631–41.
33. Lam CS, Tang WC, Tse DY, Tang YY, To CH. Defocus Incorporated Soft Contact (DISC) lens slows myopia progression in Hong Kong Chinese schoolchildren: a 2-year randomised clinical trial. Br J Ophthalmol. 2014;98(1):40–5.
34. Lam CSY, Tang WC, Tse DY, et al. Defocus Incorporated Multiple Segments (DIMS) spectacle lenses slow myopia progression: a 2-year randomised clinical trial. Br J Ophthalmol. 2020;104(3):363–8.
35. Rappon J, Neitz J, Neitz M. Novel DOT lenses from sightglass vision show great promise to fight myopia. Rev Myopia Manage. 2020;
36. Chung K, Mohidin N, O'Leary DJ. Undercorrection of myopia enhances rather than inhibits myopia progression. Vis Res. 2002;42(22):2555–9.
37. Adler D, Millodot M. The possible effect of undercorrection on myopic progression in children. Clin Exp Optom. 2006;89(5):315–21.
38. Walline JJ, Jones LA, Mutti DO, Zadnik K. A randomized trial of the effects of rigid contact lenses on myopia progression. Arch Ophthalmol. 2004;122(12):1760–6.
39. Walline JJ, Jones LA, Sinnott L, et al. A randomized trial of the effect of soft contact lenses on myopia progression in children. Invest Ophthalmol Vis Sci. 2008;49(11):4702–6.

40. Lui WO, Edwards MH. Orthokeratology in low myopia. Part 1: efficacy and predictability. Cont Lens Anterior Eye. 2000;23(3):77–89.

41. Walline JJ, Rah MJ, Jones LA. The Children's Overnight Orthokeratology Investigation (COOKI) pilot study. Optom Vis Sci. 2004;81(6):407–13.

42. Cho P, Cheung SW, Edwards M. The longitudinal orthokeratology research in children (LORIC) in Hong Kong: a pilot study on refractive changes and myopic control. Curr Eye Res. 2005;30(1):71–80.

43. Walline JJ, Jones LA, Sinnott LT. Corneal reshaping and myopia progression. Br J Ophthalmol. 2009;93(9):1181–5.

44. Kakita T, Hiraoka T, Oshika T. Influence of overnight orthokeratology on axial elongation in childhood myopia. Invest Ophthalmol Vis Sci. 2011;52(5):2170–4.

45. Santodomingo-Rubido J, Villa-Collar C, Gilmartin B, Gutierrez-Ortega R. Myopia control with orthokeratology contact lenses in Spain (MCOS): refractive and biometric changes. Invest Ophthalmol Vis Sci. 2012;53(8):5060–5.

46. Swarbrick HA, Alharbi A, Watt K, Lum E, Kang P. Myopia control during orthokeratology lens wear in children using a novel study design. Ophthalmology. 2015;122(3):620–30.

47. Kwok-Hei Mok A, Sin-Ting CC. Seven-year retrospective analysis of the myopic control effect of orthokeratology in children: a pilot study. Clin Optom. 2011;3:1–4.

48. Hiraoka T, Kakita T, Okamoto F, Takahashi H, Oshika T. Long-term effect of overnight orthokeratology on axial length elongation in childhood myopia: a 5-year follow-up study. Invest Ophthalmol Vis Sci. 2012;53(7):3913–9.

49. Rah MJ, Jackson JM, Jones LA, Marsden HJ, Bailey MD, Barr JT. Overnight orthokeratology: preliminary results of the Lenses and Overnight Orthokeratology (LOOK) study. Optom Vis Sci. 2002;79(9):598–605.

50. Van Meter WS, Musch DC, Jacobs DS, Kaufman SC, Reinhart WJ, Udell IJ. Safety of overnight orthokeratology for myopia: a report by the American Academy of Ophthalmology. Ophthalmology. 2008;115(12):2301–13. e2301

51. Bullimore MA. What can be done for my child? Optom Vis Sci. 2000;77(8):381.

52. Stapleton F, Keay L, Edwards K, et al. The incidence of contact lens-related microbial keratitis in Australia. Ophthalmology. 2008;115(10):1655–62.

53. Bullimore MA, Sinnott LT, Jones-Jordan LA. The risk of microbial keratitis with overnight corneal reshaping lenses. Optom Vis Sci. 2013;90(9):937–44.

54. Liu YM, Xie P. The safety of orthokeratology–a systematic review. Eye Contact Lens. 2016;42(1):35–42.

55. Li SM, Kang MT, Wu SS, et al. Efficacy, safety and acceptability of orthokeratology on slowing axial elongation in myopic children by meta-analysis. Curr Eye Res. 2015;41(5):600–8.

56. Fu AC, Chen XL, Lv Y, et al. Higher spherical equivalent refractive errors is associated with slower axial elongation wearing orthokeratology. Cont Lens Anterior Eye. 2016;39(1):62–6.

57. Wang B, Naidu RK, Qu X. Factors related to axial length elongation and myopia progression in orthokeratology practice. PLoS One. 2017;12(4):e0175913.

58. Cho P, Cheung SW. Discontinuation of orthokeratology on eyeball elongation (DOEE). Cont Lens Anterior Eye. 2017;40(2):82–7.

59. Anstice NS, Phillips JR. Effect of dual-focus soft contact lens wear on axial myopia progression in children. Ophthalmology. 2011;118(6):1152–61.

60. Sankaridurg P, Holden B, Smith E 3rd, et al. Decrease in rate of myopia progression with a contact lens designed to reduce relative peripheral hyperopia: one-year results. Invest Ophthalmol Vis Sci. 2011;52(13):9362–7.

61. Holden B, Sankaridurg P, Lazon P, et al. Central and peripheral visual performance of a novel contact lens designed to control progression of myopia. Invest Ophthalmol Vis Sci. 2011;52:6518.

62. Woods J, Guthrie SE, Keir N, et al. Inhibition of defocus-induced myopia in chickens. Invest Ophthalmol Vis Sci. 2013;54(4):2662–8.

63. Woods J, Guthrie S, Keir N, et al. The effect of a unique lens designed for Myopia Progression Control (MPC) on the level of induced myopia in chicks. Invest Ophthalmol Vis Sci. 2011;52:6651.

64. Walline JJ, Greiner KL, McVey ME, Jones-Jordan LA. Multifocal contact lens myopia control. Optom Vis Sci. 2013;90(11):1207–14.

65. Paune J, Morales H, Armengol J, Quevedo L, Faria-Ribeiro M, Gonzalez-Meijome JM. Myopia control with a novel peripheral gradient soft Lens and orthokeratology: a 2-year clinical trial. Biomed Res Int. 2015;2015:507572.

66. Aller TA, Liu M, Wildsoet CF. Myopia control with bifocal contact lenses: a randomized clinical trial. Optom Vis Sci. 2016;93(4):344–52.

67. Li SM, Kang MT, Wu SS, et al. Studies using concentric ring bifocal and peripheral add multifocal contact lenses to slow myopia progression in school-aged children: a meta-analysis. Ophthalmic Physiol Opt. 2017;37(1):51–9.

68. Turnbull PR, Munro OJ, Phillips JR. Contact lens methods for clinical myopia control. Optom Vis Sci. 2016;93(9):1120–6.

69. Irving EL, Yakobchuk-Stanger C. Myopia progression control lens reverses induced myopia in chicks. Ophthalmic Physiol Opt. 2017;37(5):576–84.

70. Cooper J, O'Connor B, Watanabe R, et al. Case series analysis of myopic progression control with a unique extended depth of focus multifocal contact lens. Eye Contact Lens. 2017;44(5):e16–24.

71. Ruiz-Pomeda A, Perez-Sanchez B, Valls I, Prieto-Garrido FL, Gutierrez-Ortega R, Villa-Collar C. MiSight Assessment Study Spain (MASS). A 2-year randomized clinical trial. Graefes Arch Clin Exp Ophthalmol. 2018;256(5):1011–21.

72. Chamberlain P, Peixoto-de-Matos SC, Logan NS, Ngo C, Jones D, Young G. A 3-year randomized clinical trial of MiSight lenses for myopia control. Optom Vis Sci. 2019;96(8):556–67.

73. Walline JJ, Walker MK, Mutti DO, et al. Effect of high add power, medium add power, or single-vision contact lenses on myopia progression in children: the BLINK randomized clinical trial. JAMA. 2020;324(6):571–80.

74. Rose KA, Morgan IG, Ip J, et al. Outdoor activity reduces the prevalence of myopia in children. Ophthalmology. 2008;115(8):1279–85.

75. Dirani M, Tong L, Gazzard G, et al. Outdoor activity and myopia in Singapore teenage children. Br J Ophthalmol. 2009;93(8):997–1000.

76. Guggenheim JA, Northstone K, McMahon G, et al. Time outdoors and physical activity as predictors of incident myopia in childhood: a prospective cohort study. Invest Ophthalmol Vis Sci. 2012;53(6):2856–65.

77. He M, Xiang F, Zeng Y, et al. Effect of time spent outdoors at school on the development of myopia among children in China: a randomized clinical trial. JAMA. 2015;314(11):1142–8.

78. Jones LA, Sinnott LT, Mutti DO, Mitchell GL, Moeschberger ML, Zadnik K. Parental history of myopia, sports and outdoor activities, and future myopia. Invest Ophthalmol Vis Sci. 2007;48(8):3524–32.

79. Deng L, Gwiazda J, Thorn F. Children's refractions and visual activities in the school year and summer. Optom Vis Sci. 2010;87(6):406–13.

80. Guo Y, Liu LJ, Xu L, et al. Myopic shift and outdoor activity among primary school children: one-year follow-up study in Beijing. PLoS One. 2013;8(9):e75260.

81. Guo Y, Liu LJ, Xu L, et al. Outdoor activity and myopia among primary students in rural and urban regions of Beijing. Ophthalmology. 2013;120(2):277–83.

82. Wu PC, Tsai CL, Wu HL, Yang YH, Kuo HK. Outdoor activity during class recess reduces myopia onset and progression in school children. Ophthalmology. 2013;120(5):1080–5.

83. Jin JX, Hua WJ, Jiang X, et al. Effect of outdoor activity on myopia onset and progression in school-aged children in northeast China: the Sujiatun Eye Care Study. BMC Ophthalmol. 2015;15:73.

84. Mutti DO. Vitamin D may reduce the prevalence of myopia in Korean adolescents. Invest Ophthalmol Vis Sci. 2014;55(4):2048.

85. Mutti DO, Marks AR. Blood levels of vitamin D in teens and young adults with myopia. Optom Vis Sci. 2011;88(3):377–82.

86. Ashby R, Ohlendorf A, Schaeffel F. The effect of ambient illuminance on the development of deprivation myopia in chicks. Invest Ophthalmol Vis Sci. 2009;50(11):5348–54.

87. Karouta C, Ashby RS. Correlation between light levels and the development of deprivation myopia. Invest Ophthalmol Vis Sci. 2014;56(1):299–309.

88. Smith EL 3rd, Hung LF, Huang J. Protective effects of high ambient lighting on the development of form-deprivation myopia in rhesus monkeys. Invest Ophthalmol Vis Sci. 2012;53(1):421–8.

89. Ashby RS, Schaeffel F. The effect of bright light on lens compensation in chicks. Invest Ophthalmol Vis Sci. 2010;51(10):5247–53.

90. Smith EL 3rd, Hung LF, Arumugam B, Huang J. Negative lens-induced myopia in infant monkeys: effects of high ambient lighting. Invest Ophthalmol Vis Sci. 2013;54(4):2959–69.

91. Feldkaemper M, Schaeffel F. An updated view on the role of dopamine in myopia. Exp Eye Res. 2013;114:106–19.

92. Zhou X, Pardue MT, Iuvone PM, Qu J. Dopamine signaling and myopia development: what are the key challenges. Prog Retin Eye Res. 2017;61:60–71.

93. Torii H, Kurihara T, Seko Y, et al. Violet light exposure can be a preventive strategy against myopia progression. EBioMedicine. 2017;15:210–9.

94. Rose KA, French AN, Morgan IG. Environmental factors and myopia: paradoxes and prospects for prevention. Asia Pac J Ophthalmol (Phila). 2016;5(6):403–10.

95. Schaeffel F, Smith EL 3rd. Inhibiting myopia by (nearly) invisible light? EBioMedicine. 2017;16:27–8.

96. Flitcroft DI. The complex interactions of retinal, optical and environmental factors in myopia aetiology. Prog Retin Eye Res. 2012;31(6):622–60.

97. Hua WJ, Jin JX, Wu XY, et al. Elevated light levels in schools have a protective effect on myopia. Ophthalmic Physiol Opt. 2015;35(3):252–62.

98. Ngo C, Saw SM, Dharani R, Flitcroft I. Does sunlight (bright lights) explain the protective effects of outdoor activity against myopia? Ophthalmic Physiol Opt. 2013;33(3):368–72.

99. Kakehashi NKYKNHA. Suppressive effect of combined treatment of orthokeratology and 0.01% atropine instillation on axial length elongation in childhood myopia. Invest Ophthalmol Vis Sci. 2017;58:2386.

100. Kinoshita N, Konno Y, Hamada N, Kanda Y, Shimmura-Tomita M, Kakehashi A. Additive effects of orthokeratology and atropine 0.01% ophthalmic solution in slowing axial elongation in children with myopia: first year results. Jpn J Ophthalmol. 2018;62(5):544–53.

101. Wan L, Wei CC, Chen CS, et al. The synergistic effects of orthokeratology and atropine in slowing the progression of myopia. J Clin Med. 2018;7(9):259.

102. Chen Z, Huang S, Zhou J, Xiaomei Q, Zhou X, Xue F. Adjunctive effect of orthokeratology and low dose atropine on axial elongation in fast-progressing myopic children-A preliminary retrospective study. Cont Lens Anterior Eye. 2018;42(4):439–42.

103. Dillehay S, Cooper J, Eiden S, Aller T. Determination of IOLMaster number of measurements for tracking axial length changes in myopia. Invest Ophthalmol Vis Sci. 2018;59(9):2133.

104. Si JK, Tang K, Bi HS, Guo DD, Guo JG, Wang XR. Orthokeratology for myopia control: a meta-analysis. Optom Vis Sci. 2015;92(3):252–7.

Sclera-Targeted Therapies for Pathologic Myopia

Kyoko Ohno-Matsui

Therapeutic approaches for pathologic myopia have greatly advanced in recent years; however, the therapies are still limited to treat only some kinds of macular complications, such as antiangiogenic therapies for myopic macular neovascularization (myopic MNV) or vitreoretinal surgery for myopic traction maculopathy (MTM). These treatments are useful for the improved vision in the eyes developing myopic MNV or MTM to some extent; however, it is still difficult to regain the normal vision. In addition, most of the other pathologies in eyes with pathologic myopia, such as myopic choroidal atrophy or myopic optic neuropathy, remain to have no treatment options. Thus, it would be ideal to treat the fundamental nature of pathologic myopia before developing the vision-threatening complications in the macula and in the optic nerve. The fundamental nature of pathologic myopia might be an excessive increase of axial length, a development of posterior staphyloma, and the thinning and deformity of the posterior sclera.

There are three major approaches to treat or prevent pathologic myopia. The first approach would be to identify and to regulate the neural signal which was first detected as visual blur by retinal neural cells and finally transmitted to the sclera based on the studies of experimental myopia (this approach is described in detail in Chap. 4). The second approach would be to decrease the visual blur (mainly the blur in the peripheral retina) by optical correction in the school children who could show the greatest rate of increase in axial length throughout the life (this approach is described in detail in Chap. 25). The above two approaches need to be done before or during the axial length increases, and thus, the treatment for children are required. The third approach would be to prevent and recover the scleral thinning or scleral deformity. Although it is admitted that the first trigger to cause the axial elongation exists within the neural retina, the sclera is a final target tissue which develops a staphyloma as well as eye deformity. The formation of posterior staphyloma develops in later life (after 40 years of age); thus, the third approach can also be applied to the young individual who already have high myopia in addition to children.

The sclera is a dense fibrous and viscoelastic connective tissue. It forms the outer coat frame of the eye and acts to retain the shape of the eyeball by withstanding the pressure from both outside and inside. In Eutherian mammals, by far the main component of the sclera (over 90%) is fibrous type I collagen. However, in many kinds of non-mammals like bird and fish, the sclera also contains the cartilaginous part possibly to resist the pressure outside in the water or in the sky.

Regenerative therapies have greatly advanced lately, and thus the possibility of scleral regeneration is also expected. Thus, in this chapter, we focus on sclera-targeted therapies for a pathologic myopia, and we would like to review the past, present, and future therapies targeting the sclera in patients with pathologic myopia.

31.1 Scleral Reinforcement Surgery

Scleral reinforcement has been by far the most exclusively studied treatment targeted on the sclera. Shevelev first proposed the transplantation of fascia lata for scleral reinforcement in 1930. Borley and Snyder [1] described a technique for the placement of grafts of donor sclera in 1958. Posterior scleral reinforcement surgery for high myopia has been mainly done in Russia and China, and some groups in the United States and Australia also advocate scleral reinforcement for pathologic myopia. As natural materials, autologous fascia lata [2, 3], lyophilized dura [4], strips of tendon [5], and homologous human sclera [6, 7] have been used. Curtin [7] advocated donor-sclera grafting for posterior ocular reinforcement, and Momose [4] introduced Lyodura, derived from processed cadaver dura mater, for scleral reinforcement in 1976. As artificial materials, artificial

K. Ohno-Matsui (✉)
Department of Ophthalmology and Visual Science, Tokyo Medical and Dental University, Bunkyo-Ku, Tokyo, Japan
e-mail: k.ohno.oph@tmd.ac.jp

R. F. Spaide et al. (eds.), *Pathologic Myopia*, https://doi.org/10.1007/978-3-030-74334-5_31

pericardium [8], all-dermal matrix derived from animal skin [8], and polytetrafluoroethylene [9] have been used. However, the best material for reinforcement surgery remains controversial. The biomechanical properties of reinforced material may be subjected to many factors, such as the absorption of reinforced material, and the extent of fusion between the reinforcement material and the recipient sclera and so on.

Most investigators in the United States have used homologous sclera in the form of a belt or cinch placed vertically over the posterior pole, under the inferior and superior oblique muscles, and sutured to the anterior sclera. The shape of reinforced sclera is various: single strip, X-shaped, and Y-shaped. Later, Snyder and Thompson [10] published accounts of their experiences with a modified scleral reinforcement technique. Thompson [11] offered a further simplification of Borley and Snyder's scleral reinforcement approach in 1978 (Fig. 31.1).

After years of experience with their own variations of scleral reinforcement, Thompson [12] and Momose [4] expressed satisfaction with the efficacy and safety of their series of cases. In contrast, Curtin and Whitmore [7] had negative conclusions on the outcomes for their reinforcement techniques. What makes it difficult to determine the effectiveness of this surgery is a lack of accurate measurement of refractive error and axial length pre- and postoperatively, because most studies were done before the axial length measurement by ultrasound was established. Also, most of the studies included only a small number of cases without sufficiently long follow-up. More importantly, there have been no clinical studies with appropriate control groups.

Instead of measuring the refractive error and axial length, many studies reported the improvement of the uncorrected visual acuity probably due to a decrease of myopic refraction [2, 12, 13].

Curtin [7] suggested that two problems with this surgery were the limited scleral area reinforced by narrow grafts and the possible late involvement of graft collagen in the disease process of host sclera. The present use of narrow strips of collagen materials can effectively reinforce only a small area of the typical posterior staphyloma. However, a support of wider area could cause serious complications, including an occlusion of arteries and veins in the back of the eye [14, 15]. A loss of tensile strength of the collagenous graft is also concerned, possibly because of enzymatic attack. Curtin [7] was concerned that if the pathogenetic mechanism of scleral thinning and ectasia in pathologic myopia is caused by a collagenolytic enzyme, such as collagenase or a suitable protease, the grafted collagen, when invaded by host sclerocytes, could be expected to undergo the same autolysis and weakening as the host sclera. Histological study showed that the transplanted sclera merged with recipient sclera with time [8]. It is also possible that the inflammatory reactions following the grafting material and surgical procedure could cause the

upregulation of degrading enzymes which then attack the host sclera as well as the grafted material. Thus, we suspect that it is possible that the upregulated degrading enzymes (possibly matrix metalloproteinase) secondarily attack the donor sclera in return. Curtin described that the most disappointing thing was that a staphyloma developed in reinforced eyes.

The results of the earlier studies are not consistent even among the studies which measured the axial length pre- and postoperatively. This might be because many factors (age at surgery, myopic degree, grafted material) are various. Gerinec and Slezakova [16] performed scleral reinforcement after the Thompson method on 251 eyes of 154 children with high myopia from 2 to 18 years of age using Zenoderm (porcine skin) and reported that during 10 years of postsurgical check-up, stabilization of axial length was achieved in 53.8% of eyes and the stabilization of refraction was achieved in 52.9% of eyes. The advancement of myopia in other 47% of patients has been decreased from 1.1 D/per year before surgery to 0.1D till 10 years after surgery. More recently, Ward et al. [17] reported 5-year results of scleral reinforcement (donor sclera) in a total of 59 adult eyes, with myopic refractive corrections ranging from −9 to −22 D and axial lengths from 27.8 to 34.6 mm in a follow-up of 5 years. The average increase was 0.2 mm in sutured eyes vs 0.6 mm in nonsutured fellow eyes. Zhu et al. [18] and Ji et al. [19] also reported that there is postoperative decrease of myopic refractive error (0.8D [19] and 0.59 D [18]). It seems that the effect of scleral reinforcement is limited.

Some other studies reported a lack of effect. Nesterov et al. [3] used a strip of fascia lata, and in a follow-up of 1–9 years, myopia increased. Curtin and Whitmore [7] reported an outcome of 23 patients who were followed up for ≥5 years after scleral reinforcement surgery. Of the 20 eyes that had preoperative axial measurements, 18 (90%) had increases in axial diameter of ≥0.3 mm. Progression of posterior staphyloma formation or the onset of myopic fundus degeneration was observed in ten eyes.

In addition to the little effectiveness in a long term after surgery, serious complications have been reported to occur: retinal detachment [3, 7, 20]; ocular motility disorders [7, 16]; retinal, choroidal, and vitreous hemorrhages; optic nerve damage because of circulatory decompensation; compression of the optic nerve; and compression of vortex veins [15] or cilioretinal artery [21].

With no convincing proof of the safety or efficacy of scleral reinforcement, this approach was largely unused. However recent studies reported the long-term safety and effectiveness of using donor sclera cross-linked with genipin [22–24]. A prospective study on 40 young highly myopic patients who underwent scleral reinforcement with a genipin-cross-linked donor scleral strip for one eye and the fellow eye served as concurrent control showed that in over

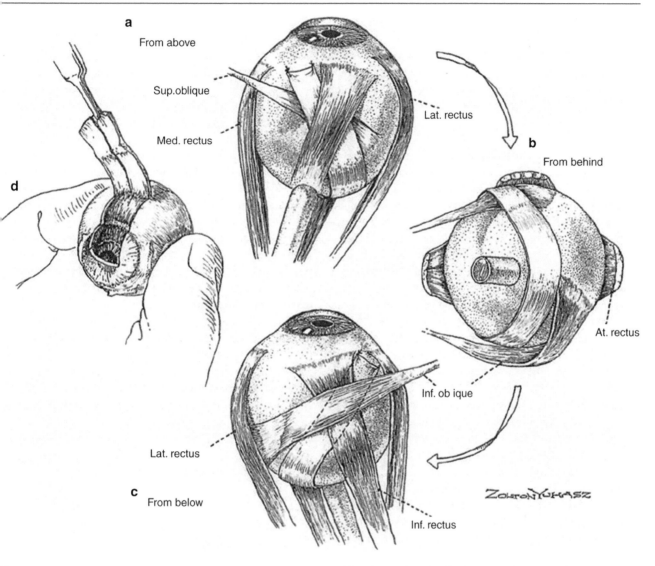

Fig. 31.1 Placement of a scleral homograft in the right eye (Cited from Jacob-LaBarre et al. [9]). (**a**) View from above showing graft placement nasal to the superior oblique muscle insertion. (**b**) Posterior view showing graft held over macular area by insertion of inferior oblique muscle. (**c**) View from below showing insertion of strip nasal to inferior rectus muscle insertion. (**d**) Donor eye showing scleral grafts being dissected and including corneal tissue to obtain sufficient length

2–3 years of follow-up, the axial elongation was significantly decreased in the treated eyes [22].

31.2 Scleral Shortening with Scleral Resection or Scleral Folding

The scleral resection operation was first reported by Leopold Miller in 1903 [25] in cases of retinal detachment in highly myopic eyes. This full-thickness scleral band resection technique was later improved by Lindner [26]. Complications such as hemorrhage and vitreous loss have been associated with full-thickness sclerectomy. A partial-thickness sclerectomy is then preferred for scleral shortening procedures owing to the decrease of intraoperative complications [27–29]. Lamellar scleral resection for ocular shortening was used as an adjunct in surgery for macular translocation as well [30, 31]. According to Borley [20], the scleral incisions are extended in depth from 1/2 to 2/3 the thickness of the sclera, and double-armed mattress sutures were inserted. The width and length of the scleral strips which were removed varied among studies; the width varied from 2 to 6 mm and the length from 20 to 35 mm. The sclera is usually removed from the temporal portion of the globe. Nakagawa et al. [32] reported that the greater the area of sclera folded, the greater the overall reduction in axial length and changes in globe appearance. However, De Almeida and Baraquer-Moner found little improvement in the refraction with resections of even 360° of the sclera.

Also, nonresected scleral invagination was used for the same purpose. However, the scleral shortening or scleral resection was reported to cause clinically intolerable regular and irregular astigmatism [33, 34].

31.3   Scleral Strengthening

Avetisov et al. [35] performed a sclera strengthening injection, in which a dose of liquid polymeric composition under the Tenon's capsule on the scleral surface. After polymerization, the composition formed over the scleral surface a layer of elastic foamed gel. Experiments on 146 rabbit eyes showed that the injected material promoted collagen formation. Gradually dissolving, the gel stimulated the growth of connective tissue on the surface of the sclera, whose stress-strain parameters improved. However, 1.5 years after the surgery, this tensile strength tended to weaken. A clinical study of 240 eyes of patients aged 8–25 years with progressive 6–10 D myopia showed that the refraction remained stable in 79.6% eyes 1 year after the injection and in 52.9% of cases 4–9 years after the injection. However, again, no detailed information of pre- and postoperative changes in refractive error and in axial length has not been provided. Cui et al. [36] showed that systemic delivery of adenosine receptor antagonist 7-methylxanthine (7-MX) increase scleral collagen concentration and diameters in form-deprived myopia in guinea pigs. Su et al. [37] reported the retrobulbar injection of the polymer networks comprised thermoresponsive poly(N-isopropylacrylamide-co-acrylic acid), customizable peptide cross-linkers cleavable by matrix metalloproteinases, and interpenetrating linear poly(acrylic acid)-graft-peptide chains to engage with cell surface receptors. This complex was a fluid as to be injectable at room temperature, but to stiffen in the body, to facilitate its retention at the injection site. A sub-Tenon's injection of a polymeric gel formulation composed mainly of polyvinylpyrrolidine [35, 37], and polytetrofluoroethylene [9] has also been reported.

31.4   Scleral Collagen Cross-linking

Collagen cross-linking was recently introduced for the treatment of progressive keratoconus [38–42]. Wollensak et al. [38] have pioneered the use of riboflavin and ultraviolet light (UVA) to cross-link collagen and enhance the mechanical properties of the cornea. By actively increasing the degree of the bonding between collagen molecules, therapeutic cross-linking could reasonably be expected to enhance corneal rigidity.

Aggregated forms of the collagen monomers are strengthened by intermolecular cross-links (Fig. 31.2). This process happens as a part of maturation but also in aging and disease. Collagen fibrils cross-link naturally as a part of their maturation process. When these fibrils are secreted, they have short segments at either end of the collagen chains (telopeptides) that do not assume the triple-helical conformation. The hydroxylysine residues in these end chains participate in cross-link formation [43]. The cross-links are formed by oxidative deamination of the ε-amino group of this single lysine or hydroxylysine in the amino and carboxy telopeptides of collagen by the enzyme lysyl oxidase. The aldehyde thus formed reacts with a specific lysine or hydroxylysine in the triple helix to form divalent bonds that link the molecules head to tail. They then spontaneously convert during maturation to trivalent cross-links [44, 45]. A second cross-linking pathway occurs during aging involving a non-enzymatic reaction termed glycation.

Oxidation is a third mechanism whereby cross-links are formed in collagen (Fig. 31.3). This type of cross-linking has been identified as being distinctive to the ones formed by enzymatic and glycation in type I collagen and can occur after the process of oxidation (O$_3$ mediated) or photooxidation (UV mediated) [46]. Outside biology,

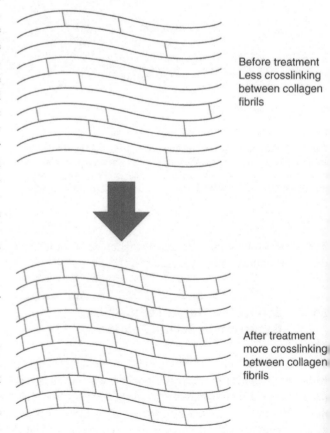

Before treatment
Less crosslinking
between collagen
fibrils

After treatment
more crosslinking
between collagen
fibrils

Fig. 31.2 A schematic illustration showing how collagen cross-linking works

Fig. 31.3 A schematic illustration showing how collagen cross-linking using riboflavin and ultraviolet works

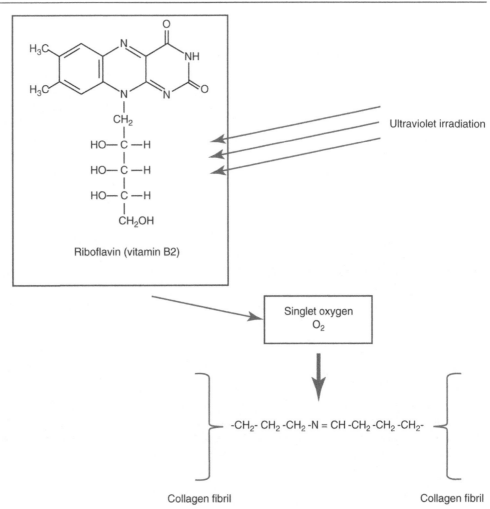

Ultraviolet irradiation

Riboflavin (vitamin B2)

Singlet oxygen O₂

-CH₂- CH₂ -CH₂ -N = CH -CH₂ -CH₂ -CH₂-

Collagen fibril   Collagen fibril

photopolymerization is a comparable process that is being used in industry to generate polymers using the free radical-generating properties of radiant energy like UV light. Photopolymerization of multifunctional monomers resulting in highly cross-linked materials suitable for applications as epoxy coatings, optical lenses, optical fiber coatings, and dental materials is in common use. A monomer substrate in the presence of a photoinitiator can polymerize by way of cross-linkage in the presence of a UV light source.

In the normal cornea, covalently bonded molecular bridges or cross-links exist between adjacent tropocollagen helices and between microfibrils and fibrils at intervals along their length [41, 47]. Collagen cross-linking method shows a promise for treatment of keratoconus, and other cross-linking approaches (e.g., glyceraldehyde and nitroalcohols) may provide stabilization of scleral shape in progressive myopia [48–50]. It has been reported that the scleral collagen contained the similar cross-linked peptides to those found in the cornea [51, 52].

Different from corneal collagen cross-linking, the scleral collagen cross-linking is still in the experimental level and no human clinical trials have been performed.

Light and electron microscopic evaluation of myopic sclera in human eyes shows not only marked thinning at the posterior pole of the eye but also a reduction in fibril diameter and a dissociation of collagen fiber bundles [53–56]. Similar observations have been found in primate models of experimental myopia [57]. McBrien and Norton [58] treated tree shrews with agents that block collagen cross-linking (β-aminopropionitrile [β-APN] or D-penicillamine [DPA]) and underwent monocular deprivation of form vision by eyelid closure to induce myopia. The results showed the amount of vitreous chamber elongation and induced myopia approximately doubled APN-treated monocular deprived eyes when compared to the saline-treated monocular deprived eyes. There was a significant increase in the degree of scleral thinning at the posterior pole in the deprived eyes of β-APN-treated animals.

For exogenous collagen cross-linking, compounds such as glutaraldehyde, glyceraldehyde [48, 59], methylglyoxal (naturally occurring Maillard intermediate), genipin (natural collagen cross-linker obtained from geniposide) [60], and nitroalcohols [50] have been used and have been shown to increase ocular tissue stiffness [61].

Wollensak et al. [48] performed scleral collagen cross-linking in rabbits with sub-Tenon injections of glyceraldehyde into the superonasal quadrant of the eye and reported that glyceraldehyde cross-linking of scleral collagen increased the scleral biomechanical rigidity efficiently as shown in stress-strain parameters and Young's modulus without having no side effects on the retina. Wollensak [62] also showed that the scleral collagen cross-linking by glyceraldehyde proved very efficient in increasing the scleral thermomechanical stability. Wollensak and Iomdina [49] reported that scleral cross-linking by the photosensitizer riboflavin and ultraviolet A (UVA) (Fig. 31.3) was effective and constant over a time interval up to 8 months in increasing the scleral biomechanical strength. Wang et al. [63] showed that both the equatorial and posterior human scleral strips were enhanced by collagen cross-linking with riboflavin/UVA irradiation.

It is difficult to know which method would be suitable to analyze whether scleral collagen cross-linking is effective for preventing ocular expansion. Young's modulus was used as an indicator of the stiffness of sclera [48, 49, 61, 63]; however, it is not certain whether an increased Young's modulus is related to the scleral strength. To overcome this concern, Mattson et al. [59] and Wong et al. [64] measured the ocular dimensions to examine a global expansion of enucleated eyes before and after collagen cross-linking under regulation of intraocular pressure.

It is considered that the scleral collagen cross-linking might be useful for preventing globe expansion in myopic children or adolescents before the sclera is markedly thinned. However, the safety and effectiveness, especially the damage on the retina, choroid, and the optic nerve, must be evaluated in more detail before going on to the human clinical trials.

drogenic, and neurogenic lineages. Seko et al. [67] found that human sclera had a chondrogenic potential, although the human sclera lost the cartilaginous part during the evolution. It might be difficult to thicken and strengthen the already thinned and deformed sclera especially in the area of posterior staphyloma. Especially for extremely thinned sclera, the cell-printing and transfer technology [68] of a sheet with cells and produced collagen would be a good option. Scaffolds based on decellularized matrices, which are mostly based on collagen, have been widely used to regenerate the bladder, the abdominal wall, and many other organs [65]. However, to insert the scaffold appropriately posterior sclera might be difficult. Among various soluble molecules that induce collagen type I expression, transforming growth factor β (TGF-β) is one of the most extensively studied [69, 70]. Jobling and McBrien [71] showed that the altered expression of TGF-β by scleral fibroblasts is important for scleral remodeling during myopia progression in animal models of myopia. TGF-β and its downstream Smad signaling have an essential function in tissue fibrosis although various different fibrogenic factors have been documented. Among the isoforms of TGF-β, TGF-β_1 is a key mediator of fibroblasts activation and has a major influence on extracellular matrix production [72, 73]. Thus, the delivery of TGF-β_1 to the sclera would be one option; however, the angiogenic effect induced by this factor is concerned. Recently, Shinohara et al. [74] reported that the sclera of rats with experimental myopia was reinforced by the newly synthesized collagen fibrils by transplanted skin fibroblasts and the axial elongation was reduced. These results can provide important information for the development of a therapy targeting myopia in humans. Further studies are necessary regarding what we use and how we deliver in regeneration of the sclera.

31.5 Regenerative Therapy Targeting the Sclera

Regeneration of scleral tissue is expected as promising future therapy. Different from the cornea, the sclera does not need to be transparent, which might make this approach a little easier.

In general, an investigator who attempts to induce regeneration at the injured site of an organ may use one or more of three types of "reactants," namely, cells, soluble regulators (cytokines, growth factors), and insoluble regulators (scaffolds) [65]. There have been only a few studies related to scleral regeneration. For cells, the use of autologous fibroblasts from other parts of the body or mesenchymal stem cells would be a good candidate. Thus, Tsai et al. [66] identified the multipotent stem cells within the mouse scleral tissue. These cells were positive for the mesenchymal markers, and the cells were able to differentiate to adipogenic, chon-

31.6 Closing Remarks

Sclera-targeted therapies have a long history, beginning from the scleral reinforcement surgery in the early twentieth century. However, up to now, we had better say that there are no established sclera-targeted treatment which is proven to be safe and to be effective to prevent or treat the myopia progression in a long term. Each treatment has many problems to solve in the future.

In addition to its extracellular matrix (collagen and elastin), the cellular components within the sclera might play some role. The presence of nonvascular contractile myofibroblasts reported within human and monkey choroid and sclera [75] raises the possibility that in vivo sclera may exhibit some active contractile behavior in addition to its passive elastic and creep properties. Scleral myofibroblasts are most concentrated subfoveally and were sparse anteriorly [75]. However, it has not been investigated whether and how scleral myofibroblasts are altered in eyes with pathologic myopia. This might be interesting to investigate.

It seems difficult to regain the cartilage, which we humans lost during the evolution. Thus, it is difficult to obtain the stiff globe which birds and fish have. However, regenerative therapies have progressed in all over the body recently. Regenerative approaches use the patients' own cells and strengthen the sclera by their own stem, or mature cells are greatly expected as a new approach.

References

1. Borley WE, Snyder AA. Surgical treatment of degenerative myopia; the combined lamellar scleral resection with scleral reinforcement using donor eye. Trans Pac Coast Otoophthalmol Soc Annu Meet. 1958;39:275–91.
2. Nesterov AP, Libenson NB. Strengthening the sclera with a strip of fascia lata in progressive myopia. Br J Ophthalmol. 1970;54:46–50.
3. Nesterov AP, Libenson NB, Svirin AV. Early and late results of fascia lata transplantation in high myopia. Br J Ophthalmol. 1976;60:271–2.
4. Momose A. Surgical treatment of myopia--with special references to posterior scleral support operation and radial keratotomy. Indian J Ophthalmol. 1983;31:759–67.
5. Scott AB. Autograft tendon for scleral buckling. Am J Ophthalmol. 1964;57:564–7.
6. Whitmore WG, Curtin BJ. Scleral reinforcement: two case reports. Ophthalmic Surg. 1987;18:503–5.
7. Curtin BJ, Whitmore WG. Long-term results of scleral reinforcement surgery. Am J Ophthalmol. 1987;103:544–8.
8. Castro LC, Duker JS. Foveoschisis without high myopia. Ophthalmic Surg Lasers Imaging. 2010;9:1–4.
9. Jacob-LaBarre JT, Assouline M, Conway MD, Thompson HW, McDonald MB. Effects of scleral reinforcement on the elongation of growing cat eyes. Arch Ophthalmol. 1993;111:979–86.
10. Snyder AA, Thompson FB. A simplified technique for surgical treatment of degenerative myopia. Am J Ophthalmol. 1972;74:273–7.
11. Thompson FB. A simplified scleral reinforcement technique. Am J Ophthalmol. 1978;86:782–90.
12. Thompson FB. Scleral reinforcement for high myopia. Ophthalmic Surg. 1985;16:90–4.
13. Coroneo MT, Beaumont JT, Hollows FC. Scleral reinforcement in the treatment of pathologic myopia. Aust N Z J Ophthalmol. 1988;16:317–20.
14. Zaikova MV, Negoda VI. Grafting of homologous sclera in progressive myopia. Vestn oftalmol. 1970;4:16–20.
15. Whitwell J. Scleral reinforcement in degenerative myopia. Trans Ophthalmol Soc U K. 1971;91:679–86.
16. Gerinec A, Slezakova G. Posterior scleroplasty in children with severe myopia. Bratisl Lek Listy. 2001;102:73–8.
17. Ward B, Tarutta EP, Mayer MJ. The efficacy and safety of posterior pole buckles in the control of progressive high myopia. Eye. 2009;23:2169–74.
18. Zhu Z, Ji X, Zhang J, Ke G. Posterior scleral reinforcement in the treatment of macular retinoschisis in highly myopic patients. Clin Exp Ophthalmol. 2009;37:660–3.
19. Ji X, Wang J, Zhang J, Sun H, Jia X, Zhang W. The effect of posterior scleral reinforcement for high myopia macular splitting. J Int Med Res. 2011;39:662–6.
20. Borley WE. The scleral resection (eyeball-shortening) operation. Trans Am Ophthalmol Soc. 1949;47:462–97.
21. Karabatsas CH, Waldock A, Potts MJ. Cilioretinal artery occlusion following scleral reinforcement surgery. Acta Ophthalmol Scand. 1997;75:316–8.
22. Xue A, Zheng L, Tan G, et al. Genipin-crosslinked donor sclera for posterior scleral contraction/reinforcement to fight progressive myopia. Invest Ophthalmol Vis Sci. 2018;59:3564–73.
23. Su Y, Pan A, Wu Y, Zhu S, Zheng L, Xue A. The efficacy of posterior scleral contraction in controlling high myopia in young people. Am J Transl Res. 2018;10:3628–34.
24. Peng C, Xu J, Ding X, et al. Effects of posterior scleral reinforcement in pathological myopia: a 3-year follow-up study. Graefes Arch Clin Exp Ophthalmol. 2019;257:607–17.
25. Muller L. Eine neue operative Behandlung der Netzhautabhebung. Klin Monatsbl Augenheilkd. 1903;41:459–62.
26. Lindner K. Heilungsversuche bei prognostrisch ungunstigen Fallen von Netzhautabhebung. Ztschr Augenheilkd. 1933;81:277–99.
27. Everett WG. A new scleral shortening operation; preliminary report. AMA Arch Ophthalmol. 1955;53:865–9.
28. Everett WG. An experimental evaluation of scleral shortening operations. AMA Arch Ophthalmol. 1956;56:34–47.
29. Chamlin M, Rubner K. Lamellar undermining; a preliminary report on a technique of scleral buckling for retinal detachment. Am J Ophthalmol. 1956;41:633–8.
30. Imai K, Loewenstein A, de Juan E. Translocation of the retina for management of subfoveal choroidal neovascularization I: experimental studies in the rabbit eye. Am J Ophthalmol. 1998;125:627–34.
31. Fujikado T, Ohji M, Saito Y, Hayashi A, Tano Y. Visual function after foveal translocation with scleral shortening in patients with myopic neovascular maculopathy. Am J Ophthalmol. 1998;125:647–56.
32. Nakagawa N, Parel JM, Murray TG, Oshima K. Effect of scleral shortening on axial length. Arch Ophthalmol. 2000;118:965–8.
33. Oshita T, Hayashi S, Inoue T, et al. Topographic analysis of astigmatism induced by scleral shortening in pig eyes. Graefes Arch Clin Exp Ophthalmol. 2001;239:382–6.
34. Kim T, Krishnasamy S, Meyer CH, Toth CA. Induced corneal astigmatism after macular translocation surgery with scleral infolding. Ophthalmology. 2001;108:1203–8.
35. Avetisov ES, Tarutta EP, Iomdina EN, Vinetskaya MI, Andreyeva LD. Nonsurgical and surgical methods of sclera reinforcement in progressive myopia. Acta Ophthalmol Scand. 1997;75:618–23.
36. Cui D, Trier K, Zeng J, et al. Effects of 7-methylxanthine on the sclera in form deprivation myopia in guinea pigs. Acta Ophthalmol. 2011;89:328–34.
37. Su J, Iomdina E, Tarutta E, Ward B, Song J, Wildsoet CF. Effects of poly(2-hydroxyethyl methacrylate) and poly(vinyl-pyrrolidone) hydrogel implants on myopic and normal chick sclera. Exp Eye Res. 2009;88:445–57.
38. Wollensak G, Spoerl E, Seiler T. Riboflavin/ultraviolet-a-induced collagen crosslinking for the treatment of keratoconus. Am J Ophthalmol. 2003;135:620–7.
39. Wollensak G. Crosslinking treatment of progressive keratoconus: new hope. Curr Opin Ophthalmol. 2006;17:356–60.
40. Caporossi A, Baiocchi S, Mazzotta C, Traversi C, Caporossi T. Parasurgical therapy for keratoconus by riboflavin-ultraviolet type A rays induced cross-linking of corneal collagen: preliminary refractive results in an Italian study. J Cataract Refract Surg. 2006;32:837–45.
41. Snibson GR. Collagen cross-linking: a new treatment paradigm in corneal disease - a review. Clin Exp Ophthalmol. 2010;38:141–53.
42. Henriquez MA, Izquierdo L Jr, Bernilla C, Zakrzewski PA, Mannis M. Riboflavin/Ultraviolet A corneal collagen cross-linking for the treatment of keratoconus: visual outcomes and Scheimpflug analysis. Cornea. 2011;30:281–6.
43. Lodish H, Berk A, Zipursky SL. Molecular cell biology. New York: W.H. Freeman & Co.; 1999.

44. Siegel RC, Fu JC. Collagen cross-linking. Purification and substrate specificity of lysyl oxidase. J Biol Chem. 1976;251:5779–85.

45. Barnard K, Light ND, Sims TJ, Bailey AJ. Chemistry of the collagen cross-links. Origin and partial characterization of a putative mature cross-link of collagen. Biochem J. 1987;244:303–9.

46. Foote CS. Mechanisms of photosensitized oxidation. There are several different types of photosensitized oxidation which may be important in biological systems. Science. 1968;162:963–70.

47. Robins SP. Biochemistry and functional significance of collagen cross-linking. Biochem Soc Trans. 2007;35:849–52.

48. Wollensak G, Iomdina E. Crosslinking of scleral collagen in the rabbit using glyceraldehyde. J Cataract Refract Surg. 2008;34:651–6.

49. Wollensak G, Iomdina E. Long-term biomechanical properties of rabbit sclera after collagen crosslinking using riboflavin and ultraviolet A (UVA). Acta Ophthalmol. 2009;87:193–8.

50. Paik DC, Solomon MR, Wen Q, Turro NJ, Trokel SL. Aliphatic beta-nitroalcohols for therapeutic corneoscleral cross-linking: chemical mechanisms and higher order nitroalcohols. Invest Ophthalmol Vis Sci. 2010;51:836–43.

51. Crabbe MJ, Harding JJ. Collagen crosslinking: isolation of two crosslinked peptides involving alpha 2-CB(3--5) from bovine scleral collagen. FEBS Lett. 1979;97:189–92.

52. Harding JJ, Crabbe MJ. Collagen crosslinking: isolation of a dimeric crosslinked peptide of alpha1-CB6 from bovine corneal and scleral collagens. FEBS Lett. 1979;100:351–6.

53. Curtin BJ. Ocular findings and complications. In: Curtin BJ, editor. The myopias. New York: Harper and Row; 1985. p. 277–347.

54. Curtin BJ, Iwamoto T, Renaldo DP. Normal and staphylomatous sclera of high myopia. An electron microscopic study. Arch Ophthalmol. 1979;97:912–5.

55. McBrien NA, Cornell LM, Gentle A. Structural and ultrastructural changes to the sclera in a mammalian model of high myopia. Invest Ophthalmol Vis Sci. 2001;42:2179–87.

56. McBrien NA, Moghaddam HO, Reeder AP, Moules S. Structural and biochemical changes in the sclera of experimentally myopic eyes. Biochem Soc Trans. 1991;19:861–5.

57. Funata M, Tokoro T. Scleral change in experimentally myopic monkeys. Graefes Arch Clin Exp Ophthalmol. 1990;228:174–9.

58. McBrien NA, Norton TT. Prevention of collagen crosslinking increases form-deprivation myopia in tree shrew. Exp Eye Res. 1994;59:475–86.

59. Mattson MS, Huynh J, Wiseman M, Coassin M, Kornfield JA, Schwartz DM. An in vitro intact globe expansion method for evaluation of cross-linking treatments. Invest Ophthalmol Vis Sci. 2010;51:3120–8.

60. Avila MY, Navia JL. Effect of genipin collagen crosslinking on porcine corneas. J Cataract Refract Surg. 2010;36:659–64.

61. Wollensak G, Spoerl E. Collagen crosslinking of human and porcine sclera. J Cataract Refract Surg. 2004;30:689–95.

62. Wollensak G. Thermomechanical stability of sclera after glyceraldehyde crosslinking. Graefes Arch Clin Exp Ophthalmol. 2010;249(3):399–406.

63. Wang M, Zhang F, Qian X, Zhao X. Regional biomechanical properties of human sclera after cross-linking by riboflavin/ultraviolet A. J Refract Surg. 2012;28:723–8.

64. Wong FF, Lari DR, Schultz DS, Stewart JM. Whole globe inflation testing of exogenously crosslinked sclera using genipin and methylglyoxal. Exp Eye Res. 2012;103:17–21.

65. Yannas IV. Emerging rules for inducing organ regeneration. Biomaterials. 2013;34:321–30.

66. Tsai CL, Wu PC, Fini ME, Shi S. Identification of multipotent stem/progenitor cells in murine sclera. Invest Ophthalmol Vis Sci. 2011;52:5481–7.

67. Seko Y, Azuma N, Takahashi Y, et al. Human sclera maintains common characteristics with cartilage throughout evolution. PLoS One. 2008;3:12.

68. Tsugawa J, Komaki M, Yoshida T, Nakahama K, Amagasa T, Morita I. Cell-printing and transfer technology applications for bone defects in mice. J Tissue Eng Regen Med. 2011;5:695–703.

69. Leask A, Abraham DJ. TGF-beta signaling and the fibrotic response. FASEB J. 2004;18:816–27.

70. Hoyles RK, Khan K, Shiwen X, et al. Fibroblast-specific perturbation of transforming growth factor beta signaling provides insight into potential pathogenic mechanisms of scleroderma-associated lung fibrosis: exaggerated response to alveolar epithelial injury in a novel mouse model. Arthritis Rheum. 2008;58:1175–88.

71. Jobling AI, Nguyen M, Gentle A, McBrien NA. Isoform-specific changes in scleral transforming growth factor-beta expression and the regulation of collagen synthesis during myopia progression. J Biol Chem. 2004;279:18121–6.

72. Border WA, Noble NA. Transforming growth factor beta in tissue fibrosis. N Engl J Med. 1994;331:1286–92.

73. Pan X, Chen Z, Huang R, Yao Y, Ma G. Transforming growth factor beta1 induces the expression of collagen type I by DNA methylation in cardiac fibroblasts. PLoS One. 2013;8:1.

74. Shinohara K, Yoshida T, Liu H, et al. Establishment of novel therapy to reduce progression of myopia in rats with experimental myopia by fibroblast transplantation on sclera. J Tissue Eng Regen Med. 2018;12:e451–61.

75. Poukens V, Glasgow BJ, Demer JL. Nonvascular contractile cells in sclera and choroid of humans and monkeys. Invest Ophthalmol Vis Sci. 1998;39:1765–74.

Index